ESSENTIALS OF LIFE & HEALTH

third edition

Consultants on the Third Edition

Richard Ahrens, *University of Maryland*
Warren Boskin, *San Diego State University*
James Calhoun, *University of Georgia*
Dennis Cryer, *University of Northern Iowa*
Jackie Estrada, *San Diego, California*
Alan Feit, *Roosevelt Hospital, New York*
Joyce Fleming, *Santa Monica, California*
Thomas G. Flora, *California State University, Chico*
Arelio Florio, *University of Illinois, Champaign*
Neil Gallagher, *Towson State University*
E. D. Glover, *University of Kansas*
Michael C. Hosokawa, *Medical School, University of Missouri*
Lois Kessler, *San Diego State University*
Marshall Krueger, *University of Utah*
Warren McNab, *University of Houston*
Aubrey C. McTaggert, *San Diego State University*
Lorraine Neisner, *University of Wisconsin*
Richard Papenfuss, *University of Wisconsin, La Crosse*
Elizabeth Ritchey, *Virginia Polytechnic Institute and State University*
Edith Roberts, *Cerritos College*
James Rothenberger, *University of Minnesota*
Michael B. Shimkin, *School of Medicine, University of California, San Diego*
Janet Shirreffs, *Arizona State University*
David Sleet, *San Diego State University*
Bertram Spector, *New York Institute of Technology*
Bonnie Spring, *Harvard University*
Jack Toohey, *Arizona State University*
T. Demetri Vacalis, *University of Texas, Austin*
Elizabeth Whelan, *American Council on Science and Health; School of Public Health, Harvard University*

reviewers

Joan Arlette, *University of Wisconsin-Milwaukee*
Pearl Bailey, *Medgar Evers College*
Robert Barnes, *East Carolina University*
Sharon Garcia, *Diablo Valley College*
Jerry Medlock, *Bloomsburg State College*
Mary Lou Pross, *Berea College*
Edgar Roulhac, *Johns Hopkins University*

Contributors to Previous Editions

S. Howard Bartley, *Michigan State University*
Barbara L. Brody, *Planned Parenthood Association, San Diego County California*
Fergus Clydesdale, *University of Massachusetts*
Stewart Dadmun, *San Diego, California*
Fitzhugh Dodson, *LaPrimera Preschool, Redondo Beach, California*
Joyce Fleming, *Santa Monica, California*
Joel Fort, Fort Help, *San Francisco, California*
Paul H. Gebhard, *Institute for Sex Research, Indiana University*
Luigi Giacometti, *National Institutes of Health, Bethesda, Maryland*
Jeoffrey B. Gordon, *Beach Area Community Clinic, San Diego, California*
Ralph Grawunder, *San Diego State University*
Seymour L. Halleck, *University of Wisconsin*
Michael C. Hosokawa, *Medical School, University of Missouri*
J. Willis Hurst, *Emory University*
O. W. Jones, *School of Medicine, University of California, San Diego*
Richard Kasschau, *University of Houston*
Robert Kavanaugh, *University of California, San Diego*
Francis C. Kenel, *University of Maryland*
Robert W. Kistner, *Harvard Medical School; Boston Hospital for Women, Boston*
Charles E. Lewis, *University of California, Los Angeles*
Marjorie Lazoff, *Wright Institute, Berkeley, California*
Purvis L. Martin, *School of Medicine, University of California, San Diego*
Aubrey C. McTaggert, *San Diego State University*
Margaret E. Neiswender, *Andrus Gerontology Center, University of Southern California*
Marvin J. Schissel, *Triboro Hospital, New York*
Michael B. Shimkin, *School of Medicine, University of California, San Diego*
Robert Straus, *College of Medicine, University of Kentucky, Lexington*
Jared R. Tinklenberg, *Stanford University*
Ian Tinsley, *Oregon State University*
Silvio S. Varon, *University of California, San Diego*
James M. Witt, *Oregon State University*

ESSENTIALS OF LIFE & HEALTH

third edition

special consultants on the third edition **ralph grawunder**
San Diego State University

b. e. pruitt
University of Oregon

writer **marion steinmann**

RANDOM HOUSE NEW YORK

Third Edition
98765432

Library of Congress Cataloging in Publication Data

Main entry under title

Essentials of life and health

Bibliography: p.
Includes Index.
1. Health I. Grawunder, Ralph, 1929–
II. Pruitt, B.E.
RA776.E78 1980 613 80-21549
ISBN 0-394-3250-2

Text design by Dana Kasarsky
Cover design by Betty Binns
Cover photo by Mitchell Funk/The Image Bank
Manufactured in the United States of America

Preface

In the several fields that *Essentials of Life and Health* surveys, the related themes of self-help and health as a matter of individual responsibility have emerged forcefully during recent years. In preparing the third edition, it thus seemed appropriate not merely to discuss these themes in a chapter or two, but to integrate them fully throughout the text and provide an aid to decision making for more healthy lives. This edition, then, places a new and strong emphasis on the "How To" of personal well-being: how to understand the relationship between health and life style (introductory chapter), how (and when) to get help for mental distress (Chapter 1), how to stop smoking (Chapter 13), how to build resistance against disease (Chapter 14), how to talk to your doctor (Chapter 18)—to name just a few of the subjects discussed. In bringing this new perspective to the fore, however, every effort has also been made to preserve the forthright manner, clear writing, and distinctive graphics that have earned such gratifying praise for the first two editions of *Essentials of Life and Health* from students and instructors alike.

New subject matter, including special boxed features, summaries, and new illustrations and photos, add greater clarity and interest to the wide range of health-related topics covered in the third edition. The chapter on Health-Care Delivery that appeared in the last edition has been redone to form the basis of Chapter 18, Health Care and the Consumer, which contains a new and valuable guide to the fundamentals of self-care. And an entirely new chapter—Chapter 2—examines both the positive and negative aspects of stress, and offers down-to-earth advice on how to avoid it—or cope with it. A helpful summary has been added at the end of each of the book's eighteen chapters.

Some material from earlier editions has been reorganized in the present volume to reflect changing concerns: for instance, Nutrition and Weight Control, subjects of increasing importance to Americans, have been broken into two separate chapters, Nutrition (Chapter 8) and Weight Management (Chapter 9), with the latter containing new material on how to develop a weight control program. The chapters on Emotional Development and Health and Emotional Problems have been combined to form Chapter 1 (Mental Health), and the chapters on Aging and Death and Dying have been merged into Chapter 7 (Aging and Facing Death). Also new to the third edition are special boxed features scattered throughout the text. These boxed materials are intended to lend support to the dual themes of self-help and individual responsibility, and students will find the information interesting and useful. The boxes are divided into three categories:

1. Focus boxes (for example, Carcinogens in the Workplace; Love and Sex; Food Fads) expand the main text with candid discussions of important and timely topics. 2. How To boxes (for example, A Guide to Sensible Drinking; Decrease Your Risks of Developing Cancer) offer useful—and usable—advice and information in a list format. 3. Viewpoint boxes (for example, Is Marijuana Safe?) highlight controversial issues.

As in past editions, special attention has been paid to the graphic and visual enhancement of the text. Among the ambitious and imaginative additions to the third edition's art program are many new charts and tables, new photographs (both color and black and white), and illustrations commissioned specifically for this edition.

For the new features and improvements in the third edition—and for providing the judgment to know when and where change would weaken rather than strengthen the text—many people deserve thanks. First and foremost are the consultants listed opposite the title page, who gave generously of their time and expertise and were instrumental in shaping this revision. Janet Shirreffs of Arizona State University deserves a special thanks for her valuable and detailed suggestions and comments on the text and illustrations. Acknowledgement must also be made to the many health educators whose contributions to earlier editions provided the foundation and framework for what has now become the leading book in the field.

The new direction for this revision was really defined by the 546 health instructors who took the time to complete a very detailed questionnaire. This revision fully reflects the changes suggested by this extraordinarily conscientious group of people, and because of their willingness to fully share their thoughts and suggestions, ESSENTIALS OF LIFE AND HEALTH will continue to be the pace setter in health education for the 1980's.

More than ever, *Essentials of Life and Health* is a book not just to be read, but to be used. Although it strives to present the latest facts, statistics, research findings, and controversies in the field of health science, this text emphasizes the practical, everyday nature of well-being. For health is not just the absence of disease. As the following pages make clear, it is above all the outcome of intelligent, informed decisions made by the people who know us best—ourselves.

Contents

Life and Health 2

OUR POTENTIAL FOR HEALTH 4

Matters of Definition 4

DETERMINANTS OF HEALTH 5

Physical Well-Being 5

Mental Health 5

Social Well-Being 5

A Hypothetical Life History 6

THE MAJOR HEALTH HAZARD 7

IT'S UP TO YOU 7

I EMOTIONAL AND SEXUAL ADJUSTMENT 8

1 Mental Health 10

THE NATURE OF EMOTION 12

EMOTIONS AND THE BODY 13

EMOTIONAL NEEDS 14

The Need for Love 14

The Need for Self-Esteem 16

Maslow's Hierarchy of Needs 16

STAGES OF EMOTIONAL DEVELOPMENT 18

Freud's Stages 18

Erikson's Stages 18

DEALING WITH EMOTIONS 20

Defense Mechanisms 21

Emotional Control 21

EMOTIONAL MATURITY AND MENTAL HEALTH 23

FACILITATING MENTAL HEALTH 23

The Human Potential Movement 26

Helping Others 26

MENTAL DISORDERS: THE PROBLEM OF DEFINITION 26

The Deviance Approach 26

The Legal Approach 27

The Adjustment Approach 27

The Issue of Labeling 27

THE MAGNITUDE AND COST OF MENTAL ILLNESS 27

CLASSIFYING THE MENTAL DISORDERS 28

Depression 29

Neuroses 30

Psychoses 32

Personality Disorders 33

Psychophysiological Reactions 33

WHEN AND HOW TO GET HELP 34

The Problems of Everyday Living 34

Signs of Mental Disorders 35

How You Can Help 37

Crisis Intervention: The Hot Line 37

Prevention 37

SUMMARY 38

2 Stress and Health 40

WHAT IS STRESS? 41

The Positive Effects of Stress 42

THE VARIETY OF STRESSORS 42

Life Changes 43

THE VARIATION IN RESPONSE 45

THE PHYSIOLOGY OF STRESS 45

Signs of Stress 45
The Stress Mechanism 46
STRESS AND DISEASE 47
COPING WITH STRESS 49
Controlling Stress Responses 50
STRESS AND LIFE STYLE 52
SUMMARY 53

3 Human Sexuality 54

GENDER IDENTITY 55
Genetic Factors 56
Hormonal Factors 56
Social Factors 57
THE REAL SEXUAL REVOLUTION 57
SEXOLOGY OUT OF THE CLOSET 58
OPTIONS OF SEXUAL ACTIVITY 59
Masturbation 59
Petting 59
Intercourse 60
OTHER PARTNER PREFERENCES 61
Homosexuality 61
Bisexuality 63
THE PHYSIOLOGY OF SEXUAL RESPONSE 63
The Female Cycle 63
The Male Cycle 66
SEXUAL PROBLEMS 68
Sexual Dysfunction in Men and Women 68
Sex Therapy 70
When a "Problem" is Not a Problem 70
THE CONTINUING EVOLUTION OF SEXUALITY 71
SUMMARY 71

II THE LIFE CYCLE 72

4 Reproduction and Health 74

THE MALE CONTRIBUTION 75
THE FEMALE SYSTEM 76
The Uterus 76
The Fallopian Tubes 76
The Ovaries 77
Feminine Hygiene 78
Menopause 78
CONCEPTION AND PRENATAL DEVELOPMENT 79
PREGNANCY 80
Pregnancy Testing 80
Visits to the Doctor 81
Blood Examinations 82
Discomforts of Pregnancy 82
Spontaneous Abortion 82
Prepared Childbirth 83
LABOR AND BIRTH 85
Midwifery and Home Delivery 87
BREAST FEEDING 88
INFERTILITY 89
Male Infertility 89
Female Infertility 89
CONGENITAL DEFECTS 89
GENETIC DISEASES 92
Sickle-Cell Anemia 92
Phenylketonuria (PKU) 93
Lipid Storage Diseases 93
Sex-Linked Genetic Diseases 93
Down's Syndrome 94
GENETIC COUNSELING 95
SUMMARY 96

5 Birth Control 98

FAMILY PLANNING AND CHILD SPACING 100
USE AND MISUSE OF CONTRACEPTION 100
METHODS REQUIRING NO MEDICAL CARE 101
Withdrawal (Coitus Interruptus) 101
Condoms 101
Foams, Creams, and Jellies 103
METHODS REQUIRING NONSURGICAL MEDICAL CARE 104
Oral Contraceptives 104
Intrauterine Devices 105
Diaphragms 105
Rhythm Method 105
METHODS REQUIRING SURGERY 106
METHODS OF THE FUTURE 106
ABORTION 107
Methods of Abortion 107
SUMMARY 109

6 Marriage and Parenthood 110

WHY DO PEOPLE MARRY 112
SELECTING A MARRIAGE PARTNER 112
Youth and Identity 112
The Lack of Facilities 114
MARRIAGE—WHAT'S EXPECTED 115
The Man's Marriage 115
The Woman's Marriage 116
Changing Ideas and Forms of Marriage 116
ALTERNATIVES TO MARRIAGE 117
Cohabitation 117
Group Marriage 119
The Single Life 119
MAKING MARRIAGE WORK 120
Personality Differences 120
Money 120
Sex 121
Children 121
Divorce 121
MYTHS ABOUT MARRIAGE 123
Marriages Are Not Made in Heaven 123
Change is Essential to a Marriage 124
Adulthood is Far from Stagnant 125
Marriage Cannot Fill All Needs 125
PARENTHOOD TODAY 125
Children: To Have or Not To Have 126
THE PARENT-CHILD RELATIONSHIP 126
Discipline 126
Adolescence 129
Child Abuse 130
CHILDREN AND DIVORCE 131
SINGLE-PARENT FAMILIES 131
ADOPTION 132
PARENTING FOR HEALTH 132
SUMMARY 132

7 Aging and Facing Death 134

THE AGING PROCESS 136
Physical changes 136
Mental changes 138
DEALING WITH AGING 139
Maturity 141
FAMILY LIFE 142
Marital Life 142
Sexuality 142
Widowhood 143
Remarriage 144
Relationships with Children 144
SOCIAL-LIFE CHANGES 144
Friendship 145
DEFINITIONS OF DEATH 146
COMMON ATTITUDES TOWARD DEATH 147
The Influence of Age 147
The Influence of Education 148
THE EXPERIENCE OF DYING 148
THE NEEDS OF THE DYING PERSON 149
The Ambulatory Dying 149
The Hospice Approach 150
Dying at Home 150
EUTHANASIA 150
STAGES OF COPING WITH DEATH 151
THE NATURE OF GRIEF 153
Anticipatory Grief 153
The Needs of the Bereaved 153
Grief Therapy 154
FUNERAL RITES 154
The Cost of Dying 155
Psychological Values 155
THIS PRECIOUS GIFT 156
SUMMARY

III THE WELL-ADJUSTED BODY 158

8 Nutrition 158

THE BASIC FOOD COMPONENTS 162
Protein 162
Carbohydrates 163
Fat 166
Vitamins 167
Minerals 167
Salt (Sodium Chloride) 167
Water 168
Fiber 168
Calories 169
A BALANCED DIET 169
The Basic Four 169
Food Labeling 172
Additives and Preservatives 172
SPECIAL NUTRITIONAL NEEDS 173
Children and Teen-agers 173
Pregnancy 174
The Pill 175
The Later Years 175

NUTRITION AND DISEASE 175
Undernutrition 175
Overnutrition 175
Simple Diet Deficiencies 177
SUMMARY 177

9 Weight Management 178
OVERWEIGHT AND OBESITY 180
Body Composition 180
Assessing Body Fat 181
CAUSES OF OVERWEIGHT 181
WHY REDUCE? 184
SUCCESSFUL WEIGHT REDUCTION 185
Planning a Weight Control Program 185
The Need for Exercise 188
Behavior Modification 188
OTHER METHODS OF WEIGHT CONTROL 189
Fad Diets 190
Sweating 192
Fat Clinics and Health Spas 192
A LIFETIME GOAL 192
SUMMARY 193

10 Physical Fitness 194
THE ROLE OF FITNESS 195
THE ELEMENTS OF FITNESS 196
EXERCISE AND HEALTH 198
Released Tension 199
Strength and Resistance 200
Support of Developmental Growth 200
HOW FIT IS "FIT ENOUGH"? 200
WHAT EXERCISE AND HOW MUCH? 202
PLANNING FOR FITNESS 203
A Few Cautions 204
Establishing A Fitness Program 206
Exercise and Aging 207
A LIFETIME NEED 208
SUMMARY 208

IV SUBSTANCE USE AND ABUSE 210

11 Drugs and Drug Use 212
WHAT IS A DRUG? 214
WHAT IS DRUG ABUSE? 214
HAZARDS AND COSTS OF DRUG USE AND ABUSE 215
The Physiological Variables 215
Drug Toxicity and Interactions 217
STAGES OF DRUG DEPENDENCE 218
Habituation 218
Tolerance 218
Physical Dependence 219
PATTERNS OF DRUG-USING BEHAVIOR 220
CAUSES OF DRUG USE AND ABUSE 221
Psychological Factors 221
Sociological Factors 222
THE PSYCHOACTIVE DRUGS 224
DEPRESSANTS 224
Major Tranquilizers 228
Antidepressants and Lithium 228
Stimulants 229
Psychedelic-Hallucinogens 231
Cannabis (Marijuana) 232
Over-the-Counter Drugs 234
Aspirin and Acetaminophen 235
Antacids 236
Antihistamines 236
Laxatives 236
Antidiarrhea Preparations 237
Emetics 237
PRESCRIPTION DRUGS 237
SUMMARY 238

12 Alcohol 240
PHYSIOLOGICAL EFFECTS OF ALCOHOL 242
Alcohol Absorption and Blood Alcohol Level 243
Other Biochemical Factors 246
PSYCHOLOGICAL EFFECTS OF ALCOHOL 246
Motivation 247
Role of Experience 247
Drinking and The Family 248
DRINKING IN AMERICAN SOCIETY 248
Drinking Among Youth 248
Intoxication and Society 250
ALCOHOLISM 251
Signs of Alcoholism 251
What Causes Alcoholism? 252
Treatment 255
Facing the Problem 255
SUMMARY 255

13 Smoking 256

THE MANUFACTURED EPIDEMIC 258
COMPONENTS OF CIGARETTE SMOKE 259
SMOKE AS A DISEASE AGENT 260
Lung Cancer 260
Other Cancers 260
Heart Disease 261
Bronchitis and Emphysema 262
Smoking and the Pill 262
Smoking and Pregnancy 262
It's Not Too Late to Quit 263
PROFILE OF THE SMOKER 263
WHY PEOPLE SMOKE 264
Social and Psychological Factors 264
Pharmacological Factors 265
A STUBBORN PROBLEM 265
The Power of the Tobacco Industry 265
KICKING THE HABIT 266
THE RIGHTS OF NONSMOKERS 267
SUMMARY 268

V DISEASE 270

14 Communicable Diseases 272

DISEASE ANALYSIS 274
CAUSES OF DISEASE 275
AGENTS OF INFECTION 276
HOW INFECTION SPREADS 278
THE COURSE OF AN INFECTION 279
BODY DEFENSES 279
IMMUNITY 281
COMMON INFECTIOUS DISEASES 282
The Common Cold 283
Influenza 284
Hepatitis 285
Mononucleosis 285
SEXUALLY TRANSMITTED DISEASES 286
Syphilis 287
Gonorrhea 289
Herpes Simplex Type 2 290
Other Sexually Transmitted Diseases 290
Prevention and Control of STDs 291
CHANGING PATTERNS OF DISEASE 292
CONTROL AND PREVENTION OF DISEASE 295
THE STATUS OF THE COMMUNICABLE DISEASES 296
SUMMARY 297

15 Cancer 298

UNCONTROLLED GROWTH 300
TYPES OF CANCER 302
DISTRIBUTION OF CANCER 302
CAUSES OF CANCER 302
Heredity 304
Diet 304
Tobacco 304
Chemicals 305
Pollution 305
Radiation 305
Viruses 305
Defective Immune Mechanisms 306
PREVENTION 306
DETECTION AND DIAGNOSIS 307
TREATMENT 308
QUACKERY 311
NEW RESEARCH 311
SUMMARY 312

16 Cardiovascular Disease 315

ANTHEROSCLEROSIS 317
HEART ATTACKS 317
Angina Pectoris 317
Myocardial Infarction (Heart Attack) 318
Faltering Heartbeat 319
Heart Block 319
Cardiac Arrest and Emergency Treatment 319
Postcardiac Rehabilitation 320
OTHER HEART PROBLEMS 320
Heart Failure 320
Congenital Heart Disease 321
Rheumatic Heart Disease 321
HIGH BLOOD PRESSURE 322
STROKES 323
Transient Ischemic Attacks 324
Treatment 324
RISK FACTORS 325
Cigarette Smoking 325
Diet 325
Exercise 326
Stress 326
The Pill 326
Factors Beyond Our Control 327

Multiplying the Risks 328
CARDIOVASCULAR SURGERY 328
PREVENTION 330
SUMMARY 330

VI HEALTH AND SOCIETY 332

17 Health in the Environment 334

THE CHEMICAL ENVIRONMENT 336
What Makes a Chemical Harmful? 336
Asbestos 336
Mercury 337
Lead 338
Pesticides and Herbicides 339
Air Pollution 341
Water Pollution 342
Solid Wastes 343
Noise Pollution 344
RADIATION AND PUBLIC HEALTH 345
Are Nuclear Power Plants Safe? 345
Biological Effects of Radiation Exposure 346
POPULATION AND HEALTH 347
Humanity at the Crossroads 347
SOLVING THE PROBLEMS OF THE ENVIRONMENT 350
INDIVIDUAL ACTION 350
SUMMARY 351

18 Health Care and the Consumer 352

HEALTH CARE AS A HUMAN RIGHT 354
THE ROLE OF COMMUNITIES 355
Future Role of the Community 356
HEALTH-CARE DELIVERY: A HOST OF PROBLEMS 356
Inefficient Distribution of Physicians 356
Inadequate Health Insurance Coverage 357
The High Cost of Health Care 357
THE QUALITY OF MEDICAL CARE 360
IMPROVING THE SYSTEM 360
Improving Distribution of Health Care 360
Group Practice 360
Health Maintenance Organizations 361
Health Care vs. Sickness Care 361
National Health Insurance and a National Health Service 363
SELF-CARE MOVEMENT 365
Limitations to Self-Care 366
THE SCOPE OF SELF-CARE 366
ACCIDENT PREVENTION 367
Motor Vehicle Accidents 367
Home Accidents 368
Evaluating Health Literature 369
Self-Care Skills 370
Taking Care of Yourself 372
YOU AND YOUR DOCTOR 373
How to Choose a Doctor 373
Physical Examinations 374
When to See a Doctor 375
How to Talk with Your Doctor 376
YOUR RIGHTS AS A PATIENT 377
MAKING CONSUMER DECISIONS 377
HOW TO RECOGNIZE QUACKERY 378
A LIFELONG RESPONSIBILITY 379
SUMMARY 379

Appendix of Common Diseases 381
Further Readings 395
Glossary 405
Index 413
Credits and Acknowledgments 423
Photo Credits 425

Boxes

Chapter 1	*HOW TO Overcome Shyness*	17
	FOCUS Who's Happy?	22
	HOW TO Help a Depressed Person	29
	HOW TO Recognize the Signals of a Potential Suicide	30
Chapter 2	*HOW TO Cope with Pressure*	50
Chapter 3	*FOCUS Love and Sex*	69
Chapter 4	*VIEWPOINT Test-Tube Babies—Miracle or Menace?*	90
Chapter 6	*FOCUS Love and Marriage*	114
	HOW TO A Guide to Parent Effectiveness Training	130
Chapter 7	*HOW TO Estimate How Long You Will Live*	140
	FOCUS The Gray Panthers	146
Chapter 8	*FOCUS Food Fads*	164–165
Chapter 9	*FOCUS A Diet to End All Diets*	191
Chapter 10	*FOCUS The Running Mania*	199
	HOW TO Develop a Daily Fitness Program	206
Chapter 11	*FOCUS Multisubstance Abuse*	219
	HOW TO Recognize a Drug Problem	221
	VIEWPOINT Is Marijuana Safe?	234
Chapter 12	*FOCUS Teen-Agers and Drinking*	250
	HOW TO A Guide to Sensible Drinking	252
Chapter 13	*HOW TO Kick the Habit—for Good*	267
Chapter 14	*HOW TO Decrease the Likelihood of Contracting a Sexually Transmitted Disease*	291
	HOW TO Build Resistance Against Disease	292
Chapter 15	*HOW TO Decrease your Risks of Developing Cancer*	307
	FOCUS Interferon Versus Cancer—A Ray of Hope?	312
Chapter 17	*FOCUS Carcinogens in the Workplace*	340
	VIEWPOINT Solar Energy—A Viable Alternative?	348
Chapter 18	*FOCUS Health Care in the Year 2003*	364
	HOW TO Perform Mouth-to-Mouth Resuscitation	366

ESSENTIALS OF LIFE & HEALTH

third edition

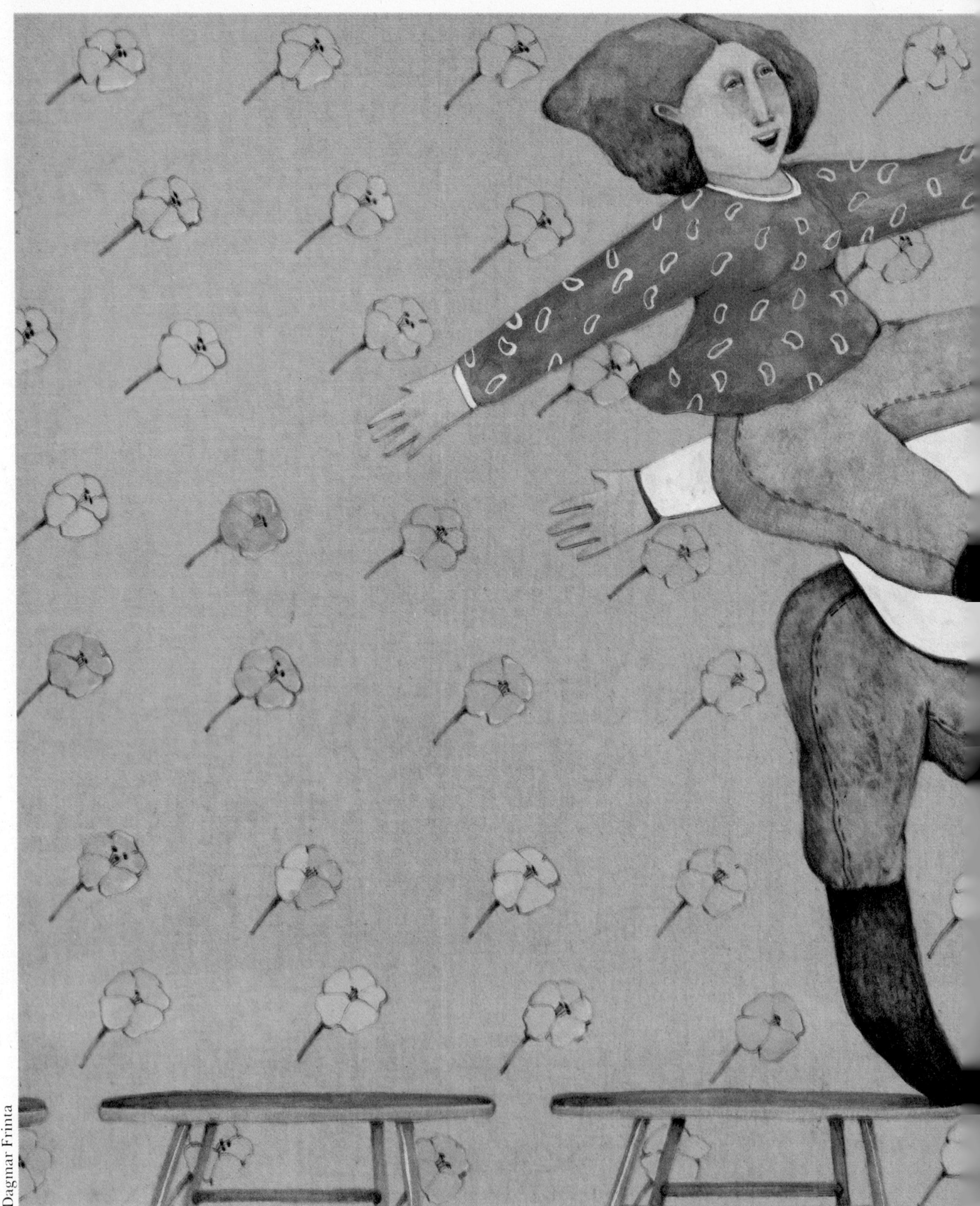

Dagmar Frinta

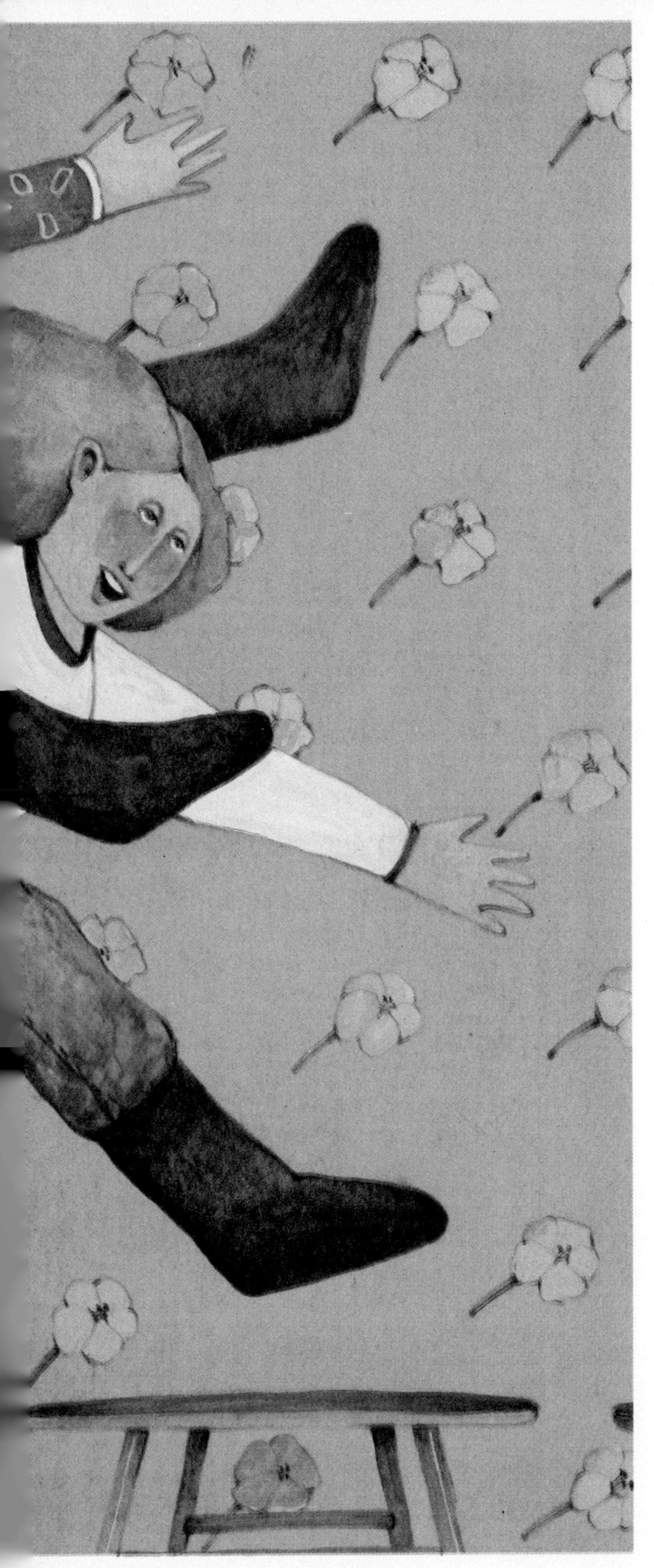

Life and Health

At birth, the average American of our time can expect to live a comparatively healthy life of seventy years or more. Most of us take this fact for granted, but just a few decades ago, such longevity was far from commonplace. An American born in 1910, for instance, had an average lifespan of just over 47 years. Every decade since then, though, advances in medicine and science have added nearly four years to our life expectancy, and today, in the words of the Surgeon General of the United States, "the health of the American people has never been better."

Indeed, during this century, the incidence of numerous life-threatening infectious and communicable diseases has been dramatically reduced or eliminated altogether. Similarly, many diseases once considered incurable can now be prevented or modified, if not cured. Thanks to remarkable strides in technology and technique, even damage to major organs (such as the kidneys or the heart) can sometimes be repaired. In fact, Americans between the ages of one and forty-two or so are more likely to die from an accidental cause than from a disease—and even the accidental death rate has been on the decline.

Not only are we Americans healthier than ever before, we are also far more health-conscious. The media bombard us with the latest medical breakthroughs, and books on diet and exercise climb the best-seller lists. Jogging has become virtually a national mania; social conversations center on fitness, and we spend our money on sports clothes and equipment. As concerned citizens, we lobby our governments about such public health issues as radiation, pollution, pesticides, and toxic wastes.

Yet despite advances in medicine, in science, in hygiene, and in health-consciousness, many Americans—rich and poor, young and old, rural and urban—are not as healthy as they might be. Why not?

OUR POTENTIAL FOR HEALTH

Many people think that health is simply the absence of disease. We can readily see the inadequacies of this view if we compare two hypothetical people with typical nine-to-five jobs. Let's say that both are thirty-five years old. One smokes several packs of cigarettes a day, has three or more drinks every evening, and is overweight and often anxious. The other does not smoke, drinks alcohol sparingly, exercises regularly, and is relaxed and confident. Both people may pass all laboratory tests and be declared free of disease, but are they equally healthy? Obviously not. Because many Americans confuse well-being with the absence of disease, they settle for less than the best possible health.

We have a great deal of information about how to promote health and avoid disease. We know about the hazards of smoking, the risks of drugs, the value of good diet and exercise. Nevertheless this knowledge does not automatically assure us good health. Good health comes only from *acting* on such knowledge; obviously, not all of us do.

Matters of Definition

The World Health Organization (WHO) in its 1947 charter defined health as "a state of complete physical, mental and social well-being, not merely the absence of disease or infirmity." Although some people criticize this definition for being too idealistic, the fact that it includes goals for mental and social well-being is extremely important. Boredom, anxiety, loneliness or general unhappiness can adversely affect the way we function. These emotional states can actually lower the body's physical resistance, making it more susceptible to disease. They can also lead to self-abusive behaviors like smoking excessively, drinking, or overeating. Not surprisingly, such behaviors often appear when basic emotional and social needs such as friendship, affection, love, and stimulation from the environment are unfulfilled.

Health professionals are now paying increasing attention to the concept of *positive health* or *optimal health,* the highest level of well-being possible. They recognize that basic human needs—physical, psychological, or social—are interdependent, and that the constant interaction of these needs influences our total health. Almost any college infirmary at final exam time will provide numerous cases in point: the combination of competitive and intellectual pressures, anxiety, and irregular sleeping and eating patterns gives rise to a long list of maladies ranging from sore gums to mononucleosis. To achieve optimal health, it is necessary to take a holistic approach to health. Holism is the concept that human beings and other living organisms are complex entities that are affected by a great number of interrelated factors. Our total health results from an interaction of many forces—genetic, physical, mental, social, environmental, economic, political, spiritual. The holistic approach involves simultaneous attention to all such forces in a person's life—all of the circumstances that might be relevant to his or her health. Thus health workers who take this approach are likely to ask not only about ordinary medical matters but also about family and social relationships and vocational plans. The ultimate

Figure 1 Positive health includes a feeling of total well being, as well as freedom from disease.

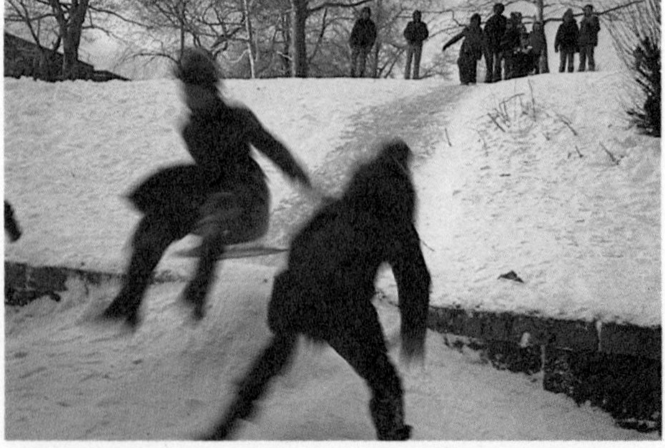

purpose of such questions, and of the holistic approach in general, is to help a person gain more control over his or her health.

THE DETERMINANTS OF HEALTH

Is complete control of our personal health possible? Obviously not: to a considerable extent our health is determined by factors beyond our control. We cannot choose, for instance, the genetic endowment that our parents pass on to us—our physique, our physical constitution, or our inborn resistance to disease. Nor do we have any say over whether we will inherit a genetic or other congenital abnormality.

Also beyond our control are many of the environmental factors that can modify our genetic potential. These include the type of family we are born into; the social, cultural and economic milieu in which we spend our formative years; and the likelihood of having an accident that leads to injury. But a closer look at the three elements in the WHO definition of health will show that many of the most important determining factors are well within our control.

Physical Well-Being

We can keep our bodies healthy in many ways by making very simple changes in our behavior. For instance, exercise can bring about a significant improvement in cardiovascular and respiratory function, and it may serve as an effective defense against heart disease. The heart is a muscle, and it will perform at less than optimal capacity if it is not kept in good shape. This is true of all our muscles and joints: if used properly and kept limber, they will remain in good condition; if neglected, they will deteriorate—even in youth.

In other ways, too, we can influence our own physical health—for better or for worse—through the choices we make or the habits we form. For example, overexposure to the sun can cause skin damage and even skin cancer. It takes just a simple decision to spend a bit less time in the sun to lessen our vulnerability. Similarly, hearing can be severely and permanently damaged by prolonged exposure to loud noises. Our vision, too, can be maintained at an optimal level through good health practices, including regular medical checkups.

Mental Health

You can consider yourself to have normal mental health if your feelings and behavior are similar to those of most other people in your culture. In American society that means, it is hoped, feeling comfortable with yourself and others; being able to love, work, and play satisfactorily; and coping successfully with the normal problems and stresses of life. Mental health does *not* mean being free from worry, doubt, fear, and guilt. There are many occasions when such feelings are justified: you *should* worry about whether your financial resources are sufficient for your needs, and you *should* feel guilty about treating other people badly.

Beyond this, a person in optimal mental health is energetic, assertive, enthusiastic, usually optimistic, relaxed, confident. Such a person may be productive and highly creative and is willing to cope with (rather than avoid) life's problems in the belief that this will provide opportunities for further development and personal growth. He or she has the capacity to deeply love and to be deeply loved, and is comfortable about his or her body. Such positive mental health is discussed in Chapter 1.

Social Well-Being

Most of us probably think that a healthy social life is an ornament to, rather than an integral aspect of, general well-being. And it is true that thus far even specialists in the health field have paid less attention to the social dimension of well-being. Yet the overall context of our lives is undeniably social: each of us lives in relationship to other people, and these relationships both create and fulfill a wide variety of needs. Being a good friend, a good neighbor, a good citizen, a good parent are all aspects of our social well-being.

At one level, then, social health simply means performing your chosen role in life in a way that satisfies both yourself and the people with whom you come in contact. At a higher level, optimal social health may involve volun-

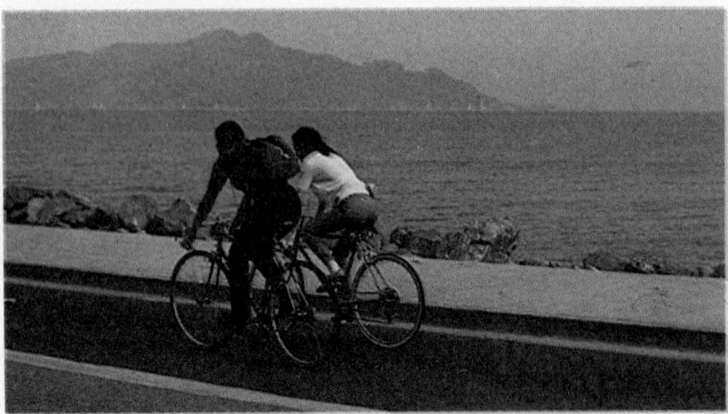

Figure 2 Bicycle riding minimizes environmental pollution and therefore contributes to social health. It is also good for your physical and mental health—and is fun.

teering your time or money to help others or to work for important causes. It may also involve a life style that minimizes waste of natural resources, conserves energy, and reduces environmental pollution. For instance, you might choose to walk or ride a bicycle rather than drive a car (which would simultaneously be good for your physical and mental health). Taking responsibility for your personal health also contributes to social health in that you are less likely to become a burden to others because of illness. Ideally, people with high levels of social health give more to the world than they take from it.

A Hypothetical Life History

Figure 3 shows graphically how these three interrelated components of health might ebb and flow over one person's lifetime. In the figure, health is shown as a continuum from optimal health at the top, through normal health (not being sick) in the middle, to illness and death at the bottom. Three colors indicate the course of a person's physical health (red), mental health (green), and social health (yellow). Some forces lift these components toward optimal levels; others push them downward toward sickness.

Tom, our hypothetical subject, was healthy at birth except for a rare heart abnormality that did not constitute a serious illness per se, but did make Tom prone to sickness during early childhood. By the time Tom was ten, the heart abnormality had resolved itself, and he began to enjoy reasonably good physical health. At just about the same time, though, Tom's parents' marriage entered a period of considerable strain, and Tom's mother became very overprotective. These two influences combined to depress Tom's mental and social development to fairly low levels.

At age twenty, Tom's physical health was normal, but his mental health had deteriorated: he was having problems at school, and his self-esteem was low. Over the next several years, Tom entered a successful marriage, got an excellent job, and enjoyed a number of close, supportive friendships; by the time he was thirty-five, his total health was at an all-time high. It remained there for ten years until Tom's physical health plummeted abruptly as a result of a nearly fatal bout of appendicitis. Then, for the following fifteen years his physical health improved, but in his mid-fifties his declining interest in his job and—ultimately—the loss of his job impaired his mental health. During these years, Tom's marriage and his close friends sustained his social health. In Tom's late sixties, his mental and social health reached another high point, despite the development of heart disease, which gave him chest pains. These components of his health remained high until Tom died at the age of seventy from a heart attack.

Figure 3 Life chart showing the interaction of positive and negative forces, and their effects, on the physical, social, and mental health of a hypothetical person named Tom. Note that at age thirty-five, Tom's health was at its peak in all three areas.

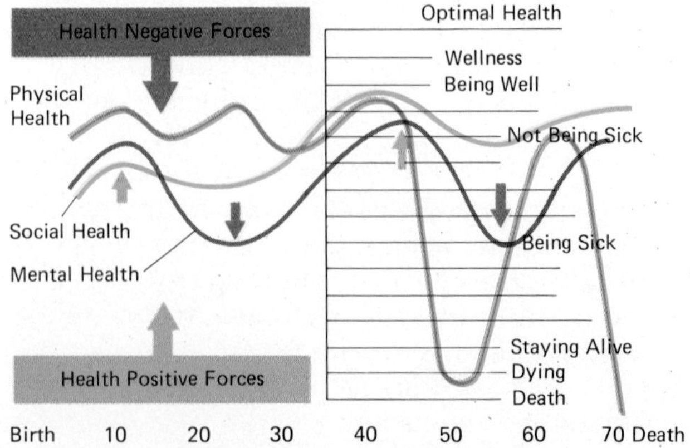

THE MAJOR HEALTH HAZARD

With all the news coverage and publicity given of late to the various health hazards that Americans face in their daily lives, selecting the most dangerous hazard would seem a difficult task. You might reasonably guess smog, food additives, toxic substances in the water supply, radiation, industrial pollution, illegal drugs, and so on. But according to a report issued recently by the Department of Health, Education, and Welfare, the major health hazard in our society is our life style.

The four most harmful components of this life style are excessive use of alcohol, excessive use of tobacco, lack of exercise, and improper diet. Together, these items contribute heavily to cancer, heart and respiratory ailments, kidney and liver diseases, and fatal accidents (particularly among young people).

Major improvements in the quality of life and health can only come about by changes in our life style. Indeed, the very large role of personal behavior in determining health was dramatically shown in a major study conducted by Lester Breslow and Nedra B. Bellock. Over a five-and-a-half-year period, Breslow and Bellock investigated the health habits of nearly 7,000 residents of Alameda County, California. The results of the study clearly demonstrate that an individual's habits strongly influence not only the amount of illness he or she experiences, but also how long he or she lives.

The specific habits associated with good health and longer survival are the following:

1. Not smoking cigarettes.
2. Drinking alcohol in moderation (no more than two drinks a day) if at all.
3. Eating breakfast.
4. Not eating between meals.
5. Maintaining normal weight.
6. Sleeping seven or eight hours each day.
7. Exercising at least moderately.

While there may be no surprises in this list, their impact on well-being is remarkable. Breslow and Bellock found, for example, that a forty-five-year-old man following six or seven of these habits lived an average of eleven years longer than men of the same age who followed three habits or less. For women, the life expectancy difference was seven years. Furthermore, men in their mid-fifties who followed six or seven habits were in about the same physical condition as men twenty years younger who followed only three or less.

The study further showed that, compared to personal health habits, income level, gender, and age had negligible effects on health. (Detailed information about the impact of these personal habits on health will be found throughout this textbook; smoking is discussed in Chapter 13; alcohol, Chapter 12; nutrition, Chapter 8; weight control, Chapter 9; and physical fitness, Chapter 10.)

IT'S UP TO YOU

We choose our general life style: the work we do, what we eat, whether we smoke or drink or use drugs, the amount of exercise and relaxation we get, the physical risks we run, and when we see a physician. In cooperation with other people, we can also exert some influence over the quality of our neighborhoods, the safety of our cars, and the pollution to which we are exposed.

It's up to you to be responsible for your own life style. This simple commitment is the first step toward a long and healthy life. No one can make this commitment for you, any more than someone else can sleep, exercise, or eat balanced meals on your behalf. Indeed, you are the only one who is in a position to take a holistic view of your own health, to know all the forces—physical, mental, social, economic, cultural—influencing your health. You are the only one who can shape your behavior in ways that affect your health.

This book will discuss the stages of the human life cycle (marriage, parenthood, aging); the major types of disease (infectious diseases, cardiovascular diseases, cancer); habits that can affect your health (smoking, the use of alcohol and other psychoactive drugs); and the health-care system and how to use it. Throughout the book, you will also find many specific, practical suggestions for maintaining your own physical and mental health and preventing illness and untimely death. In the end, however, good health grows from a series of decisions, lasting your whole life, and it's up to you to make the most of your life and health.

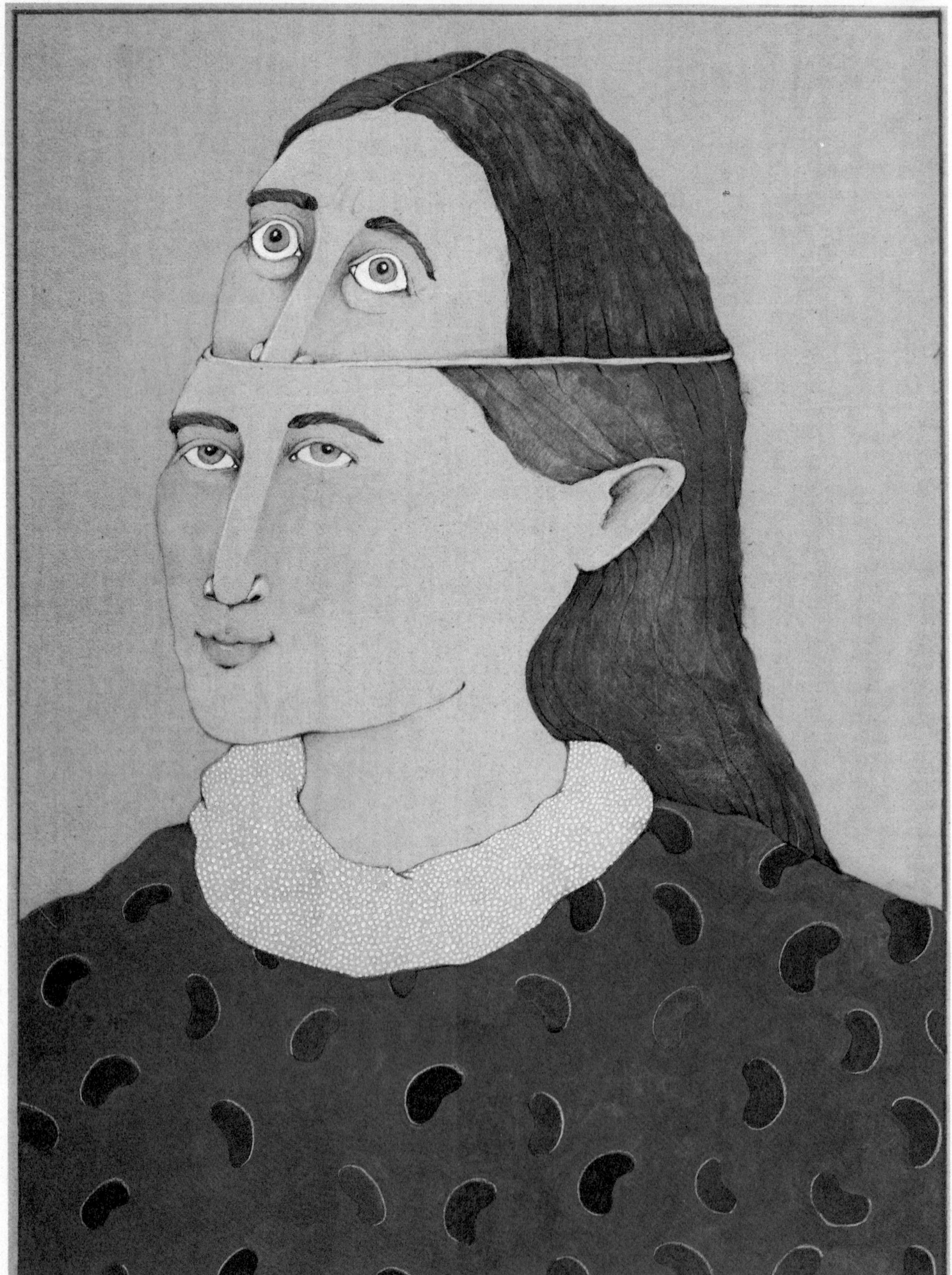

Dagmar Frinta

I EMOTIONAL AND SEXUAL ADJUSTMENT

It has long been a common axiom that a healthy mind and a healthy body go hand in hand, and medical evidence is now proving this saying true. Consider laughter. You laugh because you find something funny—a psychological judgment—but laughter is really a *physical* reaction. And the stronger your psychological reaction, the harder you laugh! This is only one example, but it is clear that physical health and mental health are intricately connected.

Part I of this book explores the nature of healthy emotional and sexual adjustment, emphasizing the interrelationships between health and the mind. Chapter 1 explains the importance of full emotional development to optimal health and discusses the compelling topic of mental disorders, which can result when people fail to understand their emotions or lose the ability to control them—or to express them.

In a fast-paced modern society such as ours, we are continually exposed to many types of stress. Stress can be a stimulating challenge, but many people find it very difficult to cope with. In Chapter 2, we look at stress, its effects on health, and how to reduce its negative effects.

Sigmund Freud believed that sexuality is the prime motivation behind all of our actions. Whether or not we agree with him, sexuality has helped many people to find deep fulfillment, while to others it has brought profound suffering. Clearly, an understanding of your own and other people's sexual behavior will contribute to your attainment of optimal health. Chapter 3 covers in detail the basic physiological and psychological "facts of life" that concern the sexually mature individual.

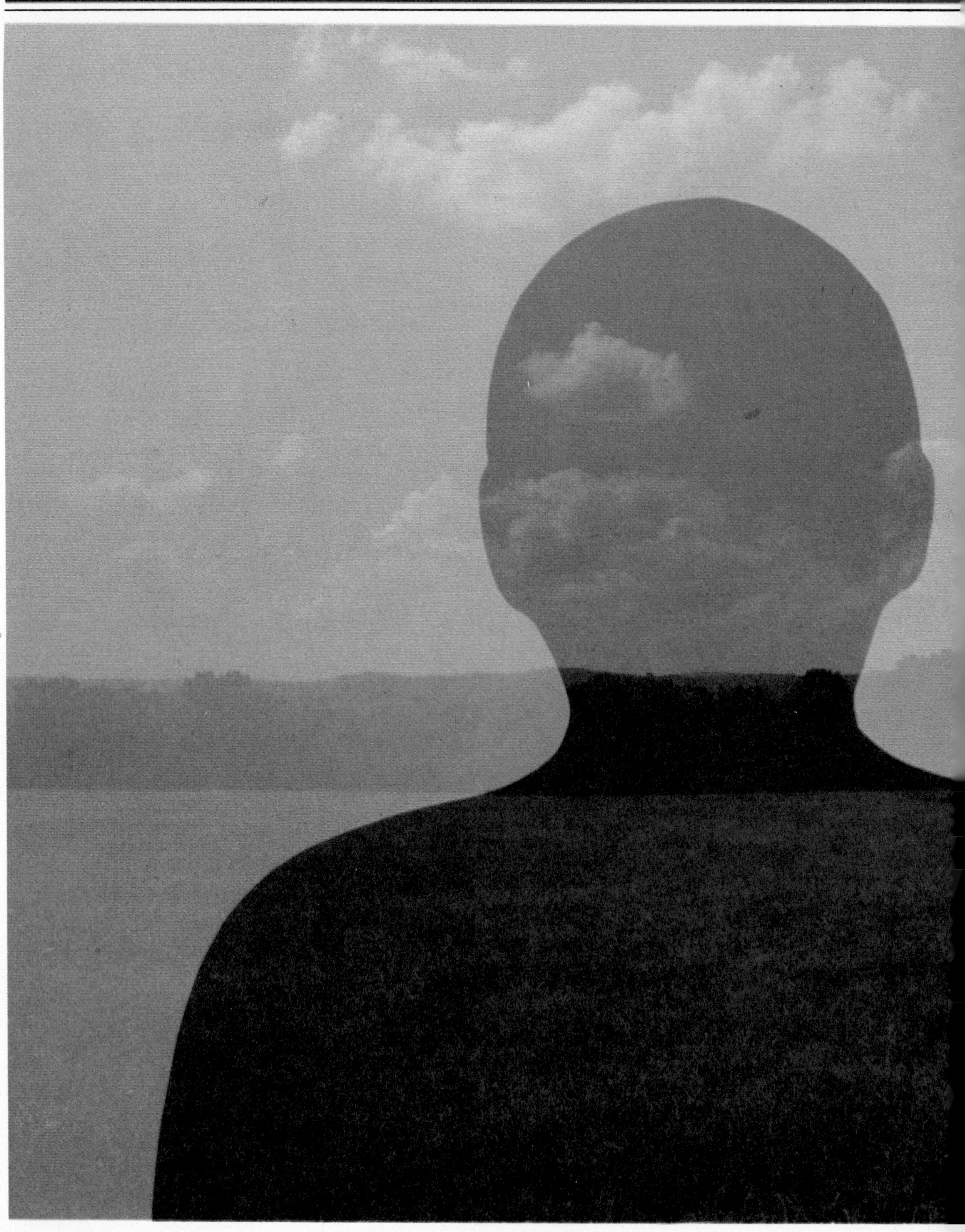

1 Mental Health

Why do we human beings behave as we do? Why do we work and play, learn and love, strive and aspire? Why are we at times lazy or mean, hostile or destructive? We behave in these ways partly because such behavior makes us *feel* better, or because it expresses how well or badly we do *feel.* The psychic and physiological aspects of such *feelings* are called *emotions.*

Other animals experience pleasure and pain, but only we humans are able to understand what we are feeling, label these feelings with language, integrate these experiences into our consciousness, and alter our surroundings—and our interactions with our surroundings—to influence what we feel and what we do about what we feel. The wonder and joy we feel when viewing a beautiful sunset, the tenderness evoked by a love story, the thrill of learning a new idea or skill, our anger at an injustice—these are all examples of emotions that enrich our lives or that can be put to constructive use.

Unfortunately, our emotions can also work against us, functioning negatively and destructively in ways that threaten our adjustment, our relationships with others, and our achievements. Emotional problems can cause a range of so-called psychosomatic reactions from mild headaches, sweating, and eyestrain to ulcers, high blood pressure, and serious digestive disorders. Conversely, physical disorders can have a major influence on psychological functioning. Vitamin B deficiency produces psychotic symptoms; syphilis can invade the brain and produce symptoms of mental illness; obesity can lead to lethargy and depression.

Our emotional and mental health and our

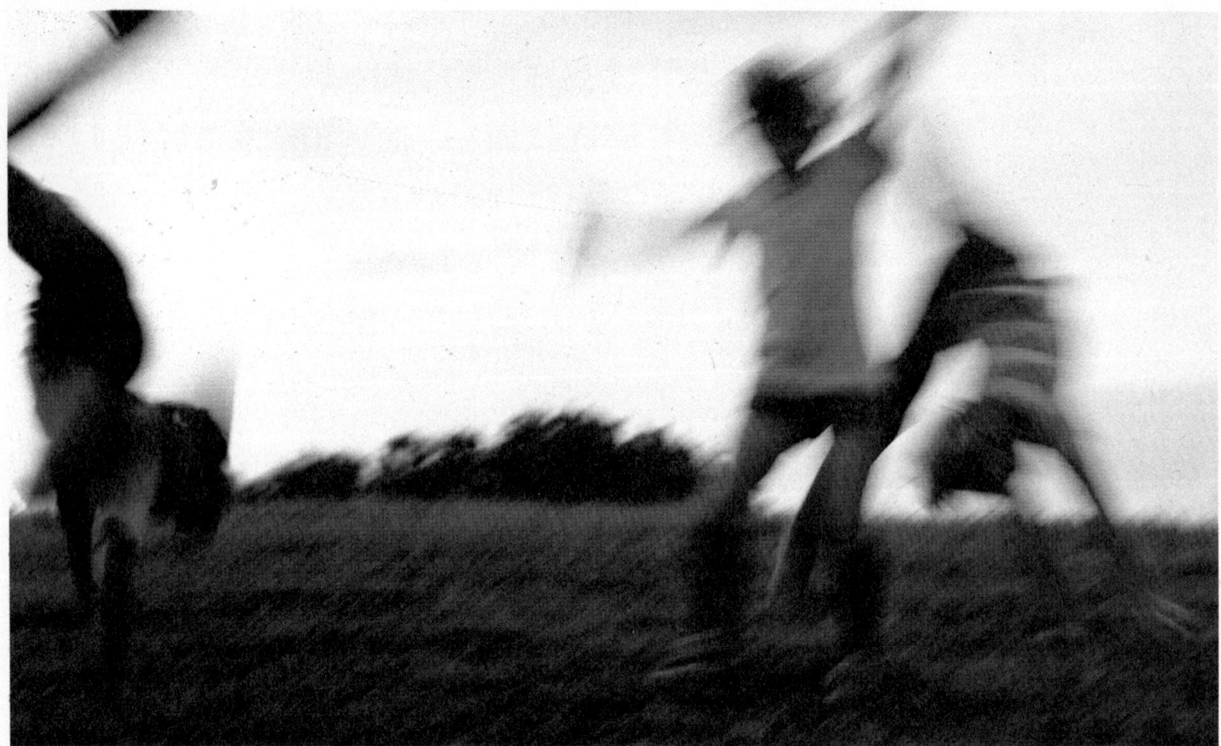

Figure 1.1 Emotional, mental, and physical health are intricately intertwined.

physical health are thus intricately intertwined. To understand one is to have a better understanding of the other. In this chapter, we will try to gain a better understanding of our emotional and mental health by looking at the nature of emotion, the ways in which emotions affect the body, how emotional maturity develops, the characteristics of the emotionally mature and mentally healthy person, and some ways in which you can facilitate emotional and mental health in yourself and others. We will also explore the compelling topic of mental disorders: how they are defined, how they are classified, and how to get help for them.

THE NATURE OF EMOTION

What are emotions? Many people would answer this question by citing examples: Emotions are such things as anger, love, fear, hope, sorrow, joy, revulsion, pity, boredom, amazement, disgust. Psychologists vary in their definitions; some describe emotions solely in terms of physical changes, while others focus on feelings as learned responses to specific situations. A growing number of psychologists are coming to agree with the definition provided by Magda Arnold: An *emotion* is "a felt tendency toward something intuitively assessed as good, favorable, beneficial or away from something assessed as unfavorable, harmful, bad." The most important word here is "assessed"; Arnold sees emotions as the results of mental evaluative processes—they don't "just happen."

Arnold carefully analyzed the sequence of events that usually occur when someone experiences and expresses an emotion. First comes *perception:* a person must perceive an object or an event before an emotion can result. (Sometimes this stage occurs in imagination, as when one becomes anxious about a possible future event.) Next comes *appraisal,* the stage at which the favorableness or harmfulness of the object or event is assessed. The third and fourth stages are the *emotion* and the accompanying *bodily changes.* (These stages are omitted if the appraisal indicates no cause for concern.) The fifth stage, *action,* may occur either alone or followed by secondary appraisal—a consideration of the bodily changes that followed the initial appraisal. An example of how these stages occur is presented in Figure 1.2.

Arnold's description of emotions is particularly valuable in that it shows emotions to be intimately linked with *thinking;* your emotional responses in a given situation are based on mental processes of which you may or may not be aware. In essence, your emotions are outgrowths of your *values*—the things that you have consciously or unconsciously determined to be good or evil, important or unimportant, useful or damaging, moral or immoral. Thus, if you value something you do not have, you feel desire; if you obtain the valued item, you feel joy. If something happens that you consider to be wrong, you feel sorrow or unhappiness; if the wrong is righted, you feel relief.

EMOTIONS AND THE BODY

Everyone has experienced the bodily sensations that accompany emotions—a racing heart, cold or clammy hands, profuse sweating, blushing, tensed muscles, clenched teeth, and so on. These are the physical events referred to in the fourth step of Arnold's emotion sequence. Why are emotional experiences so tied to observable behaviors and to bodily changes? The answer lies in the nervous system.

Of critical importance in the physiology of emotions is the *autonomic nervous system,* which controls the glands, internal organs, and involuntary muscles. The autonomic nervous system has two divisions, the parasympathetic

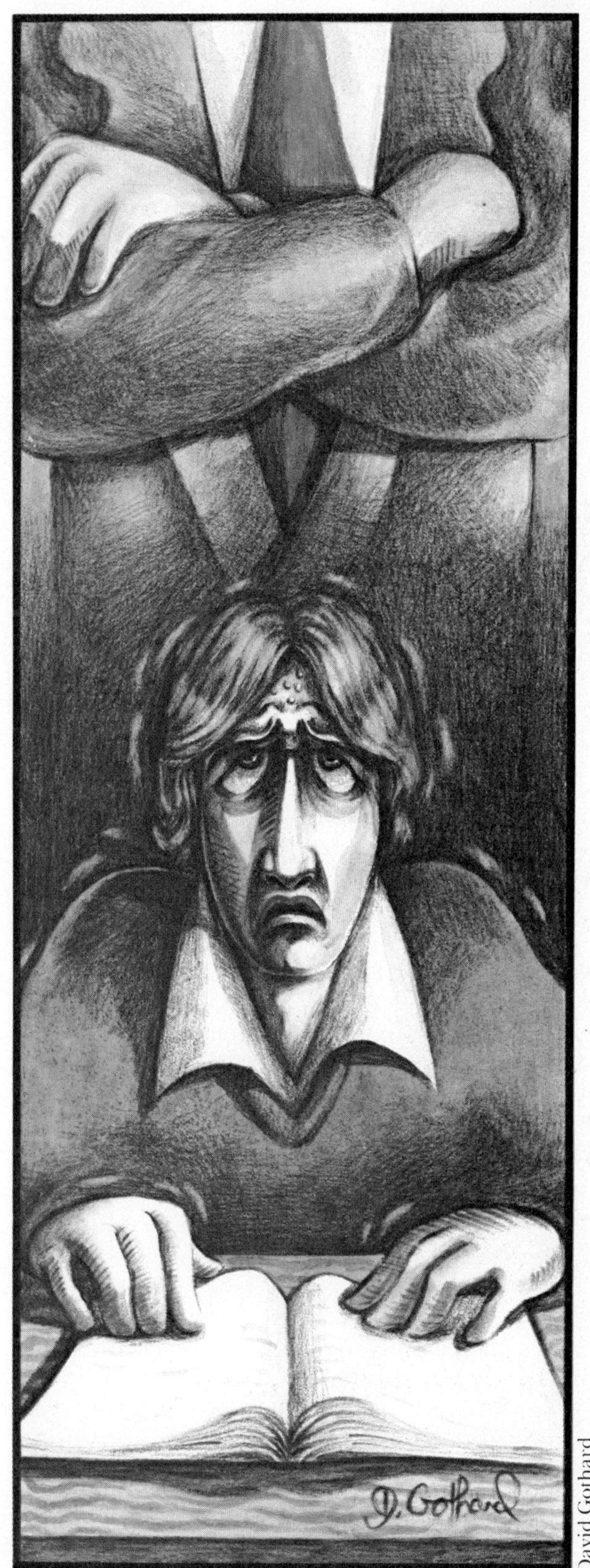

David Gothard

Figure 1.2 Michael is unprepared for his French class: an example of the sequences involved in an emotion, as described by Magda Arnold. (1) *Perception:* "The professor is going to call on me!" (2) *Appraisal:* "Boy, am I in trouble!" (3) *Emotion:* Fear. (4) *Bodily changes:* Faster heartbeat, shaking hands. (5) *Action:* "I'd better flip through my notes!"

and the sympathetic. Activation of the *sympathetic system* tends to prepare the body for dealing with emergencies or strenuous activities—speeding up the heart to hasten the supply of oxygen and nutrients, increasing the breathing rate, and dilating arteries going to the muscles and constricting those going to the digestive organs and skin, so that blood can go where it is needed most. In contrast, the *parasympathetic system* tends to conserve energy and to enhance the recuperative activities of the body. It reduces heart rate and breathing rate and routes blood to the digestive system.

These autonomic changes occur in response to the individual's external situation. The parasympathetic system, for example, would be most active after a large meal or following strenuous activity. The sympathetic system is activated by external emergencies or threats. The threat might be extreme cold, lack of food, an enemy, a coming examination, a divorce, or some other type of stress. The bodily changes instigated by the sympathetic system are designed to mobilize the body for dealing with the stress—to prepare it for fight or flight. Once the stress is dealt with, the parasympathetic system dominates, the physical reactions subside, and functioning returns to normal.

However, these bodily changes accompanying our emotions have their negative side. There are often times when a person cannot act immediately; modern society offers few threats that can be dealt with simply by fight or flight. Prolonged, unresolved stress is thought to be associated with such chronic problems as backaches, migraine headaches, asthma, high blood pressure, and stomach ulcers. But there is also a positive side to the bodily effects of our emotions. Positive emotions such as love and joy—growing out of feelings of relaxation, comfort, caring, and being cared for—tend to put the sympathetic nervous system at ease, reducing the levels of stress hormones, with their potentially damaging effects. And frequently the positive and negative effects of emotions are mixed together. Aroused emotions—with their faster heartbeat and higher levels of stress hormones—constructively motivate most human achievement, from scientific investigation to athletic excellence to esthetic creativity. (Stress and stress reduction will be discussed in detail in Chapter 2.)

EMOTIONAL NEEDS

Mental, emotional, and physical functioning are thus highly interrelated and interdependent. What is characteristic of one type of functioning is often true of the other two in a related way. It is recognized that people have certain basic physical needs that must be met in order for them to survive. They need air to breathe, water to drink, food to eat. Can it also be true that people have fundamental emotional needs, the fulfillment of which is necessary for psychological survival?

For many psychologists, the answer to this question is yes. They have proposed a number of things as being basic psychological needs—the need to love and be loved, the need to feel worthy, the need to feel safe, the need to achieve, the need to be dependent and independent, and so on. Love and self-esteem, the two emotional needs that are perhaps the most important, will be looked at more closely, and a proposed structure of needs, including both physical and psychological components, will be examined.

The Need for Love

Several studies seem to indicate that some kind of love or attention is necessary for healthy emotional development. In one of the most famous studies, Harry Harlow raised infant monkeys who had been taken away from their natural mothers at birth. Each monkey was raised with two *surrogate,* or substitute, mothers. One mother was constructed of wood and wire; the other was built similarly but was covered with soft, cuddly terry cloth. For some of the infants, the wire mother had a nipple from which the monkey could obtain milk; for other infants, food could be obtained only from the cloth mother.

The purpose of the experiment was to see which surrogate made the better mother. The results were dramatic: The young monkeys became strongly attached to the cloth mother, whether or not she gave food, and for the most part ignored the wire mother. If a frightening object was placed in the cage, the monkey would run to the terry cloth mother for security, not to the wire mother. Apparently it was the touching that mattered, not the feeding.

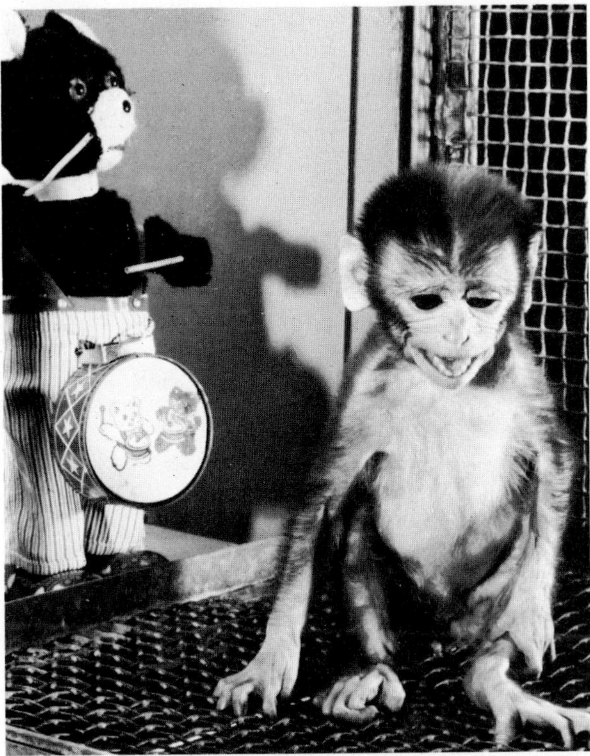

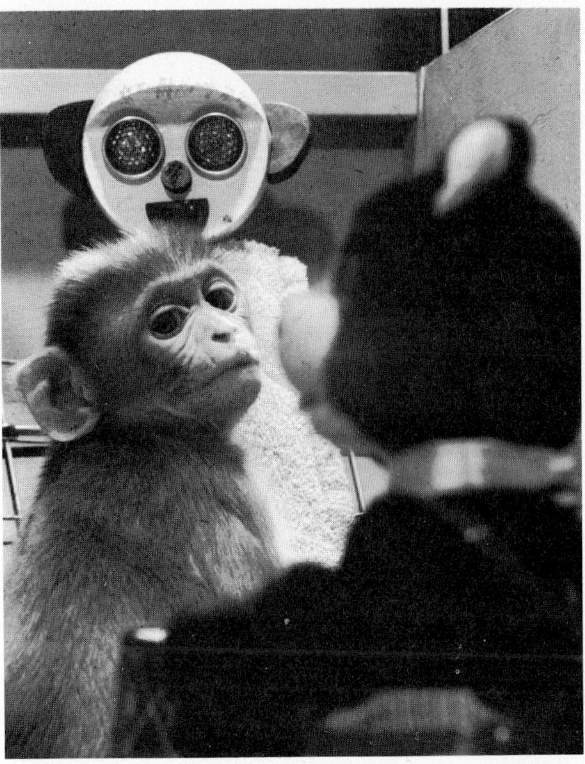

Figure 1.3 Harlow's experiments with monkeys demonstrated that love or attention is necessary for healthy emotional development. When monkeys raised by surrogate cloth mothers were placed alone in a cage with a strange object, they were frightened. But when the cloth mother was also present, they were curious.

In another set of experiments, Harlow discovered that monkeys raised without mothers grew up with serious emotional problems. As adults, they seemed not to know how to mate, even though they tried; neither did they know how to play or to defend themselves. In fact, when frightened by a strange human, they often attacked their own bodies instead of making threatening signs of aggression as normal monkeys do.

The monkeys who had cloth mothers grew up more normally than the motherless ones, but even they were not well adjusted to normal monkey life. A partially adequate substitute for a mother turned out to be *peers*—other baby monkeys. Infant monkeys that played with other monkeys like themselves grew up fairly normally, even if they never saw their mothers. To grow up completely normally, however, both mother and peers were necessary.

A number of psychologists believe that these findings can be applied to human beings. John Bowlby, René Spitz, and others have investigated cases of children who, like Harlow's monkeys, were deprived of their mothers at an early age. They concluded that severe personality problems can develop when an attachment is not formed or is forcibly broken (as by the death of the mother) before the age of seven.

Children need individual attention, warmth, comfort, security, and stimulation. Without a parent and family, they are less likely to receive this attention. Some infants in orphanages and other institutions may receive enough attention if the institution has a large staff of people who can give them love. More often, however, an institution has a cold, impersonal atmosphere in which children waste away, even though their physical needs are adequately satisfied. For full development, satisfaction of love needs is vital.

Loneliness For adults, too, the need for love and satisfying human relationships is important for both emotional and physical health. In the book *The Broken Heart: The Medical Consequences of Loneliness in America,* James J. Lynch argues that "the lack of human companionship, the sudden loss of love, and chronic human loneliness are significant contributors to serious disease . . . and premature death." Lynch points out that the mortality rates for all causes of death, including heart disease, are higher among people who are single, divorced, or widowed than among married people.

The Need for Self-Esteem

The idea that self-esteem is a fundamental emotional need has been expressed by many psychologists. Nathaniel Branden in his book *The Psychology of Self-Esteem* defines *self-esteem* as "the integrated sum of self-confidence and self-respect. It is the conviction that one is competent to live and worthy of living." According to Branden, it is important for individuals to hold themselves in high esteem, because all of their actions are aimed at benefiting the self. In order to act to achieve one's values, one must value the beneficiary of those actions. Or, as Branden puts it, "In order to seek values, man must consider himself worthy of enjoying them."

Self-esteem is a feeling that develops over the years as one grows. One's genuine opinion of oneself is rarely conscious; as Branden says, "It is a part of every other feeling it is involved in . . . every emotional response. . . . It is the single most significant key to [a person's] behavior." Without genuine self-esteem, a person would have little reason to continue to eat and dress or to attempt to stay alive. In fact, much behavior that is harmful to health or that is frankly self-destructive is motivated by a lack of self-esteem.

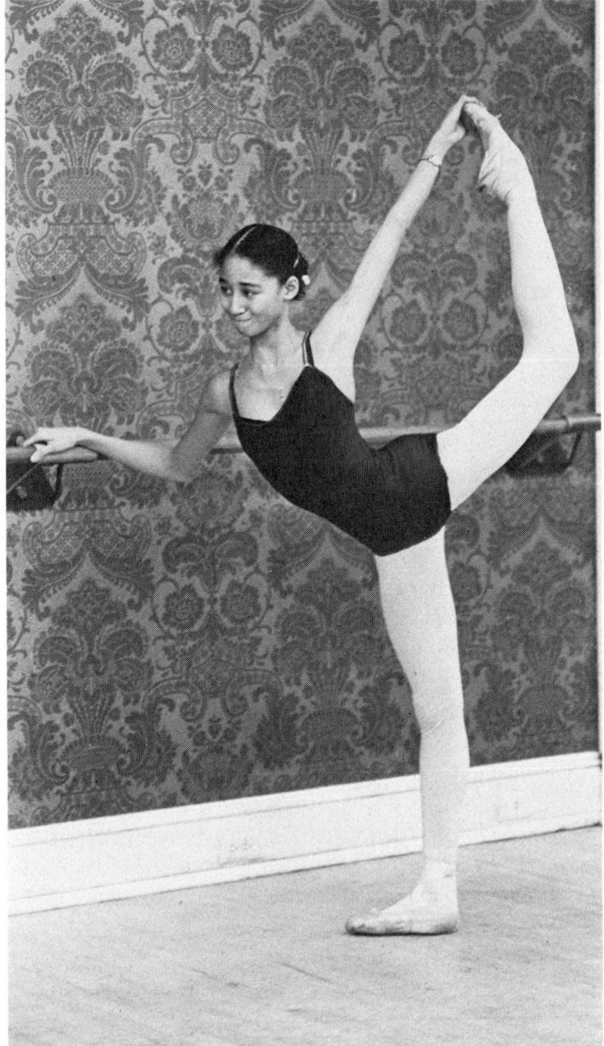

Figure 1.4 Self-esteem is the belief that you are competent and worthy of living.

Maslow's Hierarchy of Needs

The late Abraham Maslow, a great American psychologist best known for his concept of "self-actualization" (which will be discussed in detail later in this chapter), developed a list of human needs that includes not only physical requirements but also love, self-esteem, and other emotional needs. Maslow placed these needs into two categories: basic needs and metaneeds. The *basic needs* are the physiological needs for food and water and the psychological needs for affection, security, and self-esteem. These are also called deficiency needs, because if they are not met, the person will be lacking something and will seek to make up for the deficiency. The basic needs are hierarchically organized, which means that some (such as the need for food) take precedence over others. Maslow called the higher needs *metaneeds,* or *growth needs.* They include the needs for justice, goodness, beauty, order, and unity. The deficiency needs are preeminent over the

How to Overcome Shyness

Do you dread eating alone in a cafeteria or restaurant because people may think no one wants to eat with you? At a party where you don't know anyone well, do you stand uncomfortably on the sidelines because you don't know what to say to strangers? Is there someone attractive and interesting whom you would like to get to know better but avoid because you're afraid of rejection? If your answer to any of these questions is yes, you've got a case of shyness.

You're not alone! Philip Zimbardo, a psychologist at Stanford University, reports in his book *Shyness* that 80 percent of the people he studied said that they were shy at some point in their lives, and 40 percent considered themselves presently shy. This means that four out of every ten people you are afraid to meet—84 million Americans—are probably equally afraid to meet you!

Zimbardo notes that shyness has a positive side. A degree of shyness makes many people seem tactful, polite, modest, sophisticated, or intelligent. But Zimbardo stresses the fact that to many people, shyness is a crippling disorder that upsets their social lives and inhibits their everyday functioning.

How do you overcome shyness? First, Zimbardo says, get to know and like yourself. Here are a few of his suggestions:

1. Write yourself a letter whenever you need to express or clarify strong feelings. Or tape record a "state-of-yourself" message from time to time.
2. Keep a "shyness journal." Write down the date and time, what happened, your reaction, and the consequences. For example:

Tuesday, 8 P.M. Decided not to audition for play. I think acting would be fun, a good experience, and a way to meet new people, but I've never auditioned before, and I probably would have looked pretty ridiculous. Consequences—I don't know if I have any talent, or even what auditioning is *like*, and I sit in my dorm room, frustrated and annoyed with myself.

3. Build your self-confidence List your weaknesses on the left side of a page. On the right side, write down the opposite of each. Begin to think of yourself in terms of the qualities listed in the right-hand column.
4. Think of a situation that often makes you feel shy. Imagine how you would handle it if you were not shy. Think about this every day for a week. The next time the situation arises, act out what you imagined.
5. Take a risk. Do something that you want or ought to do, but have been avoiding. Write down what you intend to do and why it frightens you. Then note whether or not you did it and what happened if you did.

Next, develop your social skills. Zimbardo encourages you to strike up conversations with strangers. A good way to get people to talk is to compliment them and follow up with a question ("Your hair looks great. Where do you have it cut?"). You'll be at a real advantage if you can discuss political, cultural, athletic, or other events. Here are some of the exercises Zimbardo recommends:

1. Introduce yourself to a new person in one of your classes.
2. Invite someone who is going your way to walk with you.
3. Call someone (opposite sex) in your class about an assignment or an upcoming event.
4. Stand in line at the bank or supermarket. Strike up a conversation about the length of the line with someone nearby.
5. Chat with the gas-station attendant who is filling your tank and checking your oil.
6. Sit down next to someone (opposite sex) who looks interesting. Make an opening remark.
7. Ask three people for directions. Shift at least one of them into a brief conversation.
8. Carry a copy of a controversial book for one day. How many people can you get to start a conversation about it?
9. Throw a small party for three to five people. Invite at least one person you don't know well.
10. If you have a problem, ask the advice of someone you don't know well who lives in your dorm or neighborhood.
11. Invite someone you haven't eaten with before to go to lunch or dinner.
12. Say "Hi" to five new people today. Try to provoke a smile and a "Hi" from them.

Now, are you ready to go to that audition or ask for that date? Sure! You've practiced the skills—use them!

Source: Adapted from Philip G. Zimbardo, *Shyness* (Reading, Mass.: Addison-Wesley, 1977).

growth needs in most cases. If one is lacking food and water, one cannot attend very seriously to justice and beauty. Nor, according to Maslow, can a person who lacks basic security and self-esteem feel free to consider fairness, to feel deep reciprocal love, to be democratic, and to resist restrictive conformity. The metaneeds are not hierarchically organized; consequently, one metaneed can be pursued instead of another, depending on the particular person's life circumstances. Nevertheless, the metaneeds are real and, if unfulfilled, can lead to what Maslow called *metapathologies,* such as alienation, anguish, apathy, and cynicism.

STAGES OF EMOTIONAL DEVELOPMENT

At birth all infants seem to be capable of four basic emotions: pleasure, displeasure, excitement, and depression. As children develop, their range of emotional expression broadens and becomes more "personalized." Many complex genetic and environmental factors affect each person's specific emotional make-up. However, some psychologists believe that emotional development, regardless of individual differences, falls into a predictable stage-by-stage sequence. Erik Erikson has devised an interesting and useful description of the emotional changes and challenges that occur at each stage of development, but we should first look at the theory of Sigmund Freud, the first psychologist to suggest that emotional development occurs in stages.

Freud's Stages

Freud believed that children pass through five major stages of what he called psychosexual development: the oral, anal, phallic, latency, and genital. In each stage, the focus of the child's pleasure is a different part of the body, and in turn, the child's affections shift to a different object. For example, the focus of pleasure in the first stage, the *oral stage,* is the child's mouth, and therefore, the love object is the mother's breast. In the *anal stage,* pleasure shifts to the anus and the process of defecation. During the *phallic stage,* around the age of three to six, the focus of pleasure for a young boy shifts to his penis; for example, masturbation is very common at this age. At this time, boys begin to view their father as a rival for their prime love object, their mother. Also, what Freud calls the *Oedipal complex* develops; the young boy desires his mother and wants to destroy his rival, the father. However, the boy is afraid of his father's power—afraid that his father will retaliate and harm him in some way so as to remove him as a rival. Usually, the child resolves this conflict by repressing his desire for his mother and identifying with his father, so that he can vicariously share in his father's special relationship with his mother.

The resolution of the Oedipal conflict moves the child into the *latency stage,* where his sexual impulses are repressed, and so his love of his mother is no longer a problem, because it is nonsexual. The hormones of adolescence cause his sexuality to burst forth again, and he enters the *genital stage,* where his love object is a person of the opposite sex, and the focus of his pleasure is sexual intercourse with that particular person.

Freud felt that gratification at each successive stage, but especially through the first five years, is essential for healthy development and that the personalities or characters of certain people are the result of *fixations* at early developmental stages. For example, failure to achieve oral gratification gives rise in the adult to an emphasis on oral activities, such as chewing, smoking, and talking. Stinginess and stubbornness characterize the anal personality. Failure to resolve the Oedipal conflict results in inability to achieve normal heterosexual relationships.

Erikson's Stages

Freud's pioneering theory, with its focus on the sexual life of the male child, is controversial today. Nevertheless, it is important in that it provided a base for Erik Erikson's developmental theory. Erikson has recast Freud's stages and has added several that appear after adolescence. Erikson believes that a person's emotional make-up is the result of a series of encounters between the needs of the person and the demands of society. Erikson has outlined eight stages of development, each of which is characterized by a *psychosocial crisis;* each human must, in effect, pass eight great tests (see Figure 1.5).

Age	Stage	Result of Success	Result of Failure
Early Infancy (birth to about one year) (corollary to Freudian oral stage)	Basic Trust vs. Mistrust	Trust results from affection and gratification of needs, mutual recognition.	Mistrust results from consistent abuse, neglect, deprivation of love, too early or harsh weaning, autistic isolation.
Later Infancy (one to three years) (corollary to Freudian muscular anal stage)	Autonomy vs. Shame and Doubt	Child views self as person apart from parents but still dependent.	Child feels inadequate, doubts self, curtails learning basic skills like walking, talking, wants to "hide" inadequacies.
Early Childhood (about ages four to five years) (corollary to Freudian phallic locomotor stage)	Initiative vs. Guilt	Child has lively imagination, vigorously tests reality, imitates adults, anticipates roles.	Child lacks spontaneity, has infantile jealousy "castration complex," is suspicious, evasive, suffers from role inhibition.
Middle Childhood (about ages six to eleven years) (corollary to Freudian latency stage)	Industry vs. Inferiority	Child has sense of duty and accomplishment, develops scholastic and social competencies, undertakes real tasks, puts fantasy and play in better perspective, learns world of tools, task identification.	Child has poor work habits, avoids strong competition, feels doomed to mediocrity; is in lull before the storms of puberty, may conform as slavish behavior, has sense of futility.
Puberty and Adolescence (about ages twelve to twenty years)	Ego Identity vs. Role Confusion	Adolescent has temporal perspective, is self-certain, is a role experimenter, goes through apprenticeship, experiences sexual polarization and leader-followership, develops an ideological commitment.	Adolescent experiences time confusion, is self-conscious, has a role fixation, and experiences work paralysis, bisexual confusion, authority confusion, and value confusion.
Early Adulthood	Intimacy vs. Isolation	Person has capacity to commit self to others, "true genitability" is now possible, *Lieben und Arbeiten*—"to love and to work"; "mutuality of genital orgasm."	Person avoids intimacy, has "character problems," behaves promiscuously, and repudiates, isolates, destroys seemingly dangerous forces.
Middle Adulthood	Generativity vs. Stagnation	Person is productive and creative for self and others, has parental pride and pleasure, is mature, enriches life, establishes and guides next generation.	Person is egocentric, nonproductive, experiences early invalidism, excessive self-love, personal impoverishment, and self-indulgence.
Late Adulthood	Integrity vs. Despair	Person appreciates continuity of past, present, and future, accepts life cycle and life style, has learned to cooperate with inevitabilities of life, "death loses its sting."	Person feels time is too short; finds no meaning in human existence, has lost faith in self and others, wants second chance at life cycle with more advantages, has no feeling of world order or spiritual sense, fears death.

Figure 1.5 Erikson's eight stages of human development.

According to Erikson, the first stage of psychosocial development (comparable to Freud's oral stage) is characterized by the crisis of *basic trust* versus *mistrust.* Normally, the child acquires a basic orientation of trust—trust that the mother will return and provide comfort. If this orientation is not acquired, the child may carry for the rest of its life a feeling of mistrust toward the world. At the second stage (Freud's anal stage), the child begins to gain bladder and bowel control and to assert its individuality. If psychologically successful, the child gains *autonomy;* if not, *shame* and *doubt* result. At the third stage (Freud's phallic stage), the child becomes assertive, rivaling in fantasy the same-sex parent for the other parent. If urges are channeled into socially acceptable acts, the child acquires *initiative;* if not, a reservoir of *guilt* is built up.

Erikson's fourth stage parallels Freud's latency stage. Unlike Freud, however, Erikson thought that the early school years were important for development. The child at this time must achieve *learning* and *competence* or experience *failure* and *inferiority.*

The fifth crisis occurs at adolescence. In contrast to Freud, who emphasized the conflicts associated with intensified sexual urges, Erikson emphasizes the crisis of *identity.* The adolescent must decide who he or she is and what he or she will do later in life; otherwise *role confusion* will result. Sexual identity must be resolved, an occupation must be chosen, and life as an adult must be planned. Freud's genital stage is interpreted by Erikson—the sixth crisis—as involving a conflict between *intimacy* and *isolation.* Only after the adolescent has "found" himself or herself is he or she able to find another.

For his final two stages, Erikson discusses key crises of adulthood and old age. His seventh stage is characterized by a conflict between *generativity* and *stagnation.* A person needs more than intimacy; he or she must be productive—teaching the younger generation or working at some task worthwhile for society. The final stage in development can be reached only if the earlier crises are adequately resolved. If the person reaches the final stage, he or she achieves a sense of *integrity;* if not, *despair* is experienced, and he or she suffers the sense of a wasted life.

DEALING WITH EMOTIONS

Our emotions can trouble us in many ways: they can strike mysteriously; they can conflict with one another; they can prevent us from functioning normally. What causes troublesome emotions? How do people normally deal with them?

Much of what we base our emotions upon is buried in our unconscious mind. Therefore, we often experience feelings that we do not understand—for example, taking a sudden dislike to a new neighbor without any apparent justification. In such a situation, you might examine your attitude and discover that your neighbor reminds you of a high-school teacher you feared and disliked. Perhaps you made an unconscious judgment that all people with a particular characteristic of the teacher—such as a speech mannerism or a way of dressing—are to be feared and disliked. This unconscious judgment now emerges in the emotion you experience toward a new person with that characteristic.

In addition to mysterious emotions, people often experience *conflicting* emotions—two or more diverse responses to the same object or event. Emotional conflict often occurs when one has developed values that are incompatible. One value is often ingrained unconsciously, while another is held consciously. Many people, for instance, have buried deep within them the idea that sex is dangerous and frightening, yet they consciously believe it is healthy and desirable. When encountering an attractive individual of the opposite sex, the person feels both desire and revulsion or fear. Such conflicts are common; no one has a perfectly consistent system of values. Unconscious conflicts *are* susceptible to conscious resolution. However, it takes a lot of hard, and often painful, mental work. Some people may require professional help to resolve such unconscious conflicts.

Other kinds of emotional conflict can occur consciously. People are often faced with situations where they must choose between equally attractive alternatives—say, which of two equally good colleges to attend or which of two equally good jobs to accept. Psychologist Kurt Lewin has called such conflicting choices *approach-approach* situations. Lewin has also identified two other kinds of conflict-creating situations: *avoidance-avoidance* situations, in which the alternatives are equally unattractive (both jobs are low paying), and *approach-avoidance* situations, in which each alternative is both attractive and unattractive (one job pays well but is a dead end; the other pays poorly but might lead to something better).

Defense Mechanisms

Because it is so hard and painful to deal with them, conflicts often continue to remain a problem, and the person feels anxious, guilty, and perhaps hostile. The human mind has a number of ingenious ways of dealing with anxiety that do not remove the original problem but that do provide temporary relief from its effects. Freud termed these various methods of coping *defense mechanisms:* automatic responses that help one to alleviate or avoid the painful feelings of emotional conflict. Most defense mechanisms serve to protect a person's self-esteem by hiding or altering aspects of the self that one would consider unpleasant. Some of the more common defense mechanisms are:

1. *Repression* is "forgetting on purpose"—pushing a shameful or distasteful experience or thought out of consciousness and pretending that it does not exist. Repression is the most fundamental of the defense mechanisms. Other defense mechanisms serve to help in keeping certain ideas or perceptions repressed.
2. *Compensation* is trying to make up for failure in one area by success in another area. For example, a person who is poor in sports may become a successful team manager or sports writer.
3. *Displacement* is discharging an emotion on something other than the situation that caused it. A teen-ager questioned by police for being out at 5 A.M. might kick a neighbor's trash cans in lieu of kicking the police officers.
4. *Sublimation* is transforming "unacceptable" impulses into acceptable ones. A person who feels the socially unacceptable desire to be aggressive may enter a highly competitive career field.
5. *Escape* is running away from problems through daydreaming, fantasy, books, movies—even excessive sleep. Children who have intolerable home conditions, for example, have been known to construct elaborate fantasy worlds.
6. *Regression* is reverting to behavior more appropriate to an earlier stage of life. A woman whose husband yells at her for breaking something might revert to baby talk and call her husband "Daddy" as a way of avoiding responsibility for her actions.
7. *Reaction formation* is replacing a negative feeling with its opposite. A parent who feels hostility toward a child may react to that unacceptable feeling by being overly nice to the child.
8. *Identification* is choosing another person as an ideal and then trying to emulate that person. A teen-ager might identify with a famous rock star in order to share vicariously in the star's successes, even dressing like the star and keeping a scrapbook of his career.
9. *Rationalization* is providing a substitute reason for an occurrence. It is an attempt to cover up one's failures or mistakes—to soften the blow. Common rationalizations include: "I would have done better if I had only had more time"; "The game was rigged"; "There were too many distractions"; "That professor doesn't like me."
10. *Projection* is shifting one's negative emotions or problems to someone else in order to maintain self-esteem. A person who accuses others of lying, cheating, or bigotry is often projecting.
11. *Avoidance* is keeping away from situations that produce anxiety or bring repressed feelings to the surface. An insecure person may avoid demanding tasks. A person who is unsure of his or her sexual identity may avoid the opposite sex. A person whose self-concept is tied to family life may avoid traveling or other situations that bring separation.
12. *Denial* is refusing to perceive or accept some aspect of reality. A heavy smoker will deny scientific reports on the dangers of cigarette smoking. People who are vain about their appearance may deny that they are growing older.

Emotional Control

The defense mechanisms work internally and unconsciously, but emotions are also controlled to some extent by external or conscious forces. For example, the society or culture in which one lives places value on expression of certain emotions and suppression of others. This is particularly evident in sex roles. American society has traditionally encouraged men to be strong, aggressive, athletic, and independent and to keep their emotions under control.

FOCUS
Who's Happy?

From the time our ancestors made the pursuit of happiness a national priority, happiness has been part of the American Dream. It is something we all want and indeed expect to find. But as recent scientific studies suggest, there's no easy formula for achieving happiness and, moreover, many of our traditional beliefs about happiness are incorrect.

In an attempt to understand why some people are happy and others are not, researchers have tried to isolate the specific factors associated with happiness. In one of the most fruitful studies on happiness, Columbia University psychologist Jonathan Freedman surveyed over 100,000 people to learn exactly what makes them happy. Here are some of Dr. Freedman's conclusions as well as the findings from several other studies on happiness:

1. Social factors including marriage, family, friends, and children are the strongest predictors of happiness. Married people are happier than single people, and people who are divorced are the most unhappy group.
2. Both men and women agree that love is the single most important factor in happiness.
3. People with satisfying sex lives are likely to report an overall sense of happiness. However, 90 percent of the people surveyed said that sex is not as important to happiness as love.
4. People who are satisfied with their jobs are more likely to be happy than those who are not. Only love and marriage are more important to happiness than job satisfaction.
5. Confidence in one's personal values and the belief that it is possible to control what happens in life are much more important to happiness than success, freedom, and independence.
6. A happy childhood has a much weaker influence on adult happiness than might have been expected. Even children with serious physical or psychological problems can turn out to be happy adults.
7. People who achieve more than they expected are happier than those who achieve just what they expected.
8. Money does not buy happiness despite the fact that the lack of money often brings stress. The survey showed that rich and middle-income people are equally happy, and more than half of the low-income group said they were happy.
9. People who attend college are slightly happier than those with only a high-school degree.
10. People in good health are not necessarily happier than people in poor health.
11. Age does not affect happiness. Despite the popular belief that old people are unhappy, they are just as likely to be happy as the young and middle-aged.

In addition to all these factors, researchers have not discounted the possibility that internal biochemical factors may make one person happy and another miserable. Whatever the reasons for happiness, Dr. Freedman is convinced that the quest for happiness is a life-long commitment. He says, "People quickly get used to whatever they have, good or bad, and only deviations from the level to which they've adapted produce happiness or unhappiness."

Women, on the other hand, have been expected to be submissive, sensitive, dependent, and highly emotional. To behave differently has risked the disapproval of friends, family, and co-workers. Thus, the woman who is strong and aggressive or the man who is sensitive and cries easily has been looked upon with disdain.

These social stereotypes regarding the emotional make-up of men and women have recently come under attack as part of the general reevaluation of male and female roles in our

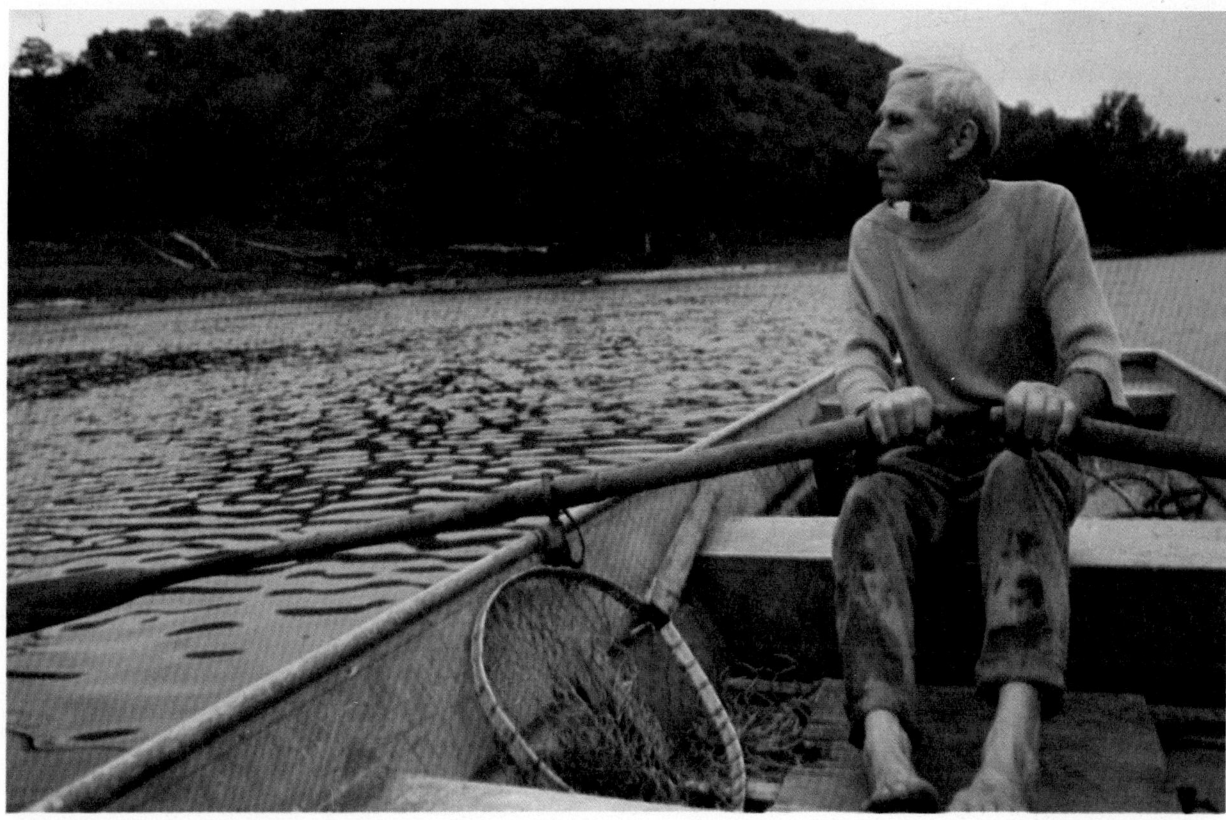

Figure 1.6 The self-actualized person is the rare individual who functions out of self-motivation and at maximum capacity. Such people are realistic, creative, independent, and unafraid of solitude.

society. Many of these ingrained ideas regarding emotional expression are changing as a result of this attack, permitting both men and women to express a wider range of emotions without fear of disapproval or rejection.

EMOTIONAL MATURITY AND MENTAL HEALTH

What do psychologists consider the characteristics of emotional maturity and mental health? Abraham Maslow used the term *self-actualization* to describe the level of development at which one functions out of self-motivation and at the peak of one's capacity. To discover the principal attributes of a self-actualized person, Maslow studied forty-nine people he considered to be self-actualized—people such as Abraham Lincoln, Henry David Thoreau, Ludwig van Beethoven, Eleanor Roosevelt, and Albert Einstein. From his study, he came up with a list of characteristics they seemed to share:

1. They are realistically oriented.
2. They accept themselves, other people, and the natural world for what they are.
3. They have a great deal of spontaneity.
4. They are problem-centered rather than self-centered.
5. They have an air of detachment and a need for privacy.
6. They are autonomous and independent.
7. Their appreciation of people and things is fresh rather than stereotyped.
8. Most of them have had profound mystical or spiritual experiences, although not necessarily religious in character.
9. They identify with humanity.
10. Their intimate relationships with a few specially loved people tend to be profound and deeply emotional rather than superficial.

11. Their values and attitudes are democratic.
12. They do not confuse means with ends.
13. Their sense of humor is philosophical rather than hostile.
14. They have a great fund of creativeness.
15. They resist conformity to the culture.
16. They transcend the environment rather than just cope with it.

By these standards, the truly self-actualized person is rare. Nevertheless, these qualities do provide a yardstick by which one can measure the extent to which one is self-actualized, and they provide an ideal that one can strive to achieve; self-actualization is an ongoing process, it is not a state of being that one can instantly attain.

Many other psychologists have formulated theories of what constitutes the emotionally mature person. Although these theories differ in many ways, there are a few qualities that seem to appear on the lists again and again as primary attributes of emotional maturity. One such attribute is the ability to be *intimate*—to give and accept love and affection. A second is the ability to be *sociable*—to have friends to whom one is devoted and whom one supports. It is also agreed that some clear, vivid *sense of self*—knowing who one is and what one's goals, values, and abilities are—is characteristic of emotional maturity. Another attribute of the mature person is an interest in and ability to do *productive work*.

FACILITATING MENTAL HEALTH

When discussing mental health, there is a tendency to emphasize emotional problems and mental illness. This is natural, because these disorders can be extremely serious, involving highly destructive behavior and requiring immediate intervention. These serious emotional and mental illnesses will be discussed later in this chapter. Here, it is important to recognize, however, that just as there are degrees of mental illness, there are also degrees of mental health.

If one's genetic make-up, environmental background, and learning experiences have been favorable, one is more likely to attain optimal mental health, in Maslow's sense of self-actualization. Such optimal mental health maximizes our potential as human beings, in our work—whether our field is music or science or religion—and in our play and our friendships. Optimal mental health is more than just the absence of mental illness. It is worth understanding and striving for in ourselves and encouraging in others.

The attainment of good mental health does not imply complete freedom from everyday problems—that is impossible. What it does mean is the ability to cope with problems and to maintain a psychological equilibrium. What can one do to try to reach this goal? How does one go about improving one's mental health? There are no easy answers; these are complex matters. Nevertheless, there are some things you can do to promote your mental health:

1. Practice liking yourself and being good to yourself.
2. Practice being alone without outside distraction some of the time and becoming comfortable with that.
3. Identify your good qualities. Be proud of them and of yourself.
4. Allow yourself the luxury of being yourself, and express this openly and honestly with others.
5. Recognize and face your fears, guilts, and hostilities. Accept these, too, as part of being human.
6. Welcome emotional experience—positive or negative—as valuable.
7. Practice sharing feelings and being intimate (including touching) with others.
8. Build friendships; love and be available for love.
9. Join in family, club, or other group activities. Share goals, values, and affection.
10. Do those things that maintain your physical health.
11. Accept responsibility for what and who you are and for what you do.
12. Develop worthwhile skills and means of expression.
13. Take advantage of opportunities for new experiences. Practice savoring good experiences.
14. Learn from successes and from failures; make full use of such experiences.
15. Be conscious of reality as the baseline of experience.

Figure 1.7 Liking yourself and treating yourself well are important to your mental health.

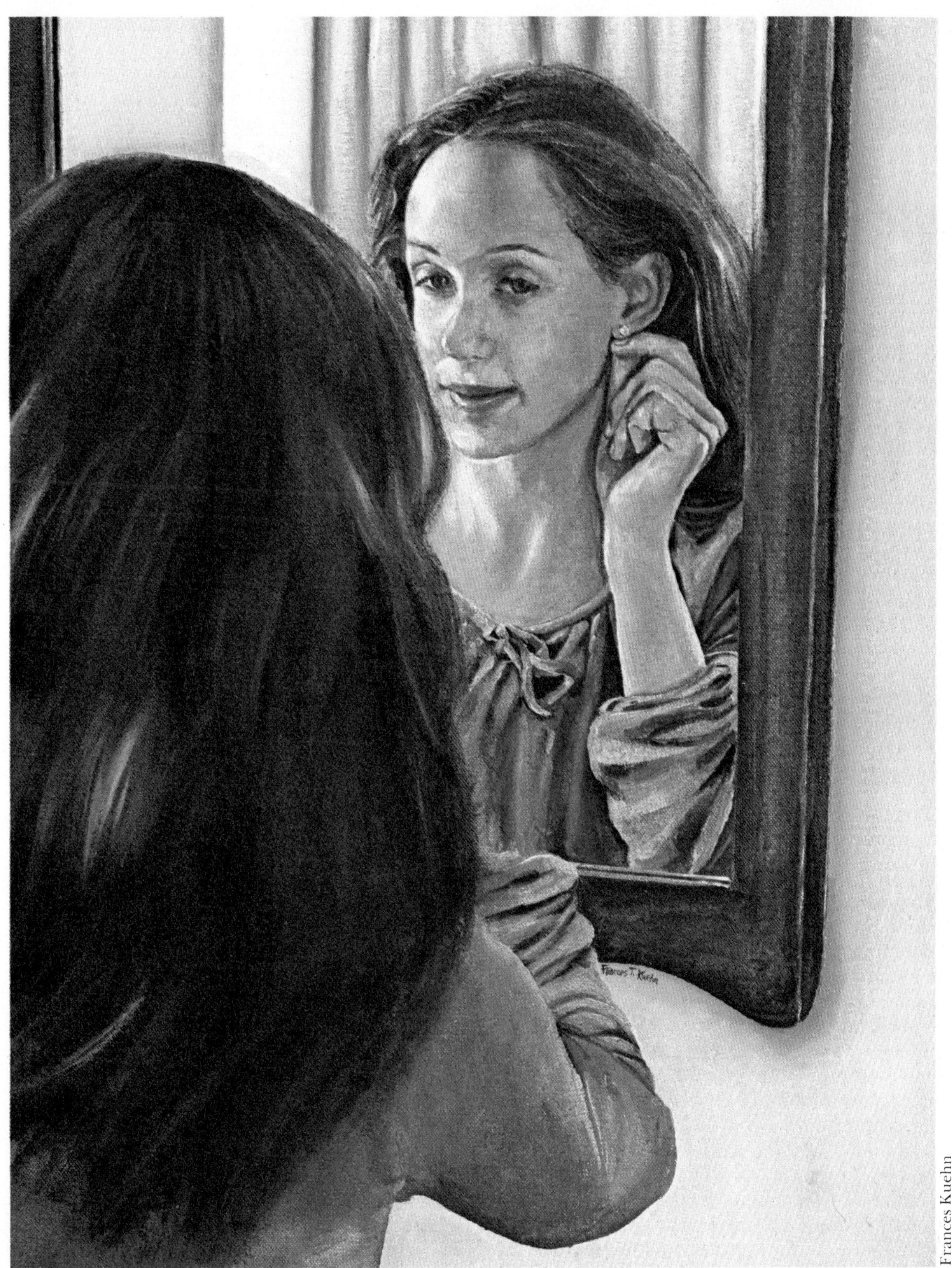

Frances Kuehn

16. Try to put yourself in the shoes of the other person. Try to view difficult experiences from the perspective of a third person.
17. Allow yourself to be pleased with what you are and excited about what you are becoming.
18. Ask for help when you feel you could use it. Accept that helping you may also be good for the person who helps you.

The Human Potential Movement

In recent years, many theories, techniques, and programs have been developed for the improvement of one's health, happiness, and effectiveness. This has been called the *human potential movement*—a term that implies both increasing and realizing one's potential. A wide variety of such programs are currently available, ranging from self-help books and single lectures to complete courses. Some emphasize activities for the mind (meditation, fantasy, problem solving); others emphasize physical activities (massage, yoga, karate and other martial arts, jogging, dancing, hiking). Other programs are designed to improve the functioning of healthy people and involve training in specific skills, such as parent effectiveness, assertiveness, prepared childbirth, cooking and nutrition, and creativity. The value of these programs varies with both the talents of the people conducting them and the readiness of the participants to learn.

Helping Others

How can you help others—your children, for instance—develop emotional maturity and mental health? First of all, you can provide warmth and security, and accept them for what they are. You can try to be a good role model. You can set realistic limits but encourage children to explore freely within those limits. You can listen to other people empathically, and show your feelings and concern about them. You can try not to judge people but instead help them to define their problems, figure out possible solutions, and face the consequences of their decisions. Finally, you can help people find constructive outlets for their emotions. You may well find that by thus helping a child or another adult to develop emotionally, you yourself will grow in your own emotional maturity and mental health.

MENTAL DISORDERS: THE PROBLEM OF DEFINITION

In the fifteenth century, Joan of Arc, a teen-aged peasant girl, believed she heard voices that commanded her to lead France to victory in its war against England. She was able to convince her king that she was divinely inspired, and she led the French armies until the English captured her and burned her at the stake for witchcraft. Today, if a teen-ager claims to hear voices or see visions, he or she is probably sent directly to a psychiatrist.

The story of Joan of Arc illustrates the problem of defining a mental disorder: no hard-and-fast line separates normal and abnormal behavior. Mental illness is not like physical illness. There are no blood tests or other laboratory tests that can invariably distinguish between a person who is mentally healthy and one who has a mental disorder. How, then, do psychiatrists and psychologists make these distinctions?

The Deviance Approach

According to the deviance approach whatever most people do is normal. Abnormality, then, would be any *deviation* from the average or from the majority. By this definition, it would be considered abnormal, for example, to take ten showers a day, find horses sexually attractive, or laugh when a loved one dies, simply because few people do these things. The popular view of homosexuality as abnormal is a result of the deviance approach. Since most people are more interested sexually and emotionally in the opposite sex, those who prefer their own sex are thus considered abnormal.

This deviance approach, however, has serious limitations. If most people are not particularly creative, was Shakespeare abnormal? Since the majority is not always right or best, the deviance approach is not generally a useful standard.

The Legal Approach

The terms *sane* and *insane* are not used much by psychiatrists and psychologists. Rather, these are primarily *legal* terms. Persons are considered legally insane if they cannot understand the difference between right and wrong, and/or if they cannot control their actions. A murderer or other criminal who is judged legally insane by a court can be acquitted of his crime on this basis. However, such a person does not go free; he serves his sentence in a mental institution rather than an ordinary prison.

This legal approach, however, is of little help in defining mental illness in the overwhelming majority of people who are not criminals, and it is difficult to apply even to criminals. There are no clear criteria for determining whether a person does indeed understand right from wrong or whether he is able to control himself. Psychiatrists not infrequently disagree about whether a given killer is mentally disturbed or not.

The Adjustment Approach

The adjustment approach says that the normal person is one who is able to get along—physically, emotionally, and socially—in the world. Such a person is able to earn a living; feed, clothe, and house himself or herself; and form friendships. The abnormal or mentally ill person is one who cannot adjust or function. This person may be incapable of holding a job or of coping with the demands of daily life, or may have so much trouble with personal relationships that he or she avoids people and lives in a lonely and isolated world. This functional definition of mental illness is one often used by psychologists and psychiatrists.

The Issue of Labeling

None of these approaches is entirely satisfactory. Indeed, the definitions of mental health and illness are somewhat arbitrary. This fact has led some theorists to conclude that labeling a person as "mentally ill" is cruel and irresponsible. The foremost spokesman of this point of view is the American psychiatrist Thomas Szasz.

Szasz argues that most people whom we call mentally ill are not ill at all. They simply have "problems in living"—serious conflicts with the world around them. Instead of dealing with these conflicts, psychiatrists label these persons "sick" and shunt them off to a hospital. Society's norms remain unchallenged, and the psychiatrist remains in a position of authority. The one who loses is the patient, who is deprived of both responsibility for his or her behavior and dignity as a human being. As a result, Szasz claims, the patient's problems intensify.

Szasz's position is a minority stand. Most psychologists and psychiatrists would agree that a person who claims to be God, Cleopatra, or Napoleon is truly disturbed. The fact that it is difficult to define mental and emotional disorders does not mean that no such things exist. It does mean that we should be very cautious about judging a person "mentally ill" just because he or she acts in a way we do not understand. We should also remember that mild psychological disturbances are extremely common. It is only when a psychological problem becomes severe enough to disrupt everyday life that it becomes an "abnormality" or "illness."

THE MAGNITUDE AND COST OF MENTAL ILLNESS

Despite these problems of definition, mental disorders are a public health problem of enormous magnitude—in terms of the number of people affected, the loss of productivity, and the economic costs, to say nothing of the human misery and the waste of human lives. It is estimated that one out of every ten Americans now needs some form of treatment for mental illness, and that one out of ten will be hospitalized for mental illness in his or her lifetime. One out of every four hospital beds is occupied by mental patients. Some 15 percent of patients' visits to doctors are for physical complaints really stemming from psychological problems. Indeed, psychological disorders are often the underlying causes of many social problems—delinquency, divorce, alcoholism,

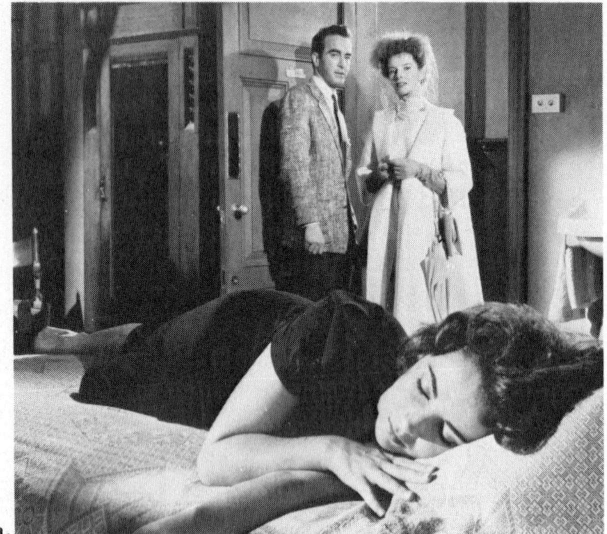
a.

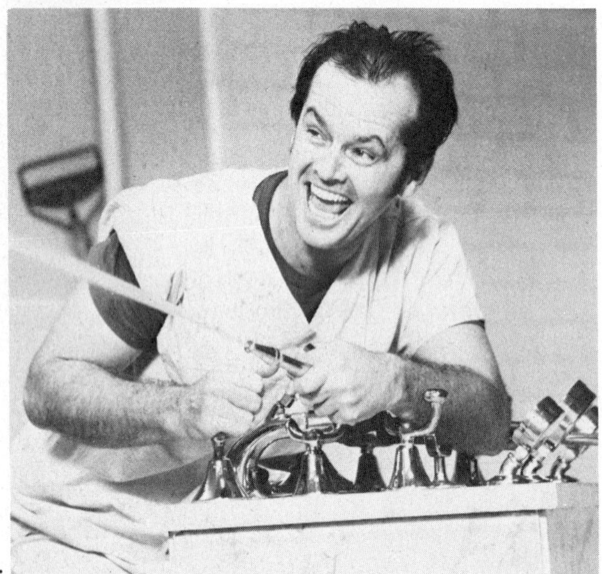
b.

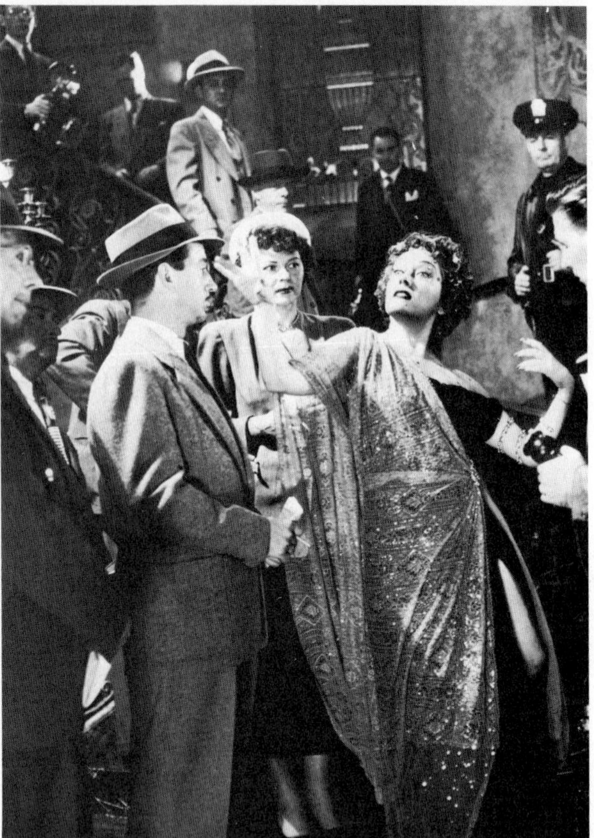
c.

Figure 1.8 Our preoccupation with mental disorders is reflected in contemporary films and literature. (a) In *Suddenly, Last Summer,* Elizabeth Taylor played a victim of amnesia—loss of memory—who is committed to a backward mental hospital by her eccentric and domineering aunt (Katharine Hepburn). (b) Jack Nicholson starred as a man hospitalized for violent and antisocial behavior in *One Flew over the Cuckoo's Nest.* (c) Gloria Swanson, in *Sunset Boulevard,* played a forgotten movie star whose obsession with making a comeback drives her into a world of delusion.

drug abuse, crime, even accidents. The economic cost of mental illness in the United States is conservatively estimated at about $40 billion a year.

And even beyond these harsh facts, there is the chilling reality that mental illness profoundly interferes with the very qualities that are most significantly human: happiness, love, achievement, creativity, motivation, and personal relationships.

CLASSIFYING THE MENTAL DISORDERS

Just as it is difficult to distinguish between mental and emotional health and illness, it is also difficult to classify the mental disorders. Human behavior is far too complex for simple categorization. The classifications of mental disorders used by psychologists and psychiatrists are not as precise or as useful as those used in general medical practice. Two therapists in the same hospital may regularly use different criteria for diagnosing schizophrenia, and a given diagnosis does not necessarily dictate a specific treatment.

Depression

Depression is considered an *affective disorder*—a disorder of "affect," or mood or feeling. It is so widespread that it is sometimes called the common cold of the mental disorders. The National Institute of Mental Health estimates that during any given year, 15 percent of adults—some 20 to 32 million people—may suffer significant depression.

Depression ranges widely in intensity, from transient feelings of the "blues"—which all of us experience from time to time and which seem to be part of the human condition—to a severe mental illness so incapacitating that it is considered a psychosis. Among the signs and symptoms of serious depression are sadness, unhappiness, crying, feelings of hopelessness and worthlessness, loss of appetite, insomnia (or, sometimes, excessive sleep), and loss of self-esteem. The most characteristic sign, however, is loss of the ability to feel pleasure; depressed people no longer enjoy the things they used to enjoy.

While the causes of severe depression are not well understood, both psychological and biological factors seem to be involved. Most often depression seems clearly related to some stressful event—the loss of a job, divorce, physical illness, the death of a loved one—but other times there is no obvious triggering event. In recent years, neuroscientists have found that moods are closely connected with brain chemistry. Within the brain, nerve impulses are transmitted by chemical substances known as *neurotransmitters.* When the amounts of specific neurotransmitters are too low in certain key parts of the brain, the person feels depressed.

HOW TO Help a Depressed Person

We all have ups and downs, and usually it's just best to accept them. But perhaps you are concerned about someone who seems to be chronically depressed. Maybe he or she never feels like doing anything and never even wants to talk. Is it best for you not to interfere? Should you just sit tight and wait for him or her to snap out of it?

There *are* ways you can help. Here are a few:

1. Get the person to *talk.* Try to get him or her to tell you not only about the depression itself, but about the fears, wishes, or losses that underlie it. This is often difficult, of course, but it can be very useful. If nothing else, it will reassure the person that someone cares.
2. *Don't* tell a depressed person that things are "not that bad." To him or her, they are.
3. Keep the person active. Depression causes apathy and lethargy, which lead to more depression, and so on. Productive or entertaining activities can help break this vicious cycle. Very often a change of scene or a vacation can be effective.
4. If you are struggling with depression yourself, make yourself do something, however trivial it may seem. Make your bed or clean up your room, for example. You'll be able to tell yourself you've accomplished *something.*
5. If serious depression persists for more than two weeks, you should begin to seek medical help.
6. If you have a depressive reaction after a major illness, surgery, or traumatic event, it's probably not depression in the clinical sense. Just get plenty of rest and wait it out.

Source: Adapted from Marion Steinmann, "Depression: Our Common Curse," *The Saturday Evening Post* (December 1975), pp. 54–55, 86.

Suicide Every year some 25,000 people in the United States commit suicide. This is the verifiable number, but the true number, according to educated estimates, may be as high as 80,000 a year. It is also estimated that there are eight to ten suicide attempts for every successful suicide.

Over the last two decades suicides among teen-agers and young adults have increased sharply. Between 1968 and 1976, the number of suicides of people aged twenty to twenty-four more than doubled. Suicide is now the third most common cause of death (after acci-

HOW TO Recognize the Signals of a Potential Suicide

There's nothing subtle about a suicide attempt. It is a dramatic plea for help or proclamation of hopelessness. And often, suicide is not a spontaneous act, but one that a person plans consciously in order to escape an intolerable existence.

Yet far too often no one recognizes the potential suicide's despair, and a person dies who really wants to live. With life at stake, you should know how to identify the warning signs of suicide. Here are some things to be aware of:

1. Watch out for extremes in mood. Suicidal people may be hopelessly depressed and withdrawn from life or so agitated that they can't eat or sleep.
2. Be alert for extreme mood swings. A person who is severely depressed one day, elated the next, and depressed again the day after may be struggling with the desire to live and the even stronger desire to die.
3. Be concerned when people start giving away the things they love. They may be telling you that they no longer have any reason to live.
4. Be alert for a crisis that may precipitate a suicide attempt. When suicidal individuals feel overwhelmed by external events—the loss of a job, the death of a parent, a pile of unpaid bills—they may feel that there is no way to cope with life as it is.
5. Listen for a suicide "plan." Suicidal people often talk about their death wish long before they try to kill themselves.
6. Take *every* suicide attempt seriously—no matter how ineffective it is. People who threaten to take their lives are crying for help. They want someone to save them from their intolerable situation.
7. Be aware that people who quickly bounce back from a suicide attempt and act as if nothing happened may try to kill themselves again within a short time unless they receive help.

Remember, most suicides really wanted to live. Suicide is preventable—if you know how to help.

Source: Adapted from *Suicides: Do They Want to Die?* (New York: St. Vincent's Hospital and Medical Center of New York, n.d.).

dents and homicides) among people between the ages of fifteen and twenty-four.

There are many theories about the causes of suicide. An insightful and useful classification has been proposed by Don Jackson, who identified three main causes. The first is self-directed aggression, which seems to encompass Freud's view of a lurking death wish and also extends to "partial" suicides, such as accident proneness, drug addiction, and excessive risk taking. The second cause is a desire for rebirth and restitution. For example, children and suicidal schizophrenics often speak of doing away with the "bad me." Third, despair, loss of self-esteem, and the real or imagined loss of love objects are frequent causes of suicide. Many suicides seem to follow a loss of some kind—of health, of financial resources, of another person, or of youth. Some authorities correlate suicide with weather or business cycle fluctuations, and others maintain that socioeconomic forces are a major factor.

People who have made suicide attempts are one of the highest-risk groups for subsequent suicide: about 70 to 80 percent of suicides have a history of suicide threats or attempts. Among young adults, particularly, suicide attempts are often a cry for help that should be heeded. Suicide attempters are frequently trying to cope with a situation they find intolerable. Unfortunately, if their suicide attempt succeeds, it is a permanent "solution" to a problem that may be only temporary. (See the How To box on the signs of a potential suicide.)

Many American communities now have suicide prevention centers and hot lines, operated by volunteers trained to counsel callers who need help in coping with personal crises (see the section on crisis intervention later in this chapter).

Neuroses

A *neurosis** is an emotional disorder in which the personality is dominated by feelings of *anxiety,* obsessional thoughts, compulsive behavior, or physical complaints without objective

*The American Psychiatric Association recently decided to drop the term "neurosis" from its official classification, yet the label is still widely used and will be retained here.

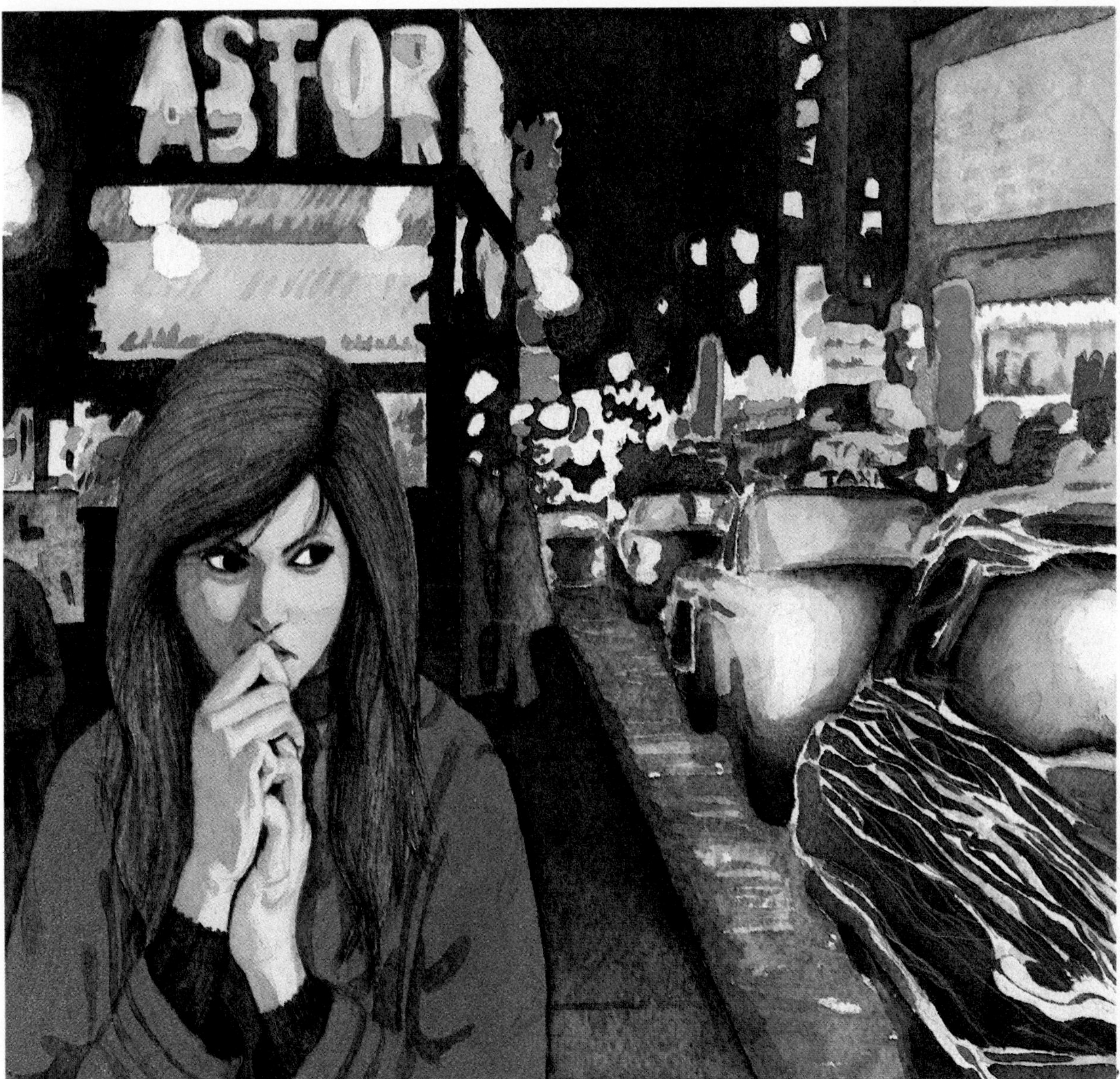

Frank Ferri / Barbara Bell rep.

Figure 1.9 Neurotic anxiety is experienced as a physiological or psychological reaction to vague, diffuse, or imagined fears.

evidence of physical disease. Anxiety is not only an unpleasant emotion; it can also affect one physiologically, disturbing breathing and increasing heart activity and sweating. Psychologically, it can involve a sense of powerlessness, an anticipation of impending danger, an exhausting alertness, and an all-absorbing apprehension that interferes with practical problem solving. Anxiety is different from fear. Fear is a frank reaction to a real danger, while anxiety usually is a reaction to vague, diffuse, or imagined dangers.

Neurotic anxiety can manifest itself either in physical symptoms or in peculiar behavior. Some anxious people feel chronically weak or tire easily. A few may develop nervous-system disorders; such symptoms as blindness, deafness, and paralysis can develop even with no organic basis. Neurotic behaviors associated with anxiety include *phobias* (intense fear of an object or situation that the person consciously recognizes as no real personal danger); *obsessive-compulsive behaviors* (the persistent intrusion of unwanted thoughts, urges, or actions that one is unable to stop even though one may perceive them as absurd); and *hypochondria* (a preoccupation with the body and with fear of disease, even though one is in good health).

Psychoses

A *psychosis* is a disorder characterized by behavior so unreasonable that it impairs a person's capacity to meet the ordinary demands of life. Sometimes psychotic behavior seems clearly related to an underlying physical or organic defect. Such an organic defect can result from circulatory disease, drug intoxication, infection, senility, epilepsy, tumors, mechanical injury or trauma, and a variety of metabolic disorders, all of which can produce either mild or severe psychological malfunctioning. Organic brain disease can interfere with a person's orientation (knowledge of time, place, and people); impair memory, judgment, and intellectual functioning; and produce instability and shallowness of feeling.

A man, for example, was jailed for violation of motor vehicle laws. He ran through a toll booth at high speed, and was twice arrested for driving without a license. He then told people that he was wealthy, that his son would be president of the United States, and he promised a hospital attendant $1 million. Physicians soon recognized that the man was suffering from an advanced case of syphilis, which had infected his brain.

Schizophrenia The most prevalent type of psychosis is schizophrenia (a word that comes from Greek and means "split mind"). It affects about 1 or 2 percent of the population, a figure that is approximately the same in every country where it has been estimated. The disorder is usually first diagnosed in people between the ages of eighteen and thirty-five, and it can seriously disrupt their education, careers, and marriages.

Schizophrenic people have severely disturbed thinking, moods, and behavior, marked by misinterpretations of reality. Often the person has *delusions* or false beliefs that cannot be corrected by logical argument. Sometimes the person *hallucinates*—perceives people or things that are not there (perhaps he or she "hears" a dead relative). Mood changes are also characteristic; the person may respond inappropriately to a situation, perhaps laughing at news of someone's death. The person may withdraw from others, become excessively active, talk incoherently, or adopt bizarre gestures or postures. Some element of paranoia (extreme delusions of persecution or grandeur) is often present.

The causes of schizophrenia are as mysterious as those of severe depression; a complex interaction of sociocultural and biological factors seems to be involved. One clear factor is social class. Studies in many countries (both Western and non-Western) consistently show that schizophrenia occurs more frequently among the lowest social classes of urban populations. Why this is so, however, is much less clear. Another factor is severe stress. A third factor is genetic predisposition; it has long been known that schizophrenia (like some other mental disorders) tends to run in families. Other evidence of biological factors comes from recent studies of the brain chemicals called neurotransmitters, discussed above. In the case of schizophrenia, overactivity of a specific neurotransmitter called dopamine seems to be involved.

Affective Psychoses Another major group of psychoses is the *affective psychoses,* which involve disorders of mood or feelings. These include the psychotic depressions mentioned above. In the so-called *manic-depressive psychosis,* the afflicted person swings—sometimes over a period of days, sometimes of years—between moods of extreme elation and hyperactivity and moods of deep despair and depression. Recent studies have shown that there is a genetic factor involved in some manic-depressive disorders. Other studies suggest that an in-

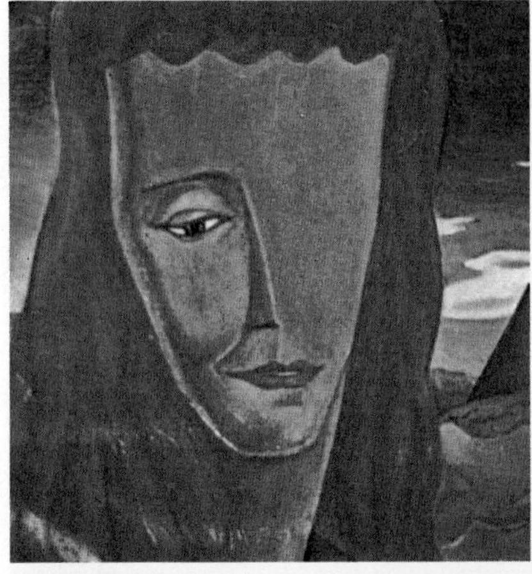

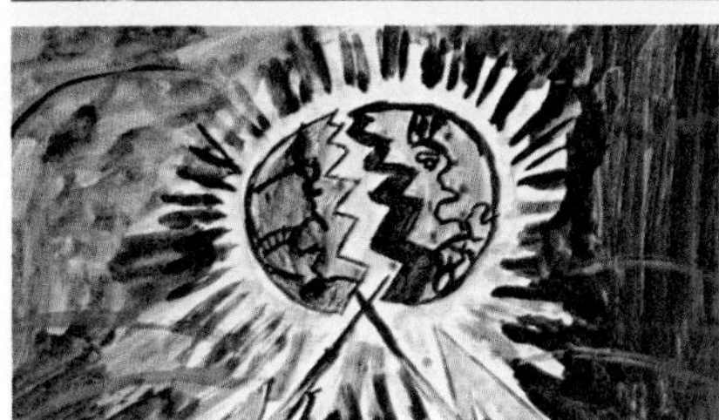

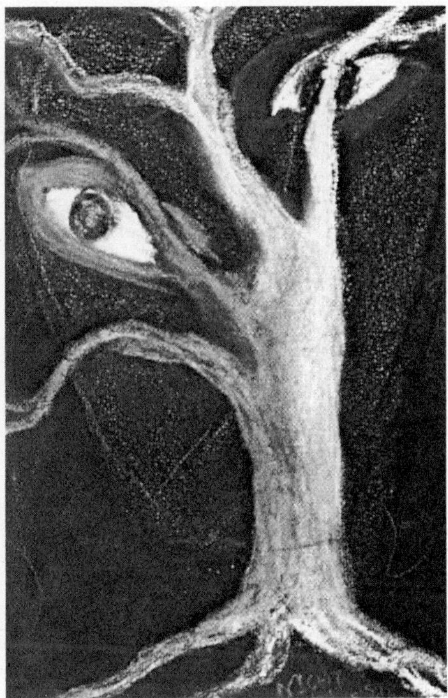

Figure 1.10 These paintings, done by a schizophrenic, reveal several patterns that are characteristic of the disorder. The portrait of a solitary, partially faceless woman in a desolate setting suggests the withdrawal and absence of emotion common in schizophrenics. The painting of a globe explosively splitting apart seems to represent the violence of the break the patient has personally experienced. The third painting conveys the sense of sinister watchfulness that frequently accompanies schizophrenia.

crease in certain neurotransmitters in the brain is associated with mania.

Personality Disorders

Some people develop characteristic, deeply ingrained, maladaptive reactions to social situations that are so consistent that the person can be classified as having a distinct personality disorder. These are diagnosed on the basis of persistent behavior patterns such as paranoia, variation in mood, withdrawal, impulsiveness, obsessiveness, or effort to find sexual gratification in ways others consider abnormal. The most common personality disorders are hysterical personality and sociopathic personality.

Some people characteristically react to minor stress by becoming excited, acting in an emotionally unstable manner, and complaining excessively about minor bodily discomforts, exaggerating their own traits to gain attention. Such people are called *hysterical personalities.* They try to control their relations with others by appearing to be sick. Generally, they deny responsibility for their manipulative behavior and act as if they cannot help themselves.

Psychopaths, individuals who have *sociopathic* or *antisocial personalities,* find themselves in repeated conflict with society. They seem, at least superficially, to be incapable of significant loyalty to persons, groups, or social values. Their frustration tolerance is low. They are often described as grossly selfish, callous, irresponsible, impulsive, and unable to feel guilt or learn from experience. In the extreme, they may be totally without conscience. The psychopathic individual is one who—knowing the difference between right and wrong—is unable to care. The desire for self-gratification takes precedence over all other values. Many criminals, particularly murderers, have been diagnosed as sociopaths.

Psychophysiological Reactions

Psychological stress often produces physical symptoms, as will be described in Chapter 20. These physiological changes may become so intense and long-lasting that a person devel-

Optimal Mental Health	Normal Coping	First Level of Dysfunction	Second Level of Dysfunction
High self-esteem	Rationalization	Worry	Intoxication
Feels good about others	Some worry	Physical "symptoms"	Incapacitating fears
Comfortable in one's environment	Daydreaming	backache	Compulsive behavior
Loving and lovable	Some anger	headache	Drug abuse
Works effectively	Some fear	nervous stomach	Self-destructiveness
Enjoys play	Some boredom	neck stiffness	Personality inadequacy
Feels and expresses emotions constructively	Some escape	Inhibiting fear	Repeated fainting
Considerate of others	Some selfishness	Sexual problems	Destructive sexuality
Feels good most of the time		Temper outbursts	
MENTAL HEALTH		MENTAL ILLNESS	

Figure 1.11 The spectrum of mental functioning, adapted from psychologist Karl Menninger's model.

ops a physical disorder. Such a person may not even be consciously aware of the emotional state contributing to the disorder. These disorders are called psychophysiological or psychosomatic reactions. Such reactions can disturb almost every bodily system. Excessive psychological stress may be a component of backaches, migraine, tension headaches, asthma, hypertension, colitis, peptic ulcer, frigidity, or impotence.

WHEN AND HOW TO GET HELP

How do you tell when someone—or you yourself—needs treatment for a mental disorder? How can you better handle your own psychological problems? How can you help someone else? And where can you turn to find professional help?

The Problems of Everyday Living

All of us face problems in our daily lives. We find ourselves in situations that challenge or frustrate us, embarrass or threaten us, or make us feel angry, guilty, afraid, or inadequate. Not to have such experiences is to withdraw from life itself. Occasionally, however, when we are called upon to meet challenges that are beyond our ability to cope, serious symptoms of psychological disturbance can occur.

Sometimes such symptoms might be avoided by the use of strategies that are within the average person's control. (1) You can try to avoid certain unreasonable problems. (2) You can sometimes alter your perceptions of some problems, and thereby your psychological response to them. (3) You can try to develop more skillful coping abilities so as to meet these problems more successfully. The more practice you get in trying different strategies—and the more successful you are—the more adjusted a person you become. Some examples:

1. It would be neither wise nor healthy to continue an academic curriculum in which you are continually unhappy, unsuccessful, or afraid. Changing to another major in which you are more comfortable and successful is a reasonable coping behavior. On the other hand, switching your major because of a minor disappointment—such as a low score on one examination—is not good coping.
2. Moving out of your parents' home to achieve more freedom and independence and to get away from what seems to be parental domination may be good for your development and mental health. Moving

Third Level of Dysfunction	Fourth Level of Dysfunction	Fifth Level of Dysfunction
Diminished control of anger and aggression Acts of violence toward self or others	Despondency and hopelessness Bizarre, erratic behavior Compulsive posturing and facial expressions Paranoia Mental confusion Mutism or incoherence	Out-of-control behavior Suicide Persistent agitated or excited behavior replaces life support behavior (eating, sleeping)

MENTAL ILLNESS

out in anger, however, and to express the rejection of your parents may create even more problems.

3. The best way to conquer an inordinate acrophobia (fear of heights), for example, is not to suddenly force yourself to walk to the edge of a precipice and peer over. Instead, you should accustom yourself to high places gradually, step by step.
4. Fear of public speaking may best be overcome in circumstances where you can speak to a group in which others not only understand but perhaps share your fear and the desire to deal with it—and where the worst that happens can be viewed as another valuable learning experience.
5. Sometimes when you feel overwhelmed by the busyness and pressures of life, it is a good idea simply to withdraw from the hurly-burly for a while, cutting down on activities and unnecessary stimuli until you feel like re-engaging yourself with the world again.

You should avoid developing coping skills that are destructive, either to yourself or to others. Kicking a person who makes you angry may express and perhaps vent the anger, but it may also cause you to feel stupid and guilty—feelings that may not be so easy to resolve. A better solution might be to express the anger verbally, openly and directly. This allows the other person to participate in resolving the issue.

Daily life, however, also involves problems that cannot always be resolved directly or immediately. Money worries, conflicts with people, deadline pressures, driving tensions, noise, crowding—all can create persistent stress. Coping with such stress may call for a strategy that does not deal with its cause but involves modifying your psychological and physiological response to it. Such strategies of stress reduction are discussed in Chapter 12.

Signs of Mental Disorders

How can you tell when such coping strategies are not sufficient? How can you distinguish between the normal disturbances that we all have from time to time and a disorder that indicates a need for help? What are the warning signs of mental disorder?

In addition to the many specific symptoms described previously in this chapter, some of the other signs are:

1. A prolonged and intense *anxiety,* a feeling that something bad is going to happen, particularly when there is no real reason for such a feeling.

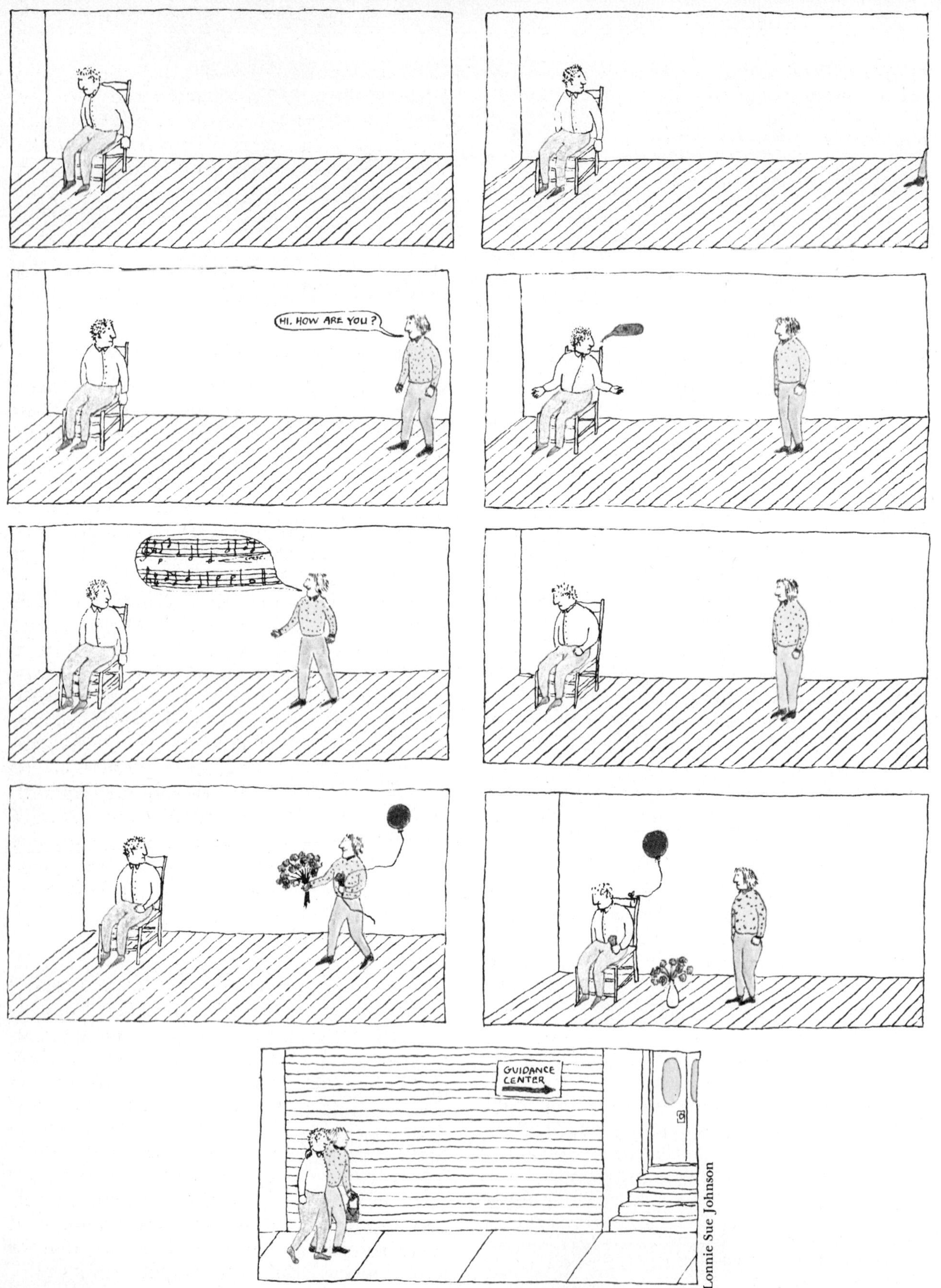

Lonnie Sue Johnson

2. A severe and persistent *depression,* in which one feels low, unhappy, uncaring. A depressed person often has little energy and motivation, withdraws completely from all relationships and activities, and finds it difficult to do anything.
3. A *sudden change* in mood or behavior that is inappropriate or inconsistent with the person's previous behavior. A relatively passive person may become very aggressive; change his or her dress, speech, or actions; and appear bizarre or reckless to family and friends.
4. One or more *physical complaints*—such as headache, nausea, pains, insomnia, shortness of breath—that continue in the absence of any medical cause.
5. A person's *performance* (in work, play, or relationships) *falling far short* of previously demonstrated potential.

How You Can Help

You can listen. If someone has a problem, it often helps him or her to talk about what's wrong with another person who will listen empathically and uncritically. Listening is most helpful if you acknowledge the person's feelings sympathetically with responses like "I can tell you are very worried," or "I've been down and unhappy, too. That can really be a terrible feeling." Usually it is better to let the person work out a strategy to resolve the problem independently rather than rushing in with advice or a pep talk. It is appropriate, however, to encourage and reassure the disturbed person.

If it becomes apparent that the person is not feeling better and the problem is not being resolved, it is time to get outside help. It is better to get such help too early than too late. In many cases, tragic outcomes of mental illness might have been prevented if the people who knew about the problems had sought outside help sooner.

One step is to reinforce whatever inclination the disturbed person has toward getting help. A good first contact might be a campus counseling service or a clergyman, a family physician, or someone else the disturbed person knows and trusts. Most communities also have mental health associations, clinics, and medical societies that can help with referral and advice. If the disturbed person has no interest in seeking help, a friend or family member can instead make this first contact and plan how the person can get help. For a summary of the leading methods of professional help for mental disorders, see Table 1.1.

Figure 1.12 How to help a friend get relief from mental distress—listen and suggest outside help if necessary.

Crisis Intervention: The Hot Line

In an emergency, if a disturbed person poses a danger to himself, herself, or others, those nearby must get professional help even against the person's overt wishes. One source of such ready help is a hospital emergency room. If the person is too violent to be taken there, one of the quickest sources of help is the police, who in most communities are trained to intervene both humanely and effectively.

Many communities have a crisis hot line, which is an instant and effective way to deal with emergency situations. People who are in trouble can telephone at any time and receive immediate counseling, sympathy, and comfort. The best known is the Los Angeles Suicide Prevention Center, established in 1958. Similar hot lines have also been set up for alcoholics, rape victims, battered women, runaway children, gamblers, and people who just need a shoulder to cry on. Hot lines also provide information on the community services available to deal with various kinds of problems.

Prevention

Mental health workers describe three types of preventive measures. *Primary prevention* consists of measures to reduce the incidence of mental disorders by preventing their development. These measures are limited by the fact that so little is known about the causes of most mental illnesses. *Secondary prevention* tries to prevent the worsening of disorders by detecting problems early and treating them before they become severe. Outpatient clinics, emergency services, and hot lines are examples of secondary prevention. Early detection of problems usually requires a trained professional,

Table 1.1 Types of Treatment*

Treatment	Characteristics
Drug Therapy	Uses drugs including *major tranquilizers, antidepressants,* and *lithium* (see Chapter 00) to treat various mental disorders by manipulating brain physiology; does not cure mental illness, only relieves symptoms.
Psychotherapy	Attempts to understand and overcome psychological causes of mental disorders; involves regular meetings between client and therapist; emphasizes the compassion and honesty that develop out of the client-therapist relationship; tries to help the client understand his or her behavior; tries to find alternative, more adaptive modes of behavior.
Behavior Therapy	Based on the view that a behavior is a response to a stimulus; concentrates on relieving specific symptoms or problems, rather than investigating causes; helps patient *unlearn* maladaptive patterns of response and learn alternate responses.
Family Therapy	Enables family members to learn how to communicate with each other; provides each member with a clear understanding of the others' problems; examines role expectations and communication patterns within a family in order to readjust restrictive roles and promote mutual support and appreciation.
Group Therapy	Concentrates on promoting better interpersonal relationships; allows patients to see themselves as others see them; may help patients to deal with a common problem such as alcoholism; enables patients to be treated at lower fees; rarely offers close relationship with therapist.

*The two major types of treatment are drug therapy and psychotherapy, and they are often used in combination.

but consultation programs with schools and law enforcement agencies can expand secondary prevention. *Tertiary prevention* tries to prevent the severe effects of major disorders on the victim and on society through treatment and rehabilitation in hospitals. These programs are designed to help people who have suffered serious mental and emotional disorders to resume their useful roles in society and to prevent the recurrence of their disorders.

SUMMARY

1. According to Magda Arnold, an emotion is "a felt tendency toward something intuitively assessed as good, favorable, beneficial or away from something assessed as unfavorable, harmful, bad." Arnold analyzed the stages of an emotion as perception, appraisal, the emotion, the accompanying bodily changes, action, and secondary appraisal.

2. Emotions affect the physical functioning of the body, and conversely, physical disorders also affect psychological feelings.

3. In addition to having certain basic physical needs, people also have emotional needs. The two that are perhaps the most important are the need for love (monkeys raised without mother love do not mature normally) and the need for self-esteem.

4. Abraham Maslow divided human needs into two categories. Basic or deficiency needs are the two physiological needs for food and water and the psychological needs for affection, security, and self-esteem. Higher needs—such as the needs for justice, goodness, beauty, order—he called growth needs or metaneeds.

5. Sigmund Freud theorized that children pass through five major stages of emotional or

psychosexual development: the oral, anal, phallic, latency, and genital stages.

6. Erik Erikson has outlined eight stages of psychosocial development, each characterized by a psychosocial crisis: trust, autonomy, initiative, competence, identity, intimacy, generativity, and integrity.

7. Some of the common emotional defense mechanisms are repression, compensation, displacement, sublimation, escape, regression, reaction formation, identification, rationalization, projection, avoidance, and denial.

8. Abraham Maslow introduced the concept of self-actualization to describe the level of development at which a person functions at his or her peak capacity.

10. There is no hard-and-fast line separating normal and abnormal behavior. When a psychological problem becomes severe enough to disrupt a person's everyday life, it is considered an abnormality or illness.

11. Mental disorders are an enormous public health problem. It is estimated that one out of ten Americans, at some time, will be hospitalized for mental illness.

12. About 20 million Americans a year suffer significant depression: feelings of unhappiness and hopelessness, loss of self-esteem, and the inability to feel pleasure. Both biological and psychological factors seem to be involved; sometimes depression is clearly related to stress. About 15 percent of depressed people commit suicide.

13. Neuroses may involve great suffering, but they do not impair a person's ability to function in most areas of life. Psychoses are characterized by behavior so unreasonable or perceptions of reality so impaired that the affected person cannot meet the ordinary demands of life.

14. The most prevalent psychosis is schizophrenia, in which people have severely disturbed thinking, moods, and behavior; misinterpret reality; and often have delusions, hallucinations, or paranoia. The cause is unknown, but both stress and a genetic predisposition seem to be involved.

15. Personality disorders are deeply ingrained, maladaptive behavior patterns. The most common are the hysterical personality and sociopathic (or antisocial) personality.

16. Among the many sources of help, for oneself or others, are a clergyman, family physician, campus counseling service, crisis hot line, community mental health centers, and hospital emergency rooms. If a person is violent, one of the quickest sources of help is the police.

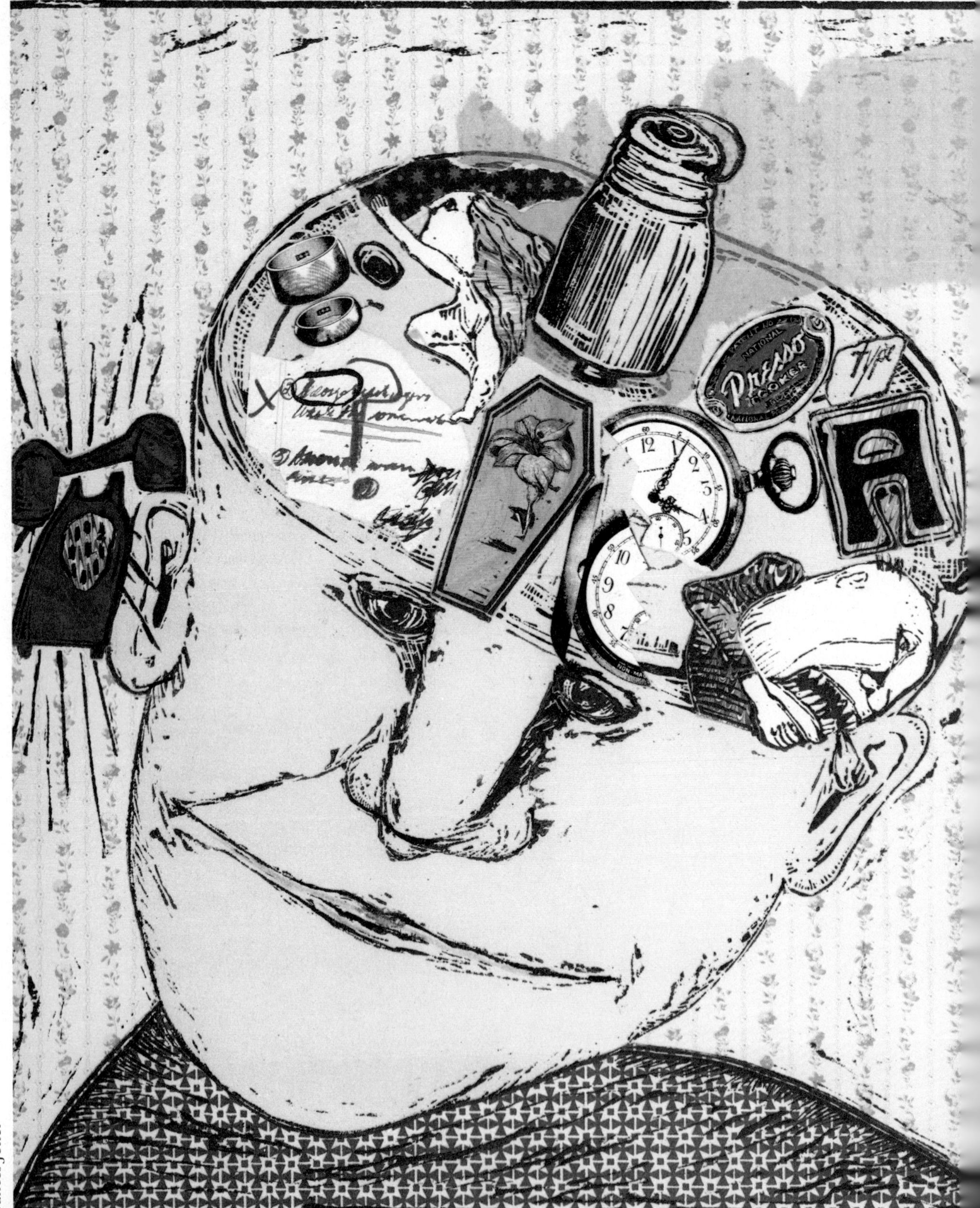

Frances Jetter

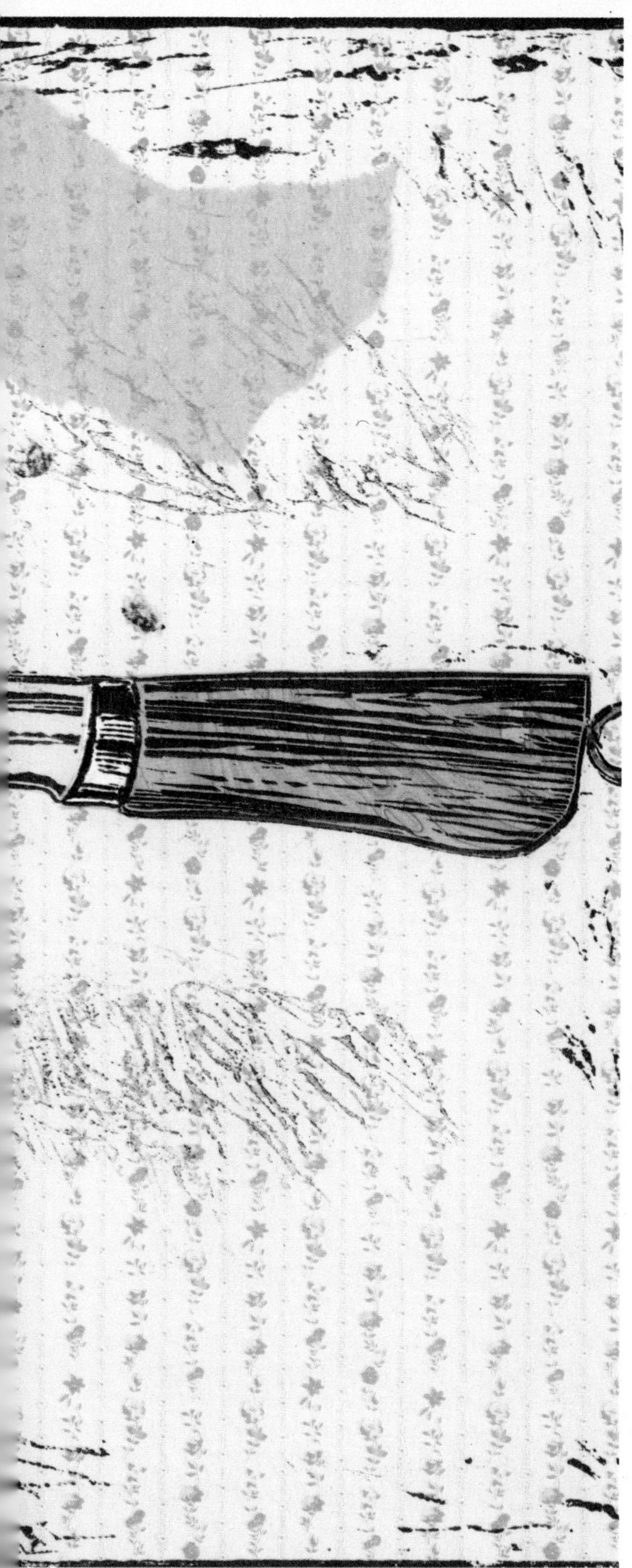

2 Stress and Health

Six months after a woman's husband dies, she develops cancer. A man wins $1,600 on a $2 bet at the racetrack; while collecting the money, he collapses and dies of a heart attack. Whenever a college sophomore thinks about an oral presentation she must make, her heart pounds and she sweats profusely; on the morning of the presentation, she wakes up tired and with a headache. Another student is so beset by anxiety that he cannot concentrate on his studies. And during exam week, the university clinic staff notices that it sees many more cases of colds, flu, and accidents.

All of these people may be victims of stress. In each case, stressful events—or a person's perception of them—have challenged his or her ability to adapt, and this attempt to adapt has disrupted the person's equilibrium and resulted in a breakdown of physical or psychological health. Yet stress is also a normal part of living; it is essential to our well-being. This chapter will discuss this paradox and also the causes of stress, how people vary in their response to stress, the physiological stress mechanism, and how stress can lead to disease. Since prevention and treatment of stress-related disease involve gaining control over our stress experiences and responses, the chapter will also explore how we can learn to cope better with the stresses of life.

WHAT IS STRESS?

The concept of stress can be confusing because different stress experts often use the word in slightly different ways. Two major meanings are relevant here. Sometimes the word is used to mean a stressful *stimulus* itself, an event or agent that produces tension—a death, the loss of a job, exam week. Other times the word is used for the *result* of such events—the psychological and physiological state aroused within the body by such stimuli. Stress researchers often use the word *stressor* when they mean a stressful stimulus and reserve the word *stress* itself for the body's internal response to that stimulus. This chapter will follow that usage.

In the mid-1930s, pioneering stress researcher Hans Selye, a physiologist at the University of Montreal, explained that part of the body's physiological response to a stimulus is specific to that stimulus: if we are exposed to extreme heat, we perspire; if we are exposed to extreme cold, we shiver. But another part of the body's physiological response, Selye discovered, remains the same whatever the stressor. This constant, *non*specific component of our body's physiological response to any stimulus or demand Selye called stress. It will be described in detail later in this chapter.

Selye's original research, which he conducted with rats, was concerned primarily with physical stressors—heat, cold, hemorrhage, X-rays, germs, forced exercise. Since then, he and other stress researchers have come to realize that the stress response is also often elicited by psychological stressors, such as the ones described at the beginning of this chapter, and that our stress response has both psychological and physiological components, which may interact with and reinforce each other.

The Positive Effects of Stress

Nevertheless, stress is not something we necessarily should try to avoid. Stress inevitably accompanies striving toward goals and meeting challenges; it is an integral component of much of the activity, achievement, joy, and meaning in life.

Indeed, stress or arousal is often useful in that it spurs us to greater efficiency and accomplishment. We are all familiar with the fact that we study and learn better under the stress of an impending exam or other challenge. Similarly, athletes and other performers know that they need to "get up" for a game or a performance. The relationship between stress and performance follows what researchers call an inverted U-shaped curve. At very low levels of stress, we are inefficient and tend to perform poorly. At moderate levels of stress, our efficiency and our performance improve; and at very high levels, they deteriorate again. The optimum level of stress (the top of the upside-down U) varies from person to person and for different types of tasks.

The challenge is for us to develop those insights and skills and to order our lives so as to minimize the destructive effects of stress while engaging in a full range of important activities and experiences. "Stress is the spice of life," says Hans Selye. Some of the most meaningful experiences of existence are also the most stressful. In any event, we cannot avoid stress. Like eating and drinking, it is a normal part of life. "Complete freedom from stress," Selye points out, "is death."

THE VARIETY OF STRESSORS

To be alive at all is to be continually encountering stressors of all kinds. The variety of stressors in modern life seems endless; they include everything, both inside and outside our bodies, that requires us to adapt, either physiologically or psychologically. As mentioned previously, some of these stressors clearly affect us physically; these include such characteristics of our environment as heat, cold, glare, pollution, and sudden or continual noise. Other stressors impinge upon us psychologically; these include those events or situations that arouse our emotions of fear, anxiety, depression, anger, joy, love.

When a stressor affects us negatively, we call it *distress.* Yet stressors are not necessarily bad; many of the good things of life are also stressors (Selye calls this positive stress *eustress*). Thus an argument with a friend or a family member is a stressor, but so is passionate love making. Worrying over financial problems is a stressor, but so is sudden wealth. An overextended schedule that leaves little time for rest or recreation is a stressor, but so are idleness and boredom.

Hard physical labor and strenuous recrea-

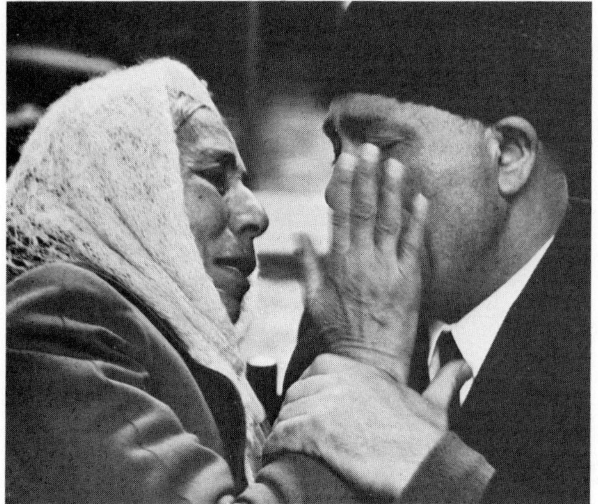

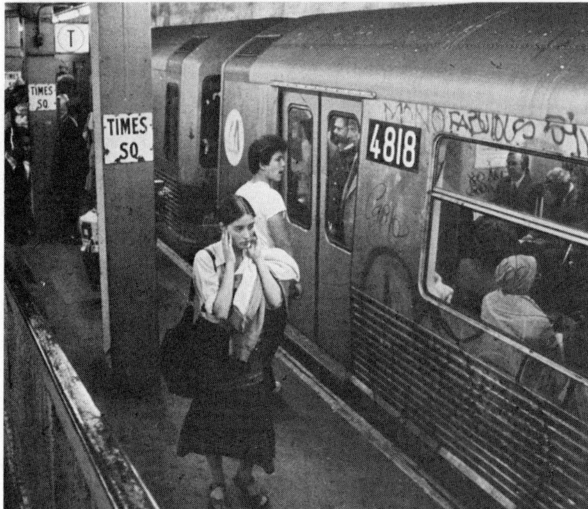

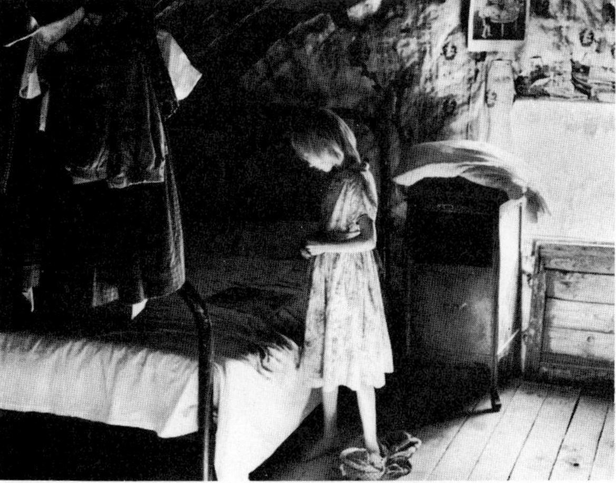

Figure 2.1 Both joyful events, as this reunion of a brother and sister, or negative situations, such as subway noise, are stressors that require significant psychological or physiological adaptation.

tional sports are both stressors. Driving an automobile in heavy traffic is a stressor, and so is watching a horror movie. Both starvation and overeating are stressors. All illnesses are stressors, both physically and psychologically; the medical treatments for illness (drugs, surgery, a change in activities) may also be stressors.

For many people, the fact that they are trying to fill a social or vocational role for which they are ill prepared or not suited is a major stressor. For others, the gap between what they expect out of life and the reality of their daily lives is a significant, continuing stressor. Women and minorities tend to experience more stress just because of their position in society.

Life Changes

Among the most significant stressors are major changes, for better or worse, in the pattern of people's lives. Dr. Thomas H. Holmes of the University of Washington, Seattle, and Dr. Richard H. Rahe of the San Diego Naval Health Research Center compiled a checklist of forty-three typical life events, ranging in intensity from the death of a spouse to taking a vacation. They then asked hundreds of people, of all ages and from all walks of life, to assign a numerical rating to these events, on a scale of 1 to 100 with marriage arbitrarily set at 50, according to the amount of adaptation and adjustment they felt each event demands. The resulting Social Readjustment Rating Scale is shown in Table 2.1.

Holmes and Rahe administered this scale to thousands of U.S. Navy officers and men serving aboard ships, where their environments and daily routines were fairly constant. The researchers found that the higher a man's score, the more likely he was to become ill. Men with scores below 150 remained in good health. Of those with scores between 150 and 300, about half became ill. And of those with scores over 300, some 70 percent became sick. Since then, investigators have administered the Holmes-Rahe scale to many other groups and have found that high scores correlate with a number of specific diseases (see the section *Stress and Disease*). While the specific value of

Table 2.1 Social Readjustment Rating Scale

Rank	Life Event	Value
1	Death of spouse	100
2	Divorce	73
3	Marital separation	65
4	Jail term	63
5	Death of close family member	63
6	Personal injury or illness	53
7	Marriage	50
8	Fired at work	47
9	Marital reconciliation	45
10	Retirement	45
11	Change in health of family member	44
12	Pregnancy	40
13	Sex difficulties	39
14	Gain of new family member	39
15	Business readjustment	39
16	Change in financial state	38
17	Death of close friend	37
18	Change to different line of work	36
19	Change in number of arguments with spouse	35
20	Mortgage over $10,000	31
21	Foreclosure of mortgage or loan	30
22	Change in responsibilities at work	29
23	Son or daughter leaving home	29
24	Trouble with in-laws	29
25	Outstanding personal achievement	28
26	Wife begin or stop work	26
27	Begin or end school	26
28	Change in living conditions	25
29	Revision of personal habits	24
30	Trouble with boss	23
31	Change in work hours or conditions	20
32	Change in residence	20
33	Change in schools	20
34	Change in recreation	19
35	Change in church activities	19
36	Change in social activities	18
37	Mortgage or loan less than $10,000	17
38	Change in sleeping habits	16
39	Change in number of family get-togethers	15
40	Change in eating habits	15
41	Vacation	13
42	Christmas	12
43	Minor violations of the law	11

Source: Reprinted with permission from T. H. Holmes and R. H. Rahe, "The Social Readjustment Rating Scale," *Journal of Psychosomatic Research,* 1967, Table 3, p. 216. © 1967, Pergamon Press Ltd.

each life event does not necessarily hold true for every individual, it is nonetheless evident that such life changes do have an impact, for better or worse, on our overall well-being.

Environmental Stressors

Until recently, people paid little attention to the stressors in such environments as homes, offices, and recreational facilities. They simply assumed that human beings could adapt to almost any environment. Now, however, increasing attention is being given to the stressful effects of noise, air pollution, glare, and insufficient light. Many people, of course, control glare by wearing hats or sunglasses. An Occupational Safety and Health Administration (OSHA) law now requires that people in noisy workplaces wear hearing protectors, and a few people choose to wear earplugs generally to reduce their exposure to noise.

Figure 2.2 The body may be subjected to a variety of environmental stressors, such as cold weather, or urban noise, or pollution.

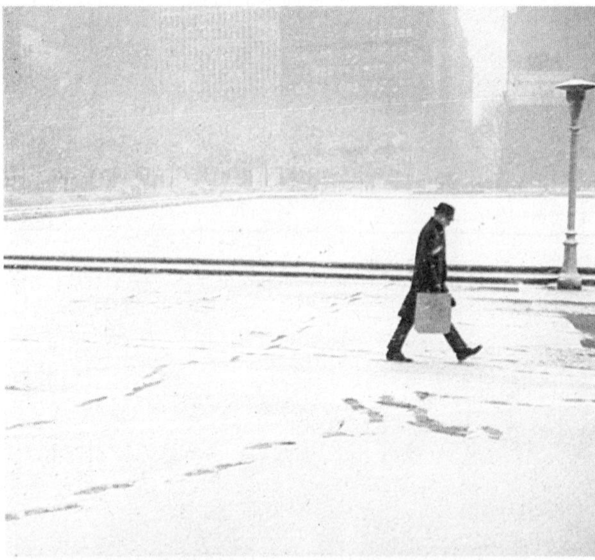

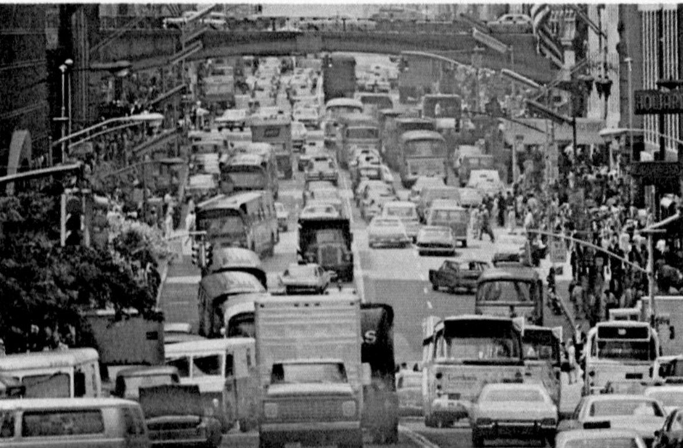

Crowding

Many social critics assume that urban crowding is one of the major stressors of modern life. San Francisco, Chicago, and Boston all have population densities of more than 10,000 people per square mile, while Manhattan has a whopping 70,000 per square mile. In 1975, however, Jonathan L. Freedman of Columbia University presented, in the book *Crowding and Behavior,* evidence that crowding is not, in fact, a significant stressor.

Using juvenile delinquency as an index of pathology, Freedman studied individual Manhattan neighborhoods—and found no relationship between crowding and delinquency. One high-density (and high-income) neighborhood had an exceedingly low delinquency rate, for example, while a low-density (and low-income) neighborhood had a very high delinquency rate. Income, Freedman concluded, was more important than crowding. Other studies in Chicago and New York have similarly failed to find any correlation between population density and such indexes of health as venereal disease, mental illness, or infant or adult mortality. What crowding does do, Freedman believes, is to intensify people's reactions to situations and other people; we may enjoy a crowded party but dislike a crowded subway.

THE VARIATION IN RESPONSE

A given stressor may have very different *effects* on different people. For one thing, people vary enormously in their *perception* of a given stressor. One student, for instance, might construe an assignment as a threat to his or her competence and worry about the possibility of failure. Another person might see the assignment as simply another piece of busywork to fit into the agenda—a nuisance or a chore, but not a challenge to self-esteem—and thus not really a stressor.

For another thing, the *impact* of a given stressor can also vary with a person's circumstances. Being fired from a job is obviously more stressful for a father with a family to support than for a student who was about to quit anyway. One criticism of the Holmes-Rahe Social Readjustment Rating Scale is that life changes actually have different impacts on people depending on many factors: their age, stage of life, cultural background, socioeconomic status, previous experiences. People's response to a stressor is also affected by how much control they have—or think they have—over the situation and the kind of social support they receive from their friends, family, and other colleagues. Thus what is a stressor for one person is often a welcome challenge for another.

THE PHYSIOLOGY OF STRESS

Whenever we respond to a stressor, whether it is a physical stressor or a psychological one, an intricate physiological stress mechanism is activated that affects our entire body. This gears us up physiologically to deal with the demands of the stressor, whatever it may be. For our prehistoric ancestors, it might have been the sight of a menacing bear, and the physiological stress response prepared them either to fight the animal or flee. For modern people, the stressor is more likely to be psychological, as we have mentioned, but the stress response still revs up our internal engines for action. Our hearts beat faster, hormones surge into our bloodstream, our blood pressure rises, and we break out in perspiration. When we can neither fight nor flee, however, as is the case with so many modern stressors, this physiological response can disrupt our body's functioning and reveal itself as one or more of many different, sometimes subtle, symptoms.

Signs of Stress

These many symptoms of stress—which can be physical or emotional or behavioral—also vary from person to person and from time to time in the same person. One person might feel stress as a pain in the neck or lower back, a loss of appetite or overeating, or insomnia or sleeping excessively or having nightmares. Someone else might have a dry mouth, or become irritable or excitable, or feel a strong urge to run from the situation. Another might be depressed, or have the urge to cry, or feel afraid without any apparent reason (so-called free-

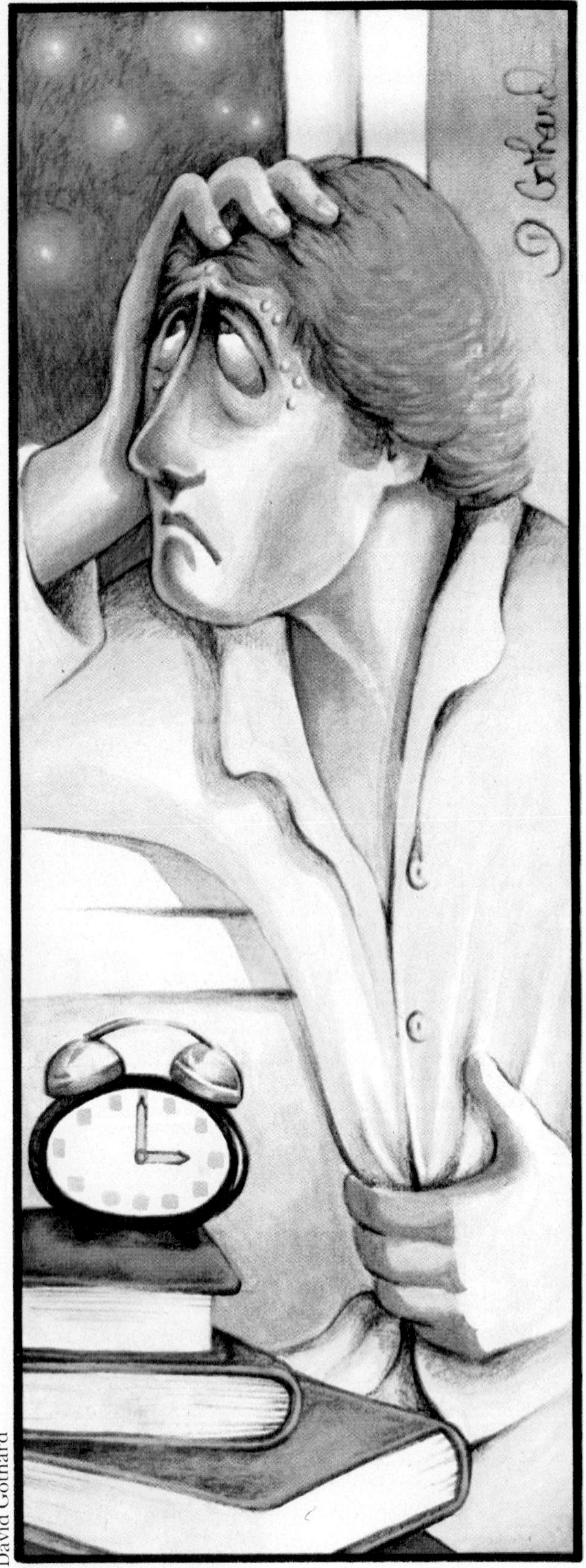

Figure 2.3 Symptoms of stress—physical, emotional, and behavioral—vary from person to person.

floating anxiety), or have feelings of unreality, or be unable to concentrate, or feel tense or keyed up. Others might feel weak or dizzy or chronically tired, or have indigestion, diarrhea, or vomiting. Still others might show stress by stuttering, trembling, laughing nervously, being easily startled, developing tics, grinding the teeth, being unable to relax, smoking or drinking alcohol or using other drugs more, becoming accident prone, or otherwise behaving inappropriately.

There is a tendency, however, for any one person to respond to stress with the same symptom or combination of symptoms. The first step in coping with stress is to become sensitive to the particular ways in which your own body responds so that you recognize when you are under stress.

The Stress Mechanism

What is going on inside our bodies that can produce so many diverse, outward signs of stress? Since Selye's pioneering research in the 1930s, many investigators have contributed to the following description of the physiological stress mechanism.

When our brain perceives a stressor, be it a menacing bear or an angry boss, the brain revs up the body by activating two interrelated physiological systems: the autonomic nervous system and the endocrine system. The hypothalamus, a key control center in the brain, activates the sympathetic division of the autonomic nervous system. The sympathetic system helps to control the involuntary muscles of the blood vessels and internal organs and also activates the endocrine glands, particularly the inner portion (medulla) of the adrenal glands, just above the kidneys. In response to the hypothalamic stress signal, the adrenal medulla pours out into the bloodstream the hormones adrenaline and noradrenaline. The hypothalamus also activates the endocrine system directly by signaling the pituitary gland, at the base of the brain, to secrete hormones that travel via the bloodstream to the adrenal, thyroid, and other glands. One of the most important of these pituitary secretions is adrenocorticotrophic hormone (ACTH), which stimulates the outer portion (the cortex) of the

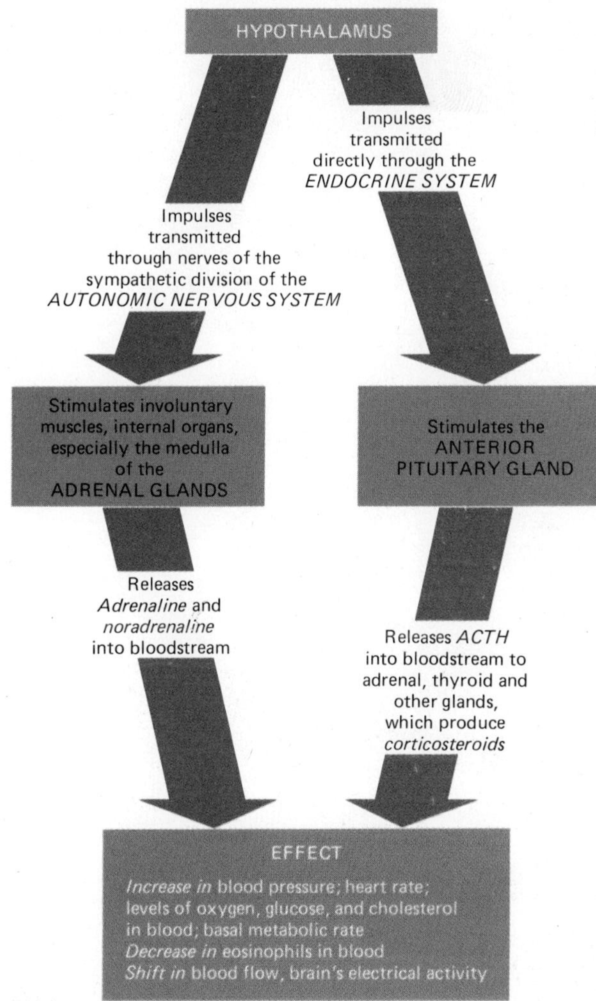

Figure 2.4 Two hormonal pathways activated during stress.

adrenal glands to produce hormones called corticosteroids.

The net effect of the activation of the autonomic nervous and endocrine systems is not only to increase the heart rate and blood pressure, but also to increase the amount of oxygen, glucose, cholesterol, and certain free fatty acids in the blood; raise the basal metabolic rate; shift blood toward the head and extremities; decrease the number of eosinophils (a type of white cell) in the blood; and alter the brain's electrical activity—changes that prepare us for fight or flight.

These initial physiological adjustments Selye calls the *alarm stage* of the biological stress syndrome. He has determined that this syndrome occurs in three stages. During the alarm stage, the body adapts to the stressor. In the second stage, the *resistance stage,* the body begins to resist the stressor. The length of this stage depends on the nature and intensity of the stressor and the body's innate adaptability. At first, stressors "may upset and alarm us, but then we get used to them," explains Selye. "In the course of a normal human life, everybody goes through these first two stages many, many times." Eventually, however, if a stressor continues, the third stage, the *stage of exhaustion,* sets in. The body's adaptation energy is used up, and the person or animal dies. At autopsy, Selye's rats showed the results of their physiological adaptation: enlarged adrenal glands, atrophied lymph nodes and thymus glands, and ulcers (see Figure 2.5, p.50).

Thus when we do resist a stressor and get used to it, this adaptation takes a physiological toll. Consider, for example, chronic exposure to noise in a large office where phones, typewriters, and other business machines ring and clatter away all day long. A new employee may, at first, be extremely conscious of this irritating environment and feel acute stress. His pulse rate and blood pressure may rise; he may feel anxious or angry. He may develop headaches or indigestion, or become prone to colds. After a while, however, the employee may adapt to the noise and become less aware of it. This adaptation will reduce the emotional component of his stress, but much of the physiological component will continue—affecting his heart, his blood vessels, the hormones in his blood, the functioning of his nervous system. In time, his health may break down and he may develop an overt, stress-related disease.

STRESS AND DISEASE

Numerous studies have shown that excessive stress is associated with a wide spectrum of diseases, both physical and psychological. People with high life-change scores on the Holmes-Rahe Social Readjustment Rating Scale, it has been found, are more likely to develop heart attacks, ulcers, diabetes, leukemia, or infections, or to die suddenly. They are also more apt to have accidents or athletic inju-

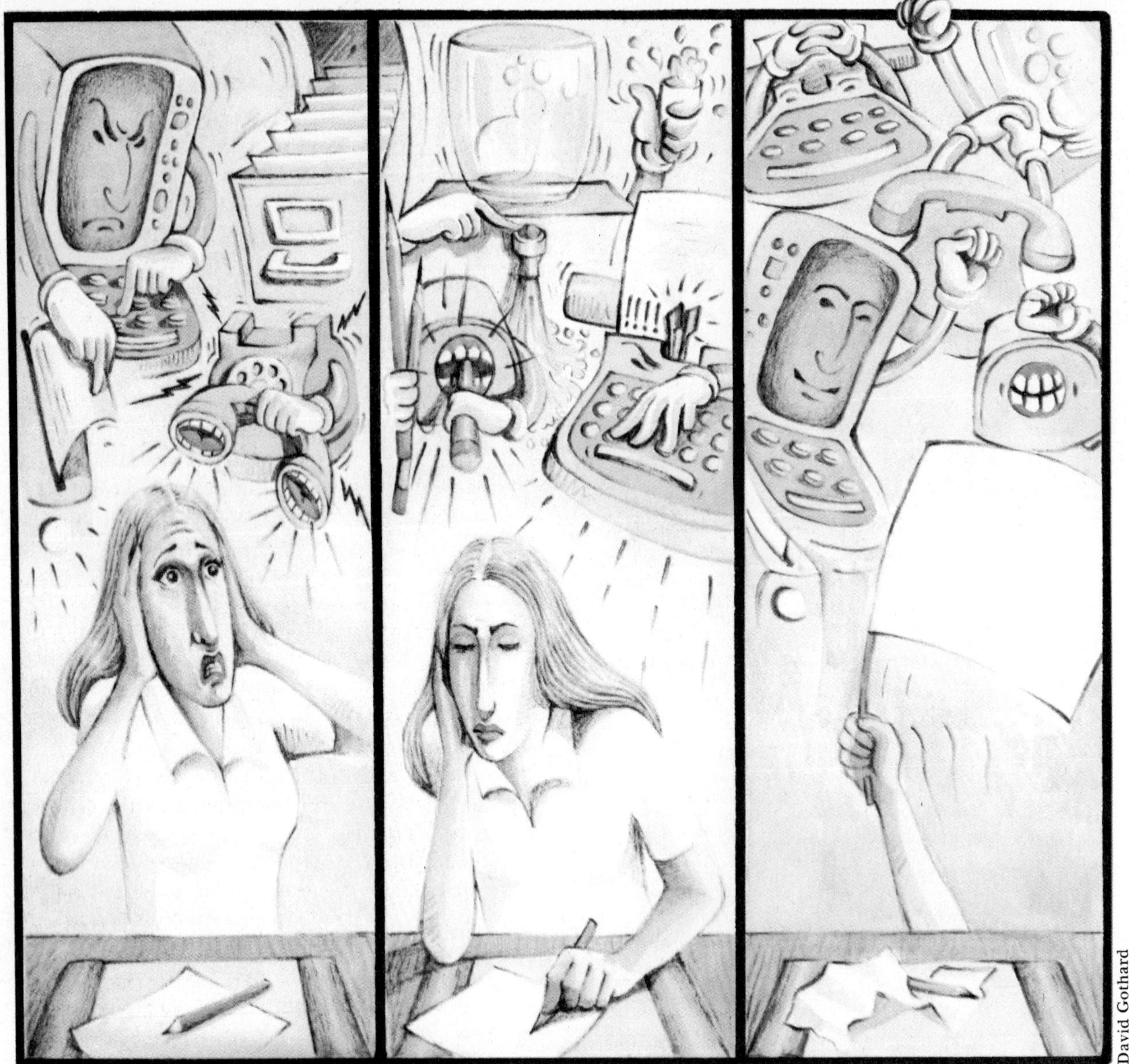

Figure 2.5 The three stages of the stress mechanism: alarm, resistance, exhaustion.

ries, be hospitalized for schizophrenia or depression, show neurotic symptoms, or attempt suicide. Holmes and Rahe have also found that people are far more likely to become ill the year following a divorce, and that ten times as many widows and widowers die the year following their spouse's death as do others in the same age group.

Sometimes stress can cause disease directly, when a person's physiological response to stress—a migraine headache, for example—is, in itself, a disease. Stress may also lower our resistance to infectious disease by interfering with our immune defense system. It can also lower our resistance to infection indirectly if we respond to stress by not eating properly, smoking and drinking too much, not exercising enough, or not getting enough sleep. Stress can also trigger almost *any* disease, as is indicated by the wide range of illnesses associated with high life-change scores.

But why should one student get the flu or a cold during exam week, while another has an accident, and others develop headaches or back pains or feel tired all the time—and most are not sick at all? Part of the reason seems to be inherited biological weaknesses. One person might have a genetic defect in a digestive enzyme that predisposes him to an ulcer. Another might have a vulnerable respiratory system, and for him or her, stress precipitates colds. Part of the reason also seems to be psychological. In some people with feelings of inadequacy, stressful situations combined with poor diet and lack of rest can produce handicapping fatigue.

Stress is a factor in every illness, since disease itself is both a physical and a psychological stressor. Our emotional response to an illness can exacerbate its course. If our fear or anger causes us to put off seeing a doctor when we suspect heart disease, cancer, or another serious disease, we reduce our chances of successful treatment. And once we have seen a doctor, if we don't follow the prescribed treatment or avoid returning for a checkup—because it is too frightening to face the fact of the illness—we complicate the treatment.

People often use the word "psychosomatic" for bodily (somatic) diseases brought on by psychological stresses. Yet this term is misleading if one takes it to imply that psychological causes are separate from physical ones. The complex interactions between mind and body work both ways; psychological factors affect our physiology, and physiological factors affect our feelings. Emotions such as love and anger evoke physiological changes. Social embarrassment may involve both brain cells that perceive the stressful situation and a shift in blood flow that causes one to blush. Conversely, a physical injury or a virus infection also elicits emotional responses. There is thus no split between mind and body; there is one mind-body.

One popular—and controversial—thesis is that people today are more susceptible to stress-related diseases than were our cave-dwelling ancestors because of the extraordinarily numerous and complex stressors of modern American society. While we have inherited a stress mechanism that gears us up for fight or flight, such a physical response is not an appropriate way of dealing with most modern stressors. Fighting or running away is not the best method of handling office noise or a heavy examination schedule or a troublesome neighbor. Our physiological stress response is thus "all cranked up with no place to go"—and stress disease results. The opponents of this thesis, however, point out that we actually have no way of knowing whether the stressors of twentieth-century civilization are greater—or less—than those of prehistoric times.

COPING WITH STRESS

Fortunately, there are many ways of learning to deal with the stresses of life and moderating the toll they can take on our health.

Investigations of people who are facing severe stress have yielded considerable insight into normal coping processes. Interestingly, it turns out that a certain amount of fear and worry over an impending stressful situation is not only normal but also essential for successful coping.

Yale psychologist Irving L. Janis has studied people undergoing major surgery—a situation, he points out, that "involves pain, a profound threat to bodily integrity, and a variety of frustrations" and is both a physical and psychological stressor. The results, Janis concludes, "clearly contradict the popular assumption that placid people—those who are least fearful about an impending ordeal—will prove to be less disturbed than others by subsequent stress. . . . Apparently, a moderate amount of anticipatory fear about realistic threats is necessary for the development of effective inner defenses for coping with subsequent danger and deprivation." If people do not do this constructive worrying beforehand, they are less likely to cope satisfactorily later.

Janis found that the surgery patients showed three different patterns of emotional response to their situation. After surgery, those who had been moderately fearful beforehand made the best emotional adjustment. Their morale was high, despite the inevitable pains and discomforts of convalescence, and they cooperated with the necessary but sometimes disagreeable treatments. The highly fearful people were much more likely to be anxiety-ridden, exhibit stormy emotional outbursts, and shrink from postoperative treatments. And those who had seemed outwardly calm beforehand now

HOW TO Cope with Pressure

Pressure is a normal part of everyday life. If you know how to deal with it, it can actually spur creativity, productivity, and healthy relationships with others. If you let it get out of hand, it can become a problem. If you have trouble handling pressure and using it constructively, here are some tips.

1. Confide in someone you can trust. Talking about a problem often helps to reduce tension, and another person can offer suggestions from his or her perspective.
2. If you're afraid of something, admit it to yourself. It's nothing to be ashamed of—*everyone* has been in the same boat at one time or another.
3. Don't try to escape a problem with lines like "I'll snap out of it" or "It's them, not me." You won't convince anyone—least of all yourself.
4. Don't take out your problems on your friends, family, or co-workers. It doesn't make you feel any better, and it makes *them* miserable, too!
5. If you're quarreling with someone, remember that it's just possible that *you* could be wrong. If you yield some ground, others will.
6. Competition induces pressure because other people become threats to you. Try cooperation instead—it's contagious! You may make life easier for several people—including yourself.
7. Don't always stick with a problem until you solve it. You may do better to let it lie and to relax or take on another task. When you return to your problem, you may find you approach it from a new and refreshed viewpoint.
8. Take your mind off your problems by doing something for someone else.
9. Take time out for fun—a baseball game, a movie, or a long walk. Relaxation absorbs pressure like a sponge, so be sure to build it into your schedule.

Source: National Institute of Mental Health, "How You Can Handle Pressure" (Rockville, Md.: U.S. Department of Health, Education, and Welfare, 1973).

tended to become much more upset than the moderate worriers. They were much more likely to be angry and resentful, display acute emotional disturbance, complain bitterly, and try to refuse routine postoperative treatment. Apparently they had been able to remain calm only by denying or minimizing the possible danger or suffering, and when they encountered the inevitable pain and discomfort, they became emotionally upset.

Further insight into coping with stress is revealed by a six-stage model, devised by stress researchers Richard Rahe of the U.S. Navy and Ransom J. Arthur of the University of California at Los Angeles, that outlines the process by which a stressful situation can lead to disease. Although this Rahe-Arthur model is most directly relevant to the stresses caused by life changes, it is also useful as a guide for controlling other kinds of stress. The six stages are:

1. *Perception of the situation.* What is challenging the person's equilibrium? The disturbance may be either positive or negative, but he or she is aware that something is different.
2. *Psychological responses.* The person marshals defense mechanisms (see Chapter 1), which often involve denying or minimizing the situation or repressing its effects.
3. *Physiological responses.* Sweating, muscle tension, elevated blood pressure, and so forth, as previously described.
4. *Protective behavior.* The person takes steps either to change the situation (redoubling efforts, say, to meet the challenge) or to alter his or her response to it.
5. *Signs of illness.* The person begins playing the sick role, misses school or work, and seeks medical attention.
6. *Frank disease.* Medical diagnosis verifies the illness, and the person becomes officially sick.

By the time a person has reached the last two stages, it is difficult to halt or reverse the progression. Rahe and Arthur suggest that both individuals and doctors can usually—and more easily—intervene to prevent illness by concentrating on the first four steps.

Controlling Stress Responses

You can deliberately develop certain skills to help you modify stress responses. Sometimes you can reduce destructive physiological stress responses by reducing your psychological responses. Often, you can get a fresh perspective on a stressful situation by taking a break from it—going away for a weekend, or even taking brief rests during the course of a day. Sometimes, by a process called *cognitive reappraisal,* you can also alter your perceptions of a situation so that it becomes less stressful. This is something you can consciously train yourself to do—that is, find other ways of interpreting potentially stressful situations. For instance, when a professor or a boss or even a friend is suddenly brusque, you might tend to become uptight and anxious about your relationship with the person. Perhaps you are in disfavor; perhaps he or she does not like you anymore. Yet consider: there may very well be another explanation. The person may be under other pressures—an illness in the family, a threat to his or her livelihood—that you do not know about. The brusqueness may have nothing whatever to do with you personally. Once having thought of these alternative explanations, you may find the person's brusqueness less stressful. And traditional psychotherapy can also sometimes help control chronic stress by helping you see other ways of perceiving situations and gain insights into your psychological stress responses.

Conversely, you can sometimes reduce your psychological stress response by reducing your physiological response. Some techniques for doing this you can learn yourself; others require professional assistance.

Drugs Physicians often prescribe drugs, such as mild sedatives and the minor tranquilizers, for people who have sought medical assistance for stress. These drugs are certainly useful for alleviating stress, but they also carry a risk of accidents, adverse reactions, and the possibility of a handicapping dependency. You should consider the use of drugs as a temporary measure to help you through a crisis rather than as a routine, day-to-day method of coping with normal stress.

Exercise Physical exercise is very useful in controlling stress because it stimulates fight-or-flight behavior and probably burns off stress hormones. Fortunately, the same continuous, rhythmic, aerobic exercise that is best for respiratory and cardiovascular conditioning is also useful for reducing stress (see Chapter 10).

Relaxation Many techniques of relaxation are widely advocated both for dealing with stress and for improving creativity. Some of these are fairly simple; others are elaborate and require extensive (and often expensive) training.

More than fifty years ago, long before the scientific study of stress, Dr. Edmond Jacobson, a Chicago physiologist, developed a technique he called *progressive relaxation* for alleviating muscle tension. Jacobson believed that in order to relax, one must first deliberately "do" (contract a group of muscles) and then "not do" (relax that muscle group). To practice Jacobson's progressive relaxation, you should first lie down in a comfortable place and then alternately tense and relax each major muscle group in turn—from the hands and arms to the head, eyes, mouth, neck, shoulders, back, chest, abdomen, buttocks, thighs, calves, and feet. Jacobson also extended his system to exercises for mental relaxation in which you alternately imagine simple sensory experiences—sights, sounds, smells, shapes, tactile sensations—and then "let go" of the images.

To relax by *meditation,* set aside a block of time (usually fifteen to thirty minutes) once or twice a day. Take a comfortable sitting position in a quiet place where there are few distrac-

Figure 2.6 Meditation is an age-old method of tension reduction that may enhance your feelings of physical and psychological well-being.

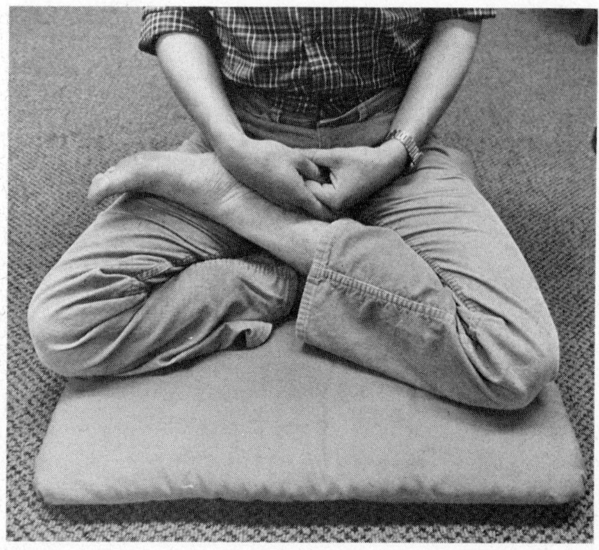

tions. Assume a passive frame of mind, in which you force nothing, and concentrate on a calming mental image or word or phrase, slowly repeating it to yourself over and over again. *Transcendental Meditation (TM)* is a form of meditation that requires special training. Studies have shown that meditation reduces both psychological feelings of stress and also some of the physiological responses: pulse rate, blood pressure, muscle tension, skin conductivity, oxygen consumption, and the level of stress hormones in the blood.

Yoga is a popular system of exercise, body control, and relaxation imported from the East. The practice of yoga varies from simple stretching exercises to elaborate, highly disciplined forms of mind-body control. Practitioners of these advanced forms of yoga are able not only to perform remarkable feats of muscle and joint flexibility but also to alter at will such physiological functions as heart rate, blood pressure, body temperature, and pain perception.

Other complex systems of relaxation are the martial arts of the Far East, such as *karate, kung fu,* and *judo.* While the apparent object of these arts is physical combat, they also require great control of one's perceptions, interpretations, and reactions, and involve learning an "inner order" that is a form of relaxation. *Tai chi* is a highly disciplined Chinese exercise system that uses slow movements of the whole body to achieve a state of physical and mental calm.

While *hypnosis* per se is not necessarily relaxing, it has been used, with varying success, to induce relaxation. The hypnotist asks the subject to go limp, feel the weight of the body pressing downward, imagine soothing sounds and tranquil surroundings, and erase all tension from the muscles.

Some anecdotal examples can show how various individuals might learn how to control or cope with different types of stressors. One young man found that he sweated profusely and got an upset stomach whenever he was to go to a social gathering where he would be meeting new people. He viewed these reactions as an illness and usually avoided such occasions because he thought he was "sick." Once he consciously identified these reactions as a stress response, he decided that these gatherings—and meeting new people—were important to him and that he would not allow this stress response to dominate him. He discovered by accident that taking a long run on the afternoon before such occasions relieved some of the sweating and stomach upset. With this new insight, he attended a dozen or so social gatherings—and the old stressful feelings virtually disappeared.

Another familiar stressful situation—a pileup of assignments at the end of a term—is shown in Figure 2.7 and analyzed in terms of a simple, three-component model. Note that the three components are interrelated in a feedback loop. In the breakdown example, stress results in illness. When the student consciously altered the components as they interacted, he achieved some success in controlling the situation, and no serious illness resulted.

STRESS AND LIFE STYLE

Perhaps the most fundamental way of controlling stress in our lives is by reordering our life styles. Some people seem to be "in tune" with their surroundings and their relationships with people and to "flow with" the forces of their environments. These people probably experience stress and its consequences less than those who are in constant conflict with their surroundings. Being in tune with the world does not mean being passive or indifferent to those problems—such as violence, injustice, or human misery—that cry for change. Instead, it means recognizing our limitations and maintaining an inner calm while working to resolve such problems. By contrast, those who are constantly in conflict with the world may often lash out crudely in ways that do not achieve success but elicit negative and stress-producing reactions from others.

Since one's health is often determined by one's ability to deal with stress, ordering one's life style to control stress is vital for approaching one's potential. Stress theorist Hans Selye has offered the following prescription for placing stress in perspective in life:

> Fight for your highest attainable aim
> But never put up resistance in vain.

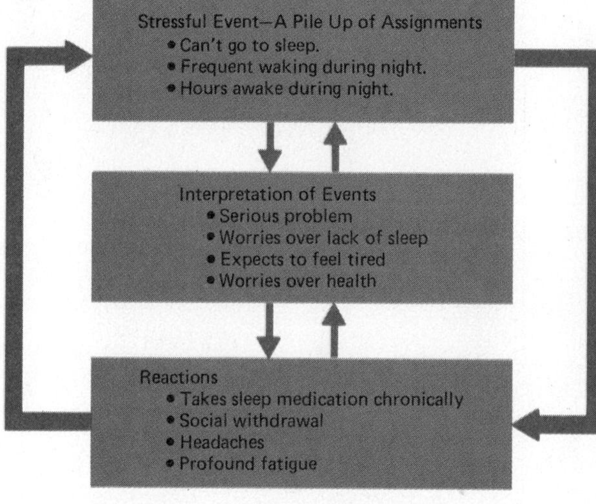

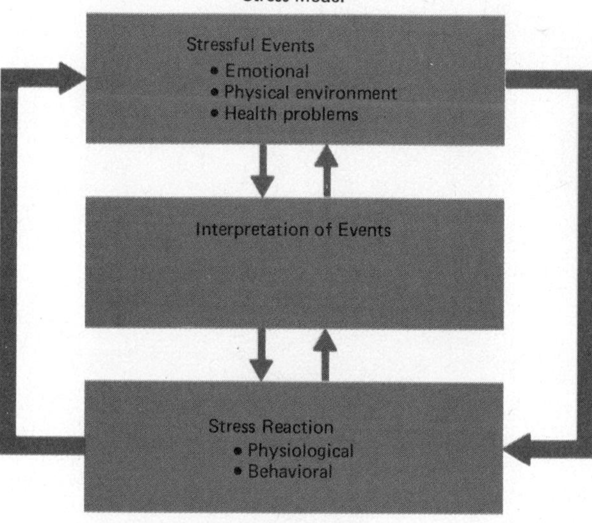

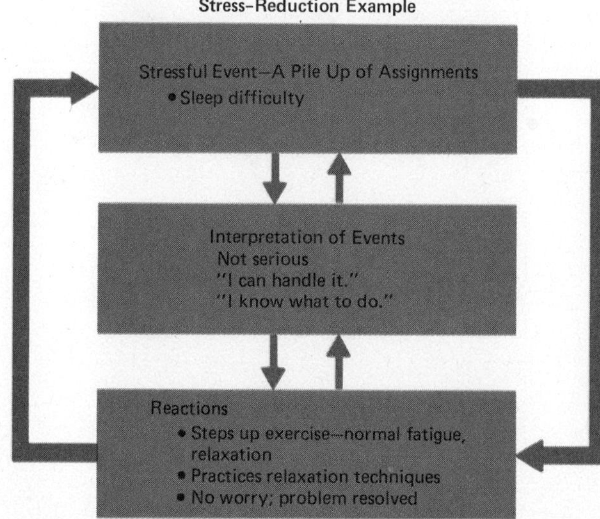

Figure 2.7 The same stressful event, if interpreted positively, can result in successful stress reduction and positive coping behavior rather than in excessive worry or physical and psychological breakdown.

SUMMARY

1. An event or agent that produces stress is called a stressor. The body's physiological and psychological response to a stressor is called stress.
2. Stress is not necessarily bad; we learn and perform better when under moderate stress. Stress is also a normal part of life; complete freedom from stress is death.
3. The variety of stressors is endless. They include characteristics of our environments, situations that arouse our emotions, overextended schedules, boredom, hard physical labor, illnesses, and trying to fill roles for which we are unsuited.
4. The Holmes-Rahe Social Readjustment Rating Scale attempts to measure the impact of stressful life changes. People with high life-change scores are more likely to become sick.
5. A given stressor may have different effects on different people, because people may perceive it differently, their circumstances may cause it to vary, and their innate anxiety levels also differ.
6. Signs of stress may include backaches, overeating, insomnia, nightmares, irritability, excitability, crying, free-floating anxiety, chronic tiredness, and accident proneness.
7. When we encounter a stressor, our brain activates two interrelated physiological systems: the autonomic nervous system and the endocrine system. The net effect is to increase our heart rates and blood pressure and to raise the levels of oxygen and glucose in our blood —changes that prepare us for fight or flight.
8. Excessive stress is associated with a wide spectrum of diseases. It can cause some directly; it can cause others indirectly by lowering our resistance; it can precipitate any disease; and it is a factor in all illnesses.
9. Among the techniques and skills for coping with stress are constructive worrying, avoiding unnecessary stressors, cognitive reappraisal, psychotherapy, drugs, exercise, and relaxation.

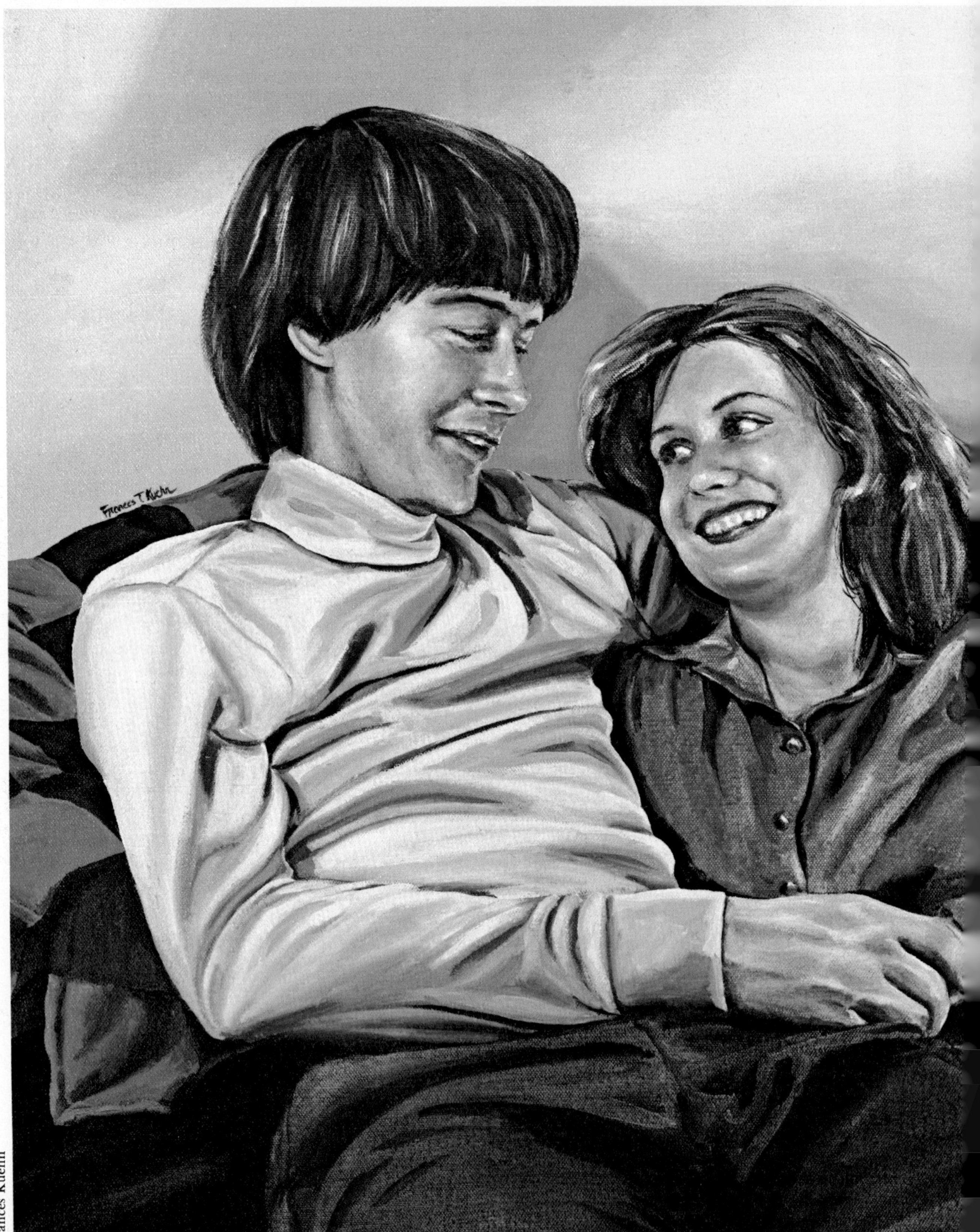

Frances Kuehn

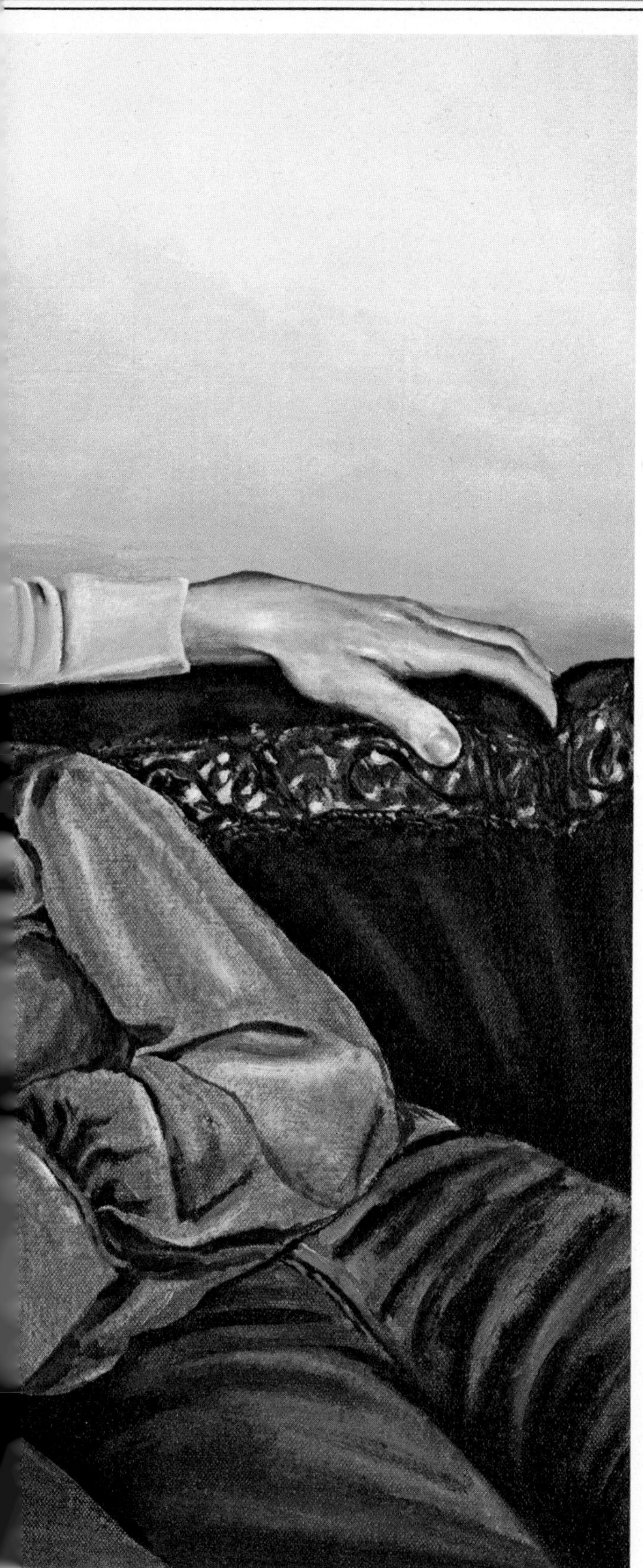

3 Human Sexuality

"It's a boy!" "It's a girl!" At the moment of our birth, we are labeled sexually with one of these glad cries, and our sexuality continues to be an integral part of our existence throughout life. Our sexuality is more than just our anatomy and what we do with it—it is central to our very identity and concept of ourselves, profoundly affecting our values and our behavior.

The sexual act, of course, has meanings far deeper than merely reproducing our species. It is not only one of the pleasures of life, but also a means of establishing and reaffirming intimacy with another person and expressing mutual love. However, it can also be a source of a great deal of hurt. Mature sex requires open and honest communication between partners, and carries with it a responsibility for the welfare, both physical and emotional, of one's partner. This chapter discusses those facts and ideas about human sexuality that will help people feel confident about themselves as sexual beings and comfortable with members of both sexes, understand the nature of the human sexual response, and make the most of their human sexual potential.

GENDER IDENTITY

One's *gender* or sex, in the biological sense of maleness or femaleness, is not a simple phenomenon but the product of a lengthy sequence of genetic and hormonal events. One's *gender identity,* or sexual identity, is a more complex concept; it is the entire sense of oneself as masculine or feminine. Gender identity is the product of a lengthy process of psychosocial

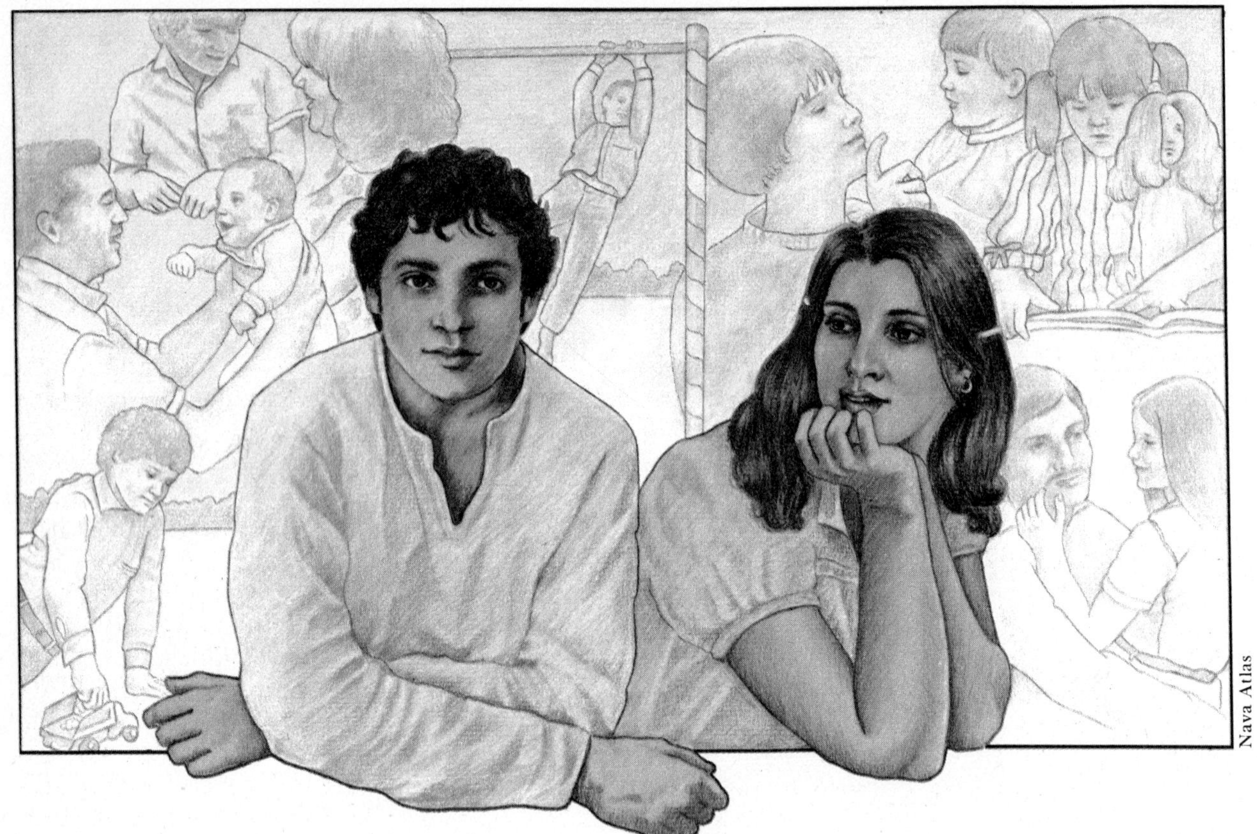

Figure 3.1 Gender identity, or sexual identity, is a complex concept, involving the entire sense of oneself as masculine or feminine. It develops as a result of social and cultural conditioning that begins at birth.

conditioning that begins at birth. A number of recent findings about human sexuality have made it possible, for the first time, to sort out the relative contributions of these various biological and psychosocial factors to gender identity.

Genetic Factors

Biological sex is determined at conception, when a sperm from the father fuses with the mother's egg (ovum). The new human being's sex is determined at that moment by the sex chromosome it inherits from the father. Eggs can contain only one type of sex chromosome, an X chromosome. Sperm, on the other hand, can contain either of the two types of sex chromosomes, an X or a Y chromosome. If the sperm fertilizing the egg contains an X chromosome, the child will be a female whose genetic sex is XX. If the sperm contains a Y chromosome, the child will be a male whose genetic sex is XY. Biological sex, however, is only the first step along the complex path of development of a person's gender identity.

Hormonal Factors

For the first six weeks after conception, male and female embryos develop in precisely the same way. It is impossible to tell them apart without examining their chromosomes under a microscope. Undifferentiated gonads (sex glands) appear along the genital ridge that runs from the embryo's umbilical cord to its tail. A genital tubercle (a small bump that will become the external genitals) and a set of genital ducts (that will become the internal sex organs) also develop along this ridge.

At about six weeks, the Y chromosome causes the undifferentiated gonads in male embryos to develop into testes, which begin secreting androgens or masculinizing hormones. The genital tubercle develops into a penis and scrotum, and the genital ducts become the seminal vesicles and the prostate. In female embryos, which lack the Y chromosome, the undifferentiated gonads become ovaries. The genital tubercle develops into the clitoris and labia; and the genital ducts into the Fallopian tubes, uterus, and vagina. The male and female sex organs are thus homologous; they arise from the same embryonic structures, and they perform corresponding functions.

Social Factors

Beginning at birth, environmental influences—social and cultural—interact with biological factors and help shape a person's gender identity and sexual behavior. These environmental influences profoundly affect how a person relates to other people, emotionally and sexually; what things will arouse him or her sexually; and much, much more.

Although there is evidence that some sex differences in behavior appear shortly after birth, these differences are not as great as people have assumed in the past. However, from that first announcement of a newborn baby's sex, society imposes a set of expectations for that particular sex. The parents give the baby either a girl's name or a boy's name and wrap it in either a blue or a pink blanket. At home, they raise the baby either as a girl or a boy, with toys and regulations they consider appropriate for its sex. From the beginning, parents behave differently with baby girls and baby boys; they tend to talk more to a baby girl and roughhouse more with a baby boy. Such different treatment contributes to the child's growing sense of masculinity or femininity—and eventually to that of the adult he or she will become. As the child behaves more like one sex or the other—displaying growing gender identity—then, more and more, this behavior elicits appropriate reciprocal behavior from others. When a small girl, for example, begins to flirt with her father, he may flirt back. Or when his small son begins to play with a ball, he may play catch with him. Such responses, in turn, further reinforce the child's gender identity. By the age of three or four, most children have developed a strong gender identity and have begun to learn their *gender roles;* that is, they have learned to imitate the behaviors their society considers appropriate for their sex.

In recent years, some research indicates that there are significant mental and behavioral differences between adult males and females. Women tend to have greater verbal abilities, to express their emotions more, to be more anxious about risking failure, and to be more likely to blame themselves if they do fail. Men tend to perceive spatial relationships more accurately, to have greater mathematical skills, and to be more likely to blame others when they fail. How much, however, of these sex differences is due to innate biological factors, and how much to social factors? Most experts now attribute *most* of these differences to this process of social conditioning that begins at birth.

THE REAL SEXUAL REVOLUTION

The continuing shift toward less inhibited sexual behavior is commonly called the *sexual revolution.* A much more important revolution—more accurately an evolution—consists of the rapid changes taking place today in gender-role expectations. Society is seriously questioning traditional assumptions about what men and women should do and what they should be. It has already been established that women can do and be most of what people formerly considered exclusively male. Likewise, men can—and many men prefer to—do and be what was formerly considered female.

This revolution is often mislabeled "women's liberation," but it is actually liberating *both* sexes from narrow and confining role expectations. This *gender liberation* gives both men and women more freedom to do and be whatever feels comfortable to them. Today, women may actively assert themselves, and men may express their nurturing side.

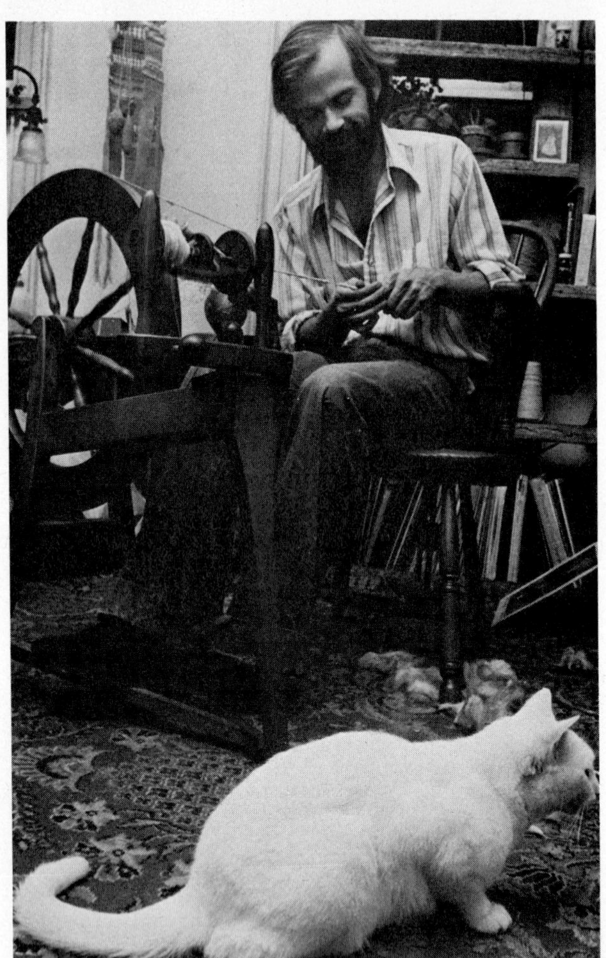

SEXOLOGY OUT OF THE CLOSET

Until fairly recently, the restrictive mores of American culture inhibited the study of—and dissemination of information about—human sexual behavior and functioning. While biologists and anthropologists could study such peripheral subjects as sexual anatomy and the process of fertilization, scientists who wanted to investigate actual sexual behavior and functioning were discouraged, even scorned and ridiculed. Fortunately, a few pioneers such as Kinsey and Masters and Johnson paved the way, and today such studies are more widely accepted. The information now being uncovered about the physiology of erotic response provides a new basis for understanding human sexuality. And studies in the behavioral sciences are contributing increased knowledge of the psychological aspects of sexual behavior.

Figure 3.2 Today's "gender liberation," which questions stereotyped sex-role expectations, allows both men and women to do and be whatever feels comfortable to them.

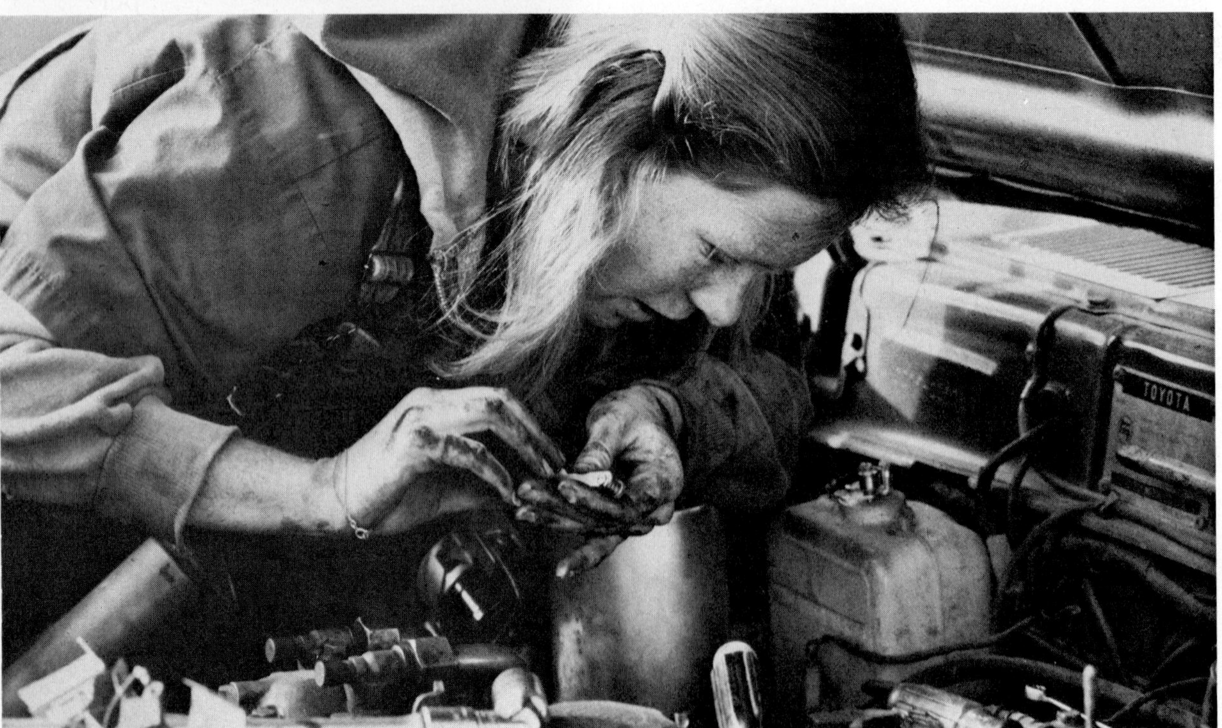

OPTIONS OF SEXUAL ACTIVITY

Human beings vary enormously in their sexual behavior, as they do in other behavior. The new studies of sexuality, while still limited, have made it clear that people learn this variety of sexual behavior within the context of their culture's gender-role expectations. This chapter will not discuss all the possible options of sexual activity.

Masturbation

Masturbation, or self-stimulation for the purpose of sexual gratification, appears to be more common among males than among females. In the United States, for example, approximately nine out of ten males have practiced masturbation, but only one-half to two-thirds of females report having masturbated. In maturity, solitary masturbation is usually replaced as the major form of sexual activity by sexual relations with other persons. It becomes a supplementary outlet, as well as one used when sexual activity with others is unavailable.

Contrary to past belief, masturbation is harmless. In fact, it can be useful in learning to respond sexually and in discovering which forms of stimulation are most enjoyable. Manual stimulation of the genitals is the most common technique of masturbation for both males and females. Insertion of an object into the vagina or insertion of the penis into an object is less common. Many people reach orgasm more quickly and easily in masturbation than in intercourse. This difference is attributed to differences in the speed and intensity of stimulation.

Orgasm or ejaculation during sleep appears to be a fairly common experience. Roughly three-quarters to nine-tenths of males and about two-fifths of females report having had this experience at some time. In males, such orgasms are most common during adolescence and tend to disappear later in life. In females, they are rare in adolescence and gradually become more frequent with age, reaching a maximum in the third and fourth decades of life. Orgasm in sleep is usually, but not always, accompanied by erotic dreams. So-called wet dreams, or nocturnal emissions, in most cases seem to be unrelated to the presence or absence of other sexual activity.

Petting

Petting is best defined as sexual stimulation not involving intercourse. In most Western societies, petting tends to follow a stereotyped sequence—hugging and kissing, followed by breast and thigh caressing, and proceeding to genital stimulation. Adolescent petting is an important opportunity to learn about sexual responses and to obtain sexual and emotional gratification without a serious commitment.

Petting techniques vary considerably, depending upon individual preference, level of sexual sophistication, and societal expectations and attitudes. Kissing is usual in Western cultures. Also common is caressing of various parts of the body other than the breasts or genitals. Manual stimulation of the female breast by the male is nearly universal, and oral breast stimulation is frequent. Manual stimulation of the genitals is common among sexually experienced individuals.

Oral stimulation of the female genitals *(cunnilingus)* is a matter on which cultures differ markedly. In some, it is prevalent; in others, it is rare or regarded as unnatural or perverse. In

Figure 3.3 Adolescent petting is an important opportunity to learn about sexual response and to gratify sexual and emotional desires without a more serious commitment.

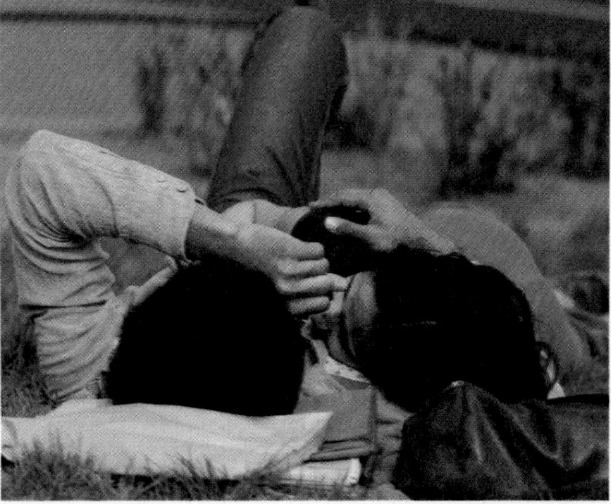

the United States, cunnilingus occurs among more than half of all married couples; however, in most states it continues to be punishable as a felony. Oral stimulation of the male genitals *(fellatio)* is equally common in the United States.

Intercourse

In every human society, intercourse is regarded as the ultimate and natural culmination of a full heterosexual relationship. Although intercourse in marriage is universally regarded as a right, or even a duty, attitudes toward intercourse under other circumstances vary greatly. For example, female premarital intercourse is officially discouraged in many societies, yet nearly all societies permit or excuse male premarital intercourse, even when illegal.

Nevertheless, actual practice may vary greatly from publicly expressed attitudes. In the United States, where premarital intercourse is—at least in theory—unacceptable and in most states is against the law, at least two-thirds of males and one-half of females engage in it. Males tend to have premarital intercourse with more partners than do females, and with less emphasis on a total human relationship.

The social and psychological significance of premarital intercourse to the individual is linked to social attitudes. In many societies, premarital intercourse is expected and serves a useful role in the selection of a spouse. In such societies, there are seldom negative psychological consequences. In societies that condemn the activity, there are possible negative consequences—rejection, guilt, and exploitation. However, the great majority of American females who have had premarital intercourse report no regrets.

Even intercourse in marriage is not wholly free of societal restrictions. In some societies, it is forbidden during menstrual flow, during part of pregnancy, or for a variable period (which can range up to many months) after childbirth. In addition, it may be forbidden before or during special ceremonies or activities.

The frequency of marital intercourse varies greatly not only among societies but among individual couples within a society. During the first years of marriage between youthful partners, a couple is likely to have intercourse frequently. As the male interest lessens later in life, however, men and women may seem to change places in respect to sexual drive. The woman, who in early marriage may feel that intercourse is too frequent, may say in middle age that it is not frequent enough.

Although age does reduce sexual activity, it need not eradicate it. If individuals are in reasonably good health and receive sexual stimulation, intercourse can continue into extreme old age. In addition to its physiological benefit and its value as one of life's great pleasures, intercourse can affirm the affection and desire that hold a relationship together. It is both irrational and unhealthy to perpetuate the notion that sexual behavior among the aged is somehow unseemly or humorous.

Figure 3.4 Individuals can continue to have intercourse into extreme old age. In fact, it bolsters both physiological and psychological well-being at all ages.

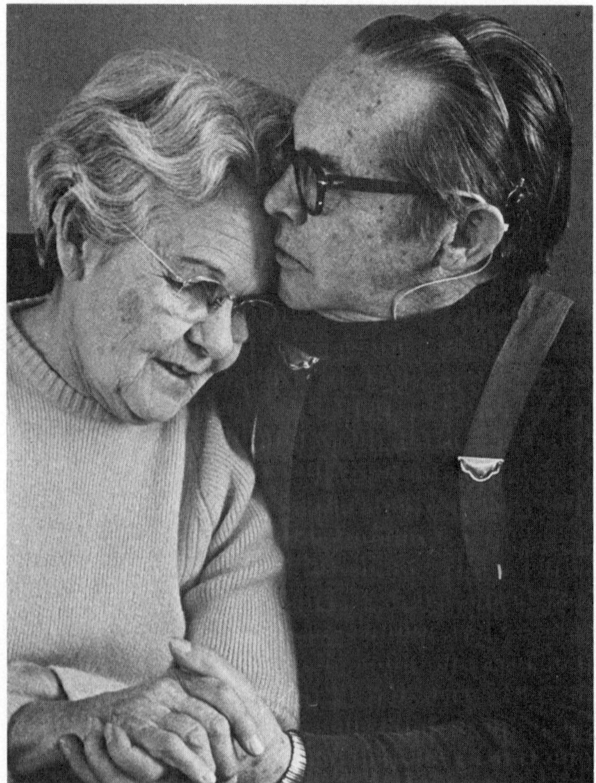

Extramarital intercourse—intercourse between a married person and someone other than the spouse—often disrupts marriages and other social relationships. Some of the complications include jealousy, conflicting emotional and social allegiances, neglect of duties, and disputed paternity. Consequently, most societies either prohibit extramarital intercourse or permit it only under well-defined circumstances. It may be allowed only with specified persons, only during certain festivities, only with the permission of the spouse, or only in extenuating circumstances. Despite social disapproval and illegality, at least one-half of all American husbands and one-third of all American wives engage in extramarital intercourse at some time.

Postmarital intercourse—occurring after a marriage has terminated but before a new one has begun—has received little attention from researchers of human behavior. Restrictions tend to be minimal. Even societies opposed to premarital and extramarital intercourse realize that persons accustomed to regular intercourse in marriage can hardly be expected to refrain after their marital status changes. This realization is well founded; the great majority of widowed or divorced persons continue to have intercourse when a partner is available.

OTHER PARTNER PREFERENCES

Homosexuality

Homosexuality is a sexual or emotional preference for persons of one's own sex. Few areas of human behavior have generated more theories or provoked more controversy than has this topic.

A number of ancient societies sanctioned homosexual behavior and in several cases made it into an established practice. This is also true of various contemporary societies throughout the world. A comprehensive study conducted some twenty years ago by anthropologist Clellan Ford and psychologist Frank Beach revealed that forty-nine of seventy-six preliterate societies either accept or actually prescribe homosexual activity.

The sexual patterns of these cultures tend to support the notion, prevalent among social scientists, that human sexual behavior has less to do with the dictates of biology than with those of society. In the United States, as in much of Western culture, society dictates an exclusively heterosexual life style. Although heterosexual and homosexual tendencies are thought to exist to some extent in every person, our society does not encourage the expression of both. As a result, most Americans apparently learn to repress the homosexual component of their nature.

No one knows for certain what factors are responsible for inducing a pattern of predominantly homosexual behavior. Some people may have a genetic predisposition toward homosexuality. Like other behavior, it is also probably largely learned. One contributing factor may be failure to identify with a parent of the same sex. Another possible factor is erotic gratification derived from self-admiration, which may lead one, through the process of projection to seek in members of the same sex an idealized image of oneself. The widely held view that seduction of a young person by a homosexual leads to later homosexual behavior has generally been contradicted by the available evidence.

Researchers do agree that incidental, temporary homosexual activity, especially during adolescent experimentation, is rather common. About one-third of the American males surveyed in 1948 and one-fifth of the females surveyed in 1952 by Alfred Kinsey reported such experiences, and a 1970 questionnaire answered by readers of *Psychology Today* revealed similar percentages.

Extensive homosexual behavior, on the other hand, is a deviation from the statistical norm. But behavior of this sort is not in itself proof of emotional or mental illness. Emotional disorders of homosexuals may stem largely from adverse self-definitions imposed on them by society, for as psychiatrist Robert E. Gould points out, "Nothing is more likely to make you sick than being constantly told that you are sick." The image of the homosexual as a sick person has begun to change. In 1973, the American Psychiatric Association removed homosexuality from its catalogue of mental illnesses.

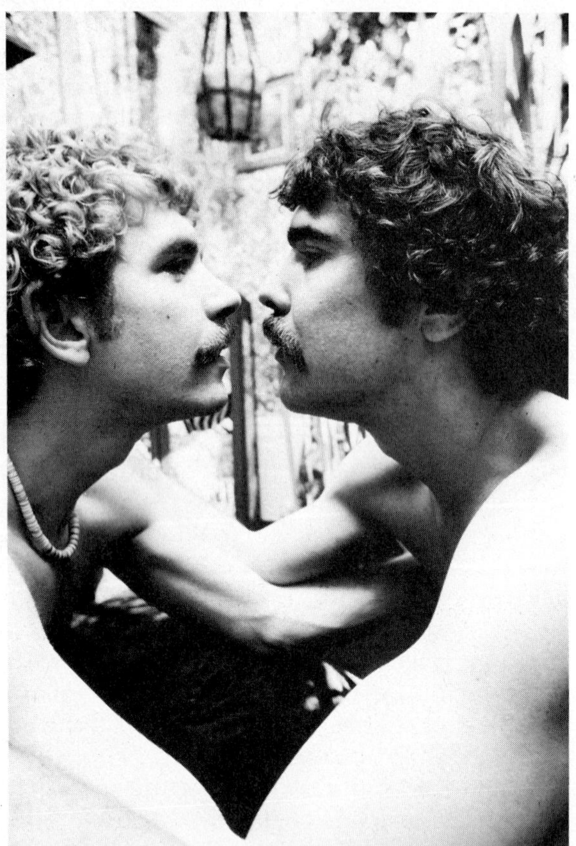

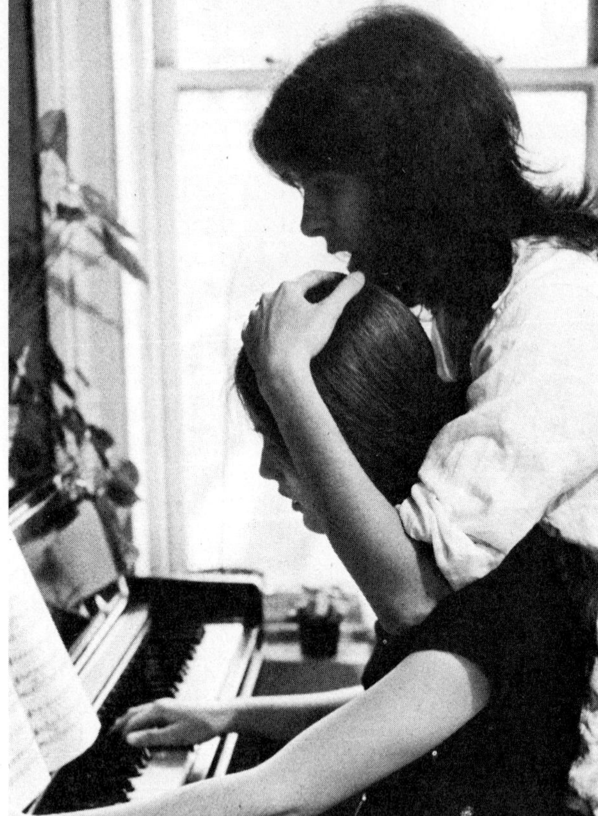

Figure 3.5 Research shows that homosexuals can lead lives that are as full and healthy as those of heterosexuals.

In 1978, Alan Bell and Martin Weinberg of the Institute for Sex Research at Indiana University published in their book, *Homosexualities,* the results of the most complete study to date of the life styles of American homosexuals. Their ten-year study involved lengthy interviews with nearly 1,000 homosexuals in the San Francisco Bay area. Their research revealed the wide diversity of life styles among homosexuals and also refuted some stereotypes about them.

Most of the male homosexuals were relatively covert about their preferences; their families, employers, colleagues at work, and heterosexual friends tended not to know that they were homosexuals. Their work histories were fully as stable as those of heterosexual men, and they tended to have more good, close friends. As with heterosexuals, the most common incidence of sexual activity was two or three times a week. Virtually all of them had had at least one affair with another man, in which the two lived together, often for several years, and felt that they were in love. Yet most "cruised" for sexual partners and reported that they had had hundreds of sexual partners, many of them strangers, in the course of their lives. They tended to have sex with these partners in the privacy of their own homes. Most had never had sex with prostitutes or minors.

Most of the lesbians, by contrast, reported fewer than ten partners in their life, almost all of whom they knew well and had sex with more than once. Nearly half lived with their current partner, combining incomes and remaining fairly faithful.

"It would appear," Bell and Weinberg concluded, "that homosexual adults who have come to terms with their homosexuality, who do not regret their sexual orientation, and who can function effectively sexually and socially, are no more distressed psychologically than are heterosexual men and women. . . . Homosexuality is not necessarily related to pathology."

Bisexuality

Researchers estimate that in the United States perhaps 25 percent of men and about half that many women are bisexual in the sense that they are attracted to and have engaged in sexual activity to the point of orgasm with both men and women at some point during their lives. In the Bell and Weinberg studies, more than a third of the lesbian women and about a fifth of the homosexual men had been married, and most of them—married or not—had experienced heterosexual intercourse.

Some people see such bisexual behavior as a threat to society, a spreading "polymorphous perversity" that will mix and weaken the physical and emotional qualities by which one sex has traditionally been distinguished from the other. Others see it as a natural and welcome outcome of relaxing our cultural constraints.

THE PHYSIOLOGY OF SEXUAL RESPONSE

Until a few years ago, little more could be said about human sexual behavior other than general statements of frequency. The research of William Masters and Virginia Johnson, at their institute in St. Louis, produced much more specific descriptions of typical physiological and behavioral processes involved in sexual responsiveness.

Because Masters and Johnson were the first to study genital physiological changes during sexual stimulation, they had to develop some new methods and equipment, particularly for examining the female response, which is difficult to observe because most of it occurs internally. They devised techniques to measure anatomical changes during different phases of stimulation, intrauterine electrodes to measure uterine contractions, electrocardiograph tracings to monitor rate and level of cardiac contractions, and equipment to measure respiration and blood pressure. They collected data during masturbation as well as during natural and artificial coitus. Plastic penises used for artificial coitus allowed direct observation and photography of the vagina's physiological responses.

The reaction patterns of both female and male were found to be essentially independent of the means of stimulation used. The sexual response cycles of both women and men apparently occur in four phases: the excitement phase, the plateau phase, the orgasmic phase, and the resolution phase. The following descriptions represent a composite of individual cycles as identified by Masters and Johnson. Individual variations are marked and usually involve duration, rather than intensity, of the response. The initial and final phases are significantly longer than the middle two.

The Female Cycle

First, it is necessary to discuss woman's physiology. The major female reproductive organs are described in Chapter 4. Here, the focus will be on the vagina and the external structures bordering it (see Figure 3.6).

The *vagina* is a responsive muscular organ, equipped to receive and clasp the male organ during intercourse. Ordinarily, the vagina is shaped like a flattened tube of toothpaste, about four inches long. It is lined with a moist, wrinkled, elastic, skinlike mucous membrane. At the inner end of the vagina lies a firm, smooth knob, the *cervix.* Encircling the vagina are the *pubococcygeous muscles,* which contract with the anal and urethral sphincters. Greater control of them can be developed by voluntary contractions that concentrate on lifting these sphincters into the abdomen. Not only does control of the contraction and relaxation of these muscles increase friction during intercourse, but maintaining the tone of these muscles is believed to reduce pelvic difficulties later in life.

In virginal females, the entrance to the vagina is often narrowed by a circular fold of tissue, much like the shutter of a camera, called

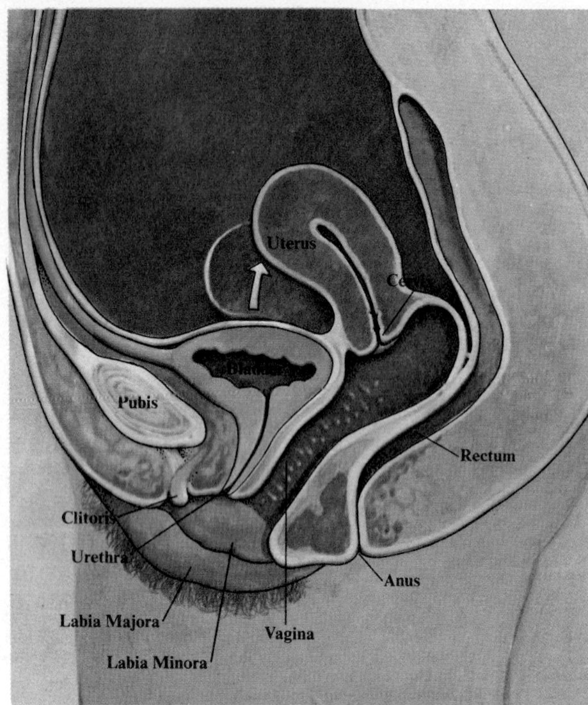

Figure 3.6 Female reproductive organs.

the *hymen.* The hymen usually has a central opening large enough to admit an examining finger or menstrual tampon. Frequently, physical activity or time obliterates the hymen, even when intercourse has not occurred. During first intercourse, it usually stretches or even tears a little with no problem. Only occasionally will the hymen be thick or tough enough to require a doctor's help in stretching it sufficiently to accommodate a penis.

Covering the vaginal opening are two soft, sensitive, wrinkled flaps of skin called *labia minora,* or smaller lips. Covering them are two broad, less sensitive, hair-covered folds of skin called *labia majora.* Just above the vaginal opening, between the labia, lies the urethra, the opening from the urinary bladder. Half an inch or more above the urethra lies a sensitive organ the size of a pea, the *clitoris.* The clitoris is usually partly hooded by a flap of less sensitive skin, the *prepuce,* formed where the labia minora join together in an arch. The clitoris, like its male counterpart, the penis, is an erectile organ comprising a head *(clitoral glans)* and a stalk *(clitoral shaft).* Lubricating glands border the vaginal and urethral openings. Most of the fluid that appears at the vaginal opening as the result of sexual stimulation, whether that stimulation is physical or emotional, comes from the vagina itself. With the stirring of sexual feelings, the vagina of a healthy woman begins to "sweat." This phenomenon is not yet understood.

All the external sexual organs participate in female sexual response. For most women the clitoris is a sort of "message center" that receives and distributes sexual sensations. Unlike the penis, the clitoris has no other apparent function. But the most important organ of all in sexual response is the brain, which is the ultimate control center that directs the human sexual response. The stages of that response are the following.

Excitement Phase Many parts of the body in addition to the genitals respond to sexual stimulation. *Myotonia,* an increase in muscular tension, is a generalized sexual response involving both voluntary and involuntary muscles. Coital position has a role in determining which muscle groups show this reaction during a particular sexual response cycle. Heart-rate and blood-pressure increases begin in the excitement phase, and blood accumulates in certain blood vessels, resulting in a phenomenon known as *vasocongestion.*

Vasocongestion is a primary response to sexual stimulation and occurs in a number of body parts, including the labia minora and the clitoris. It is instrumental in the development of the *sex flush,* which appears late in this phase. The sex flush is a superficial vasocongestive reaction that causes a temporary rash to spread from the breasts over the lower abdomen and shoulders as sexual tension increases. Vasocongestion is also responsible for other changes during this initial phase. Some internal portions of the vagina swell. The breasts may show nipple erection, a slight increase in size, or both. Expansion or swelling of the clitoral glans always accompanies the buildup of sexual tension, although it is not always observable.

Plateau Phase If sexual stimulation persists, myotonia and vasocongestion increase, the sex flush spreads, and the breasts continue to expand. The clitoral glans and shaft withdraw. The more effective the stimulation, the more marked this withdrawal is.

The expansion that affected the inner two-thirds of the vagina during the excitement phase now extends to the outer third. Both the outer third of the vagina and the labia minora are involved in a major vasocongestive reaction. Because these anatomical parts respond during orgasm, they are called the *orgasmic platform.*

Although the uterus shows partial elevation during the excitement phase, it now attains complete elevation and moves backward toward the spine. It remains in that position until the onset of the resolution phase. As sexual tension increases and orgasm becomes imminent, further increases in respiration, heartbeat, and blood pressure appear.

Orgasmic Phase Immediately before orgasm, the physiological responses reach their most intense level. Vasocongestion is widespread. The clitoris is completely withdrawn. The vagina is lubricated and extended, with the orgasmic platform well developed. The uterus is elevated. Sex flushing and breast responses, if present, are complete. Only myotonic tension will become even more intense with orgasm.

Contractions in certain organs signal the physiological onset of orgasm. The orgasmic platform is first. It displays a long contraction, lasting from two to four seconds, and then a series of shorter contractions less than a second apart. The factors that initiate this response may be neural, hormonal, muscular, or some combination of these. The platform contractions are accompanied by uterine contractions of a less definite pattern and often by contractions of the external anal sphincter. The number of these contractions is usually determined by the intensity of a particular orgasmic response. Stronger responses trigger more contractions. As indicated in Figure 3.7, unlike most men, many women have the ability to experience multiple orgasms in a relatively short period of time.

It had long been believed that orgasms resulting from vaginal stimulation (as in intercourse) were physiologically distinct from those resulting from clitoral stimulation alone (as in masturbation or manual stimulation by a partner). Masters and Johnson's data refute this view; they reveal that the orgasmic response to any stimulation is essentially the same.

This does not mean, however, that the psychological responses from the different forms

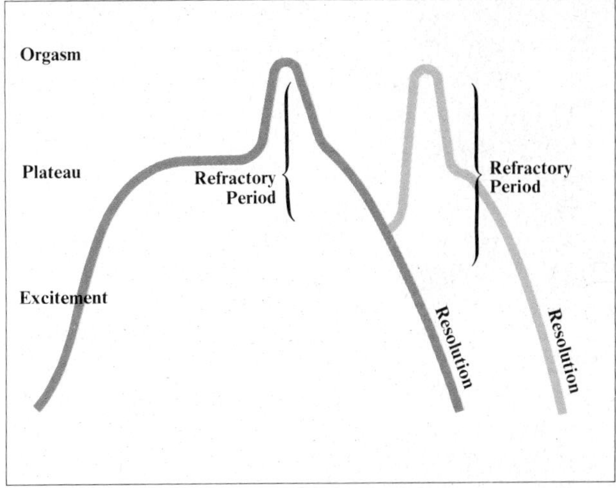

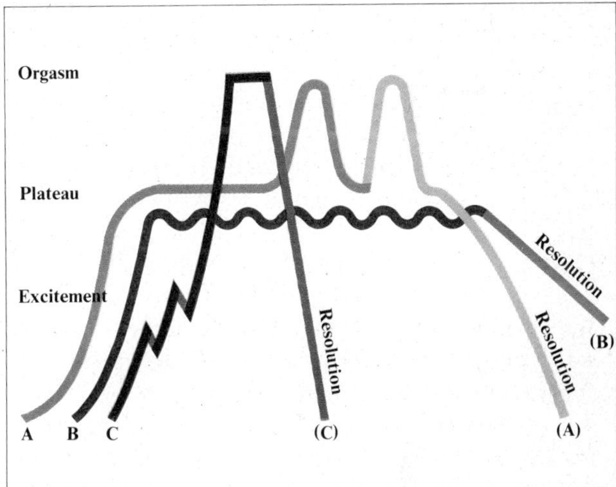

Figure 3.7 Masters and Johnson's phase graphs. *(Top)* The man's rise in sexual tension is shown diagrammatically. Once orgasm is achieved, there is a refractory period before he can have another orgasm. *(Bottom)* A woman can experience one orgasm and soon after experience another (line A). If she fails to experience orgasm, however, her resolution phase is longer (line B). Line C shows a rare kind of prolonged orgasmic experience known as *status orgasmus.*

of stimulation are indistinguishable. Sexually experienced individuals know that the psychological effects of an orgasm are a function of the context or setting in which it occurs. The context of orgasm is just beginning to be studied by sexologists. More knowledge about the effects of the setting of sexual behavior is essential to understanding the interaction between physiological and psychological factors.

Resolution Phase This phase is characterized by a return to the normal, or precoital, condition. The return is fairly rapid if orgasm has occurred. The average time is between five and ten minutes. Myotonia, sex flush, and the orgasmic platform subside quickly. The clitoris regains its normal size and position. Changes resulting from vasocongestion disappear throughout the body. This process is much slower if plateau levels of tension were reached but orgasm did not occur. Complete resolution does not occur between cycles if more than one orgasm is attained over a relatively short period.

Again, it should be stressed that the cycle described here is what Masters and Johnson see as an average cycle. Many elements may be different or missing in any particular normal cycle, but this composite picture is based on the more than 10,000 cycles they observed.

One principal finding of these studies is the great extent to which a woman's response to sexual stimulation involves her entire body. Myotonia, vasocongestion, and other specific reactions have been observed in many parts of the body. Temporary loss of sharpness of vision also often accompanies orgasm, as does perspiration.

The newly found properties of the clitoris are important to understand. The clitoris is the focal point of sensual response in the woman's pelvic area. For some women direct stimulation of the clitoris is not necessary for orgasm; they achieve full response through secondary stimulation of other parts, such as the vagina and vulva. For most women, however, direct but not constant stimulation of the clitoris is necessary for full arousal and response, but the most effective stimulation varies from woman to woman. Some women find direct touching of the clitoris irritating rather than stimulating and prefer more overall contact in the clitoral area. Others respond well to contact between the clitoris and the shaft of the penis during coitus, but many more women do not respond fully to this stimulation and require more direct stimulation of the clitoris. Each woman needs to discover which kind of stimulation works best for her and either provide it for herself during sexual activity or clearly communicate her specific needs to her partner.

The Male Cycle

A notable finding of the Masters and Johnson studies was the existence of numerous similarities between male and female sexual response patterns. The similarities are more pronounced than the differences.

Excitement Phase Many parts of the male body respond to sexual stimulation. Breast enlargement is not part of the male cycle, although the nipples may become erect. When nipple erection does occur, it usually begins late in this phase. Other extragenital responses include increased heart rate and blood pressure. Elevated tension (myotonia) in both voluntary and involuntary muscles appears early in this phase.

Early genital reactions are most visible. The penis becomes erect because of massive vasocongestion in three spongy chambers that run the length of the organ. Some myotonia is also involved. Unlike female vasocongestion, mainly arterial blood collects in the penis. Vasocongestion and thickening of the scrotal skin contribute to the elevation of the scrotal sac. Elevation of the testicles, on the other hand, results from a shortening of the spermatic cord by an involuntary contraction of the muscles near the cord. This response begins in the excitement phase but is not completed until the plateau phase.

In some men, a clear lubricating fluid may appear in droplets at the urethral opening during any phase before orgasm. This fluid often contains thousands of viable spermatozoa perfectly capable of causing conception, which is why withdrawal of the penis before ejaculation is one of the least reliable means of contraception.

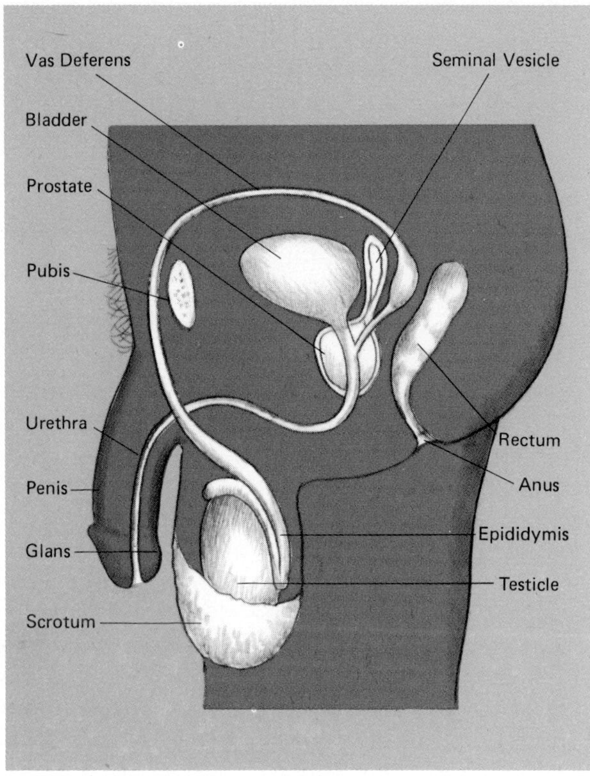

Figure 3.8 Male reproductive organs.

Plateau Phase The penis, which becomes fully erect during excitement, shows a slight increase in circumference during this second phase. This late development is restricted to its head, or *glans penis.* As the testicles rise, an increase in their size becomes apparent. Testes show about a 50 percent size increase, and if plateau levels of sexual tension continue without orgasm, an increase of up to 100 percent may occur. Like penile erection, continued testicular size increase is a vasocongestive response.

The approach of orgasm is occasionally accompanied by a sex flush similar to that in women. In men, it usually covers the chest, neck, face, and forehead, and sometimes the shoulders and thighs. Impending ejaculation is also signaled by increased heart rate, breathing rate, blood pressure, and myotonia.

Orgasmic Phase Although ejaculation and orgasm are usually considered parts of a single occurrence, they are separable. Orgasm without ejaculation—that is, without the expulsion of seminal fluids—can occur and is experienced frequently by boys before puberty.

With the exception of fluid discharge, the physiological responses that form the basis for the male and female experience of orgasm are quite similar. Both involve the loss of general muscular control as well as massive contractions in the genital area, including the anal sphincter. The contractions of the orgasmic platform in the female and of the penile urethra in the male occur at intervals of 0.8 seconds during the first part of the orgasmic experience. Heart rate, breathing, and blood pressure reach their highest levels during orgasm in both sexes.

The contractions of reproductive accessory organs (prostate, seminal vesicles, ejaculatory duct) and the resulting emission of semen distinguish the male from the female response. The total body response described for women also occurs in men, with myotonia and vasocongestion spreading throughout the body. Just as women can voluntarily contract certain muscles to enhance sexual enjoyment, some men learn to heighten the intensity of orgasm by voluntarily contracting the muscles of the buttocks, abdomen, and anus.

Resolution Phase Following orgasm, the return to the unstimulated state is usually quite rapid. The sex flush fades, and perspiration sometimes appears. *Detumescence* (loss of swelling) of the penis accompanies the end of vasocongestion, as does the descent of the testes into the relaxed scrotum. A general decrease of muscle tension then appears, usually no more than five minutes after the beginning of this phase. Nipples that were erect in the excitement phase display no additional reactions during plateau or orgasmic phases, but may require an hour to return to normal.

Myths about the male sexual response are even more numerous than those about the female response, perhaps because the male's external genitals make his reactions more obvious and more a topic of discussion than the invisible and little-known female response. Part of Masters and Johnson's research was an investigation of the validity of many beliefs about the male response.

Contrary to popular belief, *circumcision* (the surgical removal of the foreskin from the head of the penis) has no apparent influence on sexual behavior. A comparison of circumcised and uncircumcised men showed no differences in ejaculatory control, tendency toward *impotence* (difficulty in reaching erection), or sensitivity of the penis. Another fallacy was uncovered when a study of men of all ages showed that, although some difficulty in achieving erection may appear with age, impotence is in no sense an inevitable result of aging. Furthermore, this type of impotence is a reversible condition.

It has long been believed that the larger a man's penis, the better his sexual performance and the greater his partner's satisfaction. Masters and Johnson's data revealed no such correlations. Their study also failed to support the belief that a large penis expands more than a small one when erect. The small penis usually doubles its length during erection; the large one increases to one and a half times its length, so that the lengths are more comparable after erection. Therefore, penis size is not usually a significant factor in either the man's or the woman's sexual response, particularly because the vagina can accommodate a penis of any size.

SEXUAL PROBLEMS

There are times when a person cannot be aroused or satisfied sexually. This happens to everyone on occasion. However, for some individuals, it is a recurring experience that can become very upsetting. Any problem that prevents a person from engaging in sexual relations or from reaching orgasm during sex is known as a *sexual dysfunction.* It is important to recognize that this term applies only to problems in sexual response, not to sexual preferences.

Sexual Dysfunction in Men and Women

In everyday conversation, the term *impotence* is often used to describe all forms of male sexual dysfunction. Similarly, the term *frigidity* is applied to all types of female sexual problems. As popularly used, neither term tells precisely what the problem is, and they incorrectly suggest a permanent rejection of sexuality. Furthermore, these terms also incorrectly imply that the problem is either exclusively that of the male or the female. In most cases, however, sexual dysfunction involves both the male and the female, and resolution of the problem requires the loving cooperation of both partners. One of the goals of sex researchers is to replace these overgeneralized, pejorative labels with more precise definitions of specific dysfunctions.

Psychologists reserve the term *impotence* for a specific dysfunction: a man's inability to achieve or maintain an erection long enough to reach orgasm with a partner. Some men have never been able to achieve or maintain an erection (a rare condition known as *primary impotence*). Generally, though, impotent men have been aroused to orgasm with a partner in the past, but are now unable to achieve or maintain an erection in some or all sexual situations. This is called *secondary impotence.* For other men, arousal is not the problem; they may achieve an erection easily, but ejaculate before they or their partners would like. This is called *premature ejaculation,* which appears to be the most common complaint among male college students. Still other men can achieve and maintain an erection, but are unable to ejaculate during sex with a partner—a problem Masters and Johnson labeled *nonemissive erection.* At one time or another, most males experience secondary impotence, premature ejaculation, and nonemissive erection. These conditions should be considered dysfunctional only when they are extremely persistent and upsetting to the individual.

A very few women suffer from *vaginismus,* involuntary muscle spasms that cause the vagina to shut tightly, making penetration by the penis impossible or painful. Other women are able to engage in, and often enjoy, sexual intercourse, but do not experience orgasm. The term *primary orgasmic dysfunction* is used for women who have never experienced an orgasm through any means. The term *secondary* (or *situational*) *orgasmic dysfunction* is used for women who experience orgasms sometimes, with certain kinds of stimulation (such as masturbation), but not whenever they would like. This is a common complaint among female college students. As with most of the male problems, difficulties women may have in ex-

FOCUS

Love and Sex

It is a common assumption that sexual attraction between two people means that they love one another. *Not true,* stresses psychologist Erich Fromm. *Any* strong emotion—fear of loneliness, vanity, the wish to conquer or submit, *or* love—can blend with and stimulate sexual desire. But, Fromm warns, only if the two partners love one another will the union that sex seems to create be more than a fleeting illusion.

William H. Masters and Virginia Johnson deal with this issue in their book *The Pleasure Bond: A New Look at Sexuality and Commitment.* They write:

> The ability of a man and woman to become sexually committed stands or falls primarily on their willingness to give and receive pleasure in all its forms. . . . It is the willingness that flows from wishing or wanting something, of caring for someone, when the mind serves only as a catalyst and the body asserts itself in ways that the mind may not have anticipated.

To illustrate their point, they describe a young woman whose husband gave her all the material possessions she wanted. But he did not give her a loving, committed relationship or the sexual attention she craved. In fact, he often seemed totally oblivious of her presence.

After six years of trying unsuccessfully to encourage her husband to be more responsive to her needs, she realized that they were shut off from one another and that she could never trust him with her sexual or emotional well-being. She decided to look outside her marriage for a sexual partner.

She appeared to have little in common with the lover she chose—a young baker who had just come to the United States. But their differences seemed small when they were together. Their relationship was very satisfying sexually, but it was also warm and secure emotionally.

Finding herself honestly recognized and appreciated as an individual, she began to open up in a way she had never done before. Even though no vows were made, she felt she could trust her lover to be there when she needed him and to care about her welfare as much as his own. With these feelings came a depth of sexual response she had never dreamed possible. She experienced sensations in parts of her body she hadn't even known were there. In her commitment—her love—she found that her sexual identity and her personality flowered. Friends who were unaware of her new relationship commented on how obviously happy she had become.

When the woman finally left her husband to live with her lover, she thought she was making a new commitment. But, Masters and Johnson point out, her commitment had been developing along with her new-found intimacy. She had found not only physical pleasure, but mutual concern and tenderness.

periencing orgasm may be viewed as normal human variations and are not necessarily considered dysfunctional.

Psychiatrist and sex therapist Helen Singer Kaplan points out that the orgasmic reflex, just like other body reflexes, has different thresholds in different people. There are women with high thresholds who require more stimulation than others; this is a problem only if the woman herself is upset about it, does not make her needs known to her partner, or if her partner does not attempt to identify her needs.

It is not clear why some people respond freely to sexual stimulation while others do not. The research of Masters and Johnson has revealed that only rarely do sexual problems have a physiological basis. The reasons some people are unable to feel sexual pleasure are usually psychological. Some of these psychological factors involve conflicts within the individual. Therapists find that many people who seek help for sexual problems were brought up with rigid religious or moral rules concerning sex. Intellectually, they may reject the idea that sex is wrong, but emotionally, they do not. Other psychological problems may stem from having had one's anatomy "innocently" ridiculed during childhood or from having suffered outright sexual abuse. Fear of failure can also cause sexual dysfunction. After one disappointing sexual experience, a person may begin to worry about his or her sexual adequacy. The next time, this anxiety can interfere with the person's free response—thereby intensifying the self-doubt. Fear of failure can thus sometimes become a self-fulfilling prophecy. Other psychological factors involve conflicts in the relationship between the two sexual partners. And sometimes sexual problems can be due to lack of communication between partners.

Sex Therapy

During the 1970s, sex researchers evolved a number of different ways of treating people with sexual problems. In Masters and Johnson's original program, a couple had to travel to their treatment center in St. Louis and live in a nearby motel, while going through an intensive (and expensive), highly structured two-week program of daily sessions with two therapists, one a man, the other a woman, and at least one of them a physician.

Since then, other therapists have devised more flexible approaches. Sometimes a couple will visit a sex clinic once a week, say, while working on the problem. Whatever the approach, nearly all forms of sex therapy are based on seven basic principles:

1. Sexual dysfunction is a problem that concerns both partners even if only one partner has a complaint. Sex therapists usually insist upon treating both partners together.
2. Some people with sexual problems are misinformed about sex. Sex therapy includes education about sexual anatomy, function, response, and techniques.
3. Negative attitudes about sex, however deeply buried, are almost always part of the problem. Sex therapy often includes some form of psychotherapy aimed at overcoming these negative attitudes.
4. Anxiety is also often part of the problem. Some people are so self-conscious and afraid of failure that they take a "spectator" role while they engage in sex, evaluating their performance rather than enjoying themselves spontaneously. Therapy aims to reduce anxiety and make sex a pleasure, not a test of skill.
5. Sexual interaction will not improve without communication between partners. Therapy encourages couples to express their feelings and desires openly.
6. Sex takes place within the context of a couple's entire relationship. Tensions caused by disagreements over sex roles, emotional needs, even money, can interfere with sexual responsiveness. Therapy focuses on the relationship rather than on the individual with the dysfunction.
7. Sex therapists prescribe changes in sexual behavior. At the beginning of therapy, they often tell couples to forget about intercourse completely for a while and, instead, simply "pleasure" each other by caressing without touching the genitals. For specific sexual dysfunctions, such as premature ejaculation or vaginismus, they may assign specific sexual exercises.

The success rate of such sexual therapy is high. Kaplan claims that 98 to 100 percent of men can overcome premature ejaculation within a few weeks, and that about 80 percent of people with other dysfunctions can be helped.

When a "Problem" Is Not a Problem

People inevitably compare their own sexual experiences with those they encounter in popular fiction or other media. As a result, many men and women pick up fallacious ideas about sexuality. Some of the most common fallacies are that a man should be able to achieve an erection and maintain it as long as he likes without ejaculating; that a woman should always have orgasm during coitus; that all women should have multiple orgasms at least some of the time; that neither a man nor a woman can be sexually satisfied without orgasm; that all satisfactory sexual encounters have intercourse and orgasm as *the* goal; that touching, holding, and kissing should always only be foreplay for intercourse or orgasm; that sexual arousal without orgasm is somehow "unhealthy," physically or emotionally; that there is something wrong with people who find such practices as fellatio or cunnilingus objectionable or who are aroused by such stimuli as fur coats or the aroma of leather.

Such fallacies may themselves cause problems, until the person learns that he or she is still the best judge of his or her own sexual experience. For instance, simply touching, holding, and kissing may be quite satisfying without any other sexual activity. Orgasm need not be *the* goal of sexual arousal; the findings

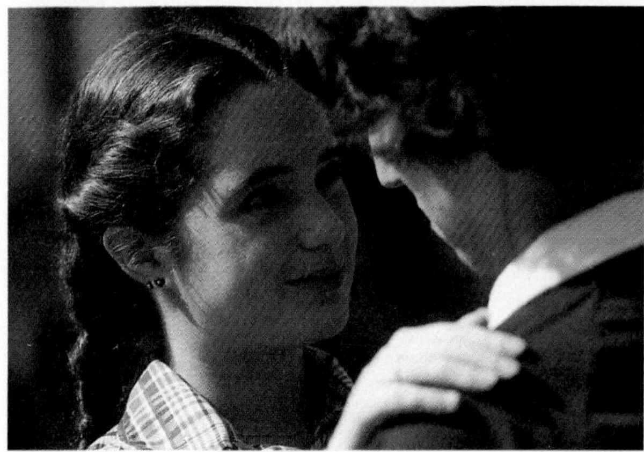

Figure 3.9 Between loving partners, sex is a means of open and honest communication.

of modern sex research should lay to rest this "touchdown" mentality. And it is perfectly normal for some people to dislike some practices or stimuli that others enjoy.

Sexual sharing can be considered a celebration of a relationship, and ultimately it is the relationship that is most important. Partners need to be sensitive to each other's desires and preferences in sexual matters as well as in other aspects of their relationship.

THE CONTINUING EVOLUTION OF SEXUALITY

Among the many reasons this is an exciting time to be alive is the unlocking of human sexual potential now taking place. As traditional, limiting stereotypes of gender roles dissolve, men and women are freer than ever before to develop fully as both human beings and sexual beings. This easing of traditional sex roles is also freeing men and women to relate to each other in deeper and more equal ways. Effective contraceptives have all but eliminated the fear of pregnancy and thus allow men and women to be more spontaneous in their lovemaking.

Research on sexual response has provided new information as a basis both for enhancing sexual pleasure and for resolving sexual problems. People are becoming more and more aware of the variety of sexual possibilities and are discovering, through their own experimentation and communication, new levels of relationship and meaning.

The continual increase in knowledge and changing attitudes toward human sexuality promise to enhance the expression of human sexuality even further. Human beings are sexual from conception to death, and, sexual behavior serves throughout life as both a means to and an expression of health.

SUMMARY

1. A person's biological sex results from a combination of genetic and hormonal influences that operate before birth. One's gender identity develops as a result of social and cultural conditioning that begins at birth.
2. The so-called sexual revolution is better termed the gender revolution. Today both men and women are more free to do and be whatever feels comfortable for them.
3. There are many options of sexual behavior: masturbation, petting, cunnilingus, fellatio, and intercourse. Other partner preferences besides heterosexuality include homosexuality and bisexuality.
4. In both men and women, the physiological response to sexual stimulation seems to occur in four phases: excitement, plateau, orgasmic, and resolution. During excitement in both sexes, heart rate and blood pressure increase, and myotonia and vasocongestion occur.
5. In women, the clitoris is the focal point of sexual response. Vasocongestion causes it to swell, the breasts to expand, and the nipples to become erect. During orgasm, the orgasmic platform and uterus contract.
6. In men, vasocongestion causes the penis to become erect. During orgasm, the genital organs contract, and ejaculation occurs.
7. In both men and women, the most important organ in sexual response is the brain.
8. Male sexual dysfunctions include primary impotence, secondary impotence, premature ejaculation, and nonemissive erection. Female dysfunctions include vaginismus, primary orgasmic dysfunction, and secondary (or situational) dysfunction.
9. Such dysfunctions are more likely to have psychological than physiological causes. Modern sex therapy, in which both partners are usually treated together, is able to overcome a high percentage of these problems.

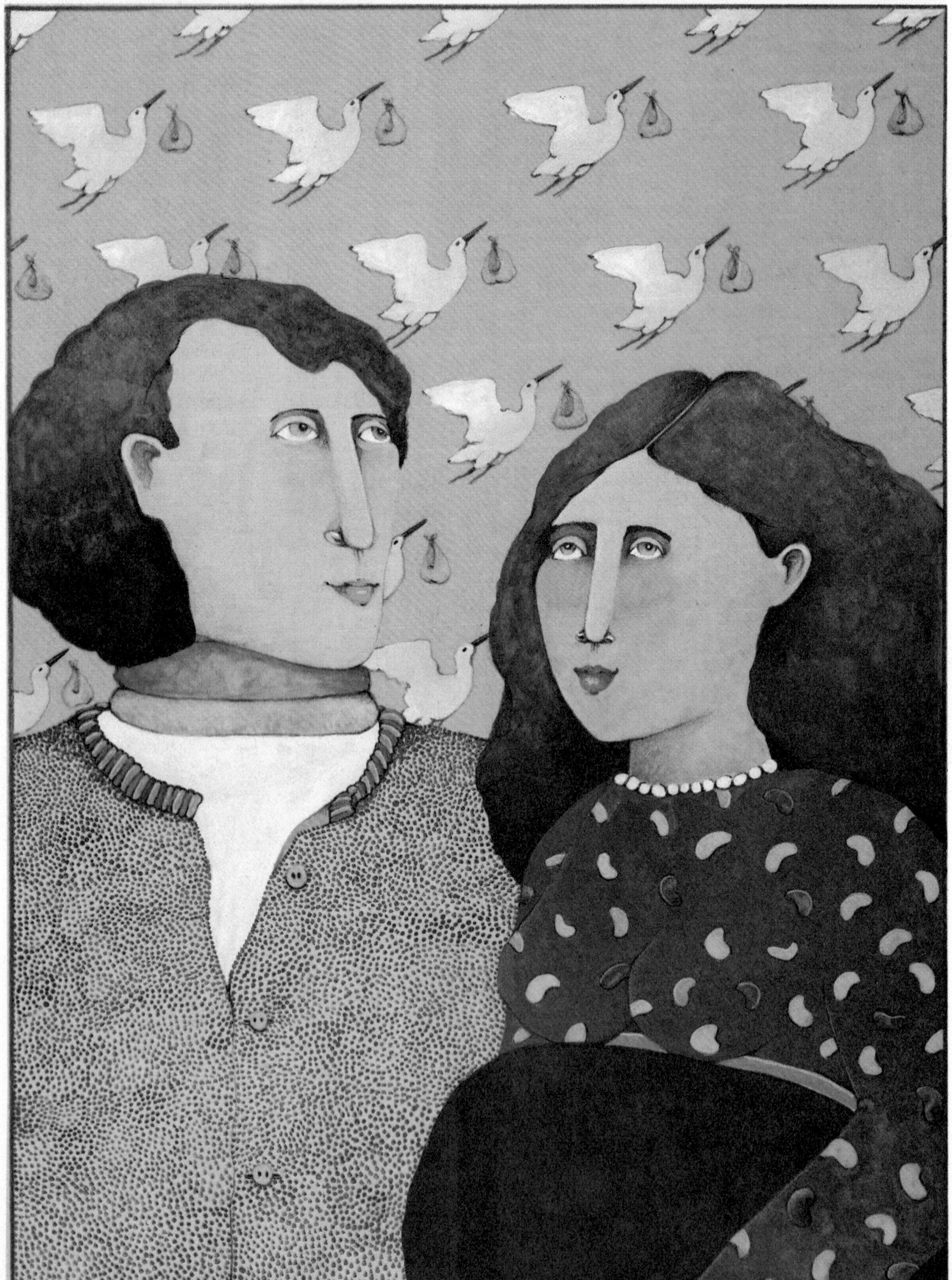

Dagmar Frinta

II THE LIFE CYCLE

Sexual maturity brings with it the chance to produce a new human being. Chapter 4 discusses this possibility in an extensive look at the process of reproduction—conception, pregnancy, birth, and congenital and hereditary defects.

Many couples today want to have small families, and a growing number do not want children at all. We now have an array of relatively safe and effective methods of birth control that make these options viable. These techniques are the subject of Chapter 5.

Although we discuss some alternative life styles that have become more commonplace and widely accepted, marriage and parenthood are still the rule rather than the exception. Why do people marry? What's expected in a marriage? What makes a marriage work? What are the "right" reasons to have children? How can parents help a child grow into a happy, healthy adult? Questions such as these are addressed in Chapter 6.

An increasing percentage of our population is over age sixty-five, and old people are becoming a major force in our society. And, partly because of the "graying" of America, death—the culmination of the life cycle—is no longer the taboo subject it once was. In Chapter 7, then, we turn to the processes of aging and facing death and the changes they can bring to physical and mental health.

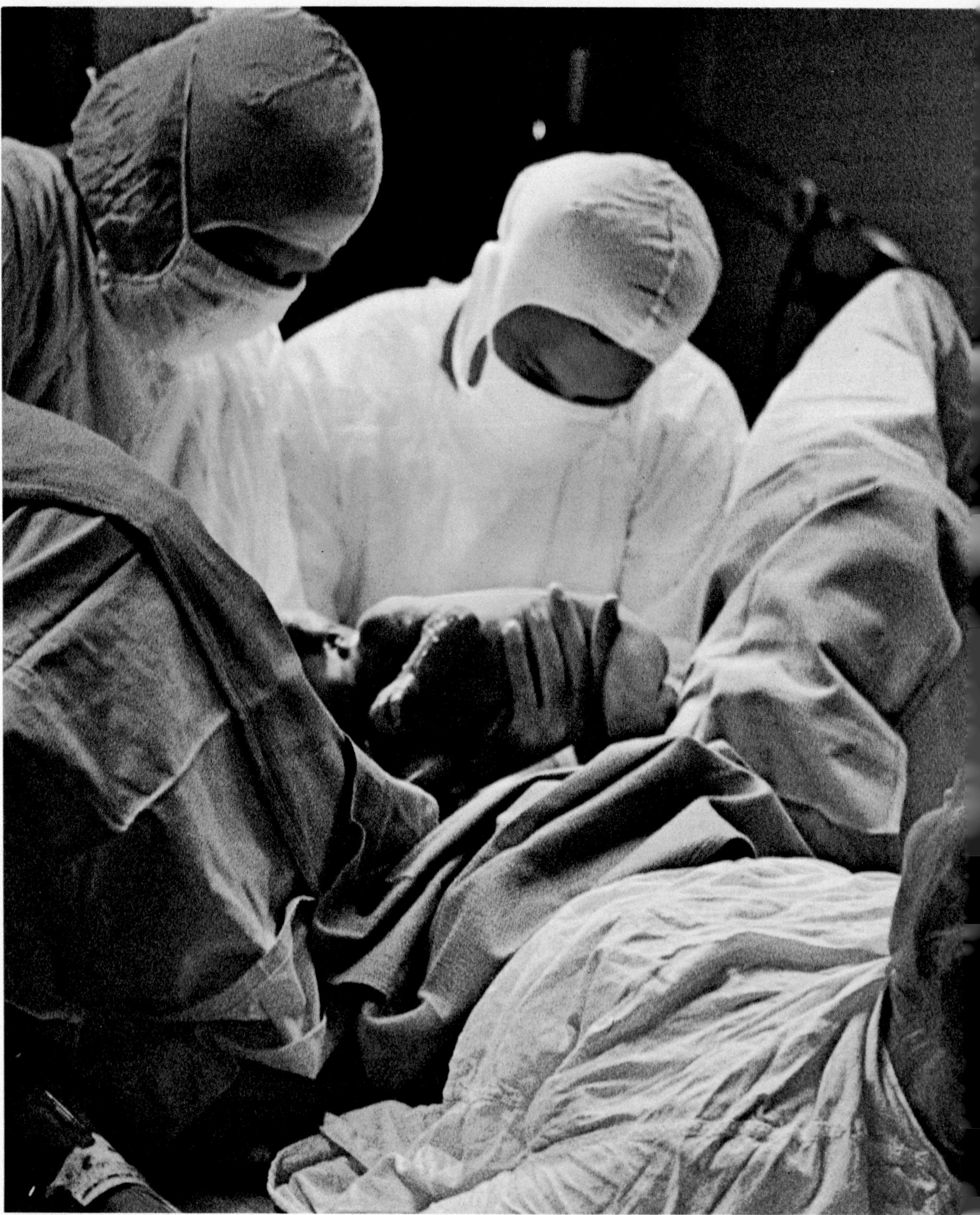

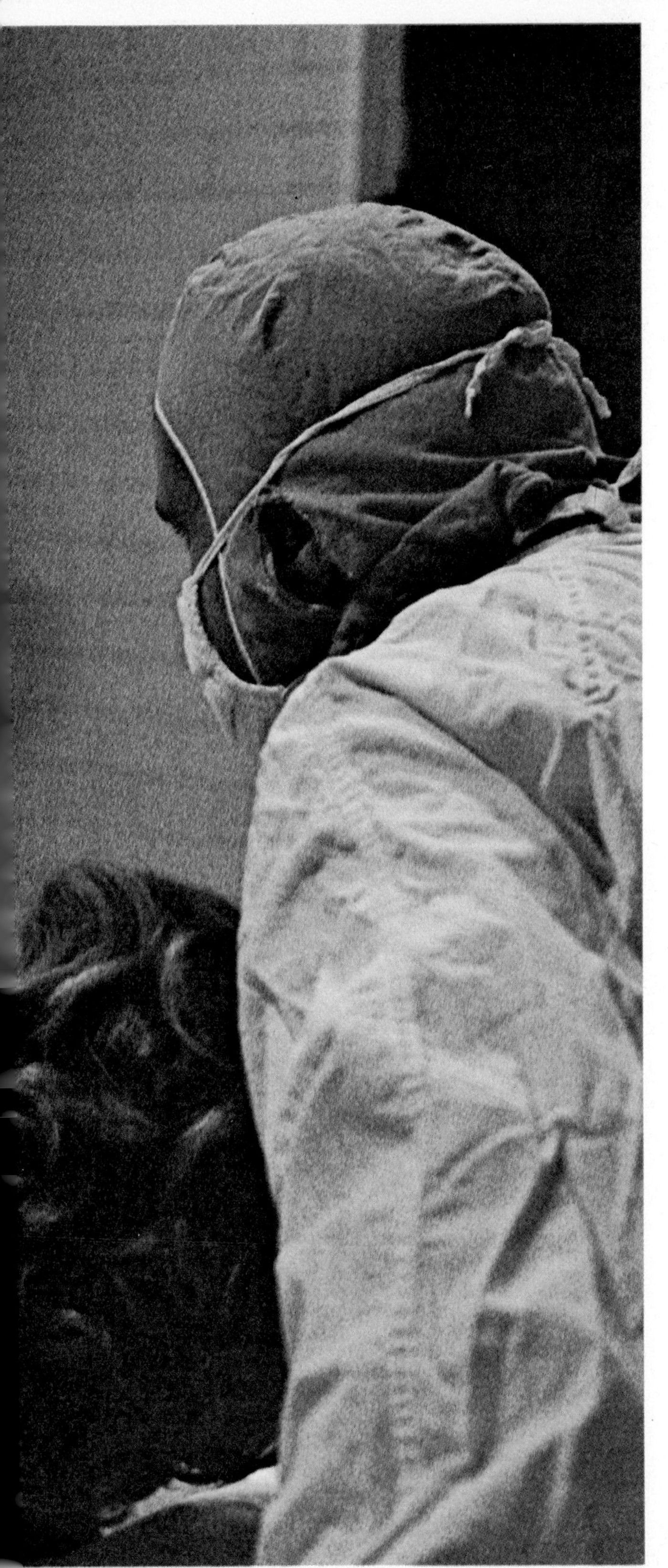

4 Reproduction and Health

Perpetuation of the human species is ensured by the instinctual drives that motivate individuals toward sexual union and by the extreme pleasure both sexes can experience during sexual intercourse. Yet with this great pleasure comes responsibility for the possible consequences—the creation of human life and the addition of another individual to the human population. In order to share responsibility for reproductive control, every man and woman should thoroughly understand the reproductive process.

The male and female reproductive systems and their role in sexual responsiveness were delineated in Chapter 3. Here emphasis will be on the processes that make possible the production and union of sex cells, or *gametes,* and the growth and birth of an individual resulting from that union. Because the essential reproductive event takes place within the female body, it is the woman's system that will be the primary focus of this chapter.

THE MALE CONTRIBUTION

Unlike women, who are born with a full set of egg cells already in their ovaries, men are not born with spermatozoa. Instead, their testes contain a number of undifferentiated cells, some of which are called *spermatogonia.* Through a process called *spermatogenesis,* which may take as long as seventy-five days, the spermatogonia undergo various changes, finally becoming *spermatozoa,* the male sex cells capable of fertilizing an ovum. A normal man's testes produce about 200 million mature spermatozoa (sperm) each day. Sperm not ejaculated disintegrate and are absorbed back into the system. Spermatogenesis is a continuous process that begins at puberty and can last into old age. Men may experience a gradual reduction in sexual interest as they age, but some remain fertile into their eighth decade.

The prostate, seminal vesicles, and bulbourethral glands constitute the accessory reproductive glands in the male. They secrete and store the *seminal fluid,* which transports the spermatozoa and provides an environment conducive to viability. Mature sperm are stored in the epididymis prior to traveling through the coiled *vas deferens* in preparation for ejaculation.

Human sperm are tiny, tadpolelike cells with oval heads and long, thin tails. Several hundred million of these sperm are contained in the fluid of a single ejaculation. However, only a small percentage can survive within the woman's body and actually find their way from the vagina through the cervix and uterus to the Fallopian tubes, where *fertilization* (the union of sperm and egg to form a zygote) occurs.

THE FEMALE SYSTEM

The woman's reproductive organs were described to some extent in Chapter 3. This section will be devoted to the internal structures of reproduction (uterus, Fallopian tubes, and ovaries).

The Uterus

The *uterus,* or womb as it is sometimes called, is a pear-shaped organ that rests on its small end (the cervix) in the center of the pelvis. The uterus has only one function: to house a growing fetus from shortly after conception until it is ready to be born. During the nine months of pregnancy, this organ grows from the size of a small pear into a huge muscular bag filling the entire abdomen—a bag that can hold not only a seven-pound baby but a quart of water and a one-pound placenta besides.

The uterus is not a sex gland. Removing it does not make a woman fat or bring on menopausal symptoms, as many people seem to believe. This fact should be clearly understood by every woman who has a hysterectomy because of uterine disease. As long as the ovaries remain, the monthly ebb and flow of ovarian hormones and corresponding feelings will go right on until the normal time for menopause.

What ceases when the uterus is removed is *menstruation.* Menstrual blood comes only from the uterus. For thirty to forty years of a woman's life, the menstrual cycle prepares and renovates her reproductive system. Each month in nonpregnant women the lining of the uterus—the endometrium—thickens, grows, and undergoes vascular and glandular changes under the influence of various hormones, preparing it to nourish a fertilized ovum. If pregnancy does not occur, the whole lining of the uterus sloughs away monthly in the bloody discharge called menstruation, named for the Latin word *mensis,* meaning "month." When pregnancy does occur, this lining remains to nourish the growing fetus. Menstruation is the only instance in nature where a loss of blood does not signify injury but is instead a sign of good health.

The onset of menstruation *(menarche)* is variable, but it usually occurs between the ages of ten and sixteen. In unusual cases, it has been reported to begin as early as two and as late as twenty years of age. Many factors, including climate, heredity, health status, and nutrition, appear to influence the age of menarche.

The average menstrual cycle lasts from twenty-seven to thirty days. Considerable variation from cycle to cycle is normal at times. Cycles that are completely irregular or bleeding that occurs at intervals of less than eighteen or more than forty-two days are considered abnormal and are often caused by lack of ovulation. Menstrual flow generally lasts from three to six days. Many women are aware of bodily changes immediately preceding their "period." They feel slightly bloated, their breasts may become sore or full, or they may have backaches, leg pains, or changes in energy level.

The Fallopian Tubes

The *Fallopian tubes,* or *oviducts,* are tiny, muscular tunnels attached by their small ends to either side of the uterus. They are connecting canals between the ovaries and uterus, serving as a passageway and meeting ground for the sperm and the egg. In order for an egg cell to develop, it must first ripen in the ovary inside what is known as a *Graafian follicle.* When the follicle is ripe, it comes up under the cover of the ovary and thins the cover into a blister, and finally the mature egg pops free from the ovary. This process is called *ovulation* (see Figure 4.1).

The process by which the egg reaches the tubes is not well understood. However, it is believed that the many-fingered fringe on the open end of the tube propels the ripened egg into the mouth of the tube. The tube is lined with tiny waving cilia, which gradually push the egg toward the first third of the tube, where, if all conditions are favorable, it will meet some spermatozoa, one of which may penetrate it. If the egg is not fertilized, it dies within a few hours and is sloughed off. But if it is fertilized, the egg moves along the tube, an ever-multiplying mass of cells, drops into the uterus, and plants itself in the lining of that organ. There it will grow to be first an embryo, then at eight weeks a fetus, and finally after about nine months a baby.

The tubes can become diseased or inflamed with a severity out of proportion to their small size. Inflammation in the tubes *(salpingitis),* often caused by gonorrhea, may leave scars and constrictions that prevent egg cells from passing through, making pregnancy difficult to achieve. Occasionally the tubes are only partially blocked, and the tiny sperm cells can wriggle past the constriction, but then the much larger egg cell cannot get down to the uterus. In this case, pregnancy in the tube may result. This situation, an *ectopic pregnancy,* is relatively rare but always serious, for it is very difficult to detect. Eventually, the tube ruptures, and immediate surgery is necessary to stop internal hemorrhage.

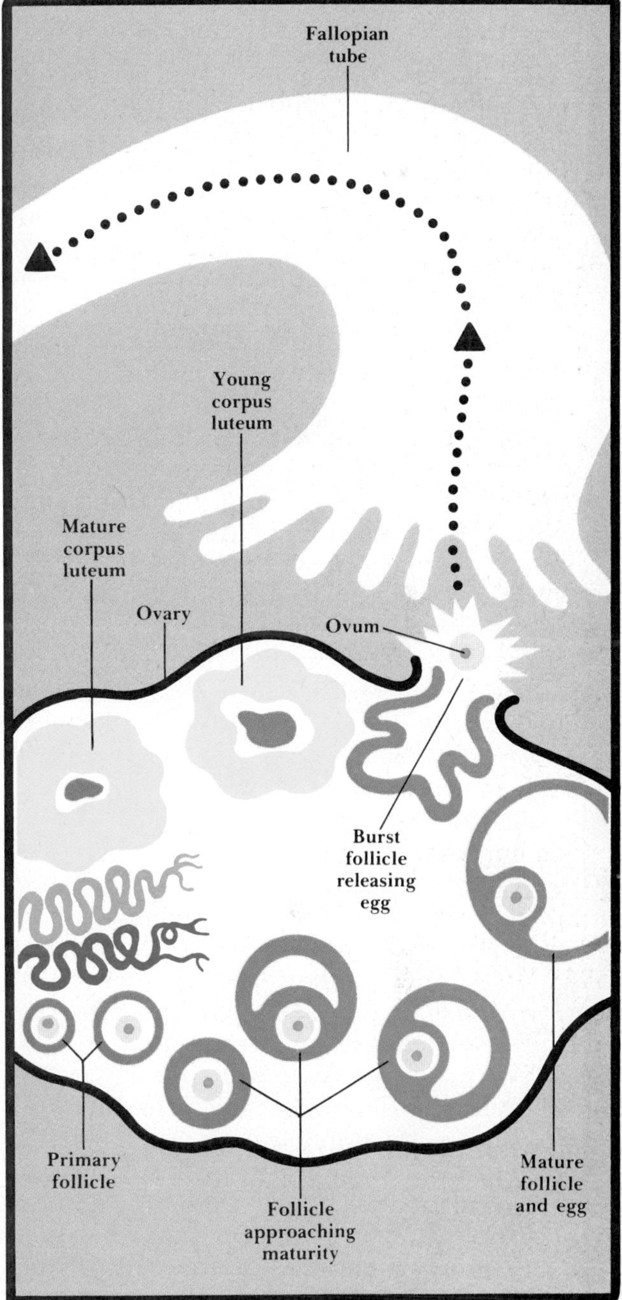

Figure 4.1 Stages of follicular maturation and ovulation.

The Ovaries

Each ovary is about the size and shape of an almond and lies close to the open end of its corresponding Fallopian tube. Each month, one or the other ovary will usually produce an egg on a day that is somewhere near the midpoint between menstrual periods. (In prolonged cycles, ovulation occurs later than midpoint. In short cycles, ovulation can take place during menstruation.) Some women can tell when ovulation occurs by the way they feel. The pelvis seems heavy, or there is a slight soreness on one side or the other or even a little pain that may last for a couple of days.

Besides making ovulation possible, the ovaries have another important purpose. They act as endocrine glands, producing the body chemicals (ovarian hormones) that regulate the menstrual cycle, and, in fact, they may influence the general emotional attitude of some women. Nervousness and tension before a period and relaxation afterward sometimes parallel the ebb and flow of ovarian hormones. One principal hormone is *estrogen,* produced mainly by certain cells of the Graafian follicle. Estrogen is responsible for the development of female characteristics as a girl matures into adulthood. Production of this hormone declines at the menopause, though female characteristics and sexual interest remain. The other principal ovarian hormone is *progesterone,* whose purpose is to prepare the uterus for the reception of the fertilized egg. Progesterone—together with more estrogen—is produced by the *corpus luteum,* a structure evolved from the residual material of the follicle after release of the mature egg.

If one ovary has to be removed or ceases functioning, the other supplies enough hormone for the body. Menstrual rhythm and ovulation remain undisturbed and childbearing may go on. But if both ovaries are removed (an *oopherectomy*) or cease functioning before the natural menopause, menstruation will cease and signs of menopause will appear.

If ovarian hormones become deficient or out of balance in relation to one another, a disturbance in menstruation often follows. In such cases, menstruation may be either too scant or too excessive, or it may stop altogether for a few months. Often, the hormone disturbance can be corrected with artificial hormone preparations, or at least an artificial balance can be achieved until the natural balance returns.

Feminine Hygiene

The healthy vagina secretes sufficient fluid to keep it moist. Used-up cells are always being shed from the lining of the vagina, and these cells mixed with fluid produce a nonirritating secretion. This secretion is clean and healthy unless it is allowed to collect in the folds of the skin surrounding the vaginal opening. Careful bathing of this area will prevent unpleasant odor from developing, since odor usually comes from the labia and outer folds rather than from the vagina itself.

When this vaginal secretion becomes excessive enough to stain clothing, or if it is yellow, irritating, watery, bloody, or smelly, then it is called a vaginal discharge, or *leukorrhea.* This type of discharge may mean infection in some part of the genital tract. It is a warning signal that should bring one to a physician for examination without delay. There are also normal causes for increased vaginal secretion, however. Sexual excitement and emotional stress may cause enough vaginal wetness to stain clothing.

Although douching seems to be a popular practice among many American women, it is not necessary for good health. The normal vaginal environment is acid, which keeps it clear of undesirable bacteria. Douching does no particular harm, provided a mild acid solution such as vinegar is used; however, alkaline or commercial chemical douches may neutralize the protective acids, allowing harmful bacteria to multiply.

Menopause

Menopause is the cessation of menstruation and of cyclic reproductive activity. The average age of occurrence is fifty, but it can begin earlier than forty or later than fifty-three. Menstrual periods usually falter for a few months and then cease altogether, at which point a woman is said to have gone through the menopause, or "change of life." This change is also known as the *climacteric,* the time that marks the end of her reproductive period.

What has happened is that her ovaries, after thirty or forty years of activity, have lost their ability to produce mature eggs. The menopausal woman may welcome her loss of fertility, but the reduced production of female hormones can create other problems.

It is not true that sexual interest and activity decline after menopause. In fact, many menopausal and postmenopausal women, no longer concerned about becoming pregnant, actually feel more sexual desire and satisfaction.

Some menopausal women tend to put on weight, primarily because they eat more and exercise less. It is not true that menopausal women become masculine, nor do they become psychotic from the climacteric. About 50 percent of women will experience "hot flashes" for a few months and sometimes for years. Hot flashes are caused when blood vessels dilate erratically due to the changing levels of hormones.

Subtle and undesirable body changes may occur after menopause as the result of hormone deficiency. The skin may gradually become drier and more wrinkled. The vagina tends to become drier and its lining thinner and more tender. The vagina may also shrink so that in rare cases intercourse becomes painful, although additional lubrication can help overcome this problem. Later, blood vessels may harden and bones may lose calcium and become more brittle.

Many American women take prescription estrogen pills for the symptoms of menopause. The Food and Drug Administration, however, says estrogens are overused for this purpose. While estrogens do help relieve hot flashes and vaginal changes, they have not been shown to be effective, says the FDA, for keeping the skin soft, helping women feel younger, or treating simple nervousness and depression. Furthermore, estrogens are risky for menopausal women. Their use is associated with a five to ten times greater incidence of cancer of the uterus and a two-and-one-half-times greater risk of gallbladder disease requiring surgery. The FDA recommends that menopausal women take estrogens in the lowest possible doses for the shortest possible periods of time, and that they be examined by their doctors at least once a year while on the drug.

CONCEPTION AND PRENATAL DEVELOPMENT

If ovulation has occurred and if sperm have been deposited in the vagina and have moved up through the uterus to the appropriate Fallopian tube at just the right time, fertilization may occur. The fertilized egg, or *zygote,* travels down the remainder of the tube into the uterus, a journey that takes about three days. During this journey, the zygote undergoes rapid cell division. After floating free in the uterus for three or four days, the cluster of cells burrows down into the endometrium (the lining of the uterine wall) in a process called *implantation.*

At the time of implantation, actual pregnancy can be said to have begun. Soon thereafter, physiological changes occur in the mother that can be detected by pregnancy tests (see below).

Within two or three days after implantation, spectacular changes occur in the endometrium around the growing organism. Specialized cells from the uterus and the now-forming embryo begin to differentiate into the *placenta,* the structure that will absorb life-giving nutrients from the mother and carry them to the developing child for the next nine months.

The events during the rest of the pregnancy constitute one of the truly amazing phenomena of life. What starts out as a single cell, a speck barely visible to the human eye, grows in a very short time into a complete and individual human being, equipped with miniature versions of all the necessary internal organs and external equipment. Table 4.1 provides a synopsis of the changes that take place each month.

Throughout its prenatal life, the developing child is enclosed in a fluid-filled sac (the *amnion*), which primarily provides protection and is attached to the placenta via the umbilical cord. As an *embryo,* the organism is less than an inch long and looks something like a curved fish. After three months, it is called a *fetus* and has developed arms and legs with perfectly shaped fingers and toes. By the end of the third month, although it is only about three inches long and weighs a mere ounce, the fetus can kick its legs, close its fingers, turn its head, and open and close its mouth. Also, by this time most of its internal organs are able to function, so that the remainder of the prenatal period can be spent in the process of growth and in putting on the finishing touches (see Figure 4.2, p.77).

At birth, the average full-term infant weighs

Table 4.1 Milestones of Prenatal Development

Period	Development
First two weeks	Zygote goes through multiple cell divisions. It attaches itself to the uterine wall, becoming an embryo—a fishlike organism floating in a fluid-filled sac.
Fourth week	Primitive heart begins beating and rudimentary organs are formed; the organism is still nonhuman in appearance.
Third month	Embryo becomes a fetus; it has a definite human appearance and is quite active; almost all internal and external physical equipment is well developed.
Fourth month	Growth of lower body parts accelerates; most bone models formed; mother feels "quickening."
Fifth month	Fetus sleeps and wakes; it has a characteristic "lie"; it is capable of extrauterine life, except that it cannot maintain respiration.
Sixth month	Eyes (fully formed) open; eye movements occur; grasp reflex present.
Seventh month	Fetus can survive outside uterus in a highly sheltered environment.
Eighth and ninth months	Fat forms over the body, and the finishing touches are put on the organs and functional capacities.

anywhere from five to twelve pounds and may be from seventeen to twenty-two inches long. The average length of pregnancy is 280 days, but babies born as early as 180 days or as late as 334 days after conception may be able to survive.

PREGNANCY

Under ordinary circumstances, the pregnant woman can do almost all the things she normally enjoys, whether it be playing, working, or having sexual intercourse. Of course, in addition to maintaining her own health, strength, and energy, she must fulfill the extra requirements of a growing baby, who for nine months depends on her for all bodybuilding materials. Excellent nutrition is required.

The medical supervision of pregnancy—ensuring that the baby's requirements are met, and watching for any complications—is called *prenatal care* and requires visits to the doctor at regular intervals. A woman in pregnancy should think of herself as an athlete in training, building up her body to the highest level of physical fitness, so that the childbirth that lies ahead will be a joy and not an ordeal. With such a plan and with the medical skills now available, she can emerge from childbirth healthier than before and with her body both strong and shapely.

Pregnancy Testing

Usually, the first sign of pregnancy is that an expected menstrual period does not occur. There may be a feeling that menstruation is about to begin but "can't quite get started." This is not positive verification of pregnancy, since it is not unusual for periods to be delayed fourteen to twenty-one days, particularly in women who are normally somewhat irregular or who are under stress (such as the anticipation—or fear—of pregnancy). A woman may also notice congested and tender breasts, increased irritability, heaviness in the pelvis, and sometimes a little nausea at mealtime.

About three weeks after the missed period, a physician can usually, by pelvic examination, be fairly certain of the existence of a pregnancy. Pelvic tissue is slightly softened, the vaginal opening becomes slightly purplish, and the uterus begins to enlarge.

There are also a number of diagnostic tests that confirm a pregnancy. A pregnant woman's system produces a hormone, human chorionic gonadotropin (HCG). In *immunoassay,* HCG in a urine sample is detected by means of antibo-

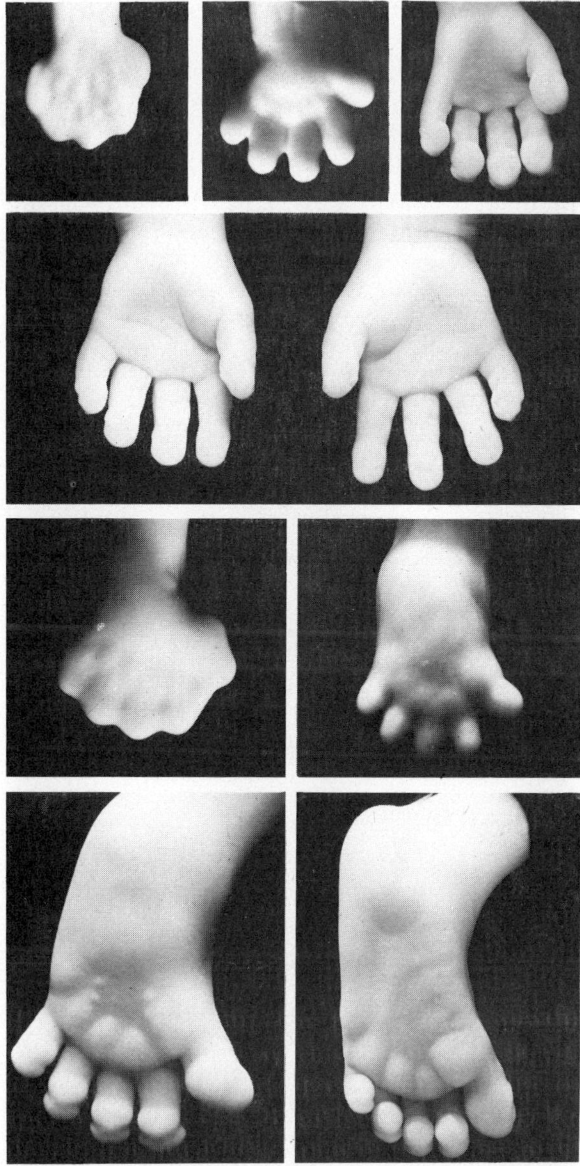

Figure 4.2 Fetal development. In the fifth week, hands are a "molding plate" with finger ridges. In the sixth week, finger buds have formed. In the seventh and eighth weeks, the fingers, thumbs, and fingerprints form; note the prominent touch pads. In the third month, the pads regress, and the hands are well formed. The feet begin to form in the sixth week and forty-eight hours later have large toe ridges. The heel appears by the end of the sixth week and grows out in the next five days. In the third month, feet are well formed.

dies that react with the hormone. A disadvantage of immunoassay is that in very early pregnancy it has a high incidence of false negatives; that is, it reports that women are not pregnant when in fact they are. In *radioreceptor assay,* HCG in a blood sample can be detected as early as the first missed period with almost 100 percent accuracy.

Radioreceptor assay is available in most cities at low cost and often requires no more than a brief visit to a clinic to leave a blood sample and a follow-up phone call for the results. Referrals for this service are available through local chapters of the Planned Parenthood Federation of America, local health departments, and county medical societies.

Immunoassay is the basis for the do-it-yourself pregnancy testing kits now on the market. These kits require fairly complicated procedures, also have a high incidence of false negatives, and are usually no cheaper than radioreceptor assays.

Visits to the Doctor

The ideal time for the first prenatal visit to the doctor is *before* pregnancy. A woman should be in the best possible general health before starting pregnancy, and it is wise for her to have a general physical examination. This should include a test to determine whether she has had German measles, which can cause birth defects if contracted in early pregnancy. If she has not, she can be immunized before beginning a pregnancy. If a woman is over thirty-five, or if there is a history of hereditary disease in either her or her husband's family, the couple can also receive genetic counseling at this time and learn about the possibilities of amniocentesis and therapeutic abortion, as will be discussed below.

If the examination has not been done before pregnancy, it should be done during the early months. Conditions that might result in complications of pregnancy, obstructed labor, or difficult delivery can then be discovered and corrected before they cause trouble. Needs for special exercise or special diet can be determined at this time.

Regular medical consultation should be provided every three to four weeks in early pregnancy and more often during the last two months. In the case of complications, more frequent visits and special tests may be necessary.

Blood pressure, weight changes, and urinalyses are important in detecting early signs of possible trouble.

Blood Examinations

Sometime during early pregnancy, a series of blood tests will be performed. Hemoglobin and red-cell counts indicate the presence of anemia. The white-cell count may reveal or rule out infection or other disorders. A blood test for syphilis is required by law.

The Rh test is always done for expectant mothers to assess the risk of Rh disease, a genetically determined blood disorder. Most people have a biochemical substance called Rh factor in their red blood cells; these people are said to be Rh positive. About 10 percent of Americans, however, lack this substance; they are called Rh negative. The disease can occur only when an expectant mother is Rh negative and the father is Rh positive, a common combination. Because the Rh-positive gene is dominant over the Rh-negative gene, there is a good chance that the developing fetus will be Rh positive and its blood be quite incompatible with that of its mother. This is no problem 90 percent of the time, and is very rarely a problem in first pregnancies. However, if the fetus's blood leaks into the mother's bloodstream (which is most likely to happen at delivery), the baby's Rh factor stimulates the mother's body to produce anti-Rh substances. In a subsequent pregnancy, these anti-Rh substances can destroy the fetus's red blood cells, necessitating a blood transfusion at birth. Sometimes the fetus may be so severely affected as to require an intrauterine blood transfusion.

The present treatment is to immunize all Rh negative mothers who are carrying Rh positive babies as soon as the fetus's blood type is known. This shot blocks the antigens that have reached the mother's circulation and prevents her immune system from "seeing" the antigen and making antibodies to it. (For a further discussion of immunity, see Chapter 14.)

Discomforts of Pregnancy

One of the common discomforts of early pregnancy is "morning sickness," so called because it appears most often soon after awakening, when the stomach is empty. This type of nausea may reappear late in the morning and late in the afternoon, each time the stomach is empty. The exact disturbance underlying this nausea is not clearly understood. It usually disappears by itself around the third month. Small, frequent meals and the use of antinausea medication usually bring relief.

"Heartburn," or acid indigestion, is a common problem in the later months of pregnancy, but relief is usually easily obtained with an antacid tablet or a change in diet. Hemorrhoids, which are varicose veins of the rectum, may also occur in the later months when the baby's head presses down in the pelvis. These frequently disappear without treatment after delivery.

Many pregnant women worry about varicose veins in the legs. If the problem produces no discomfort, it may be disregarded because it will, for the most part, disappear after delivery. If the legs ache, an elastic bandage or elastic stockings will help. Elevating the lower legs on pillows each afternoon will also help. Pains in the ligaments supporting the uterus can also be relaxed by elevating one's lower legs. This discomfort is common between the fourth and seventh months.

Spontaneous Abortion

In 10 to 20 percent of pregnancies—and perhaps even more—spontaneous abortion (commonly called *miscarriage*) is inevitable because either the developing organism was not implanted correctly or the egg or sperm was defective to begin with. Nature simply gets rid of something that has no ability to survive. Bleeding and cramps continue until the uterus expels the defective fertilized ovum. When properly managed, a spontaneous abortion is no more serious than a delivery. Future chances for childbearing are not impaired.

Spontaneous abortions are not caused by automobile trips, falls, or emotional shocks. On the other hand, they may be related to general glandular or body disorders, which is one of the reasons for having a good medical examination before starting a pregnancy. The problem of habitual spontaneous abortion, in which a woman suffers one after another, requires skilled medical treatment.

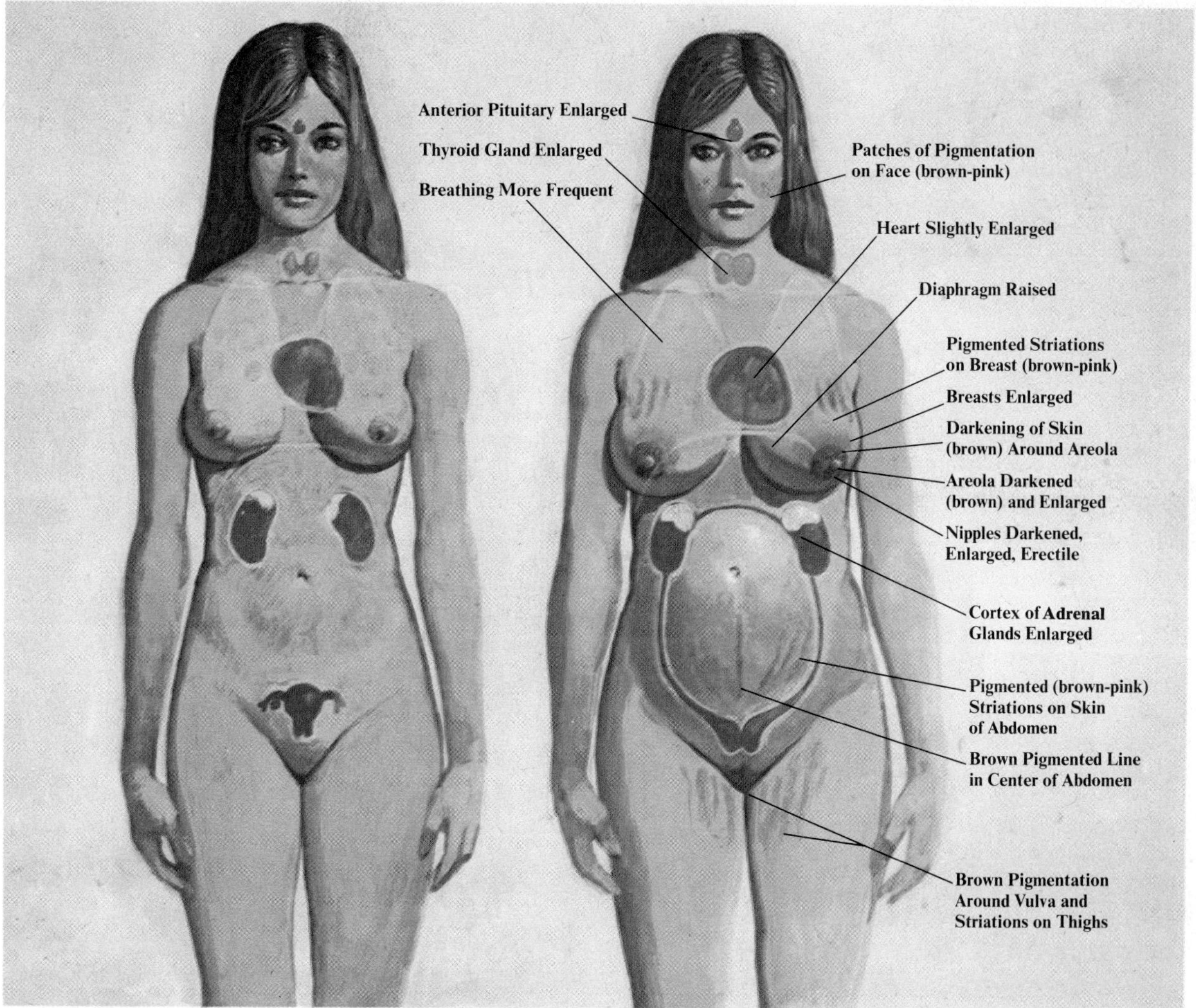

Figure 4.3 Physiological changes during pregnancy. The body is shown at conception and at thirty weeks. Some or all of these typical changes may occur.

Prepared Childbirth

Every woman has some apprehension as she approaches childbirth. To obtain the peace of mind necessary to make the birth of her baby the rich and deeply satisfying experience it should be, the pregnant woman should try to obtain as much information as she can about the birth process.

Over the past twenty years or so, more and more expectant mothers and couples have been attending classes in childbirth. The content of these classes includes physiological changes during pregnancy; nutrition; the processes involved in labor, delivery, and the postpartum period; hospital procedures; care and feeding of the newborn; and various medical means to control pain.

Prepared childbirth is often confused with unmedicated childbirth, also called "natural" childbirth. Unmedicated childbirth is an alternative that those in prepared childbirth classes can choose if it is medically indicated. In most cases, unmedicated childbirth is not painless, but it is manageable through knowledge of what to expect and through practice of special

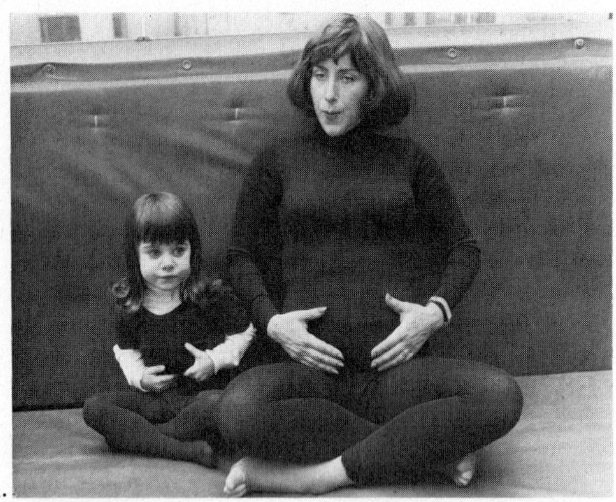
a.

Figure 4.4 Prepared childbirth. (a) An expectant mother practices special Lamaze breathing exercises. (b) A prenatal class. (c) An instruction program for pregnant women and their husbands.

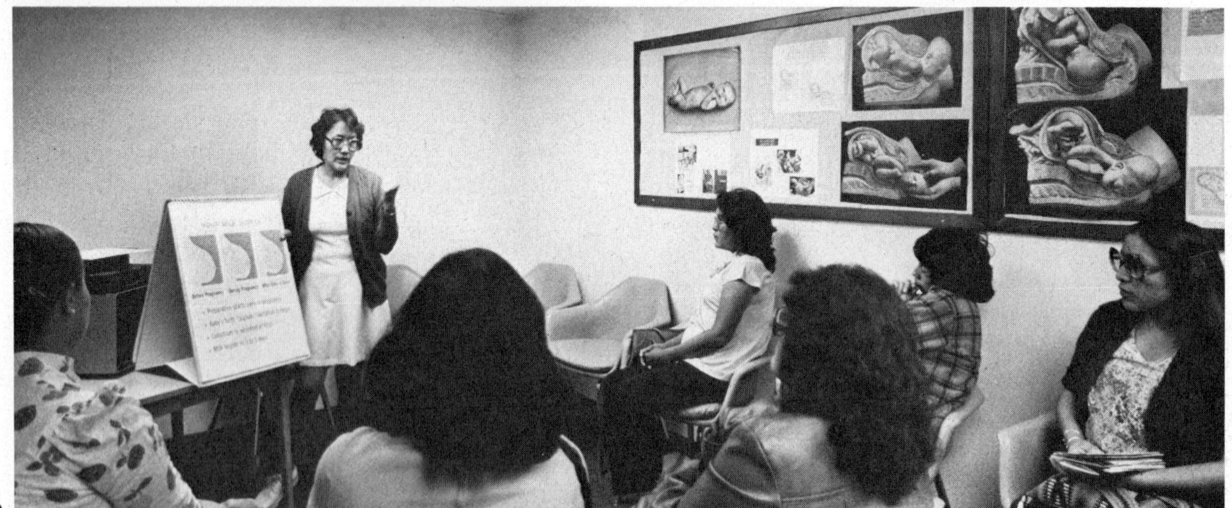
b.

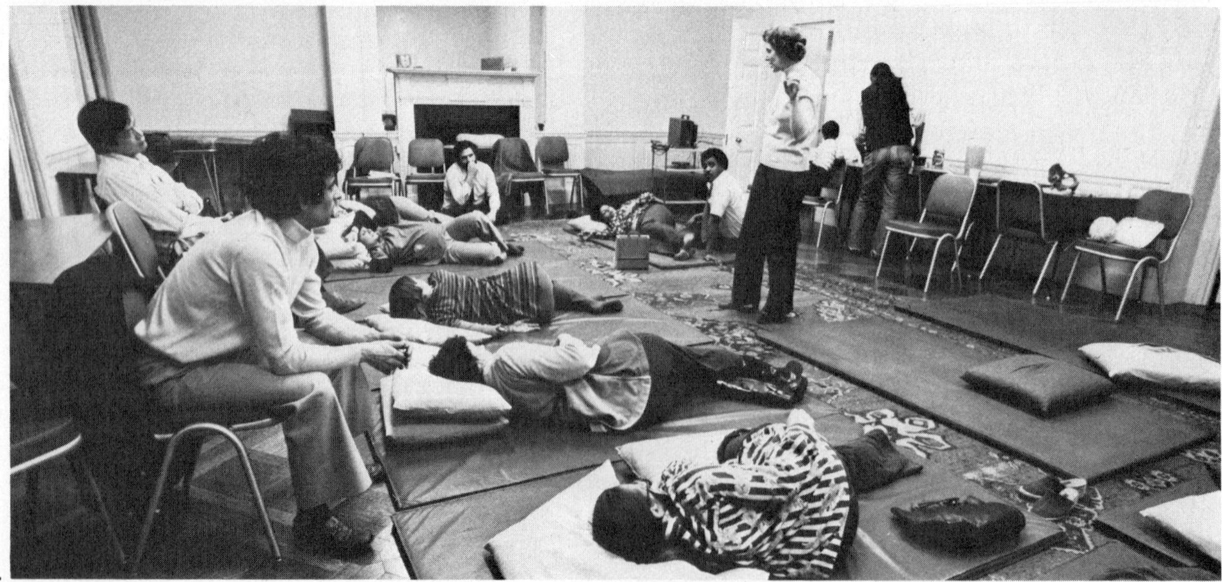
c.

exercises in breathing and relaxation. This is often referred to as the *Lamaze method.*

Prepared-childbirth classes may be sponsored by physicians, other trained professionals, hospitals, the Childbirth Education Association (CEA), or the American Society for Psychoprophylaxis in Obstetrics (ASPO). Information on courses can be obtained from the last two organizations.

The main disadvantage of prepared childbirth comes from a misunderstanding of its purpose. Those who think that the objective is unmedicated childbirth may feel they have failed if some anesthesia or other medication is needed. However, the intention of childbirth education is to provide informed choices and to enhance the childbirth experience through understanding.

There are several advantages to prepared childbirth. Foremost is that knowledge helps alleviate undue fears; the woman or couple knows what to expect and what to do to cooperate. If unmedicated or minimal medication is possible and selected, the mother can know when to push the infant out or can do so when told. In this way, anesthetic risks and recovery problems for mother and infant are minimized. And in most instances, women who have had preparation for childbirth require less medication when it is needed. Finally, women and couples who are knowledgeable and who undergo such preparation report enhanced meaning and even elation at the time of the birth.

Involving the father in the preparation for childbirth and having him present in the delivery room provide valuable emotional support for the mother and give him a greater sense of sharing and responsibility in the birth. The presence of the father in the delivery room is occurring more and more for these reasons, and health professionals and couples are requesting this option in increasing numbers.

LABOR AND BIRTH

During the last month or two of pregnancy, a woman may notice her uterus contracting at irregular intervals. These contractions are usually not painful, but occasionally they are. True labor contractions usually feel somewhat like menstrual cramps. A contraction may be felt as only a tightness in the back. Frequently, a small amount of vaginal bleeding is noticed a day or two before the onset of labor.

Near the end of pregnancy, clear fluid will drain spontaneously from the vagina, which means that the amniotic sac, or bag of waters, has broken, and labor is likely to start shortly. Contrary to some popular opinion, early rupture of the bag of waters (dry labor) does not mean that labor will be difficult or prolonged; in fact, it is likely to be faster and easier. Rupture of the amniotic membrane itself is normal and painless. True labor contractions usually start at intervals of fifteen to twenty minutes and gradually become more frequent. In some cases, however, labor sets in abruptly, with contractions coming every three to five minutes.

It is helpful for the woman to understand that each contraction of the uterus brings the baby just a little closer to birth, and that her own body relaxation can lessen the discomfort of strong contractions.

To understand what happens during a contraction, one should visualize the uterus as a big muscular bag that is upside down, with its open end emptying into the vagina. At first, this opening is almost closed by an elastic ring, the cervix. Every time the walls of the bag contract, the baby's head is pressed firmly against the cervix, and the opening dilates a little more. Finally, the cervix opens wide enough for the baby's head to pass through into the vagina.

The dilating contractions of labor may be painful, and in fact, they are often called "labor pains." If desired, medication can usually be used to relieve most of the pain and to make labor reasonably comfortable. Nevertheless, medication must be used with caution because it might slow down labor or affect the baby. The more one learns to relax the entire body during and between each contraction, the less pain there will be and the easier it will be for medication to relieve it.

When the baby's head is through the cervix and in the vagina, the woman feels a compulsion to bear down and expel the baby through the vaginal opening. First, the crown of the

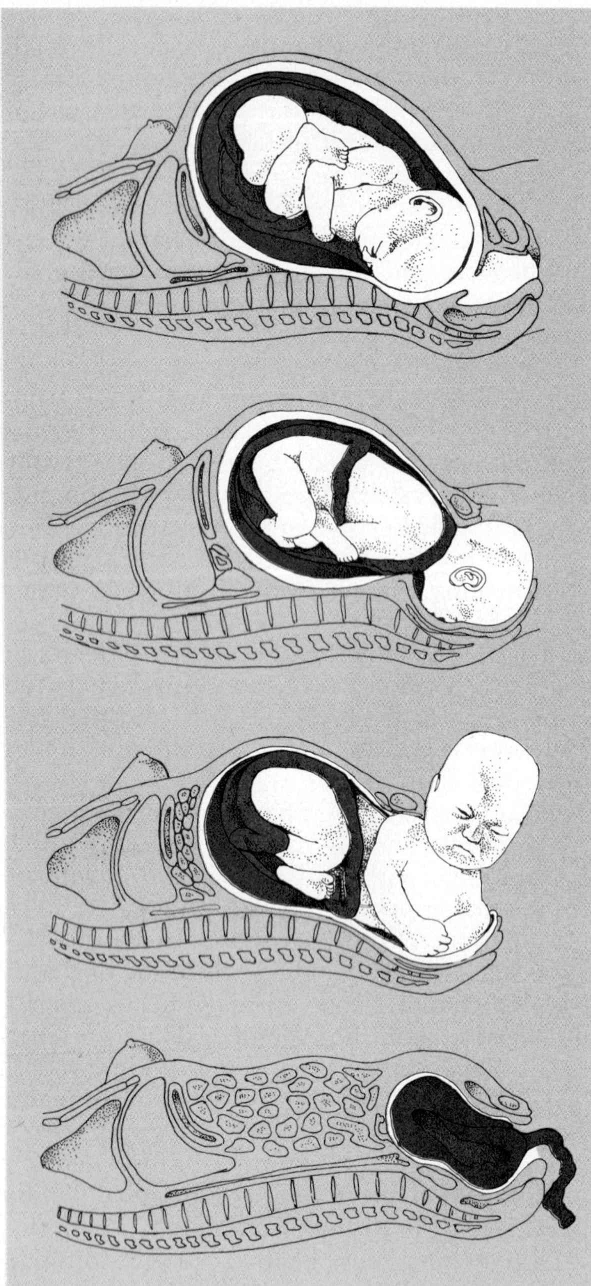

Figure 4.5 Stages of childbirth, shown diagrammatically. The baby's head lies close to the cervix, which becomes fully dilated. Strong uterine contractions begin to force the head into the birth canal (vagina). After the head appears, the shoulders rotate in the birth canal, and the rest of the body is expelled. In the last stage of delivery, the placenta and umbilical cord (sometimes called "afterbirth") are expelled.

baby's head appears, and then gradually, with succeeding contractions, the head usually slides out face down. Once the head is out, the body usually follows easily, because the head is largest in diameter. At this point, the umbilical cord is tied and severed, and the newly breathing baby is welcomed to the world. Soon afterward, the uterus contracts down into a large ball, usually expelling the placenta.

In the United States, a surgical incision called an *episiotomy* is commonly used to prevent undue tearing of the tissues around the vaginal opening. This incision is repaired with sutures, leaving the opening about the same as it was before pregnancy. Sometimes, if necessary, physicians will aid the birth with low forceps.

Sometimes women have general anesthesia, in which they are lightly asleep, during the delivery. Many women, however, have a strong desire to stay awake during delivery, and, in order to do so, forgo general anesthesia. Some have a regional anesthetic which blocks pain in only part of the body. Others are given only local anesthesia or a pain reliever like Demerol. The decision depends partly on the woman's wishes and partly on what happens during the labor and delivery.

Sometimes it becomes necessary to do a *Caesarean operation* (also called a *Caesarean section*). Instead of being delivered through the birth canal, the baby is removed through incisions in the abdomen and uterus. This operation is sometimes necessary when the mother has a pelvic opening so small in relation to the infant's head that normal delivery might be dangerous to both her and her child. Caesarean section is also sometimes used when the baby is in a poor position, when the placenta blocks the cervix (placenta previa), and if the mother has had a previous section (because of the danger of uterine rupture at the site of the previous incision).

Whatever the method of delivery, after the baby has been extracted the physician cleans the nose and mouth by means of a suction apparatus to make breathing easier. The newborn is then quickly assessed for breathing, muscle tone, heart rate, reflexes, irritability, and color to determine whether it needs further medical help.

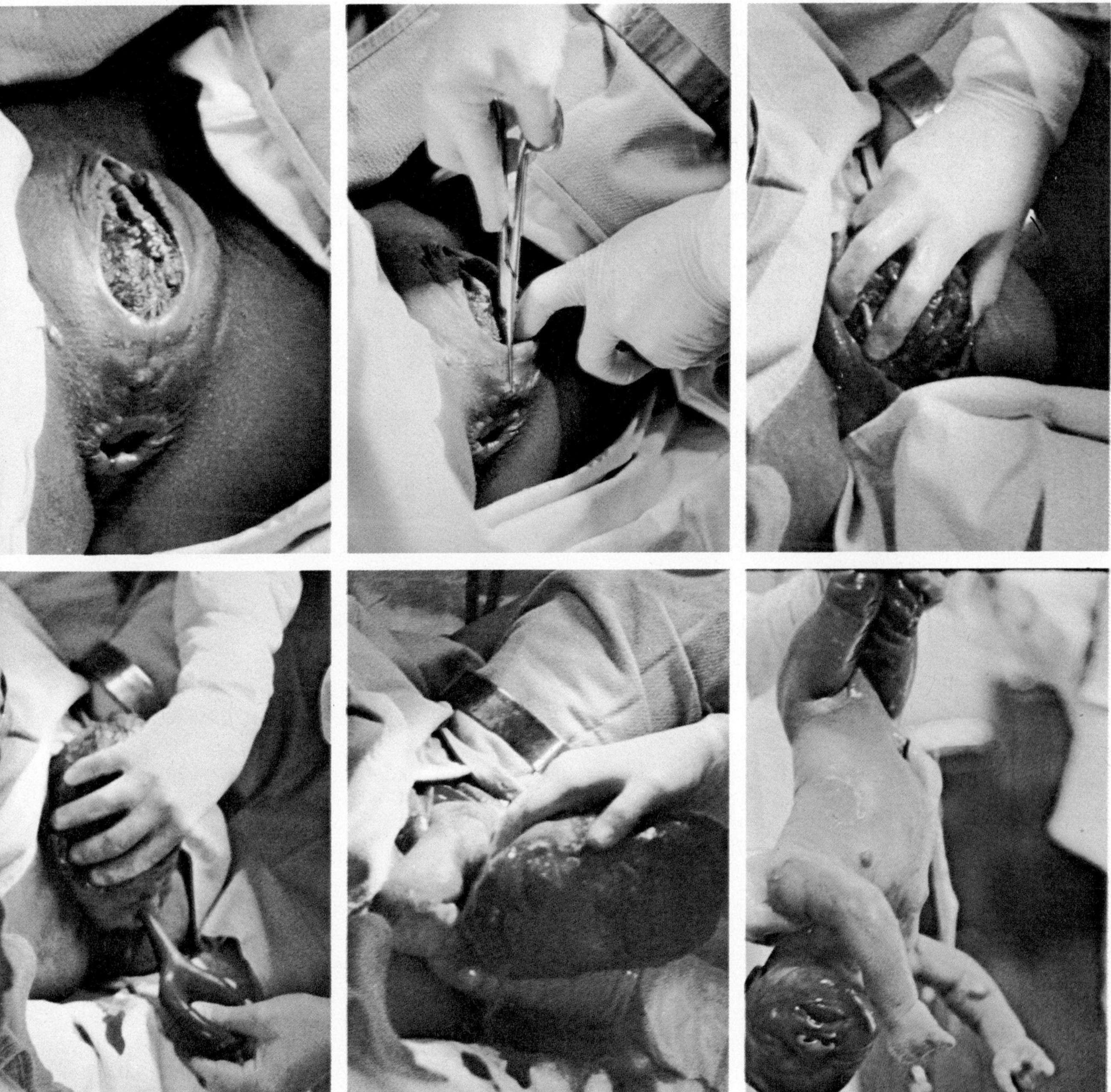

Figure 4.6 A baby is born. Note that in the top middle photograph the doctor is performing an episiotomy.

Midwifery and Home Delivery

Some 90 to 95 percent of all pregnancies and deliveries are normal, healthy events that do not necessarily need the skills of highly trained, expensive obstetricians. Today, some women are choosing instead to have their babies delivered by nurse-midwives, who are well-educated professionals trained to manage normal pregnancies and deliveries and to spot complications in time to call in an obstetrician. Nurse-midwives can practice legally in almost all states; they always work closely with obstetricians and usually in hospitals.

Some women have recently been choosing to deliver their babies at home with the assistance of unlicensed "lay midwives." This practice is extremely dangerous for both the mother and the baby. Of the 5 to 10 percent of deliveries that are not normal, about half of the problems are not predictable ahead of time but emerge only during the course of labor and delivery. There is no way to tell whether labor and delivery are normal until they are over. There are many things that can go wrong with little warning: a woman may start hemorrhaging, a baby's heartbeat may drop dangerously before it is born, a newborn may fail to breathe. And in many such cases, a physician's skills and a hospital's elaborate equipment are needed *within minutes* to save the life of the mother or baby or to prevent serious brain damage to the baby.

Some hospitals and obstetricians, recognizing the interest in home deliveries, have created homelike environments within the hospital.

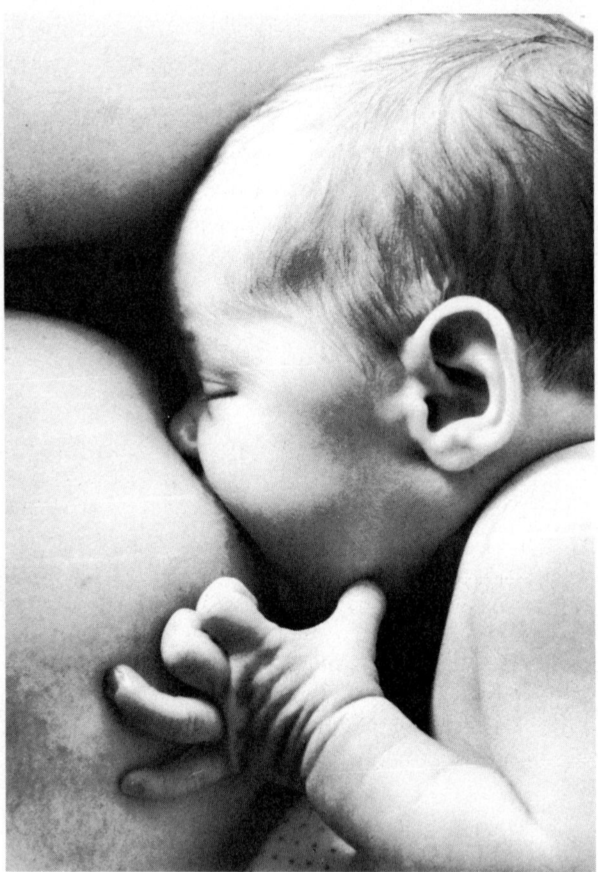

Figure 4.7 Authorities urge mothers to breast-feed their babies. Breast feeding benefits not only the child, but the mother as well.

BREAST FEEDING

The World Health Organization strongly recommends that mothers breast-feed their babies to promote harmonious physical and mental development of their children. Human milk is the natural food for infants, and modern science has not yet been able to duplicate its composition for bottle feeding.

Human milk, in comparison to bottle formula, provides the infant with greater resistance to infection through transfer of antibodies from the mother. Breast-fed infants are less likely to be obese, constipated, or have diaper rash. In addition, breast feeding is thought to minimize the tendency toward allergies, and it is also less expensive.

Breast feeding is beneficial for the mother as well. It causes the uterus to contract back to its normal size more quickly. Since production of breast milk requires more calorie output than pregnancy, women who breast-feed readily lose extra weight gained during pregnancy. In addition, special psychological benefits to both infant and mother may come from the intimacy involved in breast feeding.

Virtually all mothers are capable of breast-feeding their infants and of having an adequate milk supply, provided that the mothers have a good diet (including an extra 500 to 1,000 calories per day and an extra quart or more of liquid per day).

Formula-fed babies, however, do thrive and develop well. One advantage attributed to bottle formulas is that the mother can be away for long periods of time—for example, to go to work. Another advantage is that the father can be more involved in feeding the baby.

In a number of countries where breast feeding is encouraged, working mothers are allowed time during the workday to nurse their infants. American culture, however, has not generally supported breast feeding. Nevertheless, increasing numbers of American women, particularly among the college-educated, are adopting the practice. Mothers interested in breast feeding are being supported by physicians, understanding husbands, other women, flexible hospital schedules and routines, and education-for-childbirth groups.

INFERTILITY

In the United States today, approximately ten to fifteen of every one hundred couples try to have children without success. Difficulty in achieving pregnancy usually cannot be predicted; however, it often increases with age—a factor to consider in family planning. Adoption can be a solution to infertility for some. Fortunately, in recent years advances have been made in methods of overcoming infertility, and now it is possible for many formerly sterile couples to have children. There are many causes of infertility, and a number of tests and procedures must be carried out by a physician before all possible causes have been identified and corrected. Often a complete investigation and treatment will last eighteen months. Couples who start an infertility study should be prepared to go through the entire program. Those who see one doctor after another for superficial examinations rarely achieve success. It should be noted that there is no relationship between sexual adequacy and fertility.

Male Infertility

In one-third or more of infertile matings, the husband has an anatomical or physiological defect that is either wholly or partially responsible for the childless marriage.

Fertility in males is relatively easy to test through microscopic study of a semen specimen. Just as a low red blood count indicates anemia, so a low sperm count indicates low male fertility. Often when the cause of male sterility is found, hormone treatment is used to restore fertility.

Female Infertility

Female infertility may be caused by some minor condition that is easily corrected, but sometimes there are complicated problems in diagnosis. Because general bodily disorders, glandular disorders, and a host of conditions outside the pelvis can underlie female sterility, more than pelvic tests must be carried out. Physicians can determine whether the Fallopian tubes are open or closed by running gas through them. If the tubes are blocked, a laparoscope or X-ray may be able to locate the blockage. Another test can be performed on mucus obtained from the cervix at ovulation (determined by a rise in basal temperature) and several hours after intercourse; microscopic examination of this mucus can show whether the sperm are still alive and able to enter the uterus. (Some women's vaginas seem to contain an unknown factor that kills sperm.) Sometimes, a small sample of the uterine lining is taken to find out whether it is favorable for nourishing a fertilized ovum.

In 1978, a major advance was made toward overcoming blocked tubes, one of the major causes of female infertility, when the world's first "test-tube baby" was born in England. In this technique, a ripe ovum is removed surgically from the woman's body and mixed, in the laboratory, with the father's sperm. After the sperm fertilizes the egg, the embryo grows in an incubator for a few days and then is implanted into the mother's uterus for the normal nine months of pregnancy. (See the Viewpoint box.)

CONGENITAL DEFECTS

Most births are normal, but a significant minority of babies are born with *congenital defects* —abnormalities present at the time of birth. Some congenital defects result from genetic flaws in one or both parents (see the section *Genetic Diseases* below). Others are caused by factors that are either not genetic or still unknown; many defects in this category are directly related to the mother's health and health habits during pregnancy.

Some malformations can result from *injury* during delivery or from bungled attempts at

VIEWPOINT

Test-Tube Babies–Miracle or Menace?

On July 25, 1978, in the mill town of Oldham, England, a blonde, blue-eyed girl, Louise, was born to John and Lesley Brown. The birth attracted worldwide publicity, and complete strangers reacted with emotions ranging from joy to terror. Why?

Louise Brown was the first baby to be conceived *in vitro*—in a test tube.

Lesley Brown, the mother, seemed totally unable to bear children: she is one of the roughly 2 percent of married women whose Fallopian tubes are blocked, which prevents sperm from reaching the uterus. The blockages can sometimes be surgically corrected, but this operation did not help Mrs. Brown.

Under the care of Drs. Patrick Steptoe, a gynecologist, and Robert Edwards, a physiologist, a ripening egg was plucked from one of Lesley Brown's ovaries. The egg was placed in a test tube with sperm from John Brown, and the doctors watched as one of the sperm cells fertilized the egg. The fertilized egg was transferred to a special nutrient solution, where it split into two, then four, then eight cells. It was then reimplanted in Mrs. Brown's uterus, and, unlike previous attempts with would-be mothers, the pregnancy continued, monitored with extraordinary care. When she was born, Louise appeared to be healthy and normal.

To thousands of infertile women, the news of Louise's birth offered a glimmer of hope that one day they, too, could conceive. Approximately 30 percent of the infertile women in the United States are unable to have children because of various problems in the Fallopian tubes. And an increasing number of women who could never conceive normally are now pressing for in vitro conception.

But many scientists, philosophers, and theologians take a less enthusiastic view of the event. First, Steptoe and Edwards themselves emphasize that their procedure is still experimental—they had attempted it over eighty times previously without success. Many medical researchers believe that the birth of Louise Brown may have been due more to good luck than to science. Others fear that the baby's health is also a lucky fluke: there is no assurance that test-tube children will be genetically or physically normal. In fact, so many questions about test-tube conception are still unanswered that many doctors think it is too hazardous to attempt.

Test-tube conception also raises the menace of human control over life as we know it, a possibility that until recently was nothing more than futuristic fiction. Some of the moral and ethical issues raised are:

1. How will doctors decide which in vitro eggs to reimplant into the womb and which to discard?
2. Can we prevent the nightmare of "surrogate mothers"—women who would bear the test-tube-created fetuses of other women who have no desire to go through labor?
3. Are we close to the development of artificial wombs, which would enable children to be conceived and born without any human contact?
4. Will the technology of test-tube conception be combined with current research in DNA alteration to bring about genetically predetermined humans or clones?
5. Who will we be able to consider a true human being?

Technological advances have been so rapid that none of these questions are idle fancies any longer. But both the scientific community and large sections of the public are sensitive to the potential risks of test-tube conception, and it is being treated with extreme caution—so far.

abortion. During pregnancy, the developing fetus can be harmed by many external agents, which usually reach it via the mother's bloodstream. If the mother smokes or drinks alcohol excessively, takes even relatively harmless drugs, is X-rayed, does not eat properly, or is otherwise unhealthy, her developing child can be killed, stunted, or severely deformed. The frequency of congenital defects generally increases with the age of the mother.

Some of the most common congenital defects are deafness, microcephaly (an abnormally small head and brain), and spastic cerebral palsy, which may be caused by almost any injury to the brain before or at birth.

Timing is a crucial factor in determining whether an abnormality will appear and what it will be. Each body organ develops according to its own timetable, and if some external agent disturbs that schedule, an organ may never be able to develop fully. If development is interrupted between the seventh and tenth weeks of pregnancy, for instance, when the inner ear is being formed, the child may be born deaf.

In recent years, physicians have realized more and more that almost every substance taken by a pregnant woman can cross the placenta and enter the fetus—and that substances harmless to the mother can do great damage to the fetus. Doctors used to treat women who were threatening to miscarry with a synthetic estrogen called diethylstilbesterol (DES). Then, in the early 1970s, researchers discovered that DES taken during pregnancy was associated with the occurrence—many years later—of cancer of the vagina or cervix in daughters born of such pregnancies. The risk is estimated at about 1 in 1,000 exposures. Abnormalities of the urinary and sex organs have also been reported in sons of such pregnancies. The Food and Drug Administration advises that pregnant women should *never* take estrogens or progestogens.

The tragedy caused by the drug thalidomide is another example of the serious effects that can be caused to unborn babies by what was thought to be a harmless drug. Thousands of women in Germany and other countries abroad took the prescription drug, a mild tranquilizer, during the first few months of pregnancy. As a result, more than 8,000 children were born with *phocomelia,* a condition in which the arms and legs are stunted. Physicians recommend that mothers-to-be not take *any* unnecessary drugs (including over-the-counter drugs) during the first three months of pregnancy, when the embryo is particularly prone to congenital damage.

Excessive use of alcohol, too, can harm an unborn baby. The alcohol a mother drinks reaches the developing fetus in concentrations as high as those in her own body but because the fetus's liver is not yet mature, it cannot get rid of the alcohol as readily. Alcohol can affect a fetus very early in pregnancy and can cause a pattern of birth defects, called *fetal alcohol syndrome,* that includes stunted growth, deformation of the heart, limbs, and face, and, often, mental retardation. The Public Health Service recommends that pregnant women drink no more than the equivalent of two glasses of wine a day (see Chapter 12).

The Public Health Service also advises that pregnant women stop smoking. Mothers who smoke have twice as many spontaneous abortions and stillbirths as nonsmokers and two to three times as many premature babies. Furthermore, babies born to women who smoke during pregnancy are, on the average, 200 grams lighter than babies born to comparable women who do not smoke (see Chapter 13).

Rubella, or German measles, is another proven cause of birth defects. The disease is

The mother got over her rubella in three days.
Unfortunately, her unborn child didn't.

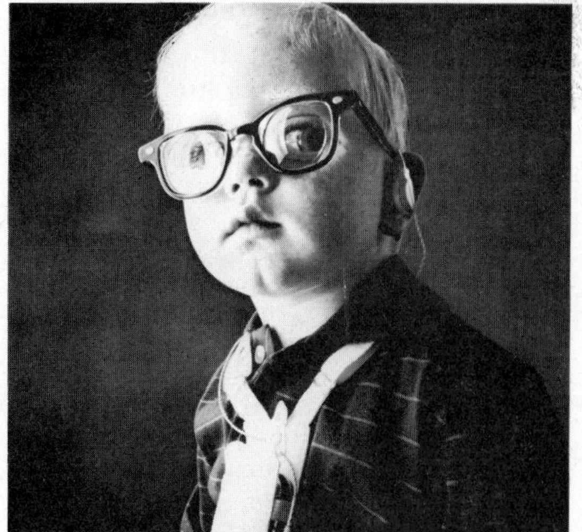

To pregnant mothers, rubella (German measles) means a few days in bed, a sore throat, a runny nose, temperature, and a rash.

But if they're in their first month when they catch it, there's a 40% chance that to their unborn babies it can mean deafness, or a heart condition, or brain damage, or cataracts which cause at least partial blindness.

Only last year, an immunization against rubella became available. But when a pregnant mother gets immunized, the prevention may be as harmful to her baby as the disease.

So if unborn babies are going to be protected, it will have to be by inoculating the kids who infect the mothers who in turn infect the fetuses.

And it will have to be done now.

You see, rubella epidemics break out every six to nine years. The last outbreak was in 1964. Which means the next one is due any day now.

In the last epidemic, 20,000 babies were deprived of a normal childhood—and 30,000 more deprived of any childhood at all—because no immunization existed.

It would be unforgivable if the same thing happened again because an immunization existed and nobody used it.

Metropolitan Life

We sell life insurance.
But our business is life.

For a free booklet about immunization, write One Madison Avenue, N.Y., N.Y. 10010.

relatively harmless to children and adults, but when it occurs in women during the first three months of pregnancy, it can be disastrous to the unborn child. In the last great rubella epidemic in the United States, in the early 1960s, some 20,000 children were born with birth defects including blindness, deafness, limb abnormalities, and mental retardation. About 30,000 more were lost by spontaneous abortions or stillbirths.

Syphilis in an expectant mother can cause abortion or stillbirth, or blindness, deafness, or other defects in her baby. Congenital blindness can also result from *gonorrhea* or *herpes simplex Type 2* in a pregnant woman (see Chapter 14).

GENETIC DISEASES

Hereditary traits are normally passed unchanged from generation to generation by *genes* in the male sperm and the female egg that fuse to form a zygote—ultimately the newborn baby. Most *genetic diseases* are the result of a *mutation*—a spontaneous change in the molecular structure of a specific gene. A mutation can be passed on for generations; in most cases, it will not manifest itself because the corresponding gene from the other parent is normal. However, if *both* parents carry the mutant gene, the defect will appear. Genetic diseases thus often occur in families of parents who are either closely related or members of the same ethnic group.

Some 2,000 specific genetic diseases have been identified so far. Most of them are extremely rare, but in the aggregate, they are a significant health problem. Genetic diseases affect 3 to 5 out of every 100 newborn babies (some 90,000 to 150,000 babies a year in the United States) and are a major cause of mental retardation.

Sickle-Cell Anemia

The hemoglobin in red blood cells is one of the most important proteins in the body, for it delivers oxygen to the body's cells and helps dispose of waste carbon dioxide. There are about eighty known hemoglobin abnormalities that result from some flaw in a gene involved in the manufacture of this vital protein. One of the best known is *sickle-cell anemia,* a genetic disease that probably originated in Africa. About 8 to 10 percent of North America's 20 million blacks carry one sickle-cell gene, and about 1 percent carry two of them.

In sickle-cell anemia, the red blood cells have a characteristic sickle or crescent shape (see Figure 4.9). These clog up the fine capillaries of the circulatory system, cutting off the oxygen supply to the tissues and causing tissue damage and severe muscle and joint pain. The disease is complicated by the action of the spleen, which destroys the abnormal sickle cells faster than the body can replace them—resulting in severe anemia. Other symptoms are weakness, general lassitude, poor physical development, pneumonia, and kidney failure.

This disease occurs only in people who have inherited *two* defective sickle-cell genes. People who have one sickle-cell gene and one normal gene have an approximately fifty-fifty mixture of the normal and abnormal types of hemoglobin in their blood. A person with one sickle-cell gene is said to carry the sickle-cell "trait" and can lead a relatively normal life. However, if such a person goes to high altitudes, where there is less oxygen in the air, he or she can become seriously ill or die. On the other hand, the single sickle-cell gene seems to protect a carrier against malaria—a distinct advantage in the part of the world where the gene is thought to have originated.

Figure 4.9 The red blood cells of people afflicted by sickle-cell anemia have a characteristic sickle or crescent shape.

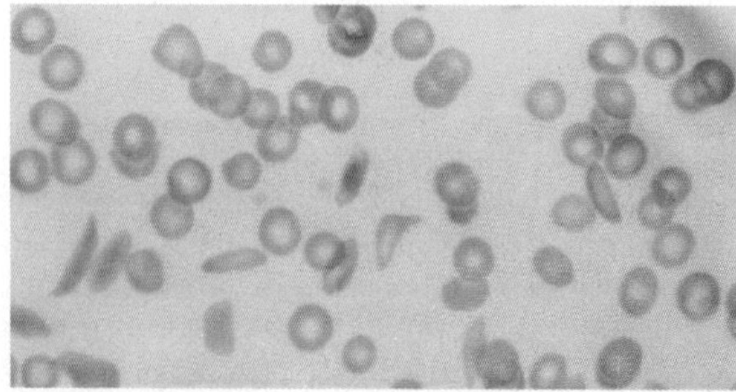

Phenylketonuria (PKU)

Many genetic diseases are caused by a gene mutation that results in a vital enzyme either being produced in an abnormal form or not being produced at all. One of the best known of these disorders is phenylketonuria, or PKU, which occurs about once in every 10,000 births. PKU victims totally lack an enzyme called *phenylalanine-hydroxylase.* This enzyme is necessary for the metabolism of the essential amino acid phenylalanine, which is common in food. Since PKU victims cannot break down phenylalanine and use it, it accumulates in their body, causing massive damage. The chief symptom is severe and irreversible mental retardation; most victims have an average IQ of about 50. Other symptoms are abnormal brain-wave patterns, epileptic seizures, skin disorders such as eczema, and a decrease in the normal pigmentation of hair, eyes, and skin.

PKU occurs when a person inherits the defective gene from both parents. People who inherit the defective gene from only one parent are able to manufacture about half the normal amount of the phenylalanine-hydroxylase enzyme, which seems to be sufficient.

In 1960, a diagnostic blood test was devised that made it possible to detect PKU soon after birth. Many states have now made this test mandatory for all newborn babies, and hospitals in every state have facilities for performing the test. This testing program has shown that PKU disease is twice as prevalent as was previously believed. More importantly, it has permitted many PKU children to lead their lives with normal or near-normal intelligence. The early detection of the disease makes it possible to control the amount of phenylalanine in the child's diet and thus prevent or slow down the course of the disease.

Lipid Storage Diseases

Another important group of genetic defects are the lipid storage diseases. In these disorders, the genetic defect interferes with the metabolism of fatty substances known as *sphingolipids.* These substances and their products thus accumulate in various body tissues, including the brain. Among these disorders are Fabry's disease, Niemann-Pick disease, Gaucher's disease, and Tay-Sachs disease.

Tay-Sachs disease is due to the genetic absence of an enzyme called hexoseaminidase A (Hex A). The resulting accumulation of sphingolipids causes blindness, convulsions, paralysis, and mental degeneration. Afflicted children inevitably die before the age of seven.

As with a number of other defective genes, the Tay-Sachs gene is largely restricted to a fairly well-defined group of people: Jews whose ancestors lived on the Russian-Polish border. The subsequent migrations of these people have spread the defective gene to many other countries. Of the people with Tay-Sachs disease, 99 percent are descendants of this group of people. More than 90 percent of American Jews have this ancestry, and each year between 100 and 200 children are born with this disease in the United States.

A blood test can easily detect Tay-Sachs carriers, who—with only one normal gene—have only about half the normal amount of Hex A in their blood.

Sex-Linked Genetic Diseases

There are a number of *sex-linked* genetic disorders that occur more frequently in men than in women because of the difference between male and female sex chromosomes.* One of the most famous is *hemophilia,* the "bleeder's" disease. In classical hemophilia, or hemophilia A, the body is unable to adequately synthesize "antihemophilic globulin," which is necessary for effective and rapid clotting of the blood. Because of this deficiency, injury or physical stress results in excessive bleeding.

A man who has hemophilia passes on the defective gene to all his daughters. However, he cannot transmit either the disease or the gene to any of his sons. His children will have normal blood, but his daughters will all be carriers. A woman who is a carrier runs a fifty-fifty chance of passing on hemophilia to each of her

*A *chromosome* is a complex structure that contains many, many genes. Normal human beings have forty-six chromosomes, or twenty-three pairs. One chromosome in each pair derives from the mother, the other from the father. The sex chromosomes, which determine gender, constitute one of these pairs.

children. There is a fifty-fifty chance that each son will have hemophilia and a fifty-fifty chance that each daughter will be a carrier. (Women who have hemophilia are extremely rare, since they must inherit the bad gene from both parents.) Thus hemophilia will usually skip a generation. A man who has it transmits the gene to a daughter (who is a carrier but does not have the disease) and, through her, possibly to some of his grandsons.

Another sex-linked, defective gene is involved in red-green *color blindness* (which is actually a group of diseases). The pattern of inheritance works exactly like that of hemophilia. If a color-blind man marries a normal woman, all their children appear normal, but their daughters are all carriers. If a color-blind woman (who must have inherited the defective gene from both parents) marries a normal man, all their sons will be color-blind, and all their daughters will appear normal but will be carriers. A color-blind female can be born only to a color-blind father and either a carrier or color-blind mother.

Down's Syndrome

About 1 in approximately 600 babies is born with *Down's syndrome,* also known as *mongolism.* It is caused by a mutation in either the sperm or the egg that creates an extra number twenty-one chromosome. The child is born

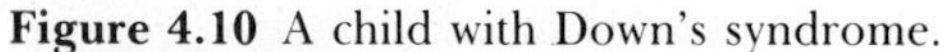

Figure 4.10 A child with Down's syndrome.

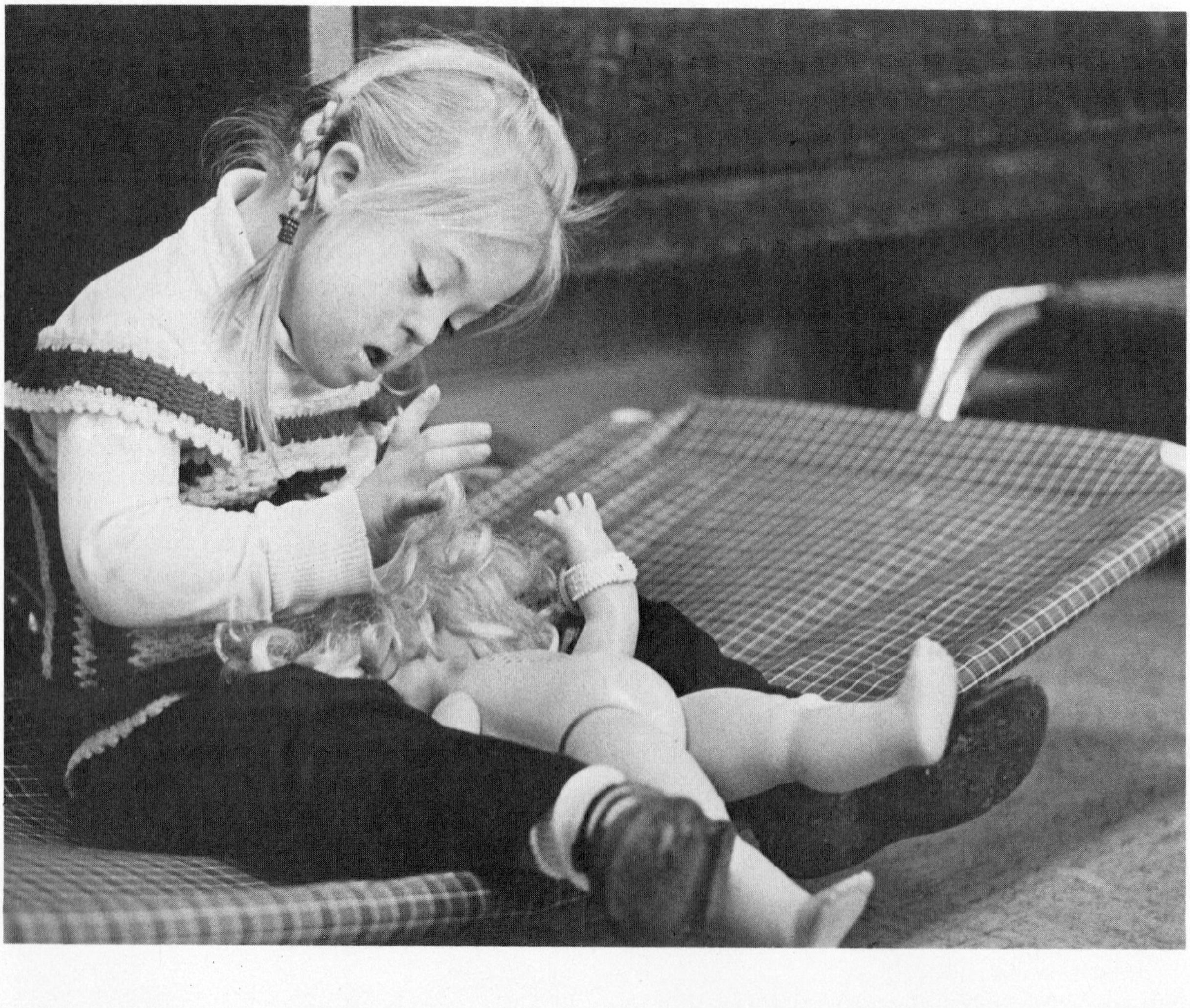

with physical abnormalities that affect almost every part of the body. The face has a characteristic mongoloid look; the torso and extremities may be shorter than normal; and the child is mentally retarded. In fact, Down's syndrome is the single most common cause of mental retardation.

Women over the age of thirty-five are much more likely to produce defective eggs that cause Down's syndrome than are younger mothers. The number of previous pregnancies and the age of the father do not seem to be relevant. For a mother younger than thirty, the odds of having a mongoloid baby are only 1 in 3,000, but for a woman over forty-four, the odds are 1 in 44.

GENETIC COUNSELING

As of now, there are *treatments* available for some genetic diseases. A special diet, as mentioned above, can help reduce the damage of PKU disease. The hormone insulin can alleviate diabetes, and for hemophilia, injections of the missing clotting factor can help control the bleeding. For the foreseeable future, however, the best that can be done for most genetic diseases is *prevention* by means of *genetic counseling* and *prenatal diagnosis.*

Genetic counselors can explain to prospective parents how a particular disorder is transmitted from generation to generation, what the odds are of the disease recurring in their family, and what the disease itself is like. In diseases like Tay-Sachs and sickle-cell anemia, for instance, parents who are carriers have a 25 percent chance of having an affected child with each pregnancy. Another factor prospective

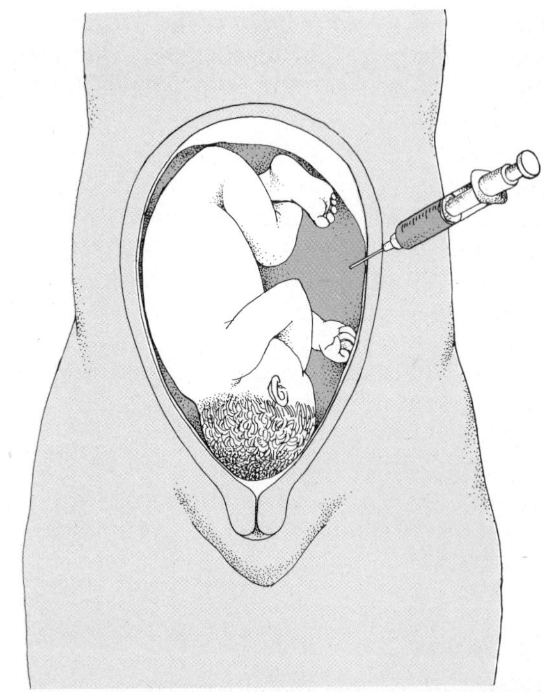

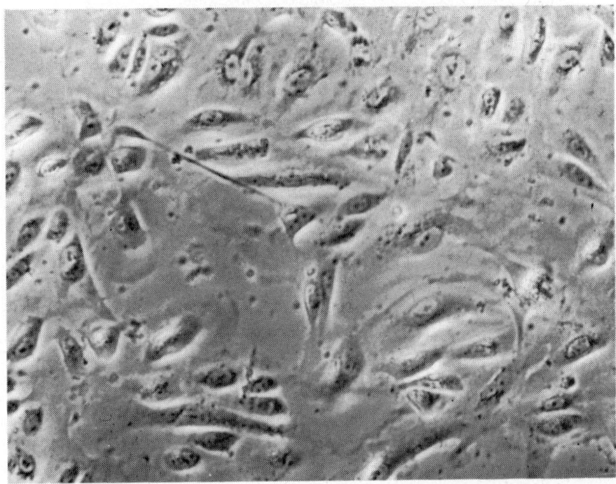

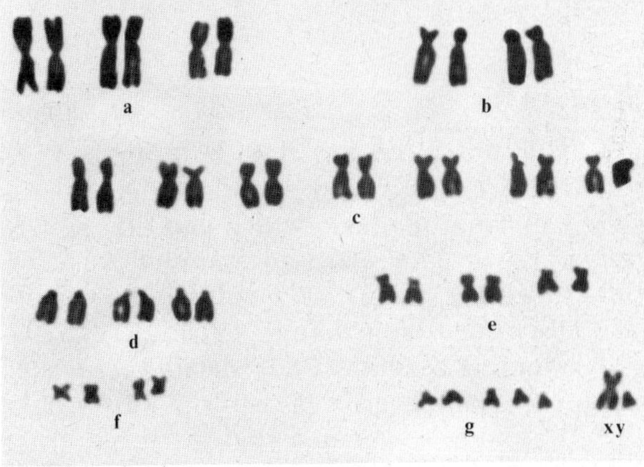

Figure 4.11 Amniocentesis. *(Top)* A sterile needle is inserted through the body and uterine walls into the amniotic cavity surrounding the fetus, taking care to avoid the placenta. A small sample of fluid is withdrawn. This fluid contains cells from the skin and lungs of the fetus. *(Center)* These cells can then be grown and studied in the laboratory to determine whether they possess the biochemical abnormalities associated with any particular genetic disease. The cells are also examined for chromosomal abnormalities such as Down's syndrome *(Bottom),* in which there is an extra chromosome in the twenty-first pair.

parents should consider is the fact that these genetic diseases vary in their severity. Cleft lip and palate is a genetic defect that can usually be repaired by surgery, while Down's syndrome is a lifelong sentence of mental retardation.

It is now possible to test a developing fetus directly for about one hundred genetic disorders as early as the fourth month of pregnancy. In a procedure called *amniocentesis,* a doctor can withdraw some of the amniotic fluid that surrounds a fetus in the womb. Laboratory tests of the fluid can then determine whether the fetus has one of these diseases. For Tay-Sachs disease, the cells in the fluid are tested for the Hex A enzyme. The sex of the unborn child can be determined—important in such sex-linked disorders as hemophilia. And an analysis of the fetus's chromosomes will show whether or not it has Down's syndrome or other chromosomal abnormalities.

Such tests are usually performed only if there is some reason to suspect that the unborn child may have a particular disease—that is, if the parents have already had one defective child or are known to be carriers of the disease. In the case of a few of these diseases—Rh disease, for one—treatments can begin before birth. Otherwise, the prospective parents have the option of considering a therapeutic abortion to prevent the birth of the defective baby. Doctors generally recommend that any pregnant woman over the age of thirty-five—whether or not she has any reason to suspect the presence of a genetic disease in her family—should consider amniocentesis.

SUMMARY

1. Human sperm are tiny, tadpolelike cells that are produced in the testes by a process called spermatogenesis, which may take seventy-five days. The prostate, seminal vesicles, bulbourethral glands, and epididymis secrete and store the seminal fluid. A single ejaculation contains several hundred million sperm.

2. To fertilize an egg, sperm must make their way into a woman's vagina, through her cervix and uterus, and into her Fallopian tubes or oviducts.

3. Human eggs, or ova, are produced in the ovaries in a process called ovulation. Women are born with a full set of egg cells. Each month one or more ripens and is released into a Fallopian tube, where it may be fertilized by a sperm to form a zygote.

4. Menopause in women is the cessation of menstruation and of cyclical reproductive activity. The average age of occurrence is fifty.

5. After fertilization, the zygote travels down the tube and implants itself in the endometrium of the uterus. Cells from the uterus and the embryo differentiate into the placenta, which nourishes the developing fetus for the next nine months.

6. A mother-to-be should get regular medical checkups every three or four weeks in early pregnancy and more often during the last two months. The physician will do blood and urine tests (including those for German measles and Rh factor), monitor blood pressure and weight changes, and spot possible complications.

7. Childbirth begins with labor contractions of the uterus that press the baby's head against the cervix, until it dilates enough for the baby's head to pass through. Once the head is in the vagina, the mother feels a compulsion to bear down and expel the baby.

8. Once the umbilical cord is cut, the newborn is quickly assessed for breathing, muscle tone, heart rate, reflexes, irritability, and color to determine whether it needs further medical help.

9. Breast feeding is beneficial, physiologically and psychologically, for both mothers and babies. It helps mothers regain their figures after pregnancy, and it provides babies with greater resistance to infection.

10. Recent medical advances can help many of the 10 to 15 percent of couples who have trouble having children. One-third of the time, the husband has an anatomical or physiological defect; this can often be determined by a simple test. In women, the problem is sometimes more complicated to diagnose.

11. Children may be born with congenital defects. A developing fetus can be harmed if the mother smokes or drinks alcohol excessively,

takes certain drugs, is X-rayed, does not eat properly, or has certain diseases. Injury before or during birth can also cause birth defects.

12. Genetic mistakes, called mutations, are responsible for a large number of genetic diseases, which affect three to five out of every one hundred newborn babies.

13. Among the most common genetic diseases are sickle-cell anemia, PKU, and Tay-Sachs disease. Hemophilia, the "bleeder's" disease, is a sex-linked genetic disorder.

14. While there are treatments available for some genetic diseases, others can be prevented only by means of genetic counseling and prenatal diagnosis. About a hundred genetic diseases can be diagnosed before birth by means of amniocentesis. Parents then have the option of considering a therapeutic abortion.

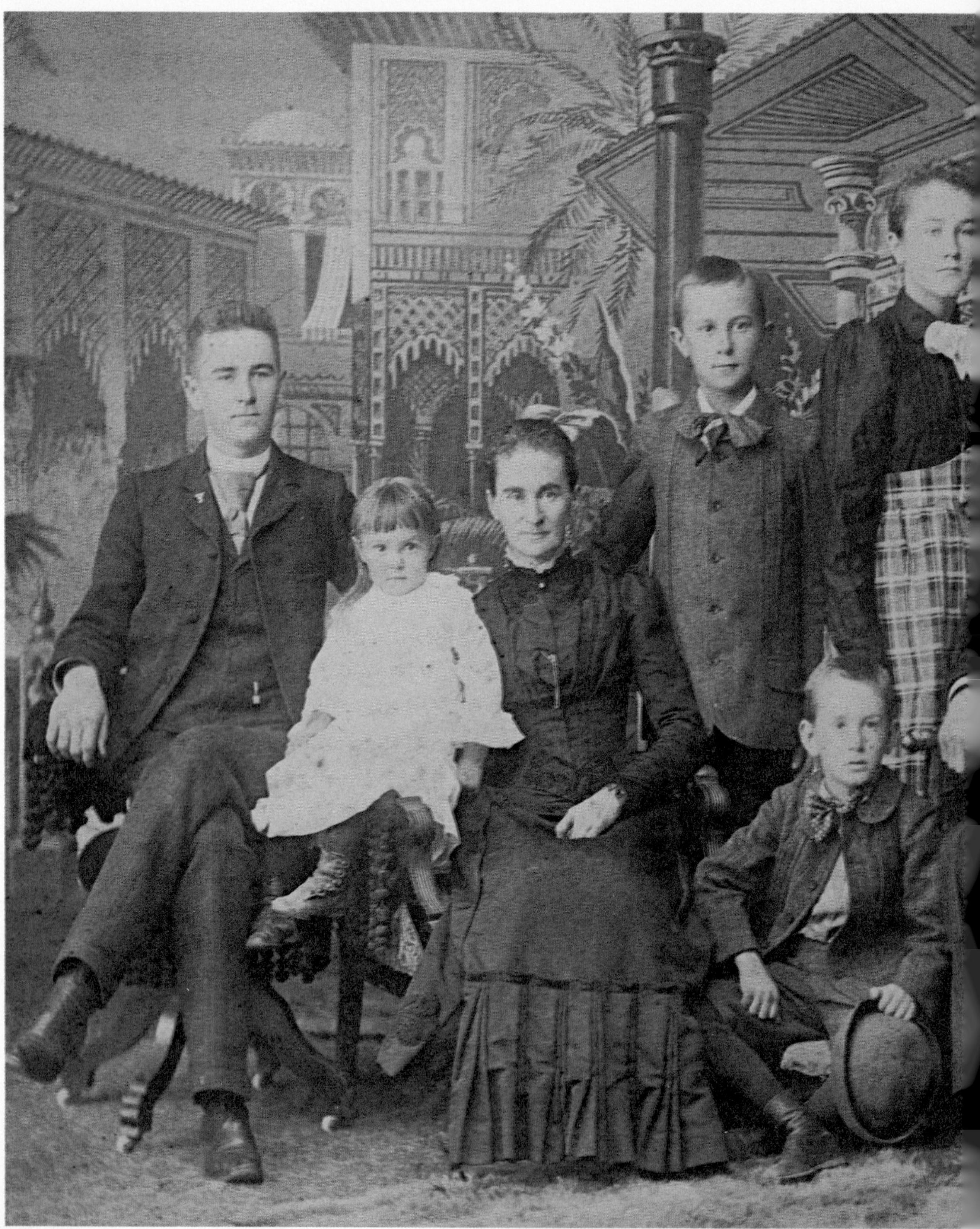

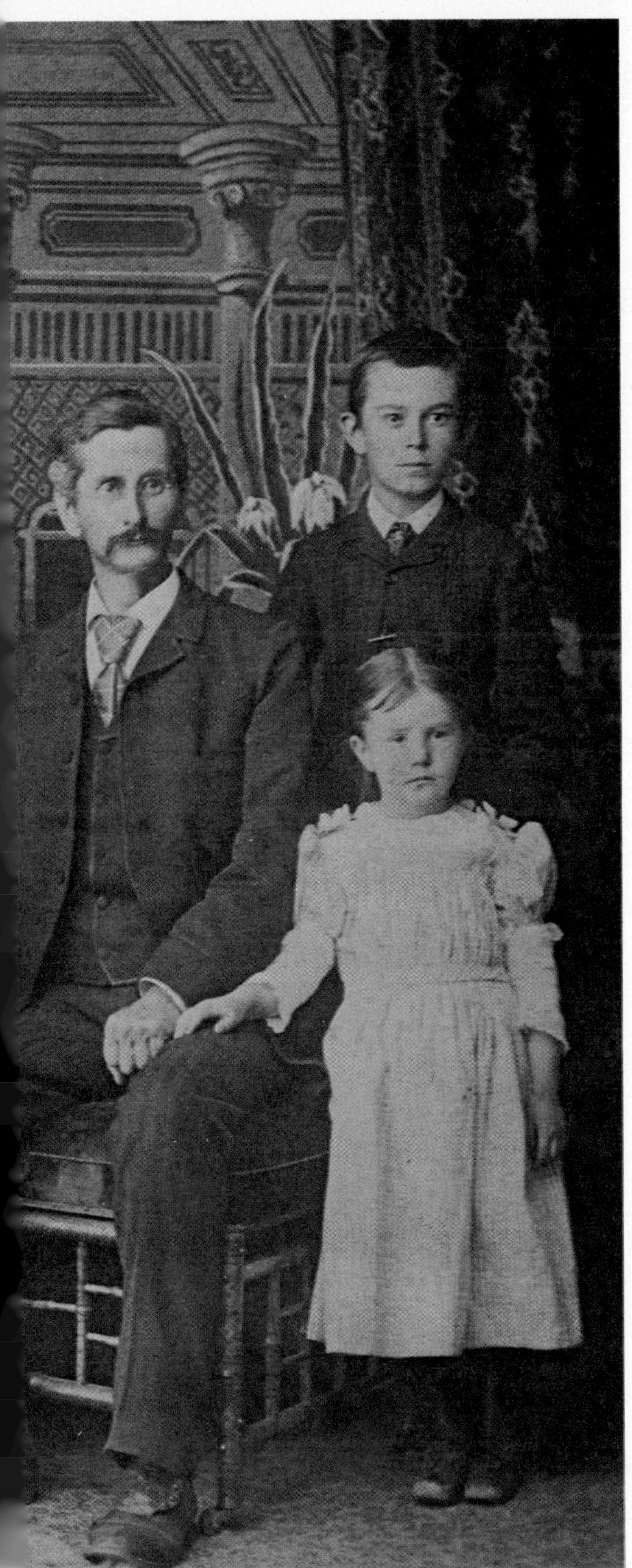

5 Birth Control

Sexual intercourse is not only a reproductive act but an expression of love. If every mating were to produce a child, the world would be overpopulated beyond our wildest imagination. In fact, the likelihood that pregnancy will result from a given act of intercourse is only 2–4 percent (the probability increases dramatically during the two days preceding ovulation, and there is a 50 percent chance of conception on the day of ovulation). We are thus provided with some degree of natural birth control.

However, since prehistoric times people have realized that this innate birth-control mechanism is both inadequate and unreliable. Societies all over the world and throughout history have tried an incredible variety of materials, devices, and techniques in order to guarantee that unwanted pregnancies will not occur. Most of these methods have been ineffective, if not downright hazardous, and some peoples have resorted to infanticide—the murder of newborn babies—to limit their populations.

In the United States today we are luckier. Thanks to modern medicine and technology, we have an array of birth-control methods that are relatively safe and effective, though not foolproof. As a result, prospective parents have the option to plan and space their families in accordance with their own personal goals. On an international level, modern birth-control methods have helped to stem the tide of rampant population growth in many parts of the world.

FAMILY PLANNING AND CHILD SPACING

Family planning means voluntary determination of the number and spacing of children in order to achieve the size family a couple desires *when* they desire it. Included in the concept of family planning is free choice of the method(s) used to accomplish these goals. Depending upon background and religion, the spectrum of available methods ranges from abstinence to abortion.

What factors should a couple consider when planning to have children? Certainly, maternal health should be a major consideration. There are health risks involved in pregnancy, including the chance of death. These risks are relative and depend on the level of health care available, the woman's general health, her genetic characteristics, and her life style. Although the chance of death is small, it is greater than the risks involved in the use of any medically supervised birth-control method, including oral contraceptives and abortion.

The child's health is another factor to consider. Women at the beginning and near the last third of their reproductive years (under seventeen and over thirty-five years of age) have a much greater chance of producing children with serious health defects. By timing births to avoid both ends of the age spectrum or by relying on prenatal diagnostic techniques (see Chapter 4), couples can reduce the chance of a baby's dying before, during, or just after birth; reduce the risk of serious genetic defects in the child; and help prevent a premature birth, which can seriously jeopardize a child's physical and mental development.

Economic factors should also be considered. It is estimated that it will cost a middle-class American family some forty to fifty thousand dollars (in 1978 dollars) to rear a child from birth through high school graduation. Personal maturity and life goals and preferences should also enter into the decision. It has been found, for example, that teen-age marriages are often burdened by children conceived before marriage and are characterized by more personal dissatisfaction, lower economic level, higher infant and child accident rates, higher child-abuse rates, and higher divorce rates than are marriages at older ages.

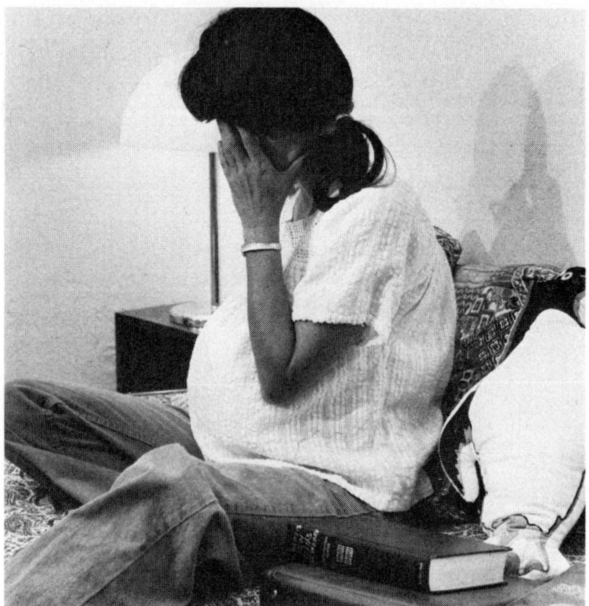

Figure 5.1 Adolescence is a stress period when an unwanted pregnancy is likely to occur.

Couples are increasingly choosing to delay having children until they fulfill other goals or until they make a decision not to have children at all. Family and social pressures to have children are not as strong as they once were, and childless couples are no longer stigmatized. Couples should examine their own preferences before making the major decisions on the number and spacing of their children.

USE AND MISUSE OF CONTRACEPTION

Workers in the field of birth control thought for some time that the answer to effective family planning was to be found in good, easy-to-obtain contraceptive methods. Although good methods and accurate information are essential, it turns out that they are not the whole answer. As Figure 5.2 shows, for many methods there is a significant difference between theoretical effectiveness and use effectiveness. In other words, human error is a huge factor in determining the effectiveness of any birth-control method.

What are some of the psychological factors involved? For many people, ambivalent feelings about sexuality and reproduction may be operating, consciously or unconsciously. Misinformed and naive beliefs about conception are also often involved. Some women believe they can feel ovulation and that they cannot conceive except at this time. Some people believe that only the first ejaculation in any one sexual encounter can cause pregnancy, or that pregnancy cannot occur unless the woman has an orgasm, or that intercourse with the woman on top is safe. Such erroneous beliefs have resulted in a great many unwanted pregnancies.

Researchers have found that contraceptive effectiveness is related to the *intent* of the couple. For example, couples *limiting* their families appear to have greater success in the use of contraception than those *spacing* their families. These findings suggest that motivation can significantly influence the outcome of contraceptive use.

Warren Miller has outlined certain changes and stress periods in women's lives that can lead to unwanted pregnancy. These critical periods include early adolescence, when fertility is just being established and may be variable; the beginning of sexual activity, before the woman has had a chance to consider the issues involved; the beginning or near the end of or during conflict in a sexual relationship; periods of change such as moving to a new community or leaving home for college, work, or other reasons; after a pregnancy; and around the time of menopause.

In order to avoid unwanted pregnancies, it would be valuable to consider the following guidelines for selecting birth-control methods and for increasing their effectiveness.

1. Recognize that no matter how effective birth-control methods are in theory, in order to be effective in practice they must be used during all acts of coitus.
2. Understand how and why the method works. Understand how to use the method correctly. Ask all your questions and keep asking until you get the answers you need.
3. Know yourself. How do you feel about the various methods? Which method seems the best for you? Is this a method you can and will use exactly as instructed for all sexual intercourse?
4. Be prepared to select alternate methods as your life changes (as with the birth of a child, a change in partners, or the approach of menopause).

METHODS REQUIRING NO MEDICAL CARE

Of the various contraceptive and birth-control methods available, those that do not require medical care are withdrawal; condoms; spermicidal jellies, creams, and foams; vaginal suppositories; and douching.

Withdrawal (Coitus Interruptus)

Withdrawal is an ancient method. As the name implies, the man withdraws his penis from the vagina prior to ejaculation. The advantage of this method is that it is readily available and costs nothing. However, there are several drawbacks. Although there may be several million sperm in one ejaculation, it takes only one, with the help of a few others, to penetrate and fertilize the egg. A few sperm are usually present in the lubricating fluids emitted from the penis during sexual excitement, prior to ejaculation.

In addition, both partners must have a great deal of will power to use this method satisfactorily. The penis must be completely withdrawn, not only from the vagina but from the external genitals as well, since pregnancy can occur from ejaculation into or on the labia. Finally, the method may create anxiety for one or both partners and may not allow sufficient satisfaction for some people.

Condoms

Condoms are thin rubber or natural skin sheaths placed on the erect penis just prior to intercourse to capture and hold seminal fluid so that sperm will not be deposited in the vagina.

The condom has been widely used throughout the world for centuries. Condoms cause no harmful physical side effects, and they are the only form of contraception that definitely aids in preventing the spread of sexually transmitted diseases. With the present epidemic of sexually transmitted diseases (see Chapter 14), this is an important consideration for men and women who are sexually active with persons who may be infected.

Condoms are available in drugstores and in some college bookstores, as well as in vending

	STERILIZATION	THE PILL	INTRAUTERINE DEVICE (IUD)	CONDOM
How it works	Permanently blocks egg or sperm passages	Prevents ovulation	Uncertain: may stop implantation of egg	Prevents sperm from entering vagina
Medical care required	Operation	Prescription and periodic checkups	Insertion and periodic checkups	None
Theoretical failure rate	Hysterectomy: 0.0001 Tubal ligation: 0.04 Vasectomy: less than 0.15	Combination pill: less than 1.0	1–5	Alone: 3 With foam: 1
Actual use failure rate	Hysterectomy: 0.0001 Tubal ligation: 0.04 Vasectomy: 0.15	2–5	6	Alone: 15–20 With foam: 5

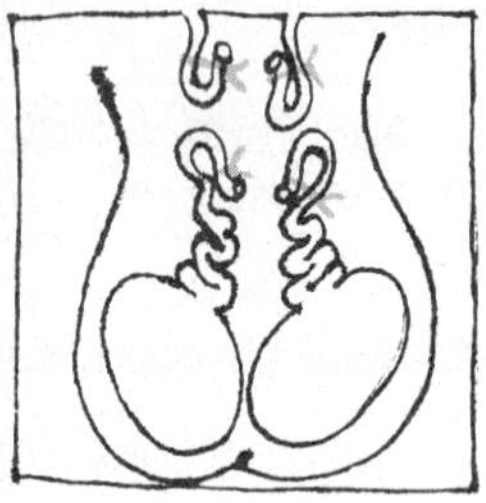

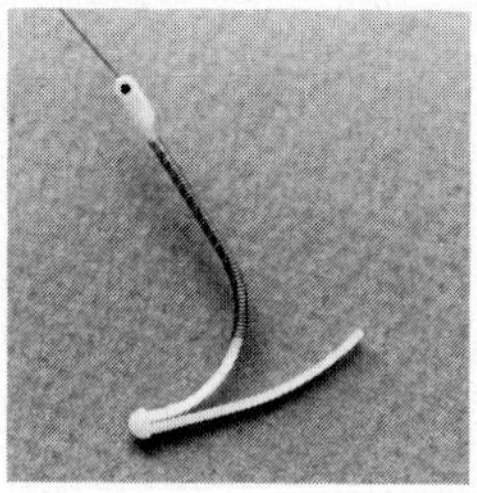

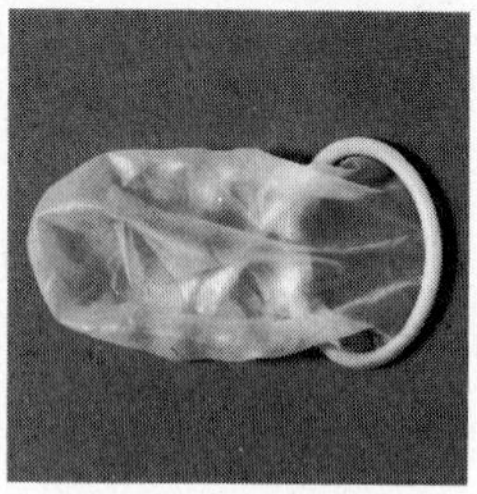

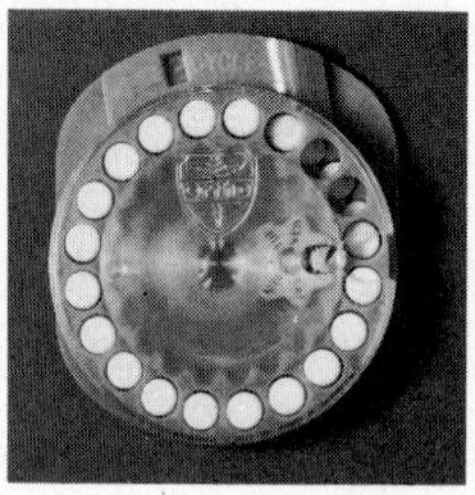

Figure 5.2 A comparison chart of various methods of birth control. Failure rates refer to the number of pregnancies per year for every 100 couples using the method.

machines in some states. Condoms come in one size and are packaged in quantities ranging from three to twelve per box. Some have reservoir ends, some are prelubricated, and prices vary. Price, however, is unrelated to effectiveness, since all condoms must by law meet the same high standards. Any additional lubricant used with condoms should be saliva or a water-soluble lubricant; petroleum jelly should never be used, because it causes deterioration of the condom and may remain in the vagina, promoting the growth of irritating bacteria.

Some individuals object to using the con-

DIAPHRAGM WITH CHEMICAL	FOAMS AND JELLIES	WITHDRAWAL	RHYTHM	DOUCHE
	PRECEPTIN CONTRACEPTIVE GEL		1 2 3 4 5 6 7 / 8 9 10 11 12 13 14 / 15 16 17 18 19 20 21 / 22 23 24 25 26 27 28 / 29 30 31	
·arrier to sperm	Barrier to sperm; spermicidal	Ejaculation occurs outside the vagina	Abstinence during fertile period	Rinses sperm from vagina
·itting	None	None	Consultation	None
	3	15	Calendar method: 15	80 (same as chance)
·–25	30	20–25	35	80

dom on the grounds that it diminishes sensation for them. For others, use of the condom results in pleasurable prolongation of intercourse. Some couples consider the putting on of the condom to be an interference, while others consider it an integral part of their sexual activity.

The condom is the leading mechanical method of birth control in the world. The importance of its easy accessibility and great effectiveness, especially when used in combination with vaginal foam, should not be underestimated; it is as effective as the IUD, when used with foam.

Foams, Creams, and Jellies

Vaginal spermicides are nonprescription foams, creams, or jellies that are inserted into the vagina against the cervix with a plastic applicator; they act by destroying sperm. There are no harmful side effects with this method, with the possible exception of rare allergic reactions that usually can be remedied by changing brands. The container of foam must be shaken well. Two applications are recommended, no more than fifteen minutes before each intercourse.

The new foams are potentially far more effective than the failure rate would indicate. Improper use is the cause of this discrepancy. The foam may be applied too long before coitus or too close to the vaginal opening instead of against the cervix; it may be applied too late or after coitus; it may be applied only once and expected to last through repeated coitus; or the supply may run out and the couple decide to take a chance. Furthermore, the woman may douche too soon after intercourse (less than six or eight hours), thereby washing away the protection. All these errors affect the failure rate. Like the condom, vaginal foam is especially useful for individuals who require a portable, simple, inexpensive, nonmedical method that can be used as often or as seldom as coitus takes place.

Spermicides used in conjunction with a condom are notably more effective than is either method alone. One advantage of combining the two methods is that both partners share the responsibility for birth control.

In addition to vaginal foams, creams, and jellies, drugstores also carry vaginal suppositories and tablets containing spermicides. However, these are considerably less effective than the foams, and they have been found to irritate and cause infection of the vagina in some women with continual use. Douching is the least effective method of birth control and cannot be relied upon. It should also be noted that feminine hygiene products, often advertised to help with "intimate problems," have no contraceptive or hygienic value.

METHODS REQUIRING NONSURGICAL MEDICAL CARE

Among the available birth-control methods that require some medical care are oral contraceptives, intrauterine devices, diaphragms, and the rhythm method. Despite technological advances, a foolproof contraceptive does not yet exist.

Oral Contraceptives

Since 1960, when the Food and Drug Administration first approved oral contraceptives for use with a doctor's prescription, well over 10 million prescriptions for them have been written in the United States alone. Through the years, investigation has shown that ovulation can be effectively prevented with much smaller doses of hormones than were originally used, which is fortunate because side effects are directly related to the amount of hormone in the Pill.

The Pill introduces into the body some synthetic equivalents of the natural sex hormones in such a way that the hormone cycle leading to ovulation is altered and ovulation is prevented. Most brands on the market today are "combination" pills; that is, each tablet contains both progestin (a synthetic progesterone derivative) and estrogen.

A consideration in using the Pill is the fact that it must be taken exactly as directed, with no omissions, and stopped while menstruation occurs. If the user forgets even one or two pills, the contraceptive effect may be lost for the cycle (including the menstrual period), and pregnancy may occur. A backup method should be used as a safeguard.

Several attempts have been made to simplify the regimen by having the user take a pill daily. Already on the market are brands containing an estrogen and a progestin for twenty-one days, with seven additional inert pills to be taken during menstruation.

The many serious side effects of the Pill include blood clots, which can impair circulation in the legs and can cause death if they travel to the lungs, heart, or brain. The use of the Pill may double the risk of a heart attack, and Pill users between the ages of fifteen and thirty-four run about an eight times greater risk of death (about 1 in 12,000) due to a circulatory disorder than do non-Pill users. These risks are increased greatly by cigarette smoking, and the Food and Drug Administration now recommends that women who use oral contraceptives should not smoke.

Pill users also run a greater risk of gall bladder disease requiring surgery; benign liver tumors, which can be fatal if they rupture; and high blood pressure. Oral contraceptives should not be taken by pregnant women, because the Pill is associated with a higher risk of birth defects involving the heart and the limbs.

Nevertheless, the oral contraceptives are the most effective method of birth control other than surgical sterilization, and the overall risk of death is low—below that of pregnancy and childbirth itself—except for women who smoke. With all oral contraceptives, continuing medical supervision is necessary in order to minimize these risks and to prescribe the appropriate pill for each woman.

There is also a "mini-Pill" on the market, which contains only progestin and is less effective than the combination pills. It is sometimes suitable for women who cannot tolerate the high hormone content of the Pill.

Intrauterine Devices

The precise mechanism of action of intrauterine devices (IUDs) is still not completely understood. IUDs do not prevent ovulation but seem to interfere in some way with the implantation of the fertilized egg in the lining of the uterus.

IUDs are made of soft, flexible plastic, molded into various sizes and shapes. Some are coated with copper. They are inserted into the uterus. The device should be sterile and should be inserted by a specially trained physician. Insertion and retention of IUDs may cause more discomfort in women who have not borne children than in those who have. Some women select the IUD because it is long-lasting, it need not be put in place every time before intercourse, and it does not alter body chemistry.

About 20 percent of IUDs must be removed because of persistent bleeding or cramps. Another major disadvantage is the high "fall-out" rate. Occasionally, the device may drop out, unnoticed by the user. Although expulsions usually occur during the first few months after insertion, there is a continuing, although low, incidence of loss. This is particularly true of women who have had many babies and in whom the cavity of the uterus is large. Some types of IUDs must be replaced every year or so. In other cases, however, IUDs remain in place indefinitely.

The most common major complication of the IUD is an unwanted pregnancy, which occurs less than 6 times per 100 women per year. Effectiveness may be correlated with size of the device—the larger the device, the fewer the pregnancies. Increased effectiveness is possible through the use of foam around the time ovulation is expected to occur. When pregnancies do occur, the incidence of abortions and pregnancies outside the uterus is higher than expected. If pregnancy is suspected, the device should be removed because of the high abortion rate with devices in place and because of the possibility of intrauterine infection.

Diaphragms

The diaphragm is a shallow rubber cup, the rim of which is a circular metal spring covered with fine latex rubber. The spring can be bent so that the entire device can be compressed and easily passed into the vagina. It is then released in the upper, large portion of the vagina, where it covers the cervix completely.

The purposes of the diaphragm are to prevent the passage of sperm and to hold spermicidal jelly or cream, which must be applied before inserting the diaphragm. The diaphragm is inserted before intercourse and removed six to eight hours afterward.

Because the dimensions of the vagina from the area behind the cervix to the pubic bone vary from woman to woman, diaphragms are available in several sizes. The distance is measured by a health professional and the proper size prescribed. Refitting is essential after each pregnancy and following a loss or gain of ten to fifteen pounds or more.

When the diaphragm is inserted properly, it will cause no discomfort and will not be noticed by the male partner. Improper insertion and use, along with forgetfulness, probably account for the most pregnancies with this method, as they do for many other methods.

Rhythm Method

The basis of the rhythm method is avoidance of coitus during the time when the woman may be ovulating. The success of this approach depends on knowledge of when ovulation will occur, the length of time the sperm remain viable in the female reproductive tract, and the length of time the released ovum is available for fertilization. Although progress is being made, medical science still has much to discover in these areas.

Utilizing the *temperature method,* a woman may try to pinpoint the time of ovulation by charting her basal body temperature daily. Ovulation is followed by a slight temperature rise that lasts until the start of the next menstrual cycle. Although this temperature change is a fairly good indication that ovulation has occurred, only pregnancy is true proof of ovulation. A slight rise in temperature may also be caused by minor colds and infections.

The *calendar method* is based on the observation that a woman usually ovulates around the fourteenth day before her next period. A year's record of menstrual periods is used to indicate the fertile period.

With the rhythm method, a period of abstinence of about a week is suggested to allow for ovulation, the viability of sperm and ovum, and a margin of error. But even a week's abstinence is no insurance, for sperm may remain capable of fertilizing the ovum for seventy-two hours or more after being deposited inside the female genital tract. It is possible, then, for intercourse that takes place two or three days before ovulation to result in pregnancy. Indeed, pregnancies have occurred after a single coitus seven days before apparent ovulation (as indicated by body temperature). If ovulation is early or late, the risks of pregnancy are greatly increased.

There is considerable variation in the length of normal menstrual cycles. To use the rhythm method effectively, medical advice is needed, at least at the beginning, in order to learn how to chart menstrual periods and daily temperatures and to calculate the "safe" and "unsafe" days.

When there is no religious objection, an alternative to abstinence is some other form of birth control, such as the diaphragm or condom in conjunction with a spermicide, around the anticipated time of ovulation.

METHODS REQUIRING SURGERY

Millions of men and women have undergone surgical sterilization. In the male, the standard technique is cutting and tying off the vas deferens, a procedure known as *vasectomy.* This is a minor surgical procedure and can be performed in a doctor's office. In the female, the standard technique is dividing or tying off the Fallopian tubes, an operation called *tubal ligation.* This is an abdominal procedure often requiring hospitalization. A new technique, *laparoscopy,* is now being used to divide the tubes with a small electrode; this method requires a small incision in the abdomen and is sometimes done under local anesthesia as an outpatient procedure. A newer technique utilizes a small plastic clip placed around the tube.

For individuals who are certain that they no longer wish to conceive, voluntary sterilization provides the closest to ideal alternative available today. It is virtually 100 percent effective (failures are due to improper technique or failure to use alternate contraceptions for six weeks following surgery) and seems to have few side effects. The popularity of vasectomy is growing, especially among educated professional families.

The effects of sterilization are usually permanent, though in recent years physicians have been attempting to devise new techniques that make it reversible in some cases. In tubal ligation, the newer plastic-clip technique is more readily reversible than some older methods. In vasectomy, new microsurgical techniques sometimes are able to restore fertility. But generally, physicians recommend, anyone undergoing sterilization should consider it a permanent procedure.

METHODS OF THE FUTURE

Scientists continue to search for better and safer methods of contraception. One line of research is investigating the possibility of injections or implants of long-lasting progestogens. Such injections might last six months to two years, and implants fifteen years or longer, unless they were removed to restore fertility. Other researchers are working on the possibil-

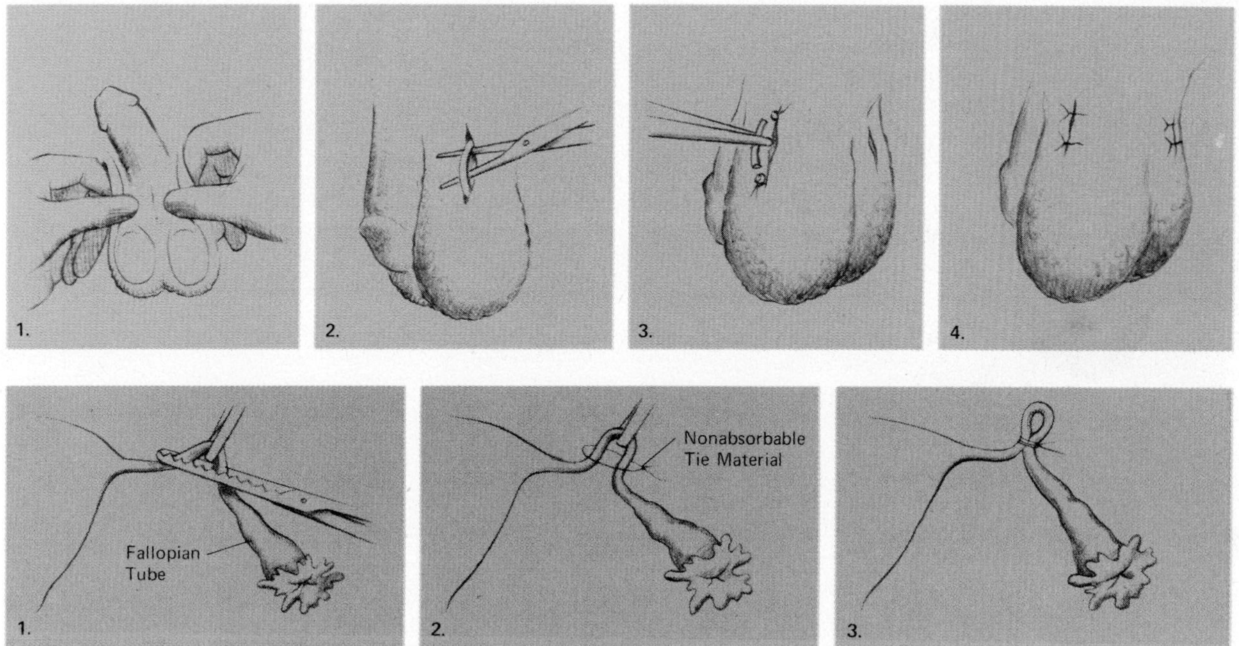

Figure 5.3 Methods of sterilization. *(Top)* Vasectomy. (1) The surgeon feels the upper area of the scrotum to locate the vas deferens. (2) An incision is made and the vas deferens is clamped. (3) A segment is removed. (4) The incision is sutured. This procedure is then repeated on the vas deferens of the other testicle. *(Bottom)* Tubal ligation. This operation is performed on *both* fallopian tubes.

ity of a tampon or suppository, containing prostaglandins, which would be used to induce menstruation each month.

Research is also underway on chemical contraceptives for men. There are many substances known that suppress sperm production but have unacceptable side effects, such as reducing potency and libido or incompatability with alcohol. Nevertheless, some progress is being made. Various combinations of male and female sex hormones and other compounds are being tested in human volunteers, and a male Pill may be on the market within the next ten years.

ABORTION

Medically, *abortion* means ending a pregnancy before the embryo or fetus can survive on its own. Though vigorously opposed by some, the right of a woman to refuse to bear an unwanted child has gradually gained ground in the United States. Public attitudes have begun to change. Factors contributing to this change include recognition that (1) abortion is now a relatively safe medical procedure, (2) early abortion involves fewer risks than pregnancy, (3) even under optimum conditions of correct and consistent use, most birth-control methods can fail on occasion, and (4) millions of dangerous illegal abortions have been taking place, with the poor suffering the worst physical consequences.

In 1973, the Supreme Court ruled that a woman's right to privacy prevailed and that in the first three months of pregnancy the decision whether to have an abortion is up to the woman and her physician. The Court specified further that in subsequent months of pregnancy the states may "regulate the abortion procedures in ways reasonably related to pregnancy" until the last ten weeks, when abortion may be prohibited except when necessary to preserve the health or life of the mother.

In 1977, under tremendous pressure from the antiabortion lobby, Congress passed legis-

THERAPEUTIC METHODS OF ABORTION	DANGEROUS ABORTION TECHNIQUES

THERAPEUTIC METHODS OF ABORTION

Methods used to about the twelfth week of pregnancy

Dilatation and Curretage (D and C) and Suction Curretage

With appropriate instruments the cervix (opening into the uterus) is dilated (stretched) large enough to accommodate forceps, curette (scraper) or suction curette (scraper connected to vacuum pump). The fetus, amnion, and placenta are suctioned or scraped from the uterine cavity. The procedure takes from fifteen to thirty minutes and rarely requires more than a twenty-four-hour stay in the hospital. Discharge is either that evening or the following morning.

Methods used between the twelfth and nineteenth weeks of pregnancy

Hysterotomy (This procedure is similar to a Caesarean Section)

An incision is made through the lower abdomen into the uterine cavity; the fetus and sac are then removed. The length of the hospital stay depends on the nature of recovery – usually five days.

(There is no removal of uterus, tubes, or ovaries. Pregnancies can occur again.)

Saline Induction

A small area of the abdomen is numbed with a local anesthetic such as novocaine. After numbing, a needle is introduced into the amniotic sac, which contains the fetus. Some fluid is withdrawn and a special salt solution is injected. After twenty-four to forty-eight hours the uterus begins to contract. After a variable amount of time the uterus will expel the fetus and placenta. A follow-up curettement (D and C) may be required to remove dead tissue that might cause infection.

DANGEROUS ABORTION TECHNIQUES

Oral Means

Ergot compounds: can cause fatal kidney damage

Quinine sulphate: can cause deformities in fetus or death to mother

Estrogen and castor oil are both useless.

Nothing that is swallowed can cause abortion without also causing death or severe disability to the mother.

Solids Inserted into Uterus

Knitting Needles	Catheters
Coat Hangers	Gauze (packing)
Slippery Elm Bark	Artist Paintbrushes
Chopsticks	Curtain Rods
Ballpoint Pen	Telephone Wire

With all of the above there is the subsequent danger of perforation of uterus and bladder and death from infection or hemorrhage.

Fluids Inserted into Uterus

Soap Suds	Lye
Alcohol	Lysol
Potassium Permanganate	Pine Oil

Administration of any of the above can result in severe burning of tissues, hemorrhage, shock, and death.

Air Pumped into Uterus

Sudden violent death from gas emboli in the bloodstream.

Injections into Uterine Wall

Ergot
Pitocin
Sodium Pentothal

Other Means:

Vacuum cleaner connected to uterus – not to be confused with vacuum aspiration – is fatal almost immediately: extracts uterus from pelvic cavity.

Physical exertion such as lifting heavy objects, running, etc., is useless.

Falling down stairs: severe injury to mother with abortion rarely resulting.

Figure 5.4 Abortion methods. Only specially trained personnel can safely use the four methods of abortion —*all* other methods can cause death but rarely induce abortion.

lation limiting the use of Medicaid funds for abortions. (Medicaid is the federal program that reimburses states for medical care costs for the poor.) The law now permits federal payment for abortions only in the case of rape or incest, or when the woman's life or health is endangered. As a result, poor women are once again turning to practitioners of questionable competence for low cost and dangerous abortions.

The issue of abortion is fraught with controversy over attitudes toward life and death, religion, and morality. For a variety of personal reasons, individuals often have mixed feelings about whether they would choose abortion, even when they are in favor of the option in principle. Similarly, there are those who oppose abortion in principle but nevertheless choose it when faced with the specific personal implications of an undesired pregnancy. And there are others who absolutely oppose abortion and do not sanction its use under any circumstances.

Even among the staunchest supporters of abortion as a free choice, many strongly advocate the use of other birth-control methods as a first course of action, with abortion as a backup measure so that no one is compelled to continue an undesired pregnancy.

Methods of Abortion

Therapeutic abortion during the first twelve weeks of pregnancy is a relatively safe procedure when conducted by a qualified physician. A simple procedure that is used during the first two weeks after a missed menstrual period is *vacuum aspiration* (sometimes called *suction curettage*). It is an office procedure and does not require hospitalization.

An operative procedure known as a "D and C"—dilation of the cervix and curettage (scraping out) of the uterine cavity—is also used up to about the twelfth week. During the past few years, most abortions have been done by dilating the cervix and then aspirating the uterine contents with a vacuum suction apparatus. This procedure is usually followed by a "D and C" to make sure that all products of the conception are removed.

After the twelfth week of pregnancy, abortion is done either by a *hysterotomy,* an operation similar to a Caesarean section and requiring an abdominal incision, or by introducing a salt solution into the uterus via a catheter inserted through the abdominal wall. This latter procedure is called a *saline abortion.*

Illegal nonmedical—and dangerous—abortions have been produced by a variety of techniques employing the insertion of a foreign object into the uterus—rubber catheters, soap solutions, irritating pastes, and various chemicals. Although these agents initiate contractions of the uterus and the expulsion of part of the products of conception, the uterus is usually not completely emptied and infection is common. Soap solutions and pastes may cause immediate death if particles enter the circulation and travel to the lung or brain. The mortality rate from legal medical abortions was 1 death per 100,000 abortions in 1976, according to the Public Health Service. The mortality rates from criminal abortions range, it is estimated, from 100 to 250 deaths per 100,000.

SUMMARY

1. When planning to have a child, a couple should consider factors including maternal health, risks to the child's health, economics, and life goals.
2. Unwanted pregnancies may result from erroneous beliefs and misuse of contraceptives.
3. Methods of birth control that require no medical care include withdrawal, condoms, and vaginal spermicides (foams, creams, and jellies).
4. Birth-control methods that require nonsurgical medical care include oral contraceptives (the Pill), intrauterine devices (IUDs), diaphragms, and the rhythm method.
5. Vasectomy is the standard technique of surgical sterilization for men; for women, the usual operation is tubal ligation.
6. Abortion, which involves terminating a pregnancy before the embryo or fetus can survive on its own, is the focus of an intense legal and moral controversy.
7. Abortion during the first twelve weeks of pregnancy is relatively safe when performed by a qualified physician. After the twelfth week, a hysterotomy or a saline abortion is required. Illegal nonmedical abortions are extremely dangerous.

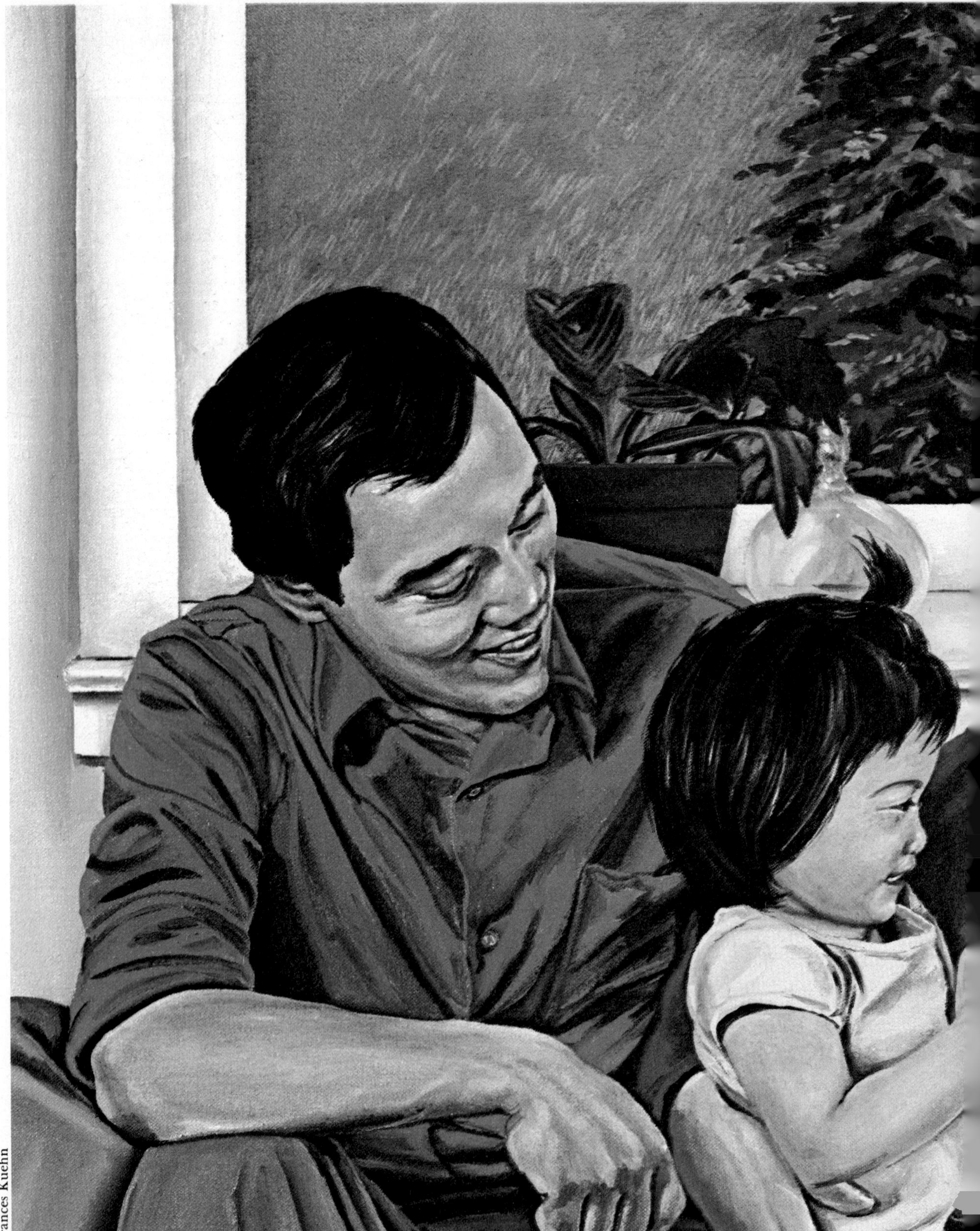

Frances Kuehn

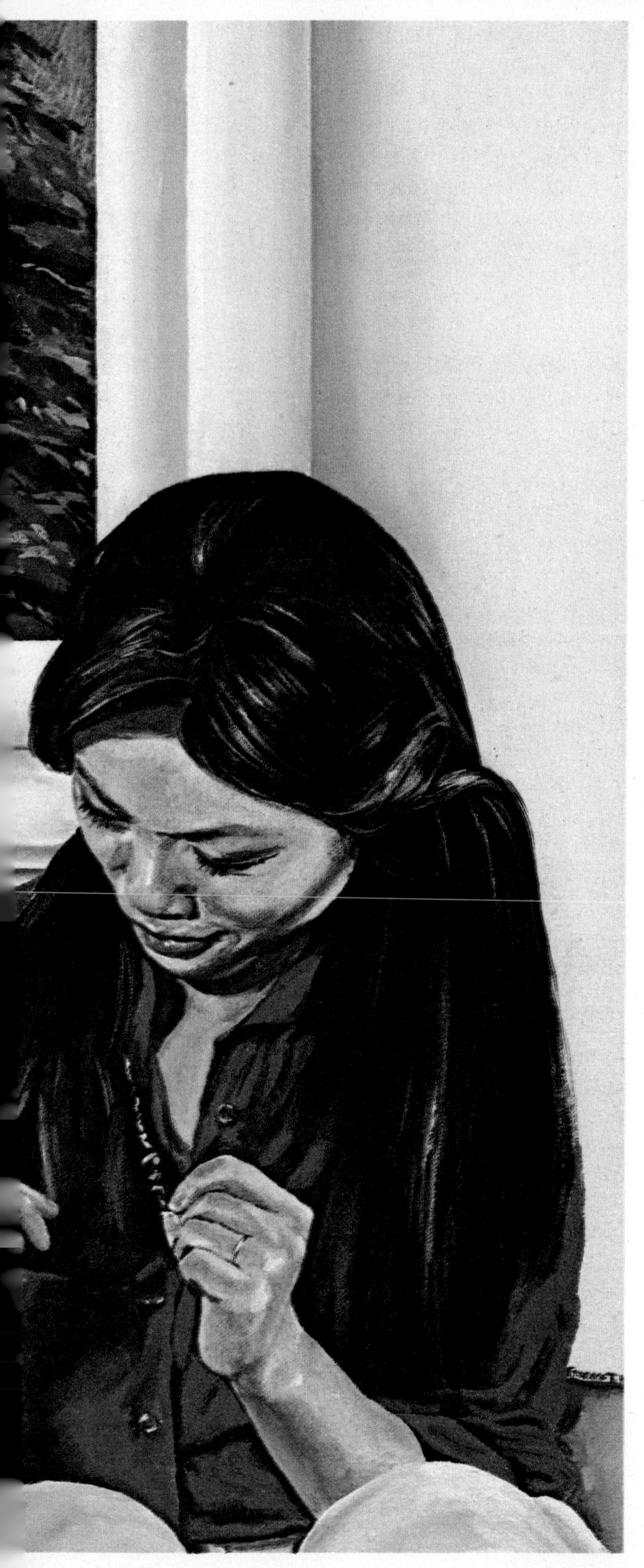

6 Marriage and Parenthood

Marriage American style attracts a lot of people. Statistics indicate that nine out of ten Americans will marry at least once and that five out of six who divorce or lose their spouses will remarry. This popularity exists despite an undependable system for meeting marriage partners, a longstanding disparity between the man's marriage and the woman's marriage, and ample opportunities to observe marriages that have failed or are "armed truces."

Although children are not essential to a marriage, parenthood is an expected component of most man-woman unions. Parents may feel a sense of challenge and accomplishment as they help a child grow into a well-functioning, mature adult. But children also bring additional difficulties, conflicts, and responsibilities, and their arrival invariably alters the relationship between parents.

In the past, society preferred all married couples capable of having children to have them. But a number of major social forces—the population explosion, the sexual revolution, and the women's movement among them—have begun to change social expectations. In 1978, for example, one-third of all American women who had ever been married remained childless, as compared with one-fourth in 1970 and one-fifth in 1960. And attitudes toward marriage have also changed, as growing numbers of people live together without marrying or choose to remain single.

But even though more and more people are opting for alternative life styles, marriage and the family remain the basic institutions of American society. Since our emotional needs continue to be met largely within marriages and families, it is important to our emotional health that we understand the ingredients that make these institutions succeed.

WHY DO PEOPLE MARRY?

Marriage tempts many people because of the promise of biological, psychological, emotional, and social advantages. Most Americans marry—or, at least, say they marry—for love, as elusive as that intriguing emotion is to define. Interestingly, there are societies where people not only do not marry for love but actually view it as an unsuitable basis for anything as serious as marriage. One Pacific island culture described by anthropologist Margaret Mead does not even have a word for love in its language.

Intimacy, sexual gratification, shared parenthood, comfortable dependency, and security are among the needs satisfied by a successful marriage. The dream of a "good marriage" or a "meaningful relationship" draws people like a magnet. The difficulties of creating and sustaining such a complex union are great, but basic optimism, the flexibility and diversity of marital patterns in the United States, and the relative ease of divorce encourage most people to try their luck at marrying.

Social pressure to marry often comes explicitly from parents and relatives and implicitly from the media and school. Besides dealing with these external social pressures, the person contemplating marriage must also grapple with his or her own motivations. Many people marry for reasons that have little to do with the desire for developing a meaningful relationship with someone. They may be escaping from an unhappy home life, marrying "on the rebound" to get even with a former lover, avoiding loneliness, looking for the security of a rich spouse, or following any number of such ulterior motives. And many couples, especially young ones, feel forced into marriage when the woman becomes pregnant.

Unfortunately, many people do not examine their motives before marrying. Indeed, many people marry who probably should never marry at all. Their personalities, values, and life styles are simply not geared to living with another person. However, American views toward marriage are undergoing some major changes, which are stimulating more and more people to examine their own ideas toward marriage, their expectations of a marriage partner, and their willingness to commit themselves to living with another person for an extended period of time.

SELECTING A MARRIAGE PARTNER

How do individuals find and select each other for such an important emotional and financial commitment as marriage? Much is left to chance. Two deficiencies in the American marriage-selection process are the early age of marriage sanctioned today and the limited facilities for finding an appropriate mate.

Youth and Identity

Erik Erikson, in *Identity, Youth, and Crisis,* describes the struggles of young adults in their late teens and early twenties as they try to develop a sense of identity and an appropriate self-concept—a difficult task in our mobile, pluralistic, technical society. As stated in Chapter 1, Erikson considers resolution of this identity problem necessary before each person can achieve true intimacy with another person.

Studies have shown that college students spend a great deal of time trying to figure out who they are and what they want to do with their lives. Much of their day is spent discussing goals and personality characteristics with friends. They put considerable effort into modifying their behavior to become more comfortable with and more acceptable to their peers.

Occasionally, students rush into marriage in order to avoid this time-consuming clarification of the self. Such marriages frequently result in dependent, immature, limited personalities, or else postpone until later years the further development of each individual's potential. Some students, marrying prematurely, choose people who harmonize with their transitory rebellious attitude toward their parents.

Other college students concentrate on their own development, finding out who they are, discovering the sort of work they want to do,

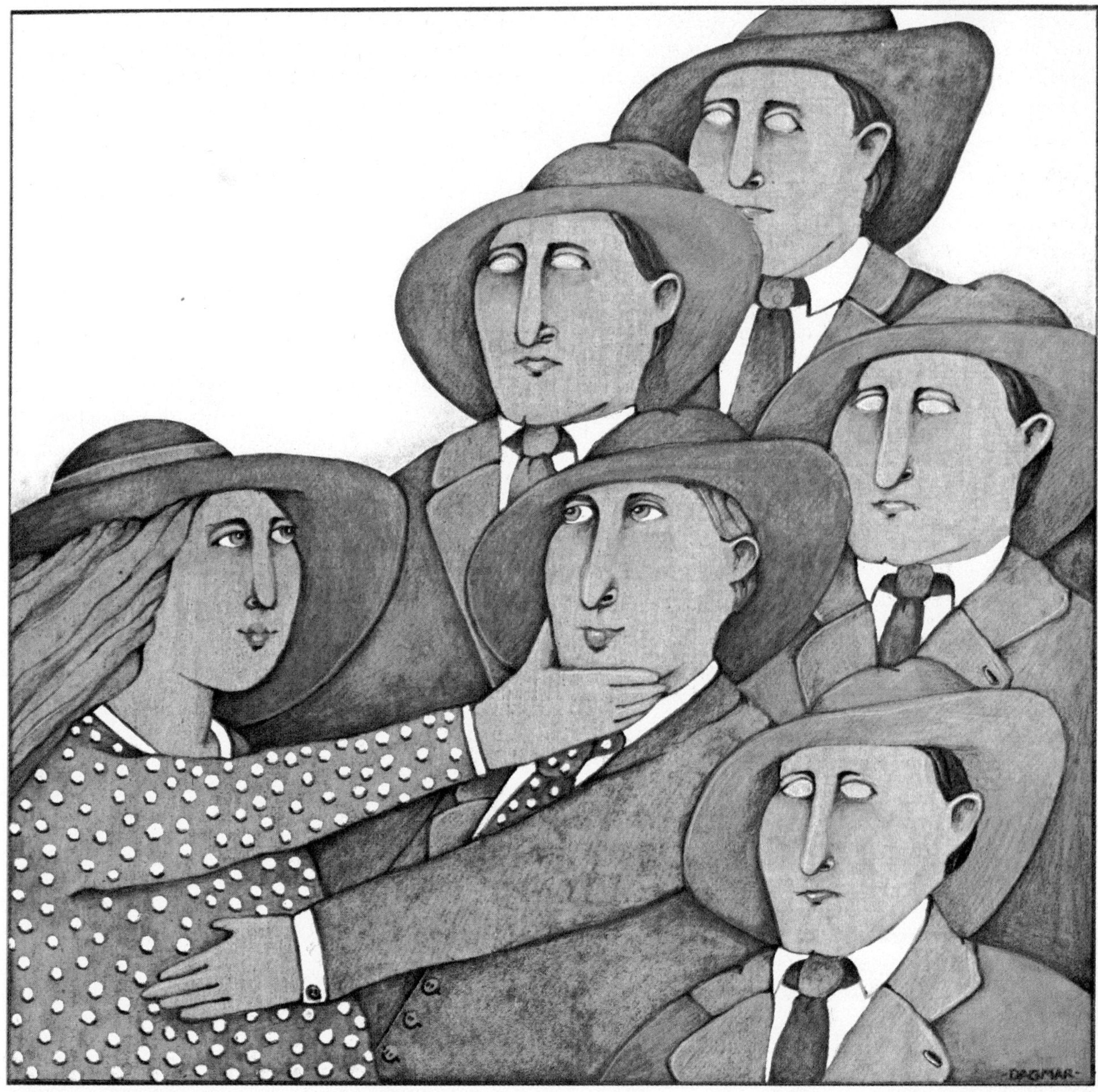

Dagmar Frinta

Figure 6.1 Selecting a partner for a happy and successful marriage results largely from achieving a clear sense of personal identity.

developing some necessary career skills, and separating themselves from dependency on their parents while developing their own independence. When these tasks are done and they have achieved a clearer sense of identity, they feel ready to move toward the selection of a mate.

This resolution of identity, or further development of a sense of oneself, does not take place in a straight line for most people. There are all sorts of detours, and one of the hazards of this period is that of making marital or occupational commitments while taking one of the detours.

FOCUS

Love and Marriage

The romantic idea of love—portrayed over and over in American television and fiction—actually dates back to medieval times in Western Europe, when gallant knights played games of courtly love with fair ladies. The distinguishing features of this idea "include the beliefs that love is fated and uncontrollable," social psychologist Zick Rubin writes in his book, *Liking and Loving,* "that it strikes at first sight, transcends all social boundaries, and manifests itself in turbulent mixtures of agony and ecstasy."

There is, however, one immense difference between this medieval idea of romantic love and its manifestations in twentieth-century America. Today, we assume that romantic love will lead to marriage, and that such love is a prerequisite for marriage. In twelfth-century Europe, however, romantic love was involved only in extramarital relationships. As one medieval countess wrote, "love cannot exert its powers between two people who are married to each other. For lovers give each other everything freely, under no compulsion of necessity, but married people are in duty bound to give in to each other's desires and deny themselves to each other nothing."

Some modern social critics believe that the adaptation of this romantic ideal to marriage "has been a colossal mistake and a key factor in precipitating the sharp rise in divorces that took place during the first half of the twentieth century." Denis de Rougement has written, "We are in the act of trying out—and failing miserably at it—one of the most pathological experiments that a civilized society has ever imagined, namely, the basing of marriage, which is lasting, upon romance which is a passing fancy." Americans, particularly, de Rougement says, tend to ignore the practical considerations that in the past helped insure successful marriages: family background, age, social level, education, material resources, temperament, intellectual compatibility.

Zick Rubin, however, argues that Americans have not really taken up the twelfth-century idea of romantic love in its pure form, that Americans—despite our apparent freedom to choose our own marital partners—actually do not ignore practical considerations. Rarely does love strike at first sight, he points out. Interviews with 226 engaged couples revealed that only 5 percent of the women and 8 percent of the men felt a strong physical attraction for their partner within the first few days of meeting. "Mates are in most cases found close to home and selected from a field of eligibles who typically share one's race, religion, social status, and important values and attitudes."

And "parents still have a surprisingly large say in determining who marries who in contemporary America. Secure in the knowledge that their children cannot marry people whom they never meet, parents often decide where to live, what schools to send their children to, and what sorts of social activities to encourage on the basis of ethnic and social class considerations. . . . one should never underestimate the ability of parents to achieve, however subtly, the end of arranged marriage in a free-choice 'romantic' society."

The Lack of Facilities

Another thing that complicates appropriate selection of a spouse is the lack of well-functioning networks for this purpose—that is, communication lines of people who concern themselves with helping single colleagues, friends, or relatives find partners. Without such facilities, the outgoing, flirtatious, gregarious individual has a strong advantage in attracting and acquiring a mate. But these are not necessarily the qualities that make for a good marriage partner. Charm and attractiveness, qualities especially favored by many young people, are not always enduring. Qualities that are more important in the long run are what the individual shows when the chips are down—good judgment, honesty, loyalty, ability to share, and imagination. And, of course, most important is liking the other person.

There are few ways for single adults to meet large numbers of other adults under circumstances that are dignified and pleasant. Rarely do single persons have the opportunity to observe and interact with a potential partner in a variety of settings—at work, at play, during meals. Colleges provide one such setting, but the impersonality and competitiveness of academic demands often prevent students from taking full advantage of the opportunity. Besides, many students are still struggling to resolve their identity problems and achieve independence.

There are limits on what individuals can do without societal help. Some single adults try to meet and learn about potential partners through communal housing, residential clubs, cruises, singles' apartment complexes, encounter groups, religious activities, and recreational clubs. Others frequent popular gathering places, join social clubs, or place newspaper advertisements in the "personals" columns.

Despite all these handicaps, people do manage to find partners. Their next task is to construct a marriage that will fulfill the needs and desires of each partner.

MARRIAGE—WHAT'S EXPECTED

In the nineteenth century, people married for practical reasons, and marriage was less concerned with personal fulfillment. Life was harder. Many women died in childbirth; many children died from diseases that are now controllable; and one or both marital partners often died before their last child reached adulthood. Men and women had only limited knowledge of other life styles, and their aspirations were narrower.

Today, with greater affluence and wider horizons, people have greater expectations of marriage. In addition to an economic partnership, they want it to be a source of emotional support and happiness; they demand a satisfying sex life; and they want more scope in their marriage for individual growth and development.

The fact that our nation is a melting pot of heritages and religious traditions from other parts of the world has introduced a variety of attitudes toward marriage into American society. Although people tend to marry within their own ethnic and socioeconomic groups, this cultural pluralism means that there is no one clear pattern to follow.

Because of these factors, the nature of marriage in America has changed and is continuing to change. This permits each couple to try to create a marriage that is harmonious with their own unique personalities and aspirations.

The Man's Marriage

Despite jokes about the dangers to men of "getting caught" or trapped into marriage, evidence is piling up to show that marriage is advantageous for many men. Jessie Bernard, in *The Future of Marriage,* shows statistically that men who marry live longer, enjoy greater physical and mental health, and are more likely to prosper in their work than men who remain single. However, the causal dimensions are not yet well understood—do healthier men marry, or does marriage make men healthy?

In the recent past, the traditional role of breadwinner provided men with advantages. Society, including religion, gave men the superior position in marriage. Most women consciously tried to attract mates whom they could "look up to," thus enhancing the man's superior position. Men had the advantage of wives who were solely responsible for the care of the home and other physical comforts. The price many men had to pay for these comforts was sexual constraint and full responsibility for the financial care of wife and children. The economic burden of marriage on men was great.

Today, with women constituting 42 percent of the American labor force, the man's traditional role as breadwinner is changing: more and more women are helping to meet the financial needs of their families. Some men, however, feel threatened by this situation; apparently their sense of masculinity is challenged by any breakdown in strictly segregated sex roles. Yet other men, with their wives playing more of an economic role, are cheerfully beginning to take on greater domestic responsibilities, including doing housework and child rearing.

The Woman's Marriage

Jessie Bernard also argues that certain aspects of the nuclear home and women's traditional role as homemaker are harmful to the mental health of many American women. Utilizing research findings from numerous sources, she shows that while marriage may be mentally healthy for men, the same is not true for large numbers of women. Married women are more likely to be depressed or anxious or show other symptoms of psychological distress than are their husbands or single women. And more wives than husbands say that their marriages are unhappy and that they regret marrying.

In America, the young woman often moves from the sociability of school or a job to the isolation of her home and then begins to wonder why she is becoming dull, irritable, and somehow dissatisfied. Raised in the myth that individuals marry and live happily ever after, she begins to wonder what is wrong with her. She has her own home, a husband, and often a child, and yet she is not happy.

The movement of women toward work outside the home seems a logical evolution of the wife's economic role. When production in the home diminished, many women moved to the world outside the home, where production took place. Before World War II, only 15 percent of American women worked outside the home. By 1950, however, almost 25 percent did so, and by 1978, nearly half of all married women—48 percent—also held paid jobs outside the home, including almost a third of all women with children under three.

This move out of the home and into the labor force has introduced new strains and conflicts into marriages and families. Many working wives still bear the major responsibility for taking care of the home and the needs of their husbands and children. Studies show that women employed full time spend an average of 4.8 hours a day on housework, while their husbands spend only 1.6 hours a day. In 1975, the United Nations International Labor Organization noted that working wives the world over have less than two-thirds the amount of free time enjoyed by husbands.

Add the fact that women still earn only 59 percent of the income of men, and it seems as if many married women are in a no-win situation. Their homes are often isolated, shrinking in function and family size, and the outside world offers them subordinate, relatively poorly paid positions and little relief from domestic responsibilities.

Changing Ideas and Forms of Marriage

As more women do work outside the home, the traditional roles of wives and husbands are also changing. Men's and women's lives and work are becoming more similar, and as a consequence, marriages are becoming more *egalitarian.* Husbands and wives are sharing household tasks and, even more importantly, are also sharing decision making more equally. And with smaller families, there is a new emphasis on companionship in marriage. Husbands and wives are expected to be best friends as well as lovers and parents. In such *companionate* marriages, the partners share mutual friends and enjoy the same sorts of leisure activities.

There is also an increase in *dual-career marriages;* that is, the wife not only works full time but pursues a professional career as seriously as does her husband. This can introduce some new and difficult issues. What happens, for instance, when the wife—but not the husband—is offered a promotion that involves moving to a different city? Does she refuse the promotion? Or does the husband quit his job to go with her?

In 1972, anthropologists Nena and George O'Neill introduced the concept of *open marriage.* The patriarchal family system of the past placed distinct limits on individual freedom and personal aspiration; such "closed marriages" were based on duty and implied self-denial, rigid role prescriptions, and total exclusivity. In contrast, open marriage is a relationship, the O'Neills write, "in which the partners are committed to their own and to each other's growth. . . . It is a relationship which is flexible enough to allow for change, which is constantly being renegotiated in the light of changing needs, consensus in decision-making, acceptance and encouragement of individual growth, and openness to new possibilities for growth."

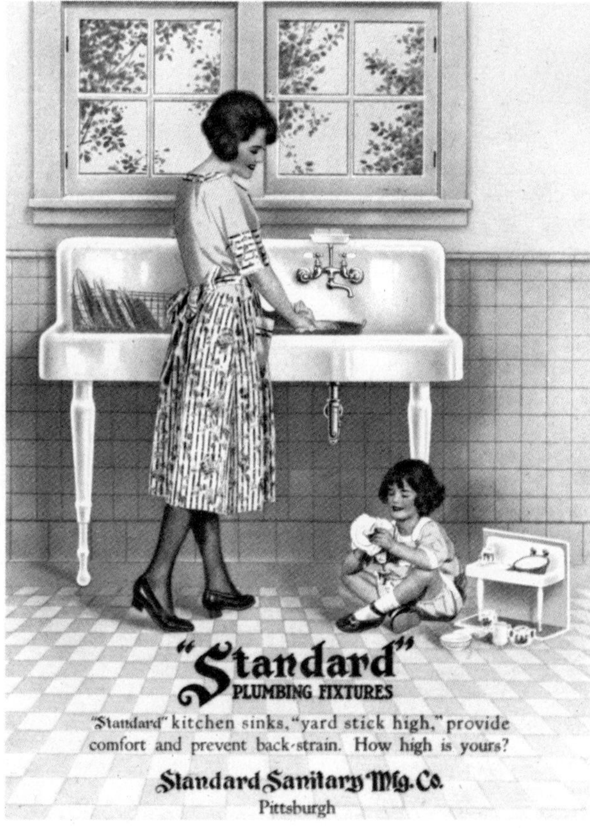

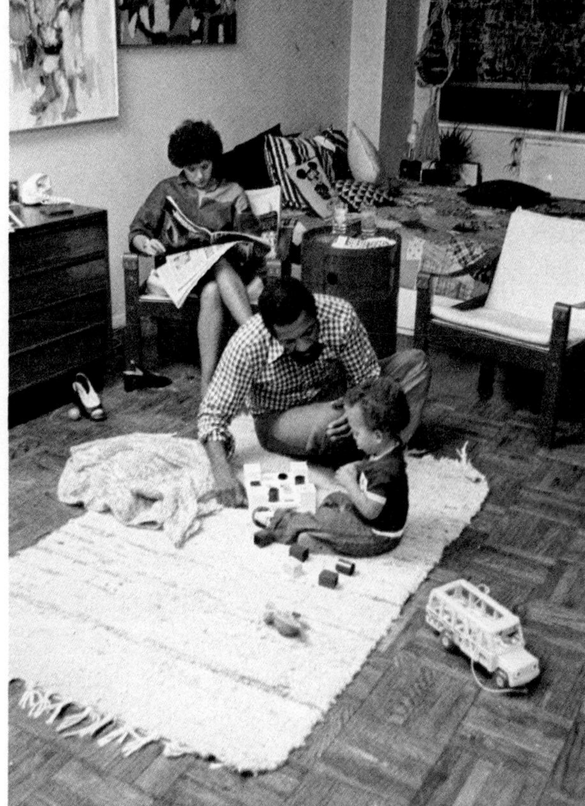

Figure 6.2 Whereas American women used to be taught from childhood to accept most of the responsibility for daily housework and child rearing, many of today's couples share these activities.

Some couples today are going so far as to draw up written *contracts* before marriage, defining the new relationship that they wish for their own marriage. Traditional marriage actually has always been a contract, with rules set not by the marriage partners but by the government. Now couples are writing their own prenuptial agreements, in addition to this legal agreement, specifying such things as the allocation of household responsibilities and expenses, sexual expectations, career priorities, whether they will have children, and if so, how many. While such a contract may or may not be legally enforceable, the process of drawing it up forces a couple to think through these crucial questions.

ALTERNATIVES TO MARRIAGE

Cohabitation

The openness with which young people live together (cohabit) these days suggests that a new social institution is in the process of developing, aided and abetted by improved contraception and a decline in emphasis on female virginity. Some young people, serious and aware of the complexities of marriage, prefer to live together before committing themselves to permanent marriage. Often, they explain, they want to find out whether they are "ready" —that is, mature enough to engage in a caring relationship with another person. Often, they

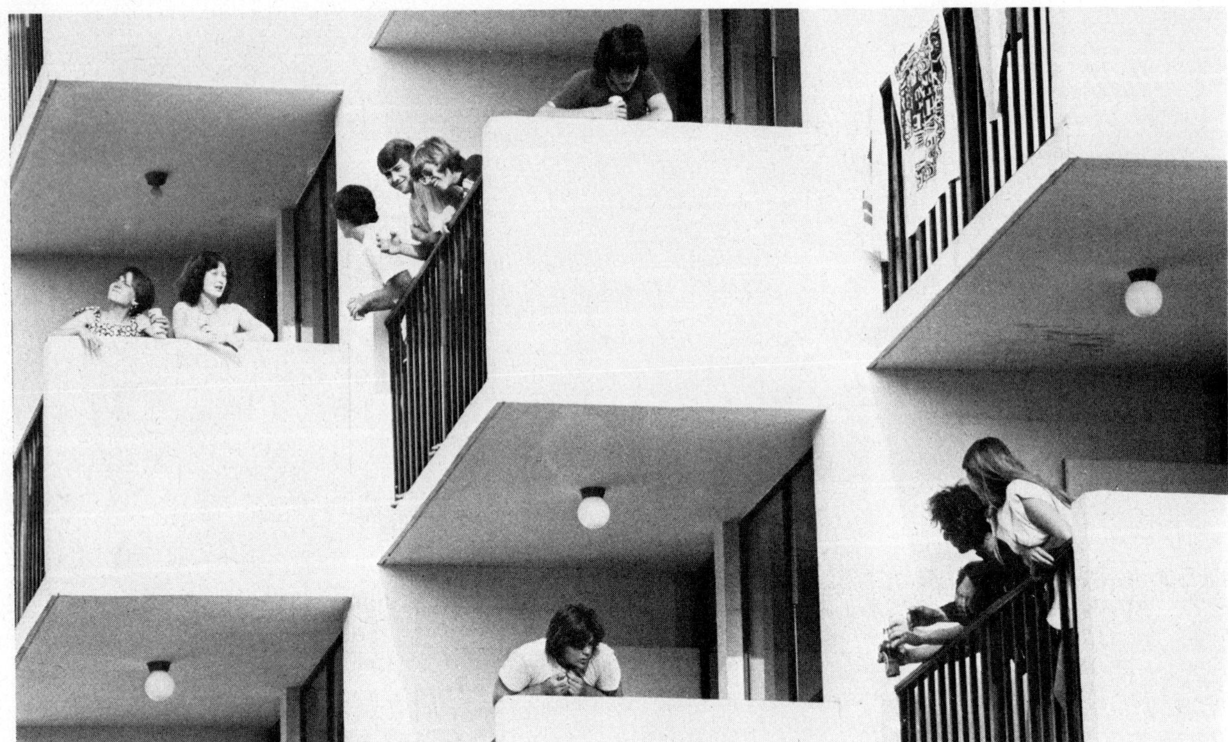

Figure 6.3 Coeducational dormitories expose students to life at close quarters with the opposite sex—creating an awareness that may facilitate successful cohabitation or marriage.

want to find out if the process of living together interferes with the personal and professional development of either partner. Not infrequently, these questions are answered satisfactorily, and the individuals make a legal commitment. Their knowledge of themselves and their needs may be enhanced by the temporary commitment of living together. When the relationship does not work out, the individuals may move with relative ease to other arrangements.

The absence of formal marriage, however, does not eliminate legal entanglements. Some courts have decided recently, for instance, that community property rights may exist for unmarried people who live together as husband and wife. And in addition to this legal liability, the breakup of such a partnership may be as painful emotionally as a divorce.

Living together outside of marriage may not be as widespread as has been presumed. A 1977 nationwide survey of 2,510 men between the ages of twenty and thirty showed that only 18 percent had ever cohabited for a period of six months or longer, and that only 5 percent were living with a woman at the time of the interview. In another study of 100,000 women, only 3 percent were living with a man to whom they were not married.

Cohabiting is not limited to young people. Because single, divorced, or widowed people who are retired sometimes lose their retirement benefits when they marry or remarry, a large number of senior citizens are also living together without formal marriage ties.

The gradual, testing approach of many young people living together may, in the long run, strengthen marriage and people. Those who move into marriage may have resolved conflicts about commitment. Those who dissolve relationships may learn their limitations as partners.

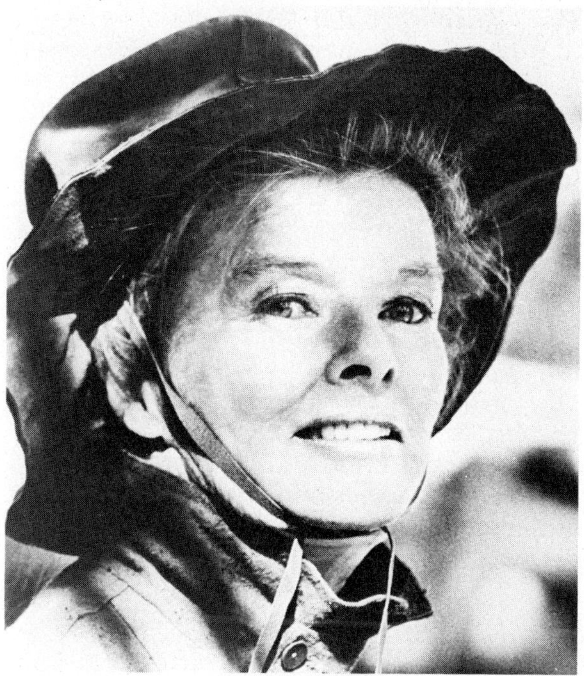

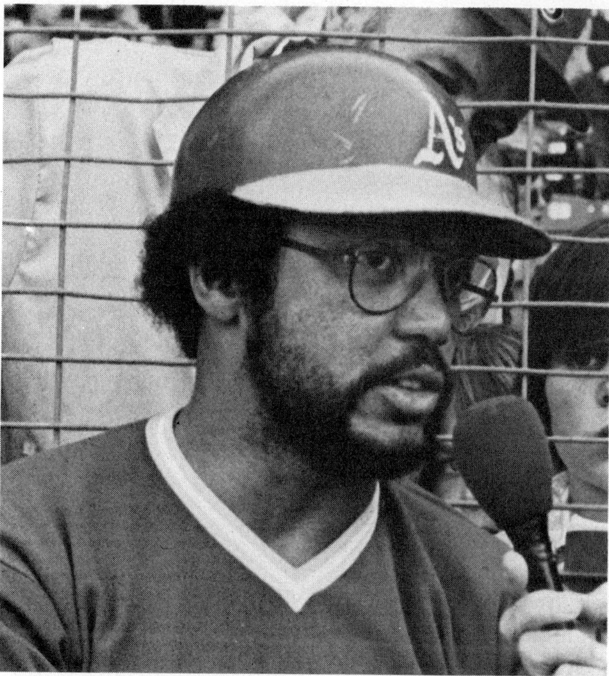

Figure 6.4 The trend toward acceptance of unmarried life styles gives both men and women the freedom to consider the option of remaining single. That people can lead fulfilling lives without marrying is demonstrated by the fascinating careers of Katharine Hepburn, an actress who has been single most of her life, and Reggie Jackson, a bachelor who is one of the richest and most publicized baseball players today.

Group Marriage

Some people have drastically reformulated marriage into communal living, or "group marriage"—in groups ranging from three to forty or more—to attempt to resolve the discontents, pressures of parenthood, and what they view as the limited opportunities for interpersonal growth of traditional monogamy. This makes for new problems, however, some of them more severe than the ones it solves. Psychologist Albert Ellis has enumerated several serious difficulties with group marriage: the near impossibility of finding three or more adults who can live lovingly and harmoniously with each other, the stubborn intrusion of love conflicts and jealousy, and the myriad difficulties of coordinating many lives. Many of the groups are quite unstable, constantly changing as people come and go. The longer-lasting group marriages are, in fact, those where couples tend to pair off in semipermanent monogamous relationships not unlike "standard" marriages.

The Single Life

Before World War II, there were many men and women who did not marry. The conventional assumption was that these individuals had been condemned to bachelorhood or spinsterhood because of family problems or obligations, personal inadequacies, or financial limitations.

Today, however, an increasing number of men and women are choosing to remain single or, at least, delaying marriage longer. In 1977, there were more than 15 million people in the United States living alone, and the number of adults under the age of thirty-five who live alone has doubled since 1970. Most of these people lead lives far different from the "swinging singles" style popularized by the media.

These are men and women who have a new awareness about marriage and value their freedom and independence. This trend is perhaps most striking among women, who—with better jobs available to them—are now more able to afford to establish households on their own.

The single state, however, has its own disadvantages. It is difficult for people who live alone to meet their own needs for intimacy, security, interdependency, sexual gratification, and parenthood outside of marriage.

MAKING MARRIAGE WORK

Numerous factors contribute to the success or failure of a marriage. Experts cite statistics showing that couples are more likely to stay married if they are of similar age, race, and religion and share the same education, social background, and socioeconomic status. These characteristics are certainly important, but a marriage that defies the statistics can still be successful.

One theory about the ingredients that make a successful marriage will be presented later in the chapter. Here, discussion will center on some areas that can lead to major problems in a marriage: personality differences, money, sex, and children.

Personality Differences

It is important that partners create a mutually gratifying life style, based on awareness of each other's differences in personality and abilities rather than on traditional sex-role expectations. One young couple has such a marriage. He is shy and reserved, and enjoys spending hours alone making and designing furniture and beautifying his garden. She is outgoing, with special skills in working with people and their problems. She has a career outside the home, and he spends his time creatively at home. Both are satisfied with their life together.

In one study of personality and marriage, researchers differentiated a group of college women on the basis of varying degrees of autonomy and conflict. The more autonomous women chose men who allowed them to develop as persons and who made demands of them that they could fulfill without interfering with their primary task of developing their own talents and interests. For example, one woman writer married another writer, and both of them shared a single teaching position. They both had strong interests in being parents, and with each sharing a half-time job, they both had time to enjoy their children and to write. Their arrangement, designed to gratify mutual needs for autonomy and creativity, permitted both of them to experience their children as a main source of pleasure and stimulation.

The college women in the study who were described as less autonomous wanted a traditional marriage in which they could play a supportive role and be protected from having to cope with the complexities of the world outside the home. They viewed the traditional role of wife, mother, and community leader as the only one that interested them. They needed a man to make this life style possible, and they were eager and willing to manage a household and care for their husband and children.

In both groups, those who came from homes in which the parents had lived in relative harmony moved into marriage with relatively little conflict and approached their life tasks with vigor and optimism. Unfortunately, those who came from conflict-filled homes frequently selected partners who tended to continue the process of conflict. The couples seemed to need therapeutic assistance to move out of this inherited pattern.

Money

A couple would be wise to consider their financial status—Do we have enough money to support the both of us?—*before* marriage. When marriages are young, partners may discount the importance of money to the stability of marriage. Yet, problems involving money cause misery and divorce in many families. In American society, having control over money means different things to different people. To some, it means freedom of choice; to others, power over people. The way a family handles decisions about finances reveals much about the relationship between husband and wife and the relative positions of the partners. Do they budget and decide cooperatively? Do partners take responsibilities on the basis of sex role or on the basis of talent in spending and saving? Is money used to enrich a mutual relationship, or is it used to define a power situation?

Handling money in a fair way to achieve short- and long-term objectives is a challenging task, especially as family finances change for better or worse. All financial decisions have meaning; they relate crucially to issues of autonomy, cooperation, and dominance. Whether funds are spent as a result of joint decisions or primarily as the privilege or responsibility of one partner indicates something about the assumption of adult responsibility by husband and wife. The reservation of some money for free, unaccounted use by each partner indicates a respect for the individuality of each.

Sex

When wives were pregnant every year or so and fear of pregnancy was a familiar part of marital sex relations, the sexual needs of men were frequently frustrated within marriage. In addition to the fact that pregnancies made the wife less available for sexual purposes, the sexual mores of Victorian times discouraged men and women from comfortably exploring their own and each other's sexuality for greater gratification. In some cultures today, as in the United States in the not too distant past, it is considered somewhat "ladylike" to view sex as one of the duties and trials of marriage rather than one of its pleasures.

Now, with current emphasis on the enjoyment of sex, both husband and wife are free to experiment, admit to sexual pleasure, and seek verification of their efforts to please each other. This new emphasis on sex, however, is also putting its own strains on marriage, as husband and wife feel pressured to "perform" sexually as frequently and as satisfyingly as they believe other couples are performing. The rising expectations of sexual enjoyment are increasing its potential for causing conflict.

In stable marriages, individuals have an opportunity to work through sexual changes. Just as adulthood is not an even, placid, unchanging period, neither is the sexuality of individuals a steady, monotonous experience. Sex between developing adults is constantly changing, provides variety, and calls for sensitivity. (Sexuality is discussed in detail in Chapter 3.)

Children

Research indicates that childless marriages, when they survive, appear to be healthier than marriages with children. There are fewer demands on the couple, and thus, husband and wife appear to be happier with each other. Research further indicates that fathers find marriage to be more restrictive and full of problems than do husbands without children. Fathers describe themselves as feeling more inadequate and dissatisfied with themselves than do childless husbands.

Children cannot help but change the structure of a marriage, sometimes for the better, sometimes for the worse. If the mother works, she must either leave her job or make complicated arrangements for child care, at least while the child is an infant. The husband and wife are no longer as free as they were—a baby sitter must be found before they can go on a simple outing to the movies. In a traditional marriage, the husband and wife come to live in two separate worlds—he in the world of his job, she in the world of diapers and baby food. Many husbands complain that their wives become duller, less fun once they become housewife-mothers, while women complain that their husbands do not take enough interest in their activities and in the children. Children may also disrupt an egalitarian marriage. In such a relationship, the time and effort required to give a child a good start in life may interfere and conflict with the personal goals of *both* parents.

Of course, in a successful marriage, children may provide a true source of pleasure and fulfillment. For a summary of the right and wrong reasons for starting a family, see the section *Children: To Have or Not To Have* later in this chapter.

Divorce

Increasingly, dissolutions of some marriages are occurring, and some probably should occur. People sometimes choose poorly; some lack the interpersonal competencies required by a continuing intimacy. Some people cannot accept or adapt to growth or change in partners. Others have unrealistic expectations of

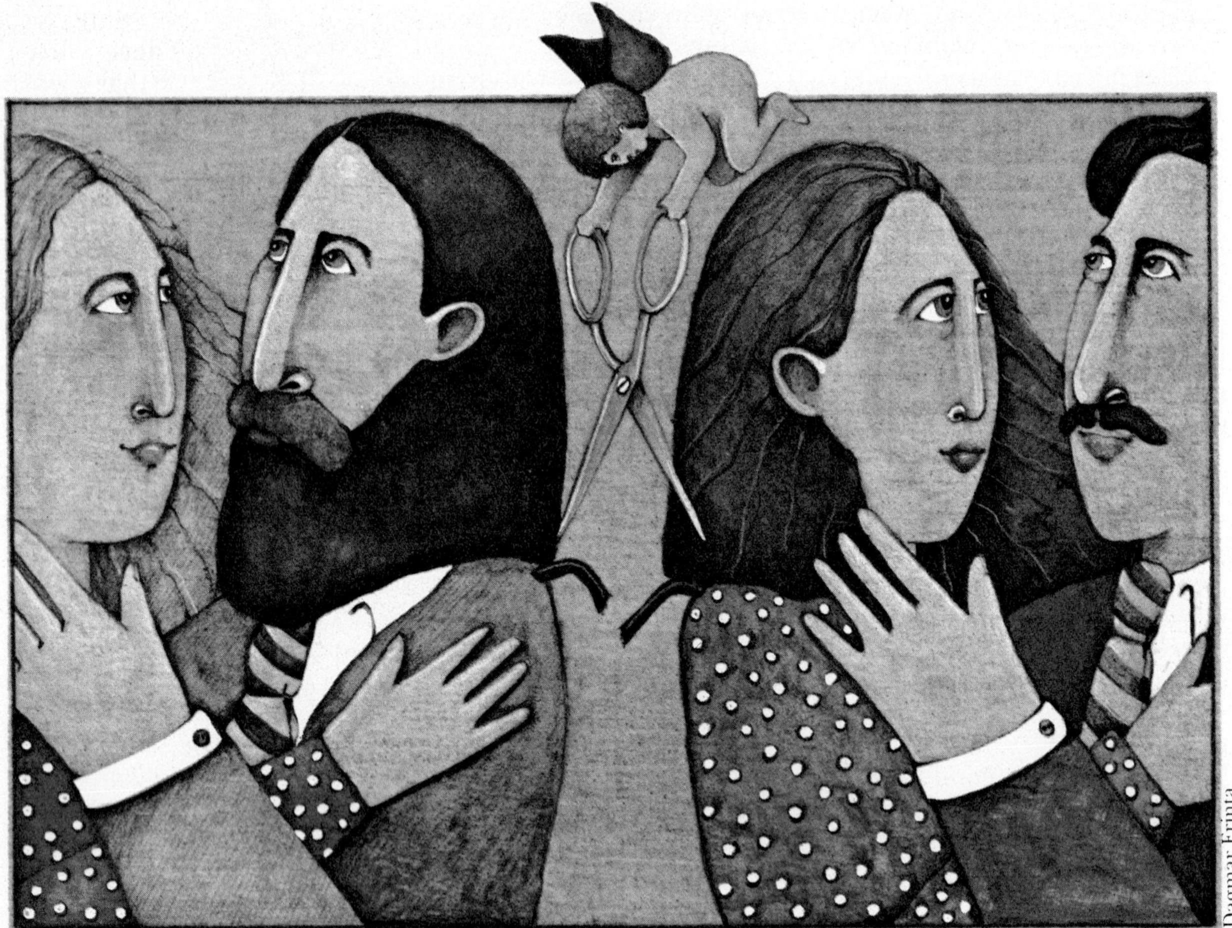

Figure 6.5 These days, divorce seems to be less a rejection of marriage than a workable cross between traditional monogamy and multiple marriage. Most people who divorce later remarry—sociologists have called this phenomenon "serial monogamy."

what marriage should be like. The availability of divorce may even encourage marriage, because the partners do not feel permanently trapped.

Far from being a radical change in the institution of marriage, divorce is actually a relatively minor modification of it. Between 1870 and 1905, both the United States population and the divorce rate more than doubled; since then, the divorce rate has increased more than four times. This has occurred not only for the reasons noted in the paragraph above but also because of increasing longevity. When people married in their late twenties and marriage was likely to end in death by the time the last child was leaving home, divorce seemed not only wrong but hardly worth the trouble. Today, however, when people marry earlier, finish raising their children, and still have half their adult lives ahead of them, boredom seems a good reason for divorce. Half of all divorces occur after eight years of marriage and a quarter of them after fifteen—most of them being the result not of bad initial choices but of disparity or dullness that has grown with time.

Divorced people, however, are seeking not to escape from marriage for the rest of their lives but to exchange unhappy marriages for satisfying ones. Whatever bitter things they say at the time of divorce, the vast majority do remarry, most of their second marriages lasting the rest of their lives. Even those whose second marriages fail are likely to divorce and remarry and, that failing, marry yet again. Divorcing people are actually marrying people, and divorce is not a negation of marriage but a workable cross between traditional monogamy and multiple marriage; sociologists have even called it "serial monogamy."

Despite its costs and hardships, divorce is a compromise between the monogamous ideal and the realities of present-day life. To judge from the statistics, it is becoming more socially acceptable every year. Although the divorce rate leveled off for a dozen years or so after the postwar surge of 1946, it has been climbing steadily since 1962, and the rate for the entire nation now stands at nearly one for every three marriages. In some areas, it is even higher. In California, where an ultraliberal law went into effect in 1970, nearly two of every three marriages end in divorce.

Divorcing couples with children face additional problems: divorce can have very upsetting effects on children, and the parents must deal with the practical problems of sharing the children while living apart. For a more detailed discussion, see the section *Children and Divorce* later in this chapter.

Marriage Counseling Some divorces probably could be prevented by *marriage counseling.* Professional marriage counselors work with troubled couples and are often able to help them resolve the conflicts threatening the marriage. Yet, counselors point out, couples too often come to them too late. Once a marriage has reached an advanced stage of disintegration, little can be done. If the same couple had come for counseling several years earlier, the marriage might have been saved.

MYTHS ABOUT MARRIAGE

There are several myths concerning marriage that need to be dispelled if people hope to achieve gratifying, companionate marriages. In this section we will explore four such myths: (1) that marriages are "made in heaven," (2) that marriages are static and uneventful, (3) that little personality change or development occurs after adolescence, and (4) that a good marriage can meet *all* of an individual's interpersonal needs.

Marriages Are Not Made in Heaven

Marriages are made by two fallible individuals, seeking by means of an inadequate process of selection the person with whom they can share and create a worthwhile and interesting life. Henry Dicks, in *Marital Tensions,* describes three clusters of variables that can be used to predict success or failure in marriage. One includes background factors, such as class, religion, education, and race. Although of decreasing importance in our mobile society, such similarity of background facilitates harmony in marriage because of the sharing of taken-for-granted values and aspirations.

The second cluster is a combination of personal norms, goals, and values that each person develops out of individual experiences and observations. It also involves conscious expectations about intimacy gained mostly through sexual experimentation, serious discussions with friends, and risk taking in moving toward closeness. In the process, individuals learn to accept both their autonomous strivings and their dependency needs.

The third cluster of variables is intangible, consisting of a sense of "rightness" about the marriage. This feeling of rightness grows out of a variety of experiences with the major figures in one's earlier life. For example, one successful marriage occurred when a man married a woman who temperamentally resembled his dynamic, imaginative mother but who lacked the mother's neurotic adaptation to a frustrating life. His chosen wife also resembled another relative, a lifetime career woman whose clarity of thinking, integrity, and gentle strength sustained a professional career, a rewarding companionate marriage, and satisfying motherhood. This man's wife resembled these two energetic women, and her husband experienced both an assuring and familiar continuity and the stimulation of uniqueness in the relationship. At the same time, the man combined for the woman the meticulousness and

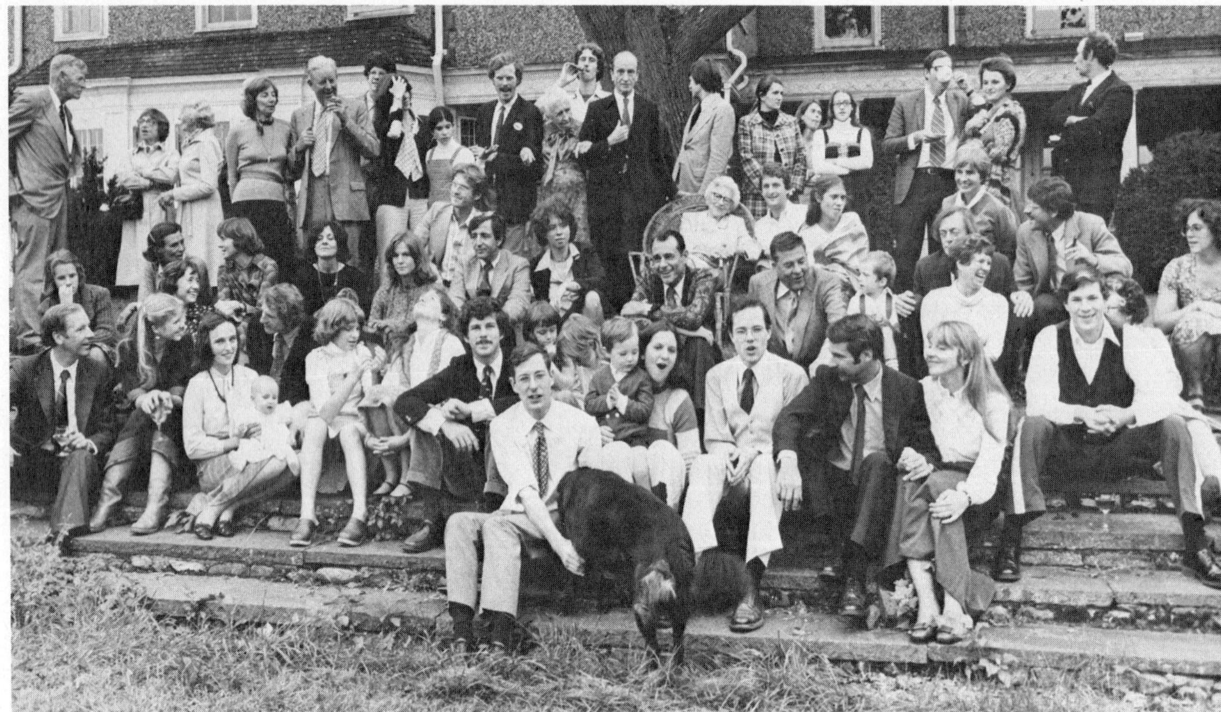

Figure 6.6 A solid marriage can provide a sense of continuity among generations as young people follow the example of parents and grandparents.

gentleness of one brother and the initiative, ambition, and aesthetic interests of a second brother.

Dicks goes on to say that if only one of the three clusters exists, the marriage or relationship will undoubtedly break up. If two of the three exist, the partnership will continue but be a rocky one. If all three exist, a happy marriage will result. According to several theorists, fewer than one-fifth of marriages and alliances constitute "happy marriages."

Change Is Essential to a Marriage

A second myth that leads to discontent in marriage is that married people live "happily ever after." It is a complex and difficult task for two persons to design a life together, and the partner is inevitably seen as a "stranger" as well as an intimate. Recognition of differences in each other produces the changes and adaptations essential to the continued vitality of a marriage.

Constructive togetherness is more a matter of the frequency, regularity, and quality of the time shared than it is of the sheer amount of time spent together. Experts suggest that couples would benefit from as little as half an hour each day spent in exclusive, uninterrupted togetherness. This time allows the partners to keep in touch with what is going on in each other's lives and to adapt to changes in each other. It also makes it easier to resolve problems immediately as they arise. This "togetherness" time—which many couples make into a ritual—also encourages daily expressions of caring and reinforcement of the relationship.

Change in a marriage is inevitable, and in a successful marriage, it is exhilarating and challenging. Living happily ever after seems, by contrast, an insipid illusion.

Adulthood Is Far from Stagnant

The third myth about marriage drops the curtain on the most interesting stage in human development. The myth holds that adulthood is a period of stagnant immutability. It derives, perhaps, from childlike ideas of maturity, suggesting Victorian taboos against close scrutiny of parental life.

Daniel Levinson, Robert Gould, and other social scientists have recently turned their attention to that large plateau of life from age twenty-two to the onset of old age. Adulthood, they have found, is a period when individuals have the greatest power and vigor, and in many ways it is more interesting than the more fully documented periods of childhood, adolescence, and old age. According to Levinson, it is a time of many stages and transitional periods, of ups and downs, of strivings, of adaptations, and of demands for flexibility and change. Complications and stress occur when one person changes and the other person does not or when changes pull them in incompatible directions. When this happens, separations occur and some seek other partners. But for many other couples, this need to change throughout the long years of marriage itself contributes to the dynamism of the long-term commitment and relationship.

Marriage Cannot Fill All Needs

Robert S. Weiss has indicated that individuals have five social-interpersonal kinds of needs. The first need, *intimacy,* is best fulfilled by marriage or a close love relationship. It is satisfied by the ability to feel unself-conscious about one's maleness or femaleness and to feel that one can trust another person sexually and with one's deep feelings.

Weiss points out that individuals who are happily married may still feel isolated if they do not *share their everyday experiences* with someone with similar activities. Often, husbands and wives, living in different worlds much of the day, can offer only a limited understanding of each other's daily experiences.

The third emotional need described by Weiss is *nurturance*—the dual need to care for and be taken care of by others. Many people feel that their lives are relatively purposeless if they are not caring for someone who really needs their assistance. A fourth need is *reassurance of worth.* This kind of self-esteem grows out of appreciation of one's behavior and values by meaningful people in one's life. The last need is that of *security*—knowing that there are people to whom one can turn for help. The family serves this function. A person who feels that there is no one to turn to in case of illness or misfortune can experience chronic anxiety and vulnerability.

Weiss's principal thesis is that a generous gratification of one need cannot substitute for the lack of another. For example, a warm and gratifying marriage cannot keep a woman happy if her self-esteem is low or if she lacks a close friend who recognizes and understands her activities. Weiss's thesis points to the conclusion that no marriage should be asked to meet all of a person's interpersonal needs.

PARENTHOOD TODAY

We have mentioned the fact that growing numbers of married couples are choosing to remain childless. Nevertheless, in most marriages, raising a family is still a primary goal. The current trend is toward small families with one or two children. Some researchers predict an imminent upturn in the national birth rate, but it appears certain that a majority of couples will continue to limit the size of their families.

Figure 6.7 Childbirth rates per 1,000 women (ages 15–44) since 1910. Note the drop in the rate since 1960.

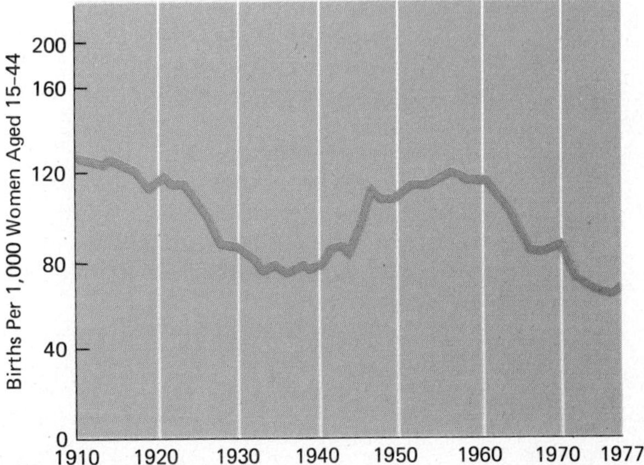

One factor that has spurred the trend toward smaller families is the changing role of women. Characteristics such as independence and initiative are now acceptable to many women, whether home-oriented or career-oriented. Such qualities have been defined as appropriate to a mentally healthy adult, and many women may thus become stronger and more self-respecting mothers. The dramatic changes going on in the lives of women today point to greater personal development for both men and women, and may thus provide a healthier, more stimulating environment for children.

Children: To Have or Not To Have

In the past, it was to people's economic advantage to have children. Sons could become hands on the farm or apprentices in a trade; daughters could help with the mother's housework and marry men who could provide additional help and income to the family.

Today, despite greater knowledge and availability of birth-control methods, people still have children, but their reasons are more diverse. Studies on why people have children have uncovered many motives, yet the reason least mentioned by parents is a love for children. There are many *wrong* reasons for couples to decide to have children. A few of them are:

1. To try to bring stability to a shaky marriage.
2. To provide objects for exercising parental dominance.
3. To give the parents immortality.
4. To substitute a love object for love missing between husband and wife.
5. To maintain family traditions.
6. To equalize the number of children of each sex in the family or to provide playmates for an only child.
7. To prove that the man is virile and the wife feminine.
8. To keep the wife out of circulation.
9. To give a bored wife something to do.
10. To project part of themselves—a chance to raise a copy of themselves who will have the things they never had and achieve the goals they never reached.
11. To exercise the only self-expression possible in a deprived socioeconomic condition —a self-perpetuating situation.
12. To provide their parents with grandchildren.
13. To provide themselves with security in old age.
14. An unplanned pregnancy compels one or both prospective parents to see it through.

What are some of the right reasons for having children? Consider the following:

1. Couple enjoys and respects children.
2. Couple has developed a strong, secure relationship, which they would like to extend and enrich with a child.
3. Couple feels good about themselves, comfortable in their environment, and confident of their success as parents.
4. Couple understands the profound change having children brings and are eager to accept the challenge.
5. Couple is interested in learning how to be good parents.
6. Couple is elated over the opportunity to participate in the creation and development of another human being.

THE PARENT-CHILD RELATIONSHIP

Because a parent is the most important teacher a child will ever have, it is important for all parents to consider their various roles in the child's life and to understand themselves and what the child means to them. It is a tremendous challenge and responsibility to provide a child with the right care and attention. Perhaps

Figure 6.8 A parent is the most important teacher a child will ever have.

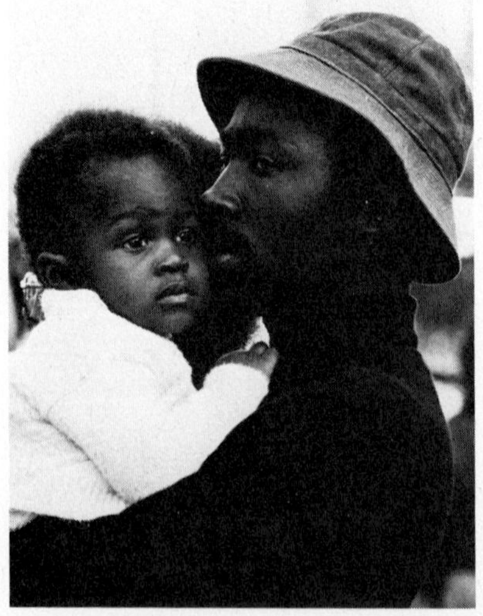

the most difficult part of being a parent involves recognizing the child as a distinct entity. The child, at every stage, must be thought of as a separate human being with individual thoughts and needs.

The ultimate goal of the parent should be to help children become responsible, mature individuals. A real child cannot be separated into segments and labeled the emotionally developing child, the socially developing child, and the intellectually developing child. A child must be treated as a whole person in whom these aspects are interacting, conflicting, growing. In addition to the child's development, parents must also take into account their *own* needs and interests. They cannot spend all their time following the child around, nor would that be desirable.

Discipline

In trying to take both the children's interests and their own into account, parents must develop rules to govern their relationship with their children. Such rules generally fall under the headings of discipline.Many parents become overly concerned about every event in their children's lives, continually asking themselves if being too strict or too permissive in a certain situation will cause a trauma that will permanently warp their children's personalities. Some parents choose to be consistently strict—sheltering children from any contact with bad parts of life by limiting their activities. Others are permissive, giving children what they want and giving in during conflicts, so that children never receive adequate guidance, never develop a sense of right and wrong, and never learn self-control. Still other parents arbitrarily mix permissive and strict actions, often in the same situation, thus giving children a feeling of helplessness; they never know what response to expect from their parents (see Figure 6.9). It is, indeed, not easy for par-

I GUESS WE COULD SPEND THE 20 BUCKS HE GAVE ME. AND WE MIGHT FIND SOMETHING TO DO UNTIL MIDNIGHT. BUT I FEEL VERY FUNNY ABOUT TAKING THE CAR.
GET DOWN FROM THERE BEFORE YOU BREAK YOUR NECK!
HEY BUDDY... LET'S SHOW THE GUYS HOW YOU CLIMB THAT BIG OLD TREE.
YOU KNOW YOU'RE ALWAYS SUPPOSED TO BE HOME FOR DINNER BY 5:22!
Saunders

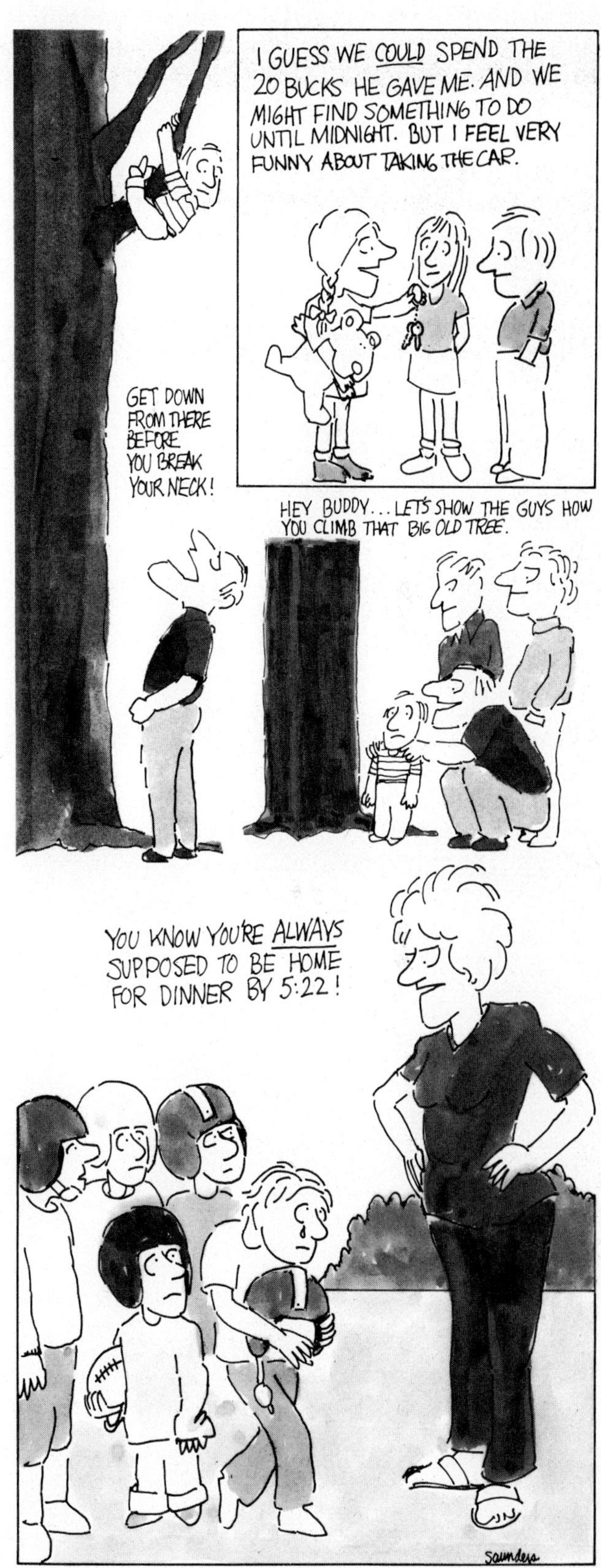

Figure 6.9 Differences in parental styles. Permissive parents run homes that are unstructured—the children are allowed to do whatever they want. Some parents are inconsistent, being strict sometimes, permissive other times, even in similar situations. Strict parents establish a great number of ironclad rules, and deal with their children by making decisions for them.

ents to strike a happy medium—setting a few essential rules and enforcing them consistently, in order to provide a sense of structure for their children's lives without being overly rigid.

Dr. Fitzhugh Dodson, a child psychologist, has come up with the following methods of discipline, all designed to help the child develop self-regulation while minimizing parent-child conflict:

1. Parents should control the child's environment to minimize the need for discipline, especially with young children. For example, a mother who tries to handle a toddler in a house full of things that must not be touched and that has few playthings will probably have to contend with needless discipline problems.
2. Parents should give children freedom to explore the environment and to assume the degree of self-regulation and responsibility suitable to their stage of development so that they build a positive self-concept. As soon as children can feed or dress themselves or turn on their own bath water, they should be allowed to do so. It is certainly faster to do these things for small children than to let them do them, but it is better for children to do such tasks themselves.
3. It is important for parents to make the distinction between feelings and actions. Children can learn to control actions; they cannot learn to control feelings. They cannot help being angry sometimes, but they can refrain from hitting or kicking; they can learn to control their actions in response to that anger. To be psychologically healthy, children should learn that feelings are natural and may be expressed in actions that do not bring dire consequences.
4. It is important for parents to set firm limits to the actions of their children, so that they know what they are permitted and not per-

Figure 6.10 The goal of discipline is to teach children a degree of self-regulation appropriate to their stage of development, while keeping parent-child conflict to a minimum.

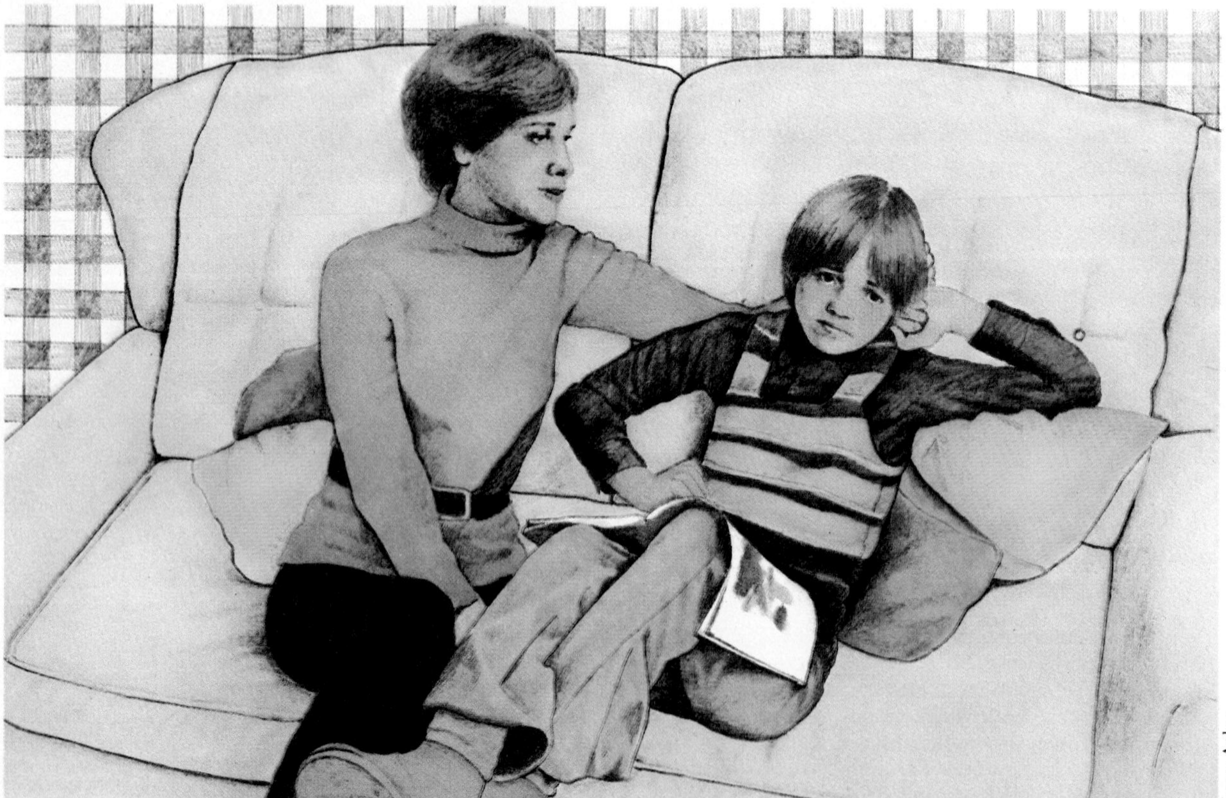

Nava Atlas

GO TO BED!
YOU WERE
JUST HAVING A
NIGHTMARE.
I KNOW HOW
SCARY MONSTERS
CAN BE. LET'S
TELL THIS ONE
TO GO AWAY SO
WE CAN GET
SOME SLEEP.

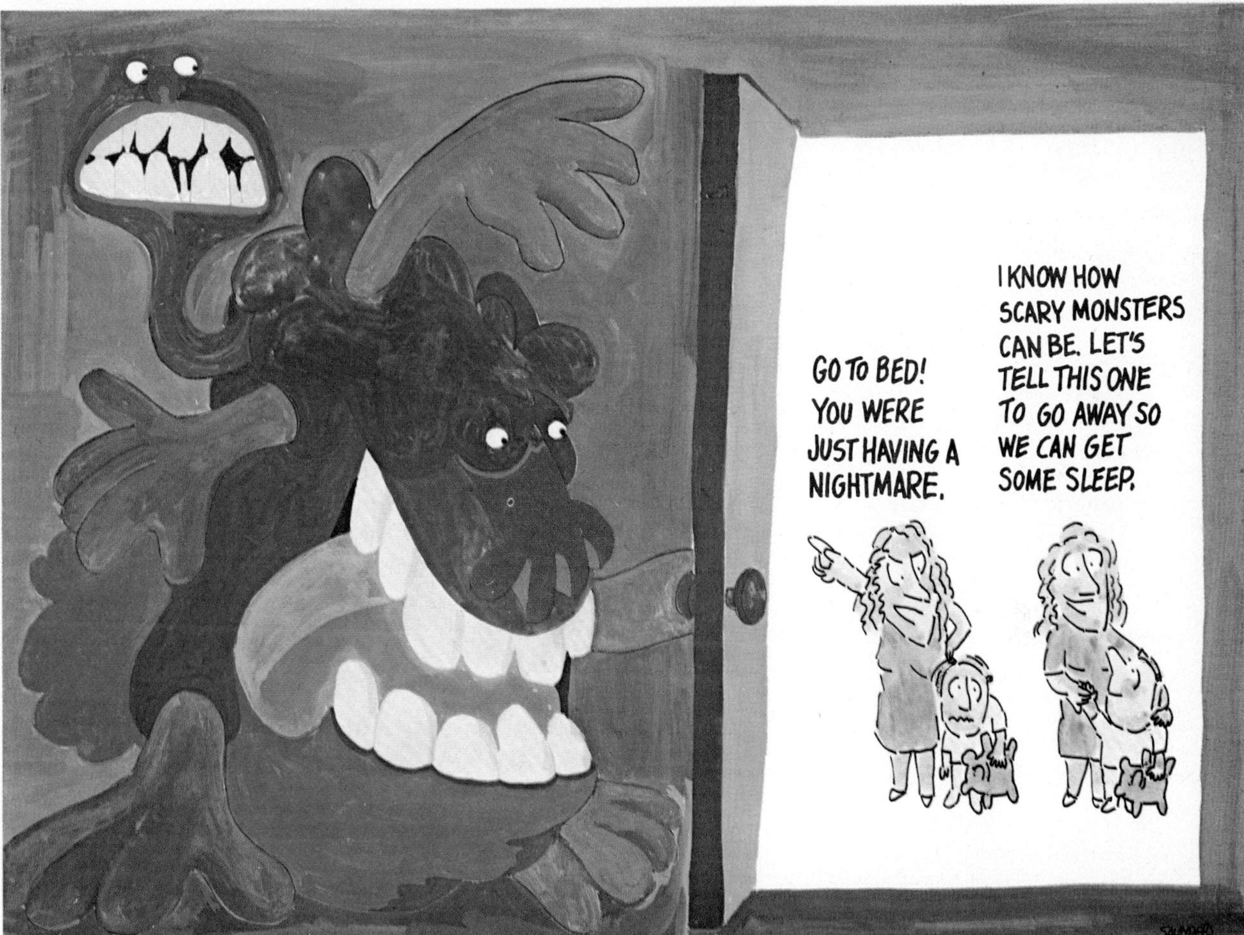

Figure 6.11 The reflection-of-feelings technique. Parents try to understand the child's fears and problems and let the child know they understand.

mitted to do. These limits should be reasonable, consistent, and suited to the children's stage of development. In addition, parents should be able to justify these limits to themselves and explain them to their children.

5. Children's feelings not only need to be talked about, they must be understood and sympathized with. When children are afraid, helpless, angry, or hurt, they want their parents to understand. A parent may make a superficial show of understanding by simply saying, "I know just how you feel," but that will not necessarily convince a child. A better way for parents to show the child they understand is to put the child's feelings into their own words and reflect them back to the child as in a mirror (see Figure 6.11).
6. Children should be praised for their efforts. Parents often reinforce bad behavior in their children by ignoring them (not rewarding them) when they are good and by punishing them (giving them attention) when they are bad.

It is inevitable that conflicts will arise between parent and child. Parent Effectiveness Training is one method that can help both be "winners" (see the How To box).

Adolescence

Adolescence, particularly, is a period of potentially explosive conflict between parent and child. An adolescent, more than ever, needs

HOW TO
A Guide to Parent Effectiveness Training

In 1962, Dr. Thomas Gordon held his first class in Parent Effectiveness Training in Pasadena, California. Today, over 250,000 parents worldwide have attended the course he devised, and Parent Effectiveness Training has helped many families that once were plagued by dissension, alienation, and hostility to find mutual respect, and cooperation.

Some parents are too strict and stifle their children, others are too permissive and get walked over, and a large number seem to waver haphazardly between these two extremes. Parent Effectiveness Training proposes a "no-lose" method that enables parents *and* children to be "winners" in family conflicts. The no-lose method consists of six steps:

1. Identify and define the conflict. (Parent to child: "Something's bothering me. I haven't been getting phone messages while I'm out. What if it were something important?")
2. Generate possible solutions. (Parent to child: "Do you have any ideas about solving this problem?")
3. Evaluate the alternatives. (Parent to child: "O.K. Now which of these ideas can we both live with most easily?")
4. Select a solution. (Parent to child: "Let's give it a try and see if it works.")
5. Implement the decision.
6. Follow up. (Parent to child: "Are you still happy with our decision? Does it seem to be working out?")

One of the most important aspects of Parent Effectiveness Training is what Gordon calls *active listening,* which enables the parent to verify the child's feelings and gives the child assurance that the parent is genuinely concerned. For example:

Child: When will dinner be ready?
Parent: Dinner will be late tonight. We won't be eating for at least two hours because Aunt Marian and Uncle Tim are coming over. Did you want to go out to play?
Child: No, I'm just hungry.
Parent: Oh. How about a peanut butter sandwich to keep you going for a while?
Child: Great! Thanks!

Here, the parent initially misread the child's interest in dinnertime, thinking that the child wanted to go out to play, but active listening provided the real reason—hunger. Of course, different problems arise at different ages, but the format remains basically the same.

Source: Thomas Gordon, *P.E.T.: Parent Effectiveness Training* (New York: Plume Books, 1975).

parents who know who they are, what they stand for, and what their values are, not only as examples to emulate or reject but as stability in a world that has suddenly become complex and full of choices. The adolescent encounters major conflicts—aspirations versus doubts of being able to achieve them, longing for independence versus the need for dependence, an idealized image of the parents versus the realization that they are human beings who can make mistakes. The adolescent's life is further complicated by increased sexual needs and the need to establish new intimacies outside the family.

The goal of the parent during this time should be to strengthen the adolescent in development without making him or her feel dependent. Parents who either attempt to retain total control or totally abdicate involvement may actually retard the adolescent's growth.

Of all the later stages of development, adolescence is the one that can most readily permit profound and benign transformations of personality. A challenging, responsive, and confirming environment can enable an adolescent to undo vast damage done in earlier childhood, to heal the wounds from parental inconsistency, ignorance, or neglect, and to move beyond these handicaps toward maturity.

Child Abuse

Physicians and hospital emergency rooms often see children who have been beaten, burned, or otherwise battered; who have been starved or sexually abused; or whose X-rays show many broken bones that have healed without being set. Accurate statistics on such abuse are hard to come by, but a 1975 nationwide survey for the National Center on Child Abuse and Neglect estimated that a million American children are abused by their parents or guardians each year. An estimated 2,000 children a year die from such treatment.

Researchers have been able to learn some things about the characteristics of abusing parents. They come from all walks of life, from all socioeconomic levels, and from all races. Their most common characteristic is that they were usually abused or neglected themselves when they were children. Abusing parents are often people who lead lonely, isolated lives; who have a strict, disciplinarian attitude toward child rearing; and who do not communicate well with their children. A stress within the family—say, the loss of a job or a household accident—frequently precipitates abuse.

All states now have laws that require physicians and other health professionals to report suspected cases of child abuse to child welfare authorities. Many communities have crisis intervention hot lines, where parents who realize that they are getting out of control can get immediate help. There is also a national organization, Parents Anonymous (analogous to Alcoholics Anonymous), where parents themselves help each other to overcome their tendencies toward violence.

CHILDREN AND DIVORCE

Each year the parents of about a million children under eighteen become divorced. By now, only about 70 percent of American children are living with both their natural parents in families undisturbed by divorce.

In the overwhelming majority of cases, the mother gets custody of the children. In a growing number of cases, however, the father does get custody, or, sometimes, custody is shared jointly in various ways between the mother and father. In some divorced families, the children live alternately with their father and mother, perhaps having a room of their own, with clothes and other possessions, in each household and switching back and forth every few days or weeks. Such a joint custody arrangement, of course, requires that the two parents live near enough to each other so that the children can continue going to a single school.

What effect does divorce have on children? One ongoing California study, by Judith Wallerstein and Joan Kelly, of sixty divorced families suggests that for most children divorce is not as devastating as some people have feared. Initially, children are upset when their parents decide to separate; it is a painful experience for adolescents as well as younger children. Extreme anger, regression to earlier forms of behavior, and physical symptoms such as asthma are not uncommon. Younger children especially seem to blame themselves; older adolescents are more often angry or ashamed. For the first few months, most children wish the separation could be repaired; they want the father or mother to rejoin the household. But within a year, most children of all ages return to a normal pattern of development and appear to be undamaged by the divorce. In the long run, it seems clear that it is usually easier for children to survive a divorce than to cope with the constant strife and irritation of unhappily married parents.

There are some things divorcing parents can do to minimize the harmful effects on their children. Parents should keep the children informed. Ordinarily, the children are better off if the parent who does not have custody still remains part of their lives. While it is not clear that any one custody or visiting arrangement is superior to another, it is important that there be some consistent pattern the children can rely upon. And the parent who does not have custody should realize that he or she contributes to the children's well-being by supporting the parent who does have custody.

SINGLE-PARENT FAMILIES

A growing number of American families are now headed by only one parent. More than 9 million children under eighteen live in single-parent families, because of divorce, separation, desertion, or death of the spouse. Or, more and more, single people are choosing to keep and raise children born out of wedlock or are adopting children themselves. The great majority of all such single-parent families are headed by a woman.

Single-parent families have a number of special problems. There are financial problems: single parents must often work full time and somehow also juggle both household responsibilities and day-care arrangements for small children. They face the impossible task of trying to be both mother *and* father to the children. They must also make social lives for themselves in a world often geared to married couples. And not least, single parents must cope with all these problems alone, without the emotional support of a spouse.

ADOPTION

Each year roughly 200,000 American couples legally adopt children either because (like 10 to 15 percent of the population) they cannot have children of their own or for humanitarian reasons or because they are concerned about overpopulation. They may have one child of their own and adopt others. The children they adopt have been born, often out of wedlock, to other parents either unwilling or unable to raise them. In recent years, because of effective contraceptives and more liberal abortion laws, there have been fewer healthy babies available for adoption, and parents who wish to adopt are more and more often taking older children, interracial children, or ones with physical or mental handicaps.

Whether a child is one's own or adopted is of little importance in the role of parenthood. However, how does adoption affect the children? A study by psychologist Barbara Tizard in England shows that sometimes they do better than children raised by their biological parents. Tizard compared a group of adopted children with another group who had lived for a while in an orphanage or residential nursery and then been restored to their natural mothers. By the time they were about eight years old, the adopted children were clearly doing better than the restored ones. The adopted children scored higher on intelligence tests and had fewer problems at home and in school.

PARENTING FOR HEALTH

Parents exert a profound influence on a child's total health, an influence that will continue through his or her lifetime. Many of our health ideas, attitudes, and practices come from our family background. Parents influence what and how much their children eat; if parents overfeed their children and they become obese, they are likely to have a lifelong weight problem. If parents themselves enjoy physically active recreation, children are also more likely to be physically active, either participating with their parents or imitating them. If parents smoke, children are more likely to become smokers. If parents misuse alcohol or other drugs, children are more likely to misuse them.

SUMMARY

1. People marry for many reasons: love, intimacy, security, sexual gratification, parenthood, to escape an unhappy home life, "on the rebound," to avoid loneliness. Unfortunately, too many people do not examine their motives before marrying.
2. Two deficiencies in the American marriage-selection process are the early age of marriage sanctioned today and the limited facilities for finding an appropriate mate.
3. In the nineteenth century, people married for practical reasons. Today, men and women have greater expectations of marriage. In addition to its being an economic partnership, they expect emotional support, a satisfying sex life, and scope for individual growth and development.
4. The traditional male role of breadwinner gives men the superior position in marriage. Married men live longer, enjoy greater physical and mental health, and are more likely to prosper in their work than single men.
5. In contrast, the isolation of the wife's traditional role as homemaker leads to poorer mental health. Married women are more likely to be depressed or anxious or to have other symptoms of psychological distress than single women or married men.
6. Among the changing forms of marriage are egalitarian, companionate, dual-career, open, and contract marriages.
7. Among the alternatives to marriage these days are cohabitation, group marriage, and the single life.
8. Couples are more likely to stay married if they are of similar age, race, religion, and socioeconomic background and have the same amount of education. Some major problem areas in marriage are personality differences, money, sex, and children.
9. The divorce rate in the United States is now nearly one for every three marriages. Divorcing people are actually marrying people. The vast majority remarry, most of the second marriages lasting the rest of their lives.
10. Common myths about marriage include the ideas that marriages are "made in heaven"; they are static; little personality change occurs during adulthood; and a good marriage can

meet all of an individual's interpersonal needs.

11. Parents have many motives for having children. Among the wrong reasons are trying to stabilize a shaky marriage or proving virility or femininity. Among the right reasons is the fact that a couple enjoys children and is eager to accept the challenges they pose.

12. Perhaps the most difficult part of being a parent is recognizing a child as a distinct human entity.

13. The ultimate goal of parents should be to help their children become self-regulating, mature individuals. Parents must develop a few rules of discipline to govern their relationship with their child. When conflicts do arise, a good way of resolving them is the no-lose method, in which parents and child together work out a solution acceptable to both so that neither loses.

14. Adolescence, particularly, is a period of potentially explosive conflict between parent and child. The goal of the parent should be to strengthen the adolescent in development without making him or her feel dependent.

15. Each year, the parents of about a million children under age eighteen become divorced. While the mother gets custody in most cases, fathers are now more often gaining custody, or there is a joint custody arrangement. For most children, divorce is less devastating than some people have feared. Generally, children are better off if both parents remain part of their lives.

16. Parents exert a lifelong effect on children's health by influencing what and how much they eat, their level of physical activity, and whether they smoke or misuse alcohol or other drugs.

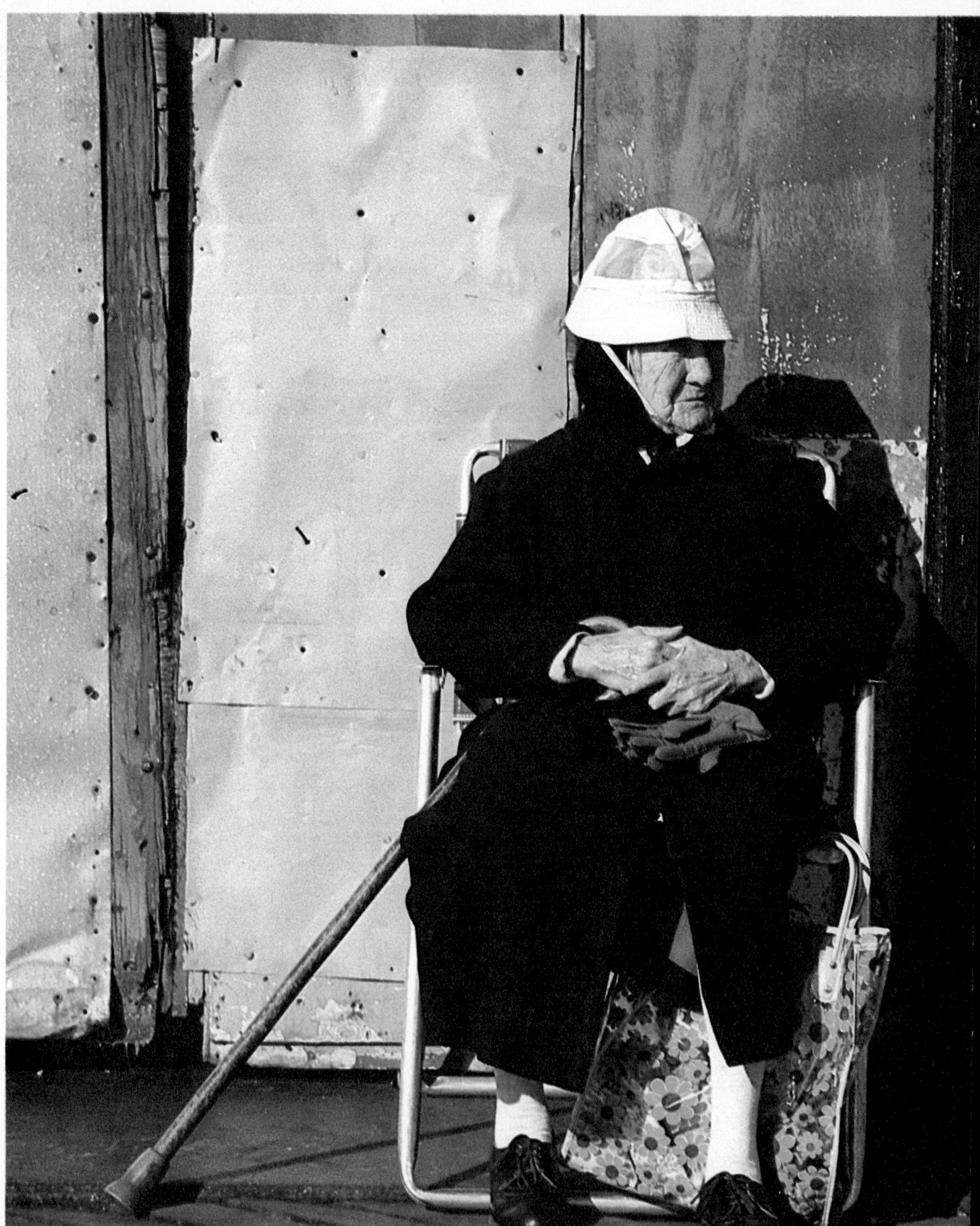

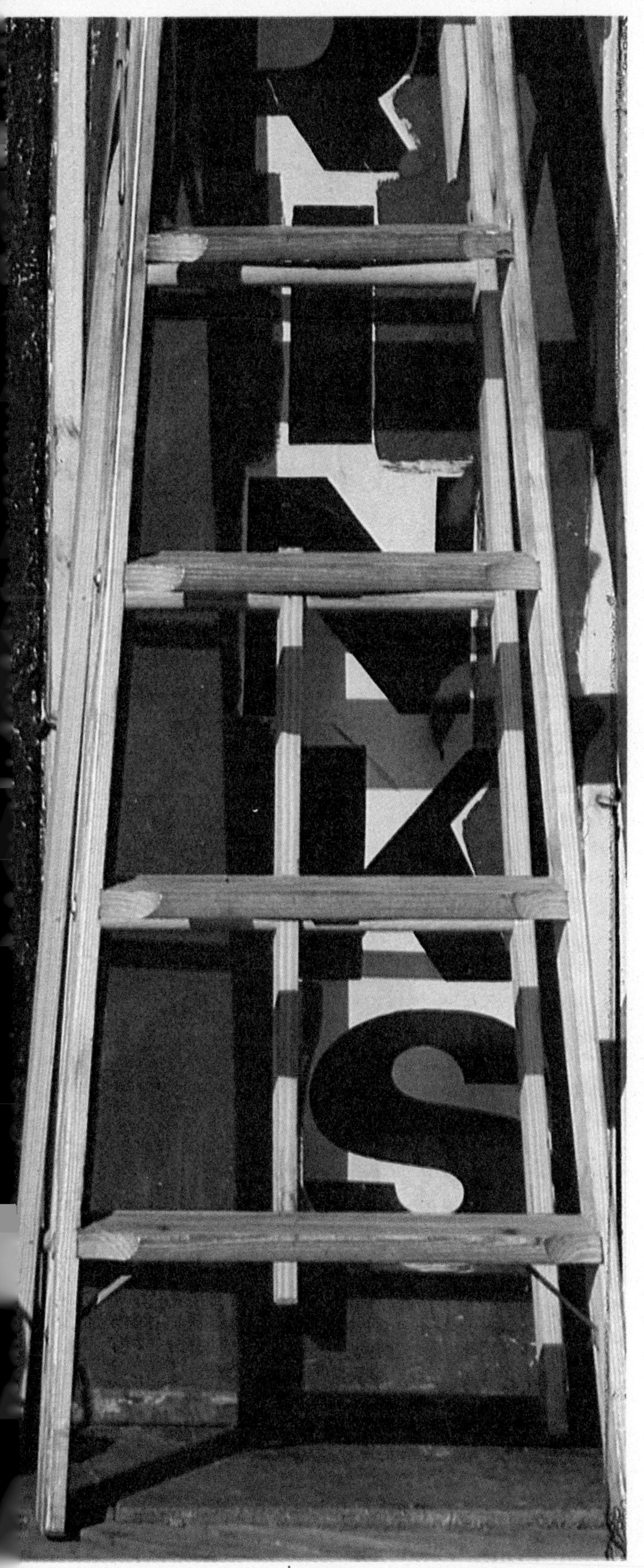

7 Aging, and Facing Death

Although we all begin to age at the moment of our conception, we usually associate the process with later adulthood. Today, better diet, better health care, and a better physical environment allow more people than ever before to reach their seventies, eighties, and even their nineties. The twentieth century's gift of extra years can be a welcome present to those who maintain their health and learn how to enjoy these later years for what they can be.

Because of declining birth and death rates, American society is now inexorably "graying." In 1900, only 4 percent of the population (3.1 million people) were sixty-five or over; today this is true of 10 percent (23.9 million people). By 2000 the aged will comprise 25 percent of the population. As their numbers grow, the elderly are increasingly becoming a group to be reckoned with socially, economically, and politically.

Many people, when they think about aging, also tend to think about death and to view both with fear. But although later adulthood is the final phase of human life, death can occur at any age.

Until recently, few but poets, philosophers, and theologians chose to dwell on the subject of death. Within the past decade, however, death has become not only an acceptable topic of discussion in many circles but a field of research as well. During the 1974–1975 school year, American colleges and universities offered more than 1,100 courses in *thanatology* (a Greek-rooted word meaning "the study of death"). This growing interest in death has been spurred in part by the fact that recent medical advances have altered our fundamental definitions of death.

This chapter will describe the aging process and various aspects of daily life in old age—marriage, sexuality, retirement, and social and intellectual activities. It will also explore the ways in which people face death—their own and their loved ones'.

THE AGING PROCESS

Biologically, aging is the increasing inability of a person's body to perform its operations and repair itself as it once did. There are many theories about the aging process. However, none of them, as yet, fully explains the underlying mechanism or mystery of how and why we age.

The "wear and tear" theory maintains that the human body simply wears out with use, as any complex piece of machinery would. The "waste product" theory proposes that damaging waste products build up within our body cells and interfere with their function. The "autoimmune theory" holds that the body's immune system, which is normally directed against foreign substances, begins to attack the body's own cells; the body ages because it can no longer distinguish between its own cells and foreign invaders. According to the "free radical" theory, highly reactive fragments of molecules—called "free radicals"—may cause aging by destroying essential body chemicals.

Or it may be that the genetic program, spelled out at conception in our chromosomes, eventually runs out, ending body functions. Another possibility is that as body cells divide and redivide, copying their DNA each time, they introduce errors into this genetic material. These errors may build up—much as nicks build up on an often-played phonograph record—until the cells can no longer function normally. Or, finally, the body may have specific pacemakers, probably in the brain, that control the aging process.

These many theories are not necessarily incompatible. It may be that several of them are essentially correct and describe different aspects of the aging process. *Gerontology*—the study of aging and the aged—attempts to shed light on this process, and as the percentage of older people in our society grows, this science will assume more and more importance.

Physical Changes

While physical changes occur throughout adulthood, they rarely have much effect on a person's everyday life during the early and middle adult years. It is only in later life that the cumulative effects of these gradual changes tend to catch up with the person and begin to interfere with daily patterns and habits.

Although there are great individual variations in the rates of aging, most people can estimate an individual's age—give or take a few years—just by appearance. During later adulthood, the hair turns white and becomes more coarse. It tends to get thinner on top of the head and starts to grow for the first time on the chins of older women. The skin loses its natural moisture and elasticity and becomes more and more wrinkled. Many people lose their teeth, which causes the lower part of the face to become shortened and brings the nose (which lengthens as the skin's elasticity decreases) nearer the chin. Eyelids thicken, and hollows develop beneath the eyes. As the skeletal structure changes, the spine bows, and many people become shorter with advancing age. The chests of men and women are no longer as full or as broad as they were thirty years before. Shoulders become narrower, and the pelvis broadens. As muscles atrophy and joints become stiff, a person's strength and movement become impaired. The dense part of the bone becomes spongy and fragile, so that bones break more easily.

Internal Changes Other changes take place inside the body; while they have no effect on appearance, they have a profound effect on physical functions (see Figure 7.2). Although the heart's structure undergoes little change, for instance, its work capacity decreases. It probably works as well as it ever did when the person is resting, but when the person is exposed to stress (as during exercise or fear), the heart does not react as fast or as well. And after stress, it takes longer for an older heart to return to its normal level of pumping.

The circulatory system no longer carries the

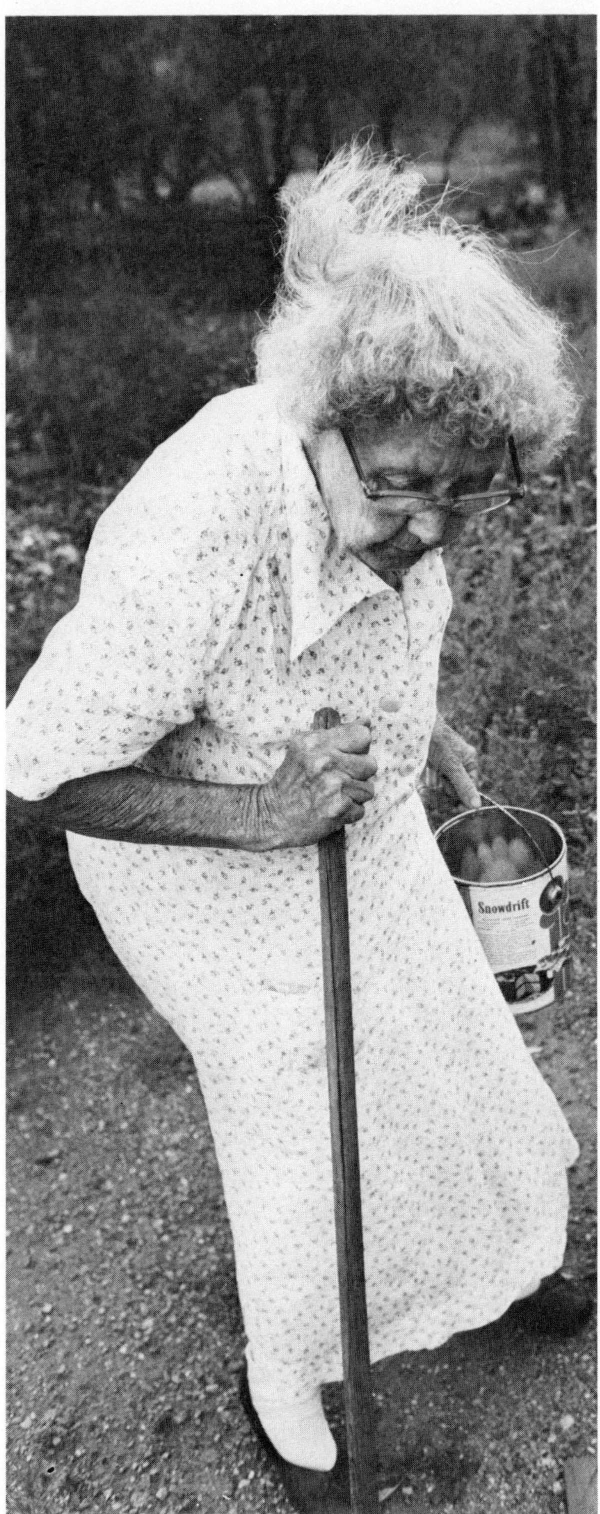

Figure 7.1 Later adulthood brings several physical changes. Hair turns white, skin becomes more and more wrinkled, the spine may bow, and strength and movement become impaired.

blood as well as it did. As circulation becomes slowed by thickening artery walls, blood pressure rises. By the time one is eighty-five, one's lungs can hold only about three-fifths of the volume of oxygen that they held at twenty-five. An older person thus generally has less energy for activity and less reserve to deal with stress. Because signals travel more slowly along the motor nerves, reactions also become slower. Digestion is no longer as efficient, nor is the process of eliminating body waste. All the senses work less well; vision, hearing, touch, taste, and smell tend to be much less sensitive. As a result, some older people may become irritable, moody, temperamental, or even paranoid because they can no longer perceive and interpret their surroundings as acutely and as rapidly as they once did.

Older people often complain that they sleep badly. They typically awaken more often during the night and sleep fewer hours. And because they sleep less, they also tend to spend

Figure 7.2 The percentage of change with age in cardiac output and certain other physiological functions, using 100 percent at age thirty as the standard. (Adapted from Nathan W. Shock, "The Physiology of Aging," copyright © 1962 by Scientific American, Inc. All rights reserved.)

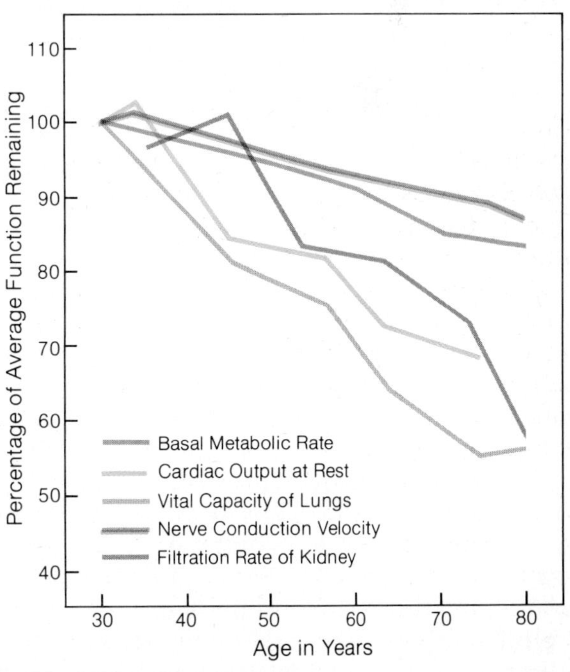

less time in deep sleep. This may be due to decreased exercise and physical activity.

Health and Disease Some older people sail through their later years active, vigorous, and the picture of robust health. Others spend these years in physicians' offices and hospitals. While old people are ill more frequently than the young, the very fact that they have survived and outlived so many of their contemporaries is an expression of their lifelong good health.

Illness in older people runs somewhat differently than it does in younger ones. In the young, illnesses tend to have quick onsets and short, stormy courses; young people tend to recover quickly and then seem to be as well as ever. In older people, illnesses are more likely to develop gradually, causing less acute distress, but lingering longer and leaving the person with a greater apparent loss of vigor.

About 80 percent of older people have some sort of chronic health problem. They thus visit doctors more and spend more days each year sick at home. Approximately one out of four people sixty-five or older is hospitalized each year, about double the proportion of those under sixty-five, and they stay there twice as long. Older people also complain more of ill-defined discomforts, such as rheumatism, arthritis, or digestive problems. On the other hand, several studies have noted that many older people who consider themselves healthy accept—as part of the aging process—conditions that physicians say are actually treatable diseases. Despite these illnesses, 81 percent of elderly people get around on their own, and only 5 percent of them live in institutions.

Older people are also particularly affected by stress. The more life changes that a person of any age undergoes in a short period of time, the more likely he or she is to experience a serious illness (see Chapter 2). Old age brings many of the most stressful life changes: personal injury or illness, sex difficulties, illness of a family member, retirement, death of a close family member, and death of a spouse. Because older people also have less tolerance for stress, their ability to handle these changes may often be tested beyond their limits, and a serious or even terminal illness may result.

While old age thus makes people more susceptible to disease, disease also tends to make people age faster. The circle is a vicious one: both processes work together and result in loss of health and, finally, death. The saying "Nobody ever dies of old age" has more than a glimmer of truth. In one study of 12,000 deaths, a pathological condition was uncovered in each case; there were no "natural deaths." In this country, the leading causes of death among older people are cardiovascular disease, cancer, and hypertension.

Mental Changes

A common stereotype about old age is that intelligence invariably declines; this is a myth. Your general health, your expectations, and how much you challenge yourself throughout life determine how well your mind will work in later years. People who expect that life after sixty-five is all downhill will usually find that this assumption is correct.

Intellectual Skills In some areas of intellectual functioning, people tend to improve well into their later years. A person's verbal skills (word use and comprehension) are better at sixty-five than at forty or twenty-five. Visual skills (such as finding a simple figure in a complex one) also keep on improving with age.

Older people are also about as flexible at shifting from one way of thinking to another as the middle-aged. However, on tasks requiring hand-eye coordination (solving a puzzle or copying words), older people do progressively worse. They also tend to do poorly on any task where speed is important. Slowness is perhaps the most characteristic mental change in the elderly.

The more stimulating a person's life has been and continues to be, the more likely that person is to gain intellectual skills during later years. In one study, men who had been bright as children showed great gains in intellectual ability during their adult years, while women who had been bright as children made fewer gains. This difference apparently came about because most of the men had stimulating jobs that forced them to think, while most of the women were housewives with fewer opportunities for intellectual challenge.

It is not true that memory declines in later years. The ability to learn and remember is likely to be as good as ever, as long as a person continues to exercise these faculties. The meaningfulness of material being learned affects how well older people remember. Younger people, particularly the well-educated, are willing to learn almost anything, no matter how irrelevant it seems. Older people, by contrast, are more likely to be unwilling or unable to learn something they judge meaningless, irrelevant, or trivial. Older people do tend to learn more slowly, but given enough time, they generally learn and remember as well as young people.

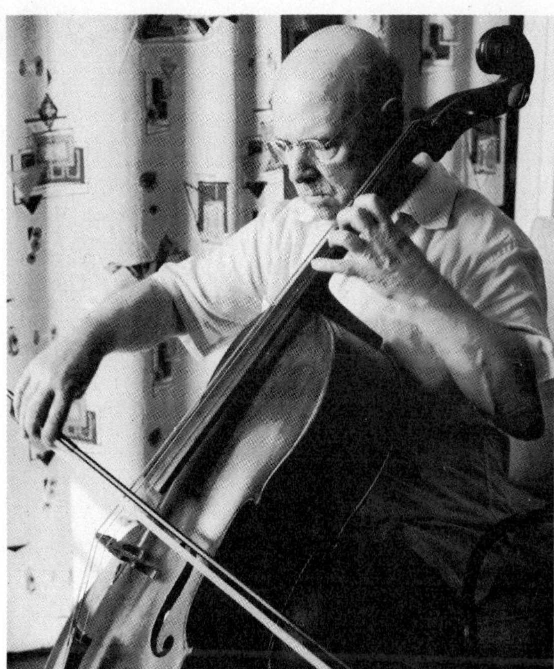

Figure 7.3 Many people remain creative and productive well into later adulthood. Cellist Pablo Casals is one exceptional example.

Creativity and Productivity The capacity for creative thought and creative work also persists into the later years. Tolstoy, Voltaire, Chagall, Picasso, and Casals all continued to produce literature, art, and music of high quality into their seventies and eighties. Creativity and productivity are likely to be the result of accumulated knowledge and experience, as well as the perspective that comes when one has relatively few years left. Wayne Dennis found that historians and inventors, for example, tend to be most productive around the age of sixty. Statesmen and Supreme Court justices are also usually older. Some people even become creative for the first time in their later years—the painter Grandma Moses, for example.

Senility Some older people do become senile. They tend to lose their memory, particularly for recent events; they may lose the ability to do simple arithmetic; and they may become disoriented as to time and place. This type of mental deterioration, it is estimated, affects about 15 percent of people sixty-five to seventy-five and about 25 percent of those over seventy-five—about 4 million elderly people altogether.

Yet "senility" is, medically, a very imprecise term. According to the National Institutes of Health (NIH), there are a hundred or more different causes of senility. Some older people who seem senile are simply depressed; older people are particularly susceptible to severe depression because of the many losses in their lives. Others are suffering from such conditions as arteriosclerosis, anemia, drug side effects, walking pneumonia, and malnutrition. Many have developed a severe organic brain disease called senile dementia, which affects perhaps half the population in nursing homes. NIH estimates that as much as 20 percent of older people who are written off as senile actually have conditions that would respond to treatment.

DEALING WITH AGING

Childhood, adolescence, and young adulthood are years for gathering experience, which is put to productive use during middle adulthood. By contrast, the major task of the later years is to clarify and deepen one's own life and to use this lifetime of experience to deal with the personal changes and losses of these years.

HOW TO Estimate How Long You Will Live

Of course, no one knows for certain how long he or she will live. However, various genetic, environmental influences, and personal habits contribute to one's longevity (or early death). Dr. Diana S. Woodruff of Temple University in Philadelphia has compiled a self-test that takes into account recent statistics on the factors that may lengthen or shorten a person's life. The results will not be scientifically accurate or prophecy, but they may help you to think about increasing your chances for a longer life.

Step one Start by adding your present age to your average life expectancy for people of your age group.

Year of Birth	Male	Female
1957–1961	57 years, 4 months	64 years, 6 months
1962–1966	62 years, 2 months	69 years, 5 months

Step two Keep a list of how many years you are to add or subtract from your life in response to the following statements:

1. Descendants of long-lived people tend to live longer themselves. Add one year for each grandparent who lived to be eighty or more.
2. Firstborn children tend to live longer. If you are the oldest or only child born to your parents, add one year.
3. Overweight is a health hazard and a killer. If you are overweight, subtract one year for each ten pounds of overweight.
4. If you do not smoke, add two years.
5. If you do smoke, subtract twelve years for two or more packs a day, seven years for one to two packs, and two years for less than one pack.
6. If you regularly go without breakfast and just have some snacks for lunch, subtract two years.
7. If you exercise at least two or three times a week (or more), add three years. Exercise can include long walks, bike riding, swimming, jogging, or any athletics as well as calisthenics.
8. If you have lived most of your life in one of the following states, add one year: North or South Dakota, Nebraska, Kansas, Minnesota, Iowa, Missouri.
9. If you have lived mostly in New York, New Jersey, or Pennsylvania, subtract one year.
10. If you live (or intend to live) most of your life in a large city, subtract one year.
11. If you live (or intend to live) most of your life in a rural area, add one year.
12. If you intend to have regular annual medical examinations throughout your lifetime, add two years.
13. If you sleep more than nine hours a night (regularly), subtract four years.
14. If you plan to get married eventually, add three years.
15. If you don't use automobile seat belts, or if you frequently drive or ride with someone beyond the speed limit, subtract one year.
16. If you do use seat belts and observe speed limits, add one year.
17. If you intend to finish college, add one year.
18. If you are planning a professional career, such as law, medicine, or science, add two years.
19. If you intend to get a job that requires you to sit most of the day and not "move around," subtract three years.
20. If you are planning a career that requires physical activity (for example, dancing or construction work), add three years.
21. If you sleep in a cool or cold room, add two years.
22. If you regularly read books or articles about good health or nutrition and try to live according to what you've learned, add five years.
23. If you're usually calm, reasonable, contented, and practical, you might be able to add up to five years.
24. If you're usually very competitive, intense, nervous, or unhappy, you might have to subtract several years—unless you seek professional help or do what you can to calm yourself and change your habits.
25. If you expect to become very rich, take a high risk job (like bomb removal, or one involving much air travel), or remain single, you may have to subtract several years.

Step three To determine your life expectancy figure combine the two results from steps one and two. This is the age to which you can expect to live unless your life style changes.

Source: Adapted from *Senior Scholastic*, vol. 110, November 17, 1977, pp. 10–11. Reprinted with permission of *Family Health* magazine.

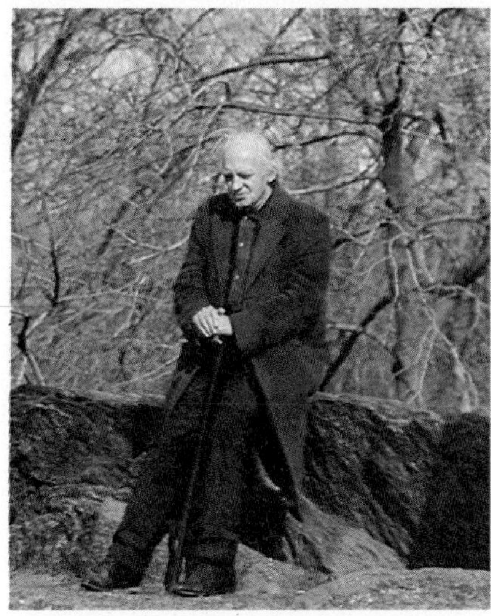

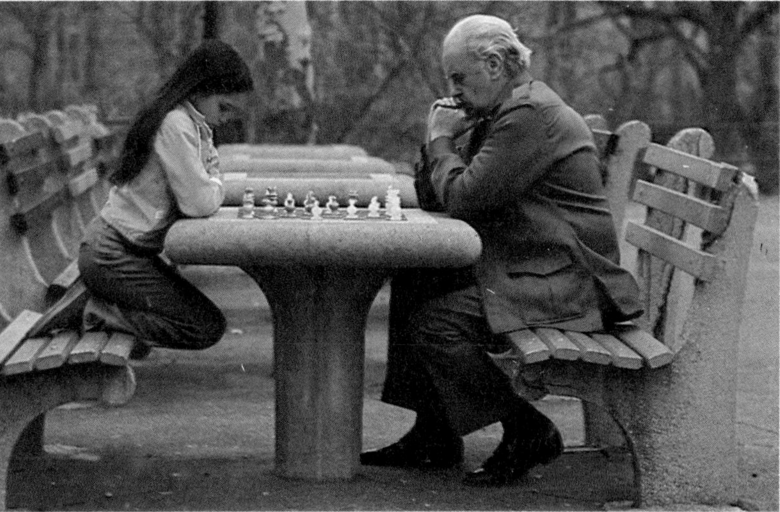

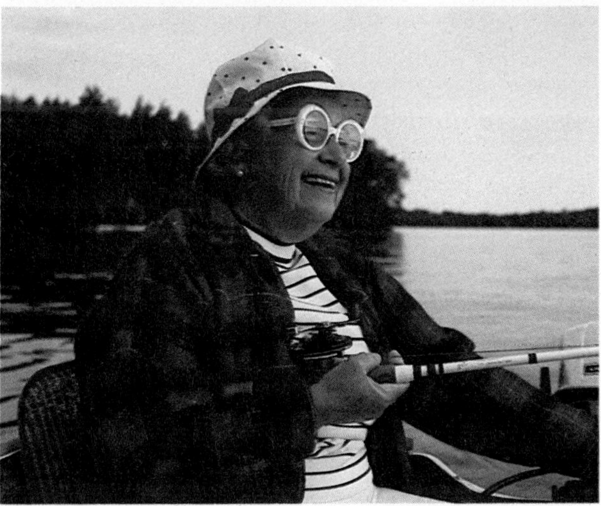

Figure 7.4 People who are unafraid of or look forward to retirement and growing older are more likely to adjust, enjoy themselves, and remain healthy.

Maturity

A mature person in the later years is able to accept his or her own life. Such a person may have achieved *integrity,* the final stage in Erik Erikson's eight stages of human development (see Chapter 1). As Erikson points out, mature people are also likely to be those who can accept the reality of death. Failure to achieve this integrity may leave older people in a state of *despair;* they have little faith in themselves, feel they would like to live their lives over again, and fear death.

People's expectations about growing old seem to be important in determining how successfully they handle the stresses and changes of later life. Those who look forward to retirement adjust to it more easily than those who find the idea distasteful. Those who look forward to growing older also tend to grow old more gracefully than those who fear old age.

Another myth about aging is that older people resist changes. The ability and willingness to change have more to do with lifelong habits and behavior patterns than with age. Studies have shown that people who challenged themselves to change and adapt earlier in life continue to do so in their later years; those who never did still do not. Mature people, because they have had a great deal of experience with change, know what to accept and what to oppose, when to sit quietly and when to fight, and they are able to accept their own limitations.

Maturity in later adulthood also means being willing to depend on others for help when it is necessary. The mature adult is also hopeful rather than helpless. Hope helps to mobilize one's energies and increases one's ability to cope with change. If a person reacts to the stresses of the later years with a sense of hopelessness and helplessness, these stresses can result in death. One who continues to hope and to have control over his or her life is not only likely to handle the events of later years successfully but also to live longer.

FAMILY LIFE

As individuals experience their own life cycles, their families undergo their own collective life cycles. Earlier in life, the family expanded as children were born. Now it contracts, as they grow up and move away. As these children marry and have children of their own, parents become grandparents and perhaps great-grandparents. And throughout all these changes, family relationships often shift.

Marital Life

The great majority of older couples say that they are "happy" or "very happy" with their marriages. The divorce rate among older couples is extremely low, partly because truly unhappy couples are likely to have divorced or separated years before and partly because being married is more desirable to an older person than living alone.

Studies indicate that many older people think their marriage is at least as good as, if not better than, before. Generally, marriages that were good to begin with tend to remain good or to improve. Apparently, once a couple adjusts to having the children gone and the husband retired, the marriage relationship is better than ever. For some, it may even be the first time that they have been able to spend time together, go at their own pace, and enjoy each other's companionship. Unhappy marriages, however, tend to become more unhappy in the later years. If the couple shared little companionship or satisfaction in earlier years, their happiness is more likely to decline.

As with younger couples, the more the relationship meets a person's needs for love, fulfillment, respect, and communication, as well as the need to find meaning in life and sense a continuity with the past, the happier the marriage is in later life (see Chapter 6). Older couples who have happy marriages tend to be more positive and more active than those who are single or unhappily married.

Sexuality

American humor spreads the myth that the years past sixty are sexless. "Definition of old age: The time of life when a man flirts with girls but can't remember why." "Description of the sexual life cycle of a man: Tri-weekly. Try weekly. Try weakly." In one study, when adolescents and young adults were asked to complete the sentence "Sex for most old people is . . . ," most answered "unimportant" or "past."

Some older people themselves accept this myth. Because they think the older years are sexless, the notion becomes a self-fulfilling prophecy. They lose interest in sex and give up sexual activity. Others, who have always found sex "dirty" or unpleasant, are glad to have an acceptable excuse for ending sexual relations.

Most people, however, continue to be sexual beings throughout their lives. Most older people still want to have intercourse almost as much as they ever did, and many continue to be active well into their later years. In one study, nearly one-half of the individuals in their eighties and nineties reported mild or moderate sexual interest.

Some changes do occur in the sexual organs and in sexual performance during later adulthood. Masters and Johnson found that these changes lead to differences in the experience of sexuality but need not lead to impotence. Among women, the vaginal tissues gradually atrophy, vaginal lubrication decreases, and the uterus and cervix get smaller. Among men, there is a steady decline in the production of testosterone. It may take an older man two or three times longer to achieve an erection, but he can preserve it without ejaculating much longer than he could in earlier years. Older men also usually experience less intense orgasms, and it takes longer for them to be restimulated after an ejaculation. Thus, although the capacity for sexual response gradually slows down, reasonably healthy men and women have the capacity for sexual activity well into their later years.

Frequency of sexual satisfaction, not surprisingly, is related to marital happiness. While the average frequency of intercourse among older people is about once a month or less, in one study 28 percent of happily married older women reported that they made love with their husbands more than once a week. Older men generally report more sexual activity than older women. The reason for this may be the

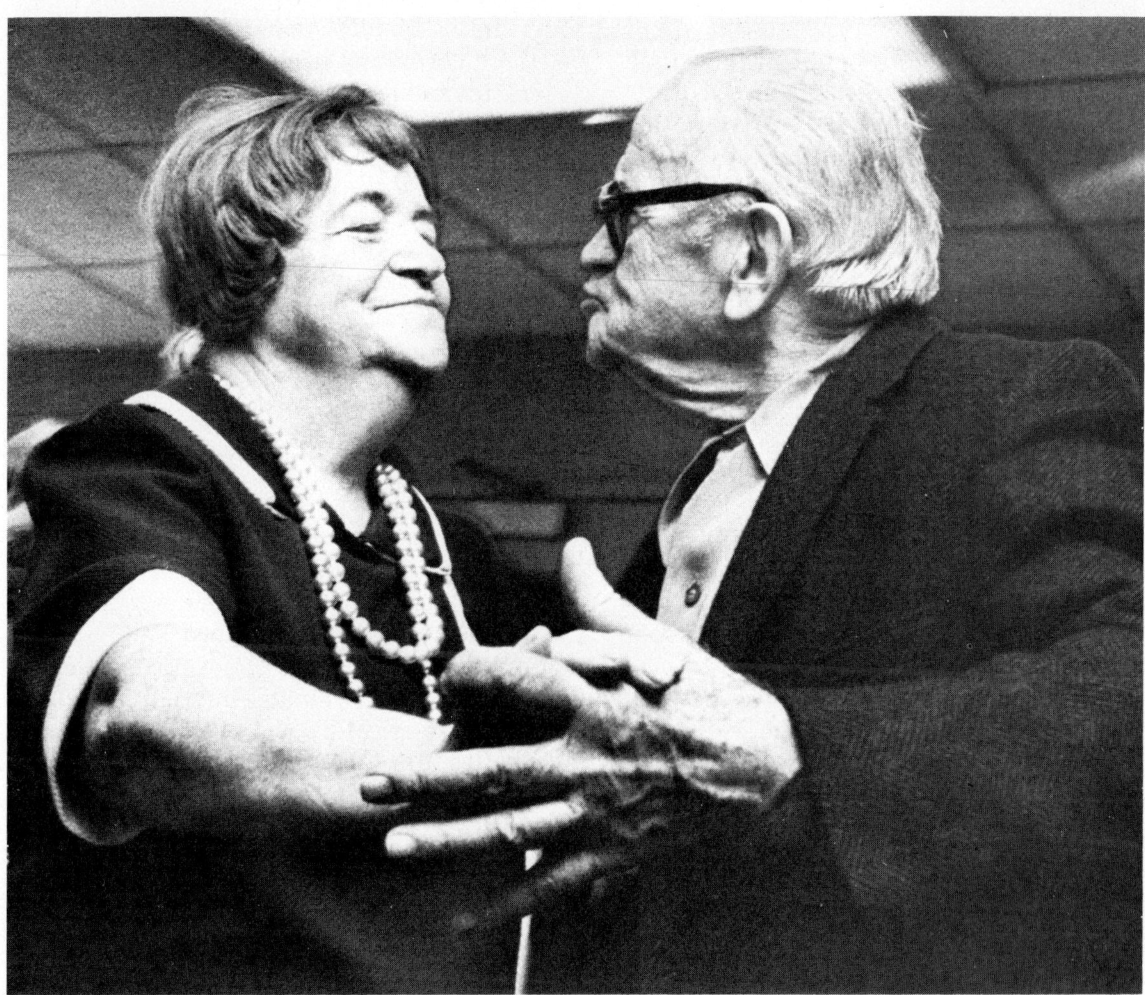

Figure 7.5 Sexual interest and activity usually continue throughout a person's lifetime.

fact that older women are less likely to be married and therefore less likely to have a sex partner. Lack of a partner may lead many older people to turn to masturbation.

The myth of the "dirty old man" who is an exhibitionist or a child molester, however, is completely unsupported. Exhibitionism is rare among people over forty, and older people are the least likely of any to be involved in child molesting.

According to Masters and Johnson, only four criteria appear to be necessary for a long and active sex life: an interesting and receptive partner, regular sexual activity, reasonably good health, and a healthy mental attitude toward aging. Thus the richer and happier your sexual life has been, the more likely you are to continue being sexually active into the later years.

Widowhood

Three times as many older women as men become widowed. Among people sixty to sixty-four, 25 percent of the women have been widowed but only 6 percent of the men. Among women seventy to seventy-four, half are widows. It is not until fifteen years later, when they are eighty-five or older, that half of men are widowers.

The loss of a spouse is a major blow to either a man or a woman. Many women who lose their husbands also lose their social status, their source of emotional support and intellectual stimulation, and often their financial security. Grieving over this loss is a necessary part of the process of adjustment (as we will discuss later in the chapter). Many older people find it impossible to deal with widowhood. It is not uncommon for a widowed person to die soon after a spouse's death, and both suicides and mental disorders are more frequent among widowed people than among married people.

Widowed persons must often develop a new social identity, learning to see themselves in a new way and relating to other people—particularly those of the opposite sex—differently. Widowhood often means learning to live alone, perhaps for the first time. Many feel socially marooned. Friends and even relatives may avoid a widowed person, because they do not know what to say or because the person rearouses the pain of the loss or because they need to deny that they too are also getting older. Once the grieving is over, however, and widows and widowers learn to deal with their new status, many also find a new sense of freedom.

Remarriage

Far more older widowers remarry than do older widows. Each year, some 35,000 men over sixty-five marry, compared to only 16,000 women over sixty-five—although, in this age group, women outnumber men by 3 million. Because society approves of an older man marrying a younger woman while frowning on the reverse, an older widower has many women to choose from while an older widow has less choice. Widowers rarely wait more than a year or two before remarrying; widows are likely to wait about seven years.

Like younger people, older people tend to marry those with similar economic, social, and religious backgrounds; and the groom is usually a little older than the bride. There is one major difference, however, between the marriages of older and younger people. Over half the older people have known their new spouses for a long time, often for most of their lives. Some couples had dated when they were young; others are friends or neighbors. The courtship is usually short and sweet, and the marriage ceremony itself simple.

The advantage of remarriage, of course, is that it makes it possible to avoid living alone, living with a friend, or moving in with the children. And most couples marrying late in life have highly successful marriages.

As mentioned in Chapter 6, an increasing number of older men and women are living together without marrying, because remarriage could mean a substantial reduction in their pension benefits.

Relationships with Children

Long before we ourselves reach old age, we are confronted directly with the realities of aging as we watch and take care of our parents as they grow old. Despite the changes in American families in recent decades, studies show that grown, middle-aged children and their elderly parents do remain mutually involved with each other. More than 80 percent of the elderly live an hour or less away from at least one of their children; 30 percent are ten minutes or less away; and they see each other frequently.

In the majority of families, the two generations continue to exchange advice, services, gifts, and financial assistance. Most older people, however, get more from their families than they give. About two-thirds report that they receive support from their families in the form of money or gifts. And nearly one-third depend on children or other relatives to help with housework, meals, or shopping. The older a person is, the more likely he or she is to live with children.

The importance of these family relationships is shown by the fact that older people who have no relatives or family alive or living near them (about 10 to 20 percent) are the ones who tend to have inadequate financial resources and who must turn to the various social agencies.

SOCIAL-LIFE CHANGES

There are many other changes, in addition to the ones already discussed in this chapter, that affect the elderly—and to which they must adjust. Often, one of the most significant changes is retirement. A man finds himself without his job or career and without daily contacts with fellow workers. If his wife has been working and retires at the same time, she loses both her income and her independence; if she continues to work, the couple can face other problems. While retirement means more time for leisure activities, it also makes some people feel useless and question who they are, in a kind of second identity crisis. This is more likely to happen to a person who has centered his or her life on work.

Only about 30 percent of older people, however, report difficulty in adjusting to retirement. Those who look forward to retirement, who choose to retire early, and who have many identities other than their work identity tend to adjust most easily. Also, people with many friends and who are actively involved in family, church, and social organizations generally find the transition to retirement an easier one.

Older people do tend, however, to lose their former social roles. One study found that the number of social roles (living with another person, keeping in contact with relatives, going to church, being a friend) remained fairly stable for both men and women until they reached sixty-five. After that, people had fewer social roles. Men tended to lose their formal roles not only as workers but also as members of organizations. Women were likely to lose both their formal roles and also their roles as spouses and members of households.

How older people use their leisure time depends heavily on the interests and activities of their middle years. The person who developed many ways to spend free time during earlier adulthood will probably continue these activities. With increasing age, the tendency to participate less actively and to watch others increases. Older people's participation in clubs declines, and older women, particularly, are likely to spend more time around the house and in solitary activities.

Nevertheless, older people continue to participate in the political process. They are generally well informed and actively discuss political issues. People over sixty vote as often as the middle-aged and more often than younger people. Added to the fact that there are now so many more older people, this means that the elderly—if they were organized—could wield a great deal of political power. Some older people have begun to assert themselves politically by organizing an activist group called the Gray Panthers (see the Focus box).

Old age often brings changes in living arrangements. A retired couple may sell a house that has become too large for them and move to a smaller house or an apartment. Some move into retirement communities inhabited exclusively by older people. In these communities, a couple may find themselves far from grown children and old friends. They must learn to live in a new town, among new people, and perhaps in a new climate. Some appear to thrive in these retirement communities, where planned activities may fill every minute. Others find that the absence of younger people cuts off an important source of intellectual stimulation.

The chances of an older person having to live in a home for the aged, nursing home, or other institution are, according to a Duke University study, only about one in four. The people most likely to become institutionalized are those who live alone or have few or no children to help take care of them.

Many older people have serious financial problems. Retirement generally cuts a couple's income in half; a greater proportion must thus go for necessities such as food, housing, and medical expenses. Inflation drastically reduces the real value of savings and fixed-income pensions. And lengthy illnesses with high hospital costs can rapidly deplete the financial resources of even those people who, in their middle years, providently set aside for their old age what seemed like sufficient funds. As a result, while the elderly form only one-tenth of the United States population, in 1975, one-sixth of them had incomes below the official poverty line.

Friendship

Research suggests that if an older person has at least one intimate friend with whom to share the details of life and discuss personal problems, he or she will adjust more easily to the changes and stresses of the later years. This

FOCUS
The Gray Panthers

In 1970, Maggie Kuhn, an energetic Philadelphia woman, was forced to retire at sixty-three after twenty-five years of service with the Presbyterian Church. Angered by this policy, she and five friends who were also retiring from religious and social-work organizations decided that it was time to unite to combat *ageism*—discrimination against and stereotyping of old people. Kuhn's idea took hold, and her group began to attract followers. They were called—in jest, at first—the Gray Panthers.

The name has stuck, and so has the movement. Today there are 10,000 Gray Panthers in the United States; about 25 percent are under thirty years old. Their interests have broadened, and they define themselves as "a group of people—old and young—drawn together by deeply felt common concern for human liberation and social change." But they are still essentially committed to the fight against ageism.

The Gray Panthers seek to protect the rights of old people, and their major legislative concern is the removal of the mandatory retirement age. Due largely to the work of the Panthers, this age has been raised from sixty-five to seventy, but the group hopes to abolish it altogether. They regard the mandatory retirement age as an imaginary line that bears no relation whatsoever to competence, productivity, or creativity, but perpetuates the myth that old people are "useless." Kuhn also points out that the number of old people in the United States is growing steadily. She says, "If we continue to waste the experience and talent of the older population, we will become a dying society."

The Gray Panthers have been active, often in coalition with other groups, on several related legislative fronts. They have helped to bring about a good deal of nursing home reform, with particular emphasis on the patient's rights; they successfully pressed for the passage of the "Living Will" in the California legislature, enabling a person to refuse to prolong his or her life with artificial treatments if death is clearly imminent; they fight for consumer rights and have been instrumental in protecting the hearing impaired from being misled or defrauded by hearing aid companies.

The Gray Panthers are also working to change the image of the old person in American society. They believe that the mass media are among the foremost promoters of ageism, and a group of Panthers established Media Watch to keep track of specific complaints. Volunteers watch television to look out for youth-oriented advertising, negative stereotypes of old people in programming, and representation of old people as emcees or newscasters. Research shows that old people watch more TV than any other age group, and the Panthers feel that TV should present them more often in more favorable, less stereotyped ways.

The Gray Panthers hope to replace common ageist misconceptions with positive attitudes toward old people. Maggie Kuhn sums up, "We must give old people new images of themselves as functioning individuals of value to society."

confidant does not have to be a mate, nor does it matter whether the person is male or female. A man most frequently names his wife as his best friend, while a woman is more likely to name a child or a friend. She seldom names her husband even if he is still alive. The fact that women are more likely than men to have a close friend other than their spouse may help give women an advantage in survival and adaptability.

Having a close friend to talk with becomes important when one must face death—either one's own or that of a loved one. Being able to confide in another person helps one to come to terms with one's life and the imminent end of it. As Erikson has pointed out, one of the major tasks of old age is successful preparation for death.

DEFINITIONS OF DEATH

Formerly, a person was considered dead when he or she stopped breathing and the heart ceased to beat. Today, however, medical technology is able to keep respiration going and the heart beating in people who otherwise

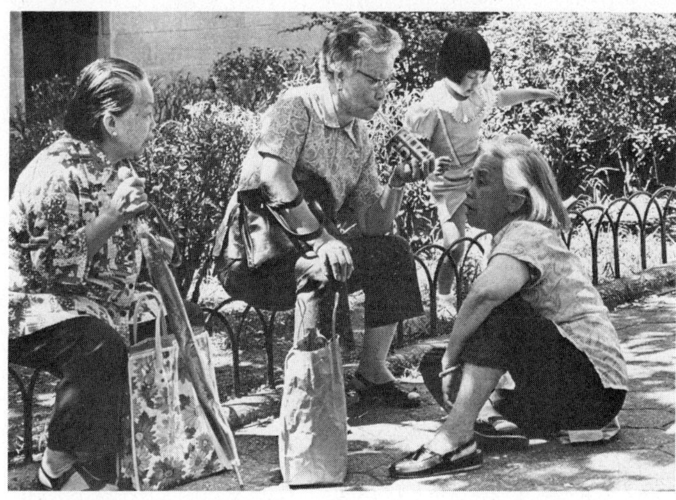

Figure 7.6 Research suggests that older people who have at least one intimate friend can cope more easily with the stresses and changes of the later years.

would be dead. And today it is also important to determine when death occurs because of the need for body parts (such as kidneys) to transplant into—and save the lives of—other people. In 1968, a committee of the Harvard Medical School offered a new definition of death based on brain death. A person would be considered dead if he or she is unreceptive and unresponsive, is in an irreversible coma, does not move or breathe off a respirator, has no reflexes, and has a flat electroencephalogram (EEG), indicating no brain waves. This definition is now widely accepted medically, and a number of states have written it into law.

COMMON ATTITUDES TOWARD DEATH

The current interest in thanatology may represent a shift in prevailing attitudes toward death. At present, however, it is only a slight shift. Most Americans, like most members of Western society, tend to avoid thinking about death—thereby denying its reality—until that reality confronts them directly. When one does happen to think of death, one usually tends to back away as quickly as possible, moving to safer areas of thought. Sometimes the death of a friend or relative brings the subject home, but soon—if not immediately—the subject becomes too threatening for the mind to bear. Indeed, many people feel that in order to remain sane and healthy, they must avoid thinking about death and keep at a comfortable distance the unresolved crisis of one's own inevitable death.

The Influence of Age

People's attitudes toward death are related to their age. Many young Americans, for instance, have grown up with little talk of death. One survey of 30,000 young adults found that one-third did not recall any discussion of death during their childhood; one-third recalled discussion of the subject but in an uncomfortable way; and only one-third said death was talked about openly. Most first became aware of death between the ages of five and ten, and for nearly half, the death of a grandparent was their first personal involvement with mortality.

For a child, especially a child under ten, death is a difficult idea. By the time they are eight or nine, most children know that it happens to everyone. But they are less sure about the fact that it is final: they may wait for a squashed bug to revive or not understand that someone who has "gone away" will not someday come back. Researchers have also found that some children may see death as a form of punishment, as something that happens to a person who has done wrong. Realizing that death has physical, not psychological, causes; that it comes to everyone; and that it is final depends both on age and stage of development.

In childhood and adolescence, death may be puzzling, but it is basically an abstract idea.

Experience with death is rare, and it seldom touches the young person's life in a deep or lasting way. The middle years of life bring a heightened awareness of death as a personal possibility. The middle-aged person is likely to have experienced the death of one or both parents and may have seen the death of friends and colleagues. As they see these other people die with their goals and projects unfinished, middle-aged people may become apprehensive about dying when they are not ready for it. One national survey of more than 1,500 adults found that middle-aged adults were most fearful of death and more likely than either the young or the old to believe that "death always comes too soon."

The same survey found that older people were least likely to think this and most likely to have made plans for it. Death is generally less frightening to older people, and they tend to think of it more often and talk about it more. There are a number of possible reasons for this diminished fear of death among older people. Because they have finished many of their life projects, and may be facing ill health or having financial problems, they may place less value on life, or become more realistic about their *own* mortality. If they have survived beyond their allotted time span, they may feel that they are now on "borrowed" time. And as older people live through the deaths of friends and relatives, they may become more used to the idea of their own deaths.

Death also has special meanings for older people. The fact that they know themselves to be close to death alters their perception and use of time. Older people tend not to plan as far ahead as do younger people. In one survey, when people were asked what they would do if they had only six months left to live, older people were less likely than younger people to say they would change the way they lived and were more likely to say they would spend their remaining time in quiet contemplation.

The Influence of Education

How people view death is also likely to depend in part on their education. People with little education are likely to think often of death and have negative views of it. They are more likely to agree that "death always comes too soon" and that "to die is to suffer," and are least likely to have made any plans for their death. The more education a person has, the more likely he or she is to have talked with others about death, to have made a will, and to have discussed funeral arrangements. People's views of death are also likely to be strongly influenced by their religious beliefs. Dealing with death and dying is likely to be easier for those who are religious and are regular church-goers.

Although it is considered morbid to dwell on the subject of death, most people have a great deal of curiosity about it and want to know "what it's like to die." Such curiosity usually includes equal parts of excitement and dread: people want to know, yet fear knowing for certain. Death, after all, remains throughout one's lifetime an unknown factor, and fear of the unknown is a universal human trait.

THE EXPERIENCE OF DYING

Despite fears of a painful, lingering death, few people spend many months seriously ill before they die. Most people can expect only a few days or weeks of terminal illness requiring special care. Even most terminally ill patients avoid a painful death, and older persons often die more easily than younger ones. In one study of dying patients, 45 percent of those under fifty had pain or other unrelieved physical distress. Among patients between fifty and seventy, those with unrelieved pain dropped to 32 percent, and only 10 percent of those over seventy experienced such discomfort.

As death approaches, people are likely to feel increasingly drowsy and be quite unaware of what is going on around them. The disease, the drugs, and the psychological distancing of the dying patient from the world all tend to contribute to this drowsiness. Only about 6 percent of dying patients are conscious shortly before death, and the moment of death is only rarely distressful. There is even some evidence that, as death approaches, the brain releases a chemical that makes the moment of death pleasant instead of painful.

People who have narrowly escaped death say the experience is not painful and may even be peaceful and blissful. One study of more than 35,000 deathbed observations by doctors and nurses concluded that fear was not common among dying patients who were conscious just before their deaths, and that a great many reported seeing visions of heaven, beautiful pastures, or lush vegetation.

Raymond Moody interviewed more than fifty people who had been resuscitated after having been pronounced dead or who had narrowly escaped death by accident. He found considerable similarities in their reports. Common elements of these brushes with death included overhearing a doctor pronounce one dead; pleasant sensations; noises, the feeling of being drawn quickly through a dark, enclosed space; the feeling of watching one's body from some point outside it; encounters with close relatives or friends who had died; visions of a radiant and benevolent being of light; a partial or total review of one's life; the feeling of approaching a border or limit.

Although many first made desperate attempts to get back into their bodies and felt sad that death had come, they soon felt a sense of timelessness, peace, and tranquility, and were unwilling to return. Most reported that, as a result of their encounters with death, their attitudes toward life and death had changed. They were no longer afraid of death, they valued and enjoyed life more, and they were more philosophical about existence.

THE NEEDS OF THE DYING PERSON

One of the first people to study the needs and responses of terminally ill patients was the Swiss-born psychiatrist Elizabeth Kübler-Ross. In her now famous book *On Death and Dying,* published in 1969, Kübler-Ross reported research she had conducted in the United States with more than 200 dying people of varying ages and backgrounds.

Her most consistent finding was that terminal patients are usually willing, and often eager or anxious, to discuss their situation. The patients she and her students interviewed persuaded her that the majority of people who are about to die need to talk frankly with people who can listen to them without pretense, without judgment, and without signs of terror or despair.

Whether or not a dying person should be told explicitly of his or her condition should really depend on the person's own wishes. In one study, 80 percent of cancer patients said that they wanted to be told that their illness was fatal. Knowing that they were going to die permitted them to get their affairs in order and plan for their deaths. It also helped them, they felt, to understand their illness and gave them peace of mind. Not every person, however, who says he or she wants this information actually means it. Closeness to death may make some people less eager to know the truth.

A problem exists when the patient, doctor, hospital staff, and family all know that a person is dying but are unwilling to discuss it. Although this pretense may provide dignity and privacy to the dying patient, it also keeps him or her from having warm and supportive family relationships and from being able to deal openly with any concerns about death. When these can be talked about openly, the patient finds it easier to face death and the family finds it easier to cope with the patient's condition.

The Ambulatory Dying

The ambulatory dying—such as some cancer patients whose death may be certain but is being deferred by radiotherapy or chemotherapy—have the same needs as people dying in hospitals or other institutions, but they also have other concerns. Because their daily lives may seem on the surface the same, for them death and dying have a special unreality. They may hesitate to face death squarely by talking about their condition, for fear of losing their friends or jobs. They may weigh the idea of shortened life against the wisdom of saving it to provide for a possibly prolonged dying. As death approaches, these people may be sentenced to an island of isolation, created partly by their own personal fears and partly by the uneasiness that many acquaintances cannot help displaying in their presence.

Those who feel especially clumsy or inarticulate near a dying friend need to remember that all human beings are gifted with a talent for psychological deafness. A dying person is quite likely to block out unwanted truths or postpone digesting them. Remembering this can help alleviate the worry of professionals and laymen alike in talking with the dying.

The primary psychological state of most dying patients can best be described as ambivalence: a constant wavering between opposites, sometimes needing the presence of people, sometimes abhorring their presence; sometimes angry, sometimes serene; sometimes openly confronting the fact of their dying, sometimes denying it.

The Hospice Approach

With the increasing complexity of medical care, more and more people are dying in hospitals or other institutions. In New York City, for example, in 1955, 66 percent of deaths occurred in institutions. By 1967, the proportion had risen to 73 percent. Only 24 percent of deaths took place at home.

In recent years, people with fatal illnesses (and also those who are still healthy) have begun to emphasize their desire to have some say over the time and place of their death. The *hospice* movement has been one response to this demand. The aim of the hospice is to provide a humane, dignified environment where people can die gracefully without the indignity of extraordinary measures—such as respirators, transfusions, and intravenous feedings—to prolong life. Hospices offer the dying person a warm, homelike atmosphere in which he or she can face death.

The first hospice, St. Christopher's, was established in England by Cicely Saunders. The patients at St. Christopher's know they are there to die. Medical treatment is available to ease discomfort and relieve pain, and friends and family can visit at any hour. The institutional setting is played down, so that patients can feel they are surrounded by ongoing life. About forty other hospices have been established in England, and the movement is now spreading to the United States.

Dying at Home

As another response, in some places, physicians are releasing patients from hospitals so that they can die at home. In a number of hospitals, for example, children who are dying of cancer are allowed to go home. It has been reported that the parents of these children feel less guilty than parents of children who die in hospitals, and they are pleased that they can satisfy their children's wishes to be at home. When a family member dies at home, death can become less mysterious and frightening for the whole family.

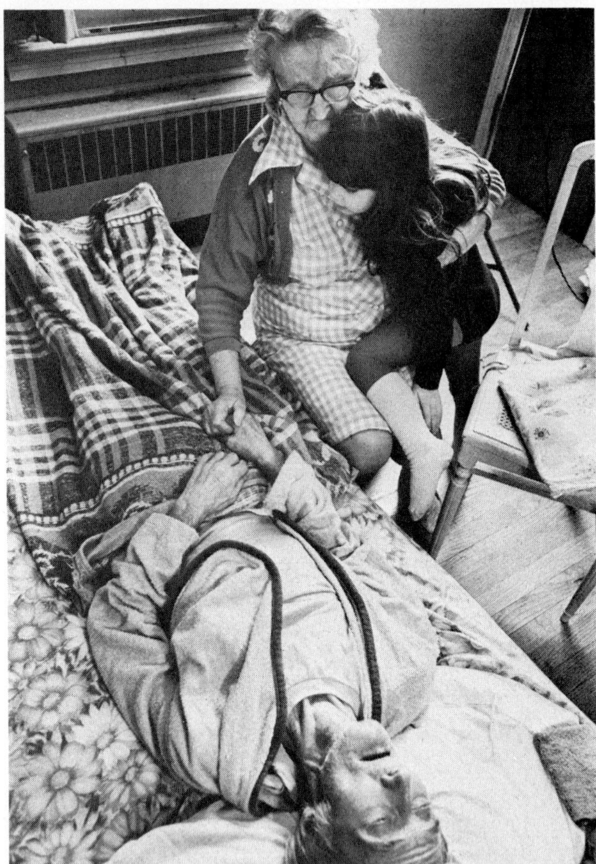

Figure 7.7 This man chose to die with dignity at his home surrounded by the loving support of his wife, children, and grandchildren.

EUTHANASIA

The fact that dying people can now sometimes be kept "alive" almost indefinitely by respirators and other medical technology has introduced new complexities to the controversial question of *euthanasia* or "mercy killing." Should a person who is brain-dead and virtually a vegetable be maintained on a respirator for months or even years? Or should someone "pull the plug"? And if someone does, is the act euthanasia? Or is it murder? Or is it simply stopping useless treatment on a person who is, in fact, already dead? And who should decide whether to pull the plug? The physician? The person's family? Or a court of law?

In discussing such questions, ethicists draw a distinction between *active* and *passive euthanasia.* In active euthanasia, death is hastened by the use of drugs or some other simple procedure. In passive euthanasia, everything possible is done to ease pain and discomfort, but extraordinary life-prolonging measures are eliminated. One's life is not extended by the use of machines, drugs, transfusions, or intravenous feedings.

Most Americans admit to a belief in passive euthanasia. It is not uncommon in medical practice, although doctors rarely acknowledge it for fear of legal complications. Passive euthanasia has considerable authoritative backing, including that of the late Pope Pius XII, who declared that no extraordinary means need be taken to prolong human life.

The number of people who actually practice active euthanasia is difficult to ascertain. Some physicians admit privately that they have done so, either directly, by administering a lethal drug, or indirectly, by allowing either the patient or the family to cause the death.

On the other hand, many people believe that all possible efforts should be made to prolong the life of seriously ill patients as long as possible. Those who take this stance maintain that any tampering with human life is a form of playing God and that the result is either murder or, if the patient concurs, murder combined with suicide.

Increasingly, dying people themselves want to be involved in such life-and-death decisions. To some, the prospect of a life filled with pain or considerable physical or mental damage is less preferable than death. Legally, people generally can refuse medical treatment even when it might prolong their lives; the tough questions arise when a dying patient is comatose or otherwise incompetent to make such decisions. A number of people have begun to write "living wills," documents that give them an opportunity to set forth their wishes at a time when they are well enough to make reasonable decisions. A living will specifies the circumstances in which the writer would choose death over life and expresses a preference for active or passive euthanasia. Although the will is not legally binding, it gives physicians and families some guidance at a time when their decisions can affect the quality of a loved one's death.

STAGES OF COPING WITH DEATH

Kübler-Ross has identified five psychological stages that patients go through in the course of coping with the reality of a terminal illness.

Denial and Isolation The beginning stage is characterized at first by denial, a temporary defense mechanism that buffers the unwelcome news. Later in this stage comes isolation, a mechanism by which patients can drop their denial long enough to talk about the illness and at other times can talk about their lives as though the illness does not exist.

Anger When patients can no longer deny the fact of their illness, they move to a second stage, consisting of resentment and anger. Neither family nor medical personnel are able to help much at this stage, since the anger tends to be directed at everyone in sight, including them. Those who come to visit patients during the anger stage usually find the encounters painful.

Bargaining The third stage is the bargaining stage, during which patients may offer their talents or their very lives in exchange for a bit more time. A typical bargain consists of the promise to live one's life "in the service of the church."

Depression When complications set in, such as added symptoms, increased financial burdens, and a growing inability to function, dying patients generally experience a sense of loss and depression.

Directive to Physicians

Directive made this ______ day of ______________________________ (month, year).

I ______________________________, being of sound mind, willfully, and voluntarily make known my desire that my life shall not be artifically prolonged under the circumstances set forth below, do hereby declare:

1. If at any time I should have an incurable injury, disease, or illness certified to be a terminal condition by two physicians, and where the application of life-sustaining procedures would serve only to artificially prolong the moment of my death and where my physician determines that my death is imminent whether or not life-sustaining procedures are utilized, I direct that such procedures be withheld or withdrawn, and that I be permitted to die naturally.

2. In the absence of my ability to give directions regarding the use of such life-sustaining procedures, it is my intention that this directive shall be honored by my family and physician(s) as the final expression of my legal right to refuse medical or surgical treatment and accept the consequences from such refusal.

3. If I have been diagnosed as pregnant and that diagnosis is known to my physician, this directive shall have no force or effect during the course of my pregnancy.

4. I have been diagnosed and notified at least 14 days ago as having a terminal condition by

   ______________________________, M.D., whose address is ______________________________

   ______________________________, and whose telephone number is ____________________.
   I understand that if I have not filled in the physician's name and address, it shall be presumed that I did not have a terminal condition when I made out this directive.

5. This directive shall have no force or effect five years from the date filled in above.

6. I understand the full import of this directive and I am emotionally and mentally competent to make this directive.

Signed ______________________________

City, County and State of Residence ______________________________

____

The declarant has been personally known to me and I believe him or her to be of sound mind.

Witness ______________________________

Witness ______________________________

This Directive complies in form with the "Natural Death Act" California Health and Safety Code, Section 7188, Assembly Bill 3060 (Keene).

Figure 7.8 The directive to physicians allows a terminally ill person to instruct his or her doctor not to use artificial methods to extend the natural process of dying.

Acceptance Those who have enough time in the course of their illness to work their way through the other four stages eventually reach the stage of acceptance, during which they seem neither depressed nor angry about the imminence of death. Acceptance, observes Kübler-Ross, is not a happy stage, but a period that is nearly void of feelings. During this time, patients tend to be quiet and calmly reflective. Often, they prefer to have few visitors or none at all.

Other authorities have questioned the existence of these stages, saying the only state that appears to be universal to dying people who are aware of their condition is depression.

Kübler-Ross emphasizes that the stages described here do not necessarily occur one after the other; some stages may exist together, side by side, for a while. Some, especially denial, may return unexpectedly. And persisting throughout all of them, she says, is hope.

> In listening to our terminally ill patients, we were always impressed that even the most accepting, the most realistic patients left the possibility open for some cure, for the discovery of a new drug or . . . "last-minute success in a research project."

THE NATURE OF GRIEF

Grief is a normal human response to the loss of anyone or anything to which a person has an emotional attachment. The intensity of grief varies with the importance of the loss and the circumstances in which it occurred. The more closely a loss affects the daily lives of the survivors, the more disruptive its impact is likely to be.

Whenever a person suffers any major loss, it is natural to experience a variety of emotions. At the death of a loved one, a person usually feels shock, disorganization, hopelessness, frustration, anger, guilt, loneliness, isolation, terror, and relief. Colin Murray Parkes has identified four phases of the emotion of grief: first, a period of numbness; a time of yearning, characterized by the desire to recover the lost one; a period of despair, when the reality of the loss sets in; and finally, a period of reorganizing one's way of life to adjust to the loss.

Physical ailments—such as headaches, backaches, insomnia, loss of appetite, dizziness, nausea, and diarrhea—often accompany grief. Death rates among widows are higher during the first year of widowhood than among married people the same age. In acute cases, grief can manifest itself in bizarre symptoms ranging from hallucinations to suicidal impulses. Such acute grief sometimes occurs among survivors of accidents that killed friends or loved ones. In such cases, the survivors' loss is intensified by guilt that they escaped with their own lives only by a quirk of fate.

In normal grieving, physical and emotional problems tend to disappear as the intensity of grief recedes. Since each person copes with loss at an individual pace, there is no time limit on a normal recovery. To the extent that mourners grieve openly and share their feelings candidly, the more crippling effects of grief may either fail to appear or dissipate more rapidly.

Normal grief is resolved when the needs supplied by the lost relationship are gradually supplanted by new relationships or met within the self. One of the surest signs that grief is moving toward resolution is the ability to reach out to a fellow griever without reliving and retelling the entire grief experience. Research indicates that grievers are less than adequate consolers to one another until individual grief nearly subsides. Before that, grievers in a group concentrate on their own hurts to the exclusion of sympathy for others.

Anticipatory Grief

When people learn that a loved one is dying, they often begin to prepare themselves for the impending death. In this *anticipatory grieving,* people deal with their feelings about death before the person actually dies. Thus, loved ones may have completed much of their mourning before the death occurs. When this happens, mourning afterward may be shorter and easier.

According to Kübler-Ross, when family members anticipate the death of a loved one, their reactions go through a sequence similar to that felt by the dying person—denial, anger, bargaining, depression, acceptance. Kübler-Ross believes that the most difficult time for the family is likely to be when the dying person is becoming detached from the world. Although this detachment is a normal way of dealing with one's own death, it tends to make the family feel rejected.

THE NEEDS OF THE BEREAVED

In hospitals, after a person dies, the staff may pay more attention to permission for an autopsy than to the needs of the bereaved. Rarely are the bereaved given more than perfunctory attention—perhaps some tranquilizers or sleeping pills. Few hospitals have waiting facilities that allow or encourage more than stoic bravery when a death is announced. Also, it is usually the custom to treat all bereaved persons the same, whether their loss has been sud-

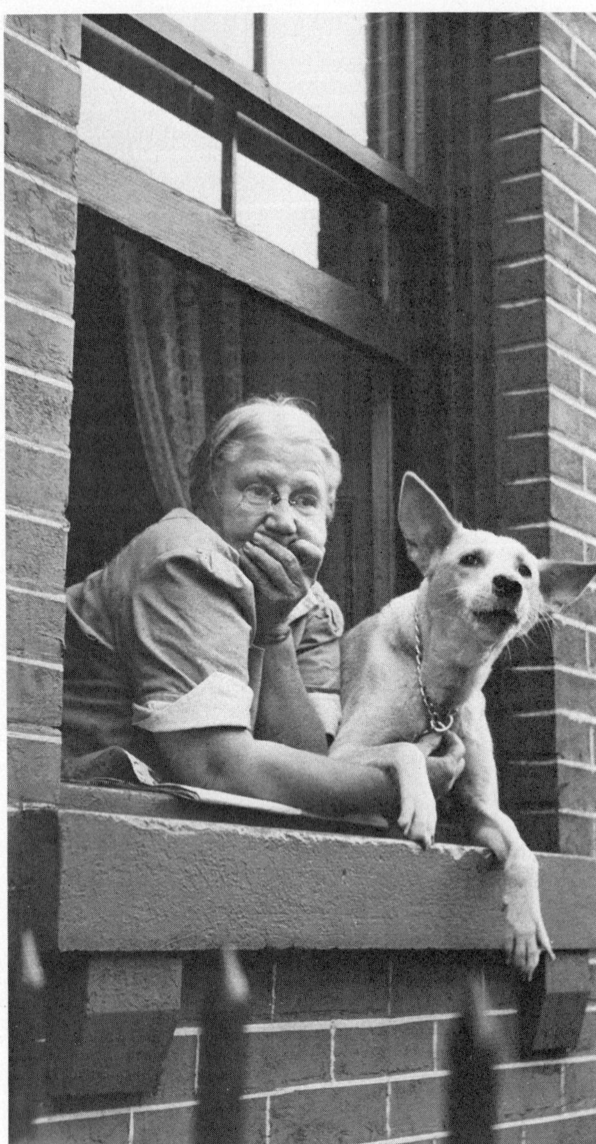

Figure 7.9 Even after the initial phases of grief have passed, people need the comfort of companionship, which can be provided by a loving pet.

den or has followed a prolonged and tedious dying. In cases of lingering death, where grief is anticipatory, the needs of grievers are greatest during the time when they must await that loss. After such a death, the need of the bereaved is for support in beginning life anew.

In the event of a sudden death, time alone can adequately dull the force of the loss. Whatever the cause of death and the age of the deceased, both the crippling and the remedial aspects of grief may surface months later, long after friends have stopped coming or have grown too impatient to listen.

Animals, especially cats and dogs, often play an important role in the lives of grieving people. Many a lonely bereaved person finds needed companionship in an animal during the days of declining grief.

Grief Therapy

For some people, grieving becomes a way of life. For others, the problem is an apparent inability to mourn. Such people consciously or unconsciously resolve not to admit their loss. They may refuse, for example, to alter the personal belongings of the deceased.

Both grief and lack of grief are now considered treatable illnesses. Like other forms of psychotherapy, grief therapy usually consists of "talking out" the patient's problems. Most experts agree that one should try to talk out, feel out, and act out one's grief—if possible, during the initial weeks of bereavement. Sometimes, what David Dempsey refers to as "a little curbstone psychotherapy" by a minister or friend can help a bereaved person regain equilibrium during this difficult period.

Research shows that the people most in need of grief therapy tend to be those who have suffered a sudden loss. Such people face a shock that is made more intense by its unexpectedness.

FUNERAL RITES

When death finally comes, with it comes the necessity for some sort of parting ceremony. This ritual occurs, in one form or another, in every human society (see Figure 7.10). Like other rituals, it satisfies deep-seated human needs. Just as weddings are planned primarily for the benefit of the spectators, so funeral services are designed and conducted for the benefit of the survivors.

For most Americans, funeral customs have changed very little through the years. Most people (82 percent in a recent poll) prefer burial as the form of final disposition. Usually the dead person is placed in a casket, eulogized

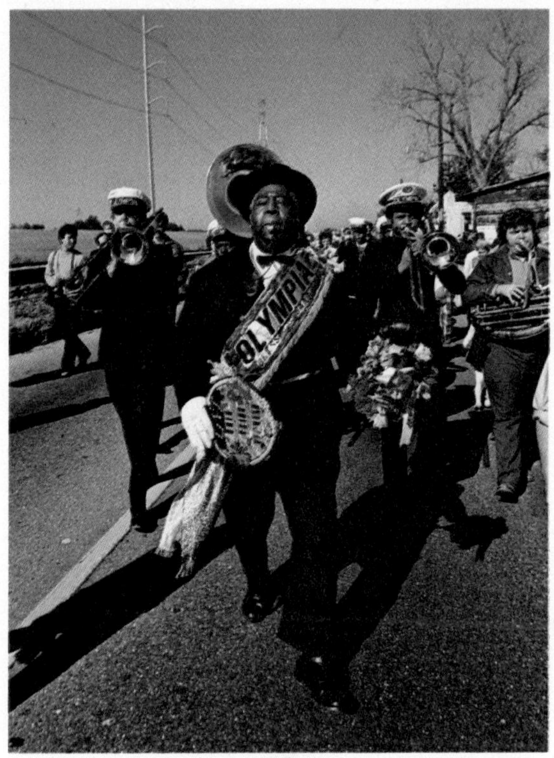

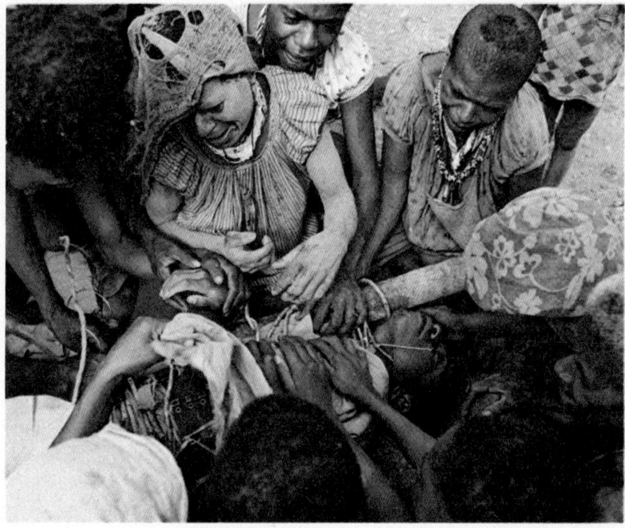

Figure 7.10 In every human society, the dead are granted ceremonial recognition by their family and immediate community.

during a brief service, carried to a cemetery, given religious blessings, and buried in the earth or in a mausoleum.

Although people are beginning to consider new rituals and differing modes of disposition, tradition encourages Americans to dispose of their dead with a degree of dignity and ceremony. Tradition also favors some manner of preserving the remains and of making survivors remember the impact of important family and community members.

The Cost of Dying

The traditional funeral is a sizable expense for many people (see Figure 7.10). As a ceremonial expenditure, it ranks second only to the amount Americans spend each year on weddings. Simple, inexpensive funerals are rare. For example, the average total bill for a 1974 funeral in the Washington, D.C., area was $1,886, excluding the cost of the grave plot.

No American business has been more criticized for both its costs and its practices than the funeral industry. In her best-selling book *The American Way of Death,* Jessica Mitford drew national attention to widespread industry practices that she considered deceptive or unscrupulous.

It should be noted, however, that most Americans questioned in numerous surveys have indicated their approval of both funerals and funeral directors. In fact, though funeral directors are the most publicly maligned of all death-related professionals, they continually score much higher in client satisfaction than doctors, nurses, or clergy.

Psychological Values

Despite the costs of traditional services, there is evidence that full-scale funerals, with all their cumbersome ceremonial trappings, may be of psychological value to the survivors. In particular, the tradition of viewing the body or casket in the funeral home prior to the service is thought to be important as a means of "giving up" the deceased. Research suggests that

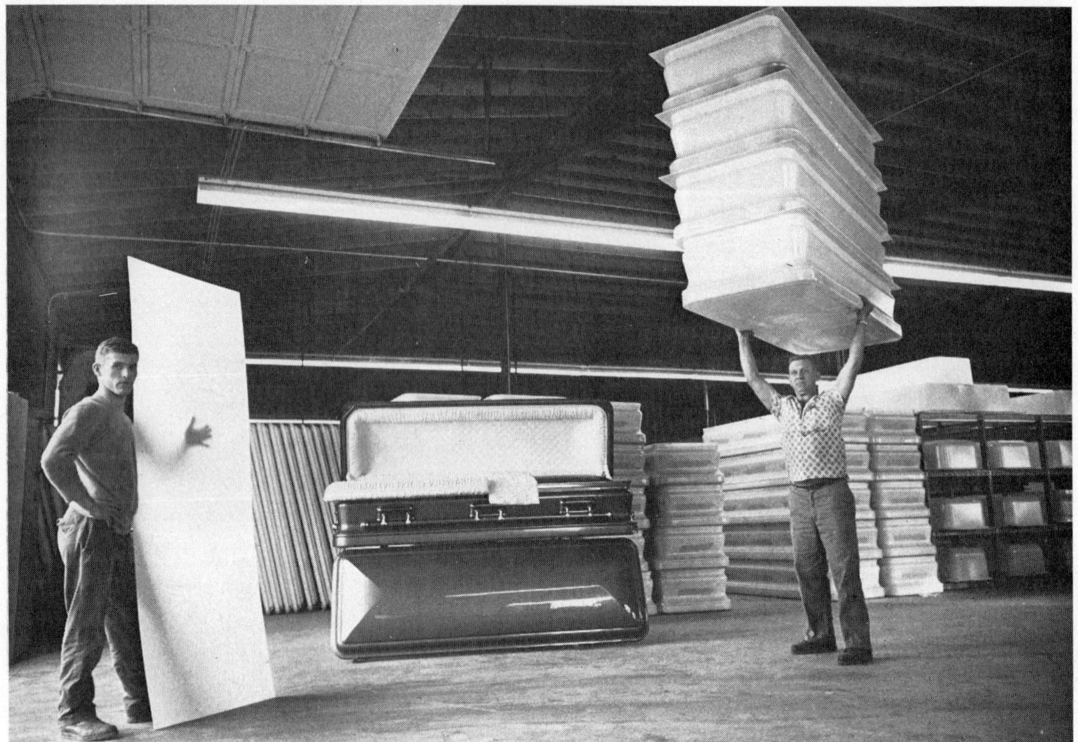

Figure 7.11 Death is a multibillion-dollar business for the funeral industry.

survivors who view the body or casket and then see it laid to rest are less likely to experience serious problems of adjustment than those who do not partake of these ceremonies.

THIS PRECIOUS GIFT

As it must to all living creatures, death will eventually come to each of us. Life, after all, is in itself a terminal condition.

When someone close to us—a grandparent, a parent, a relative, or a friend—is going through the process of dying, we should endeavor to help them in any way we can: supporting them emotionally, performing small services, lending a sympathetic ear whenever they need it. When our own turn comes, hopefully there will be someone near to do the same for us, and help us accept the reality of our own death with grace and dignity.

It is, after all, our awareness of this biological inevitability and the transience of our lives that distinguishes us from the other animals on this earth and heightens our appreciation of this precious gift of life.

SUMMARY

1. Both the number and the percentage of older people in the United States are steadily increasing. In 1900, 4 percent of the population (3.1 million people) were sixty-five or over. Today this is true of 10 percent (23.9 million people).
2. There are many theories (none fully satisfactory) about the cause of aging: that the body simply wears out; that waste products build up; that the immune system causes the body to attack itself; that free radicals destroy essential chemicals; that the genetic program runs out; that errors in DNA accumulate; that specific pacemakers control the process.
3. Some of the external physical changes of aging are thinning, whitening hair; wrinkled

skin; loss of teeth; shorter stature; stiff joints; atrophied muscles; and more fragile bones. Some of the internal changes are decreased work capacity of the heart; slower circulation; and reduced lung capacity.

4. Elderly people are sick more than younger people. About one out of four is hospitalized each year, and they stay twice as long. About 80 percent have a chronic health problem.

5. Aging per se does not diminish intelligence or memory. Verbal and visual skills improve with age, and the capacity for creative thought and work persists. Older people do slow down mentally, however, and hand-eye coordination diminishes. About 25 percent of those over seventy-five, however, do show signs of senility.

6. Mature elderly people may achieve "integrity," the final stage in Erik Erikson's eight stages of development. If not, they may be in the state Erikson calls "despair."

7. Most older couples are happy with their marriages and continue sexual activity. Three times as many older women as men become widowed, but more than twice as many men over sixty-five as women that age marry each year.

8. Among the many other changes that older people may face are retirement, loss of social roles, different living arrangements, institutionalization, and seriously reduced income.

9. Most people tend to deny the reality of death until it confronts them directly. Children find it hard to conceive of death's finality; younger adults tend not to think of death as something that affects them personally. Middle-aged people are likely to be the most fearful of death, while older people find death less frightening and are most likely to have planned for it.

10. Death usually comes quickly, painlessly, and peacefully. Most people are terminally ill, requiring special care, for only a few days or weeks.

11. Research by Kübler-Ross found that most terminal patients need to talk frankly about their situation with people who can listen without pretense, judgment, terror, or despair. Whether or not a dying person should be told of the condition should depend on his or her own wishes.

12. In passive euthanasia, life is not prolonged by the use of extraordinary measures. More and more people are writing "living wills" that set forth their own wishes at a time when they are still well.

13. Kübler-Ross has identified five psychological stages that patients go through in the course of coping with the reality of a terminal illness: denial and isolation, anger, bargaining, depression, and acceptance.

14. Grief is a normal human response to the death of a loved one. It is often accompanied by physical ailments, such as headaches, backaches, insomnia, loss of appetite, dizziness, nausea, and diarrhea.

15. All societies have some sort of ritual parting ceremony at death. While the traditional American funeral is expensive, it offers psychological values, which are of both sociological and therapeutic importance, to the survivors.

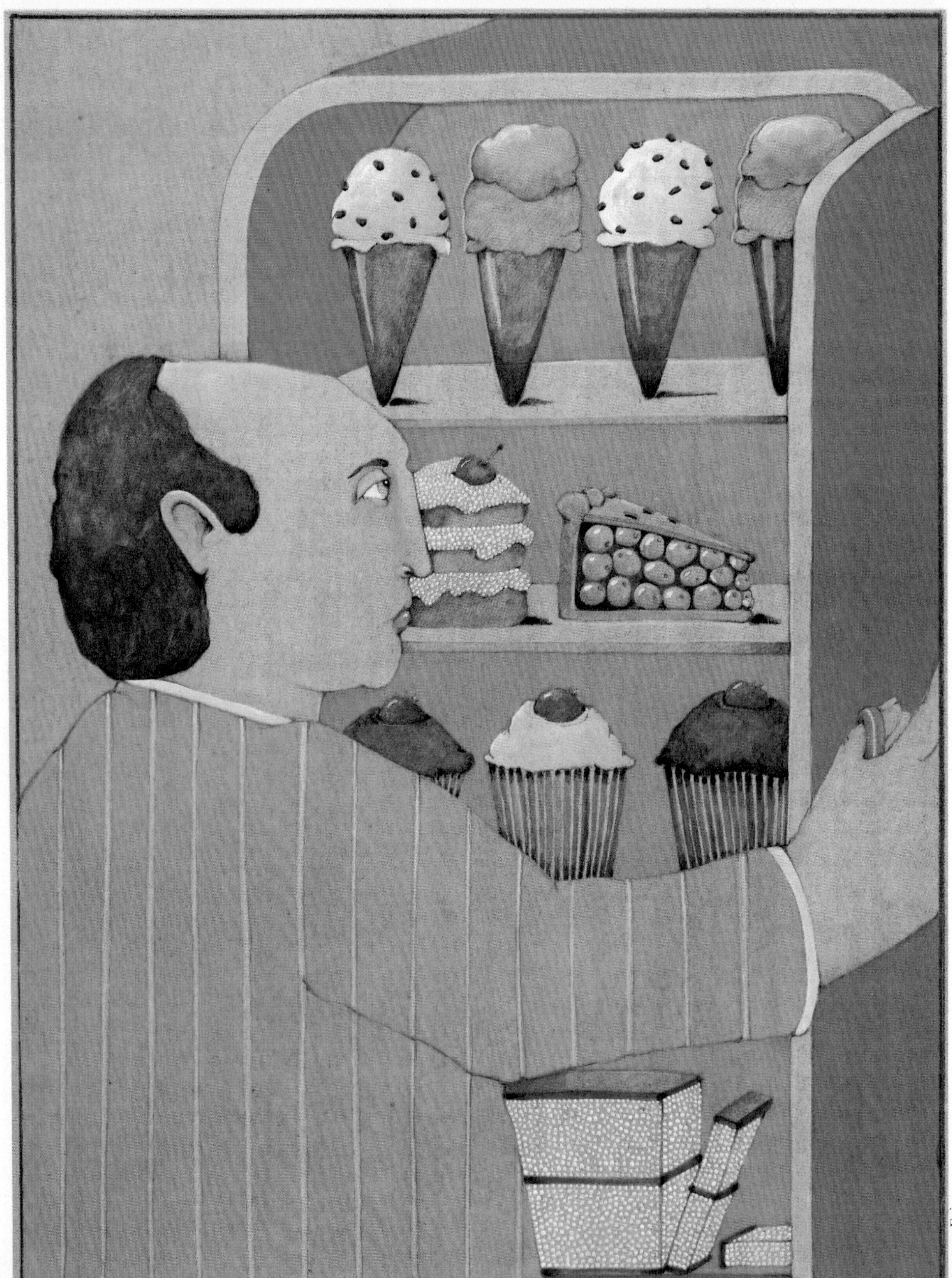

Dagmar Frinta

THE WELL-ADJUSTED BODY

To a certain degree, the state of your health is a product of forces beyond your control—your genetic make-up and where you were raised, for example. But to a great extent, your health is in your hands, and you can improve your chances for optimal health by making sensible decisions about your nutritional and exercise habits.

A well-adjusted body—which is largely the result of the foods you eat and the physical activities you undertake—can significantly enhance your life and health and free you from at least some illness and unhappiness.

Part III covers some areas of personal care that can make big differences in the way you look and feel. Chapter 8 presents the basics of nutrition: what you should eat to stay healthy and how poor eating habits can increase your chances of becoming sick.

Americans today are preoccupied with physique and weight control. Many of us practically starve ourselves to attain an "ideal" figure, but are we damaging our health in the process? Just why is it wise to keep your weight under control? Such questions are discussed in Chapter 9.

Finally, feeling healthy largely depends on being physically fit. Chapter 10 examines physical fitness, emphasizing the components of fitness, the benefits of fitness, and how to tailor a fitness program to your individual needs and limitations.

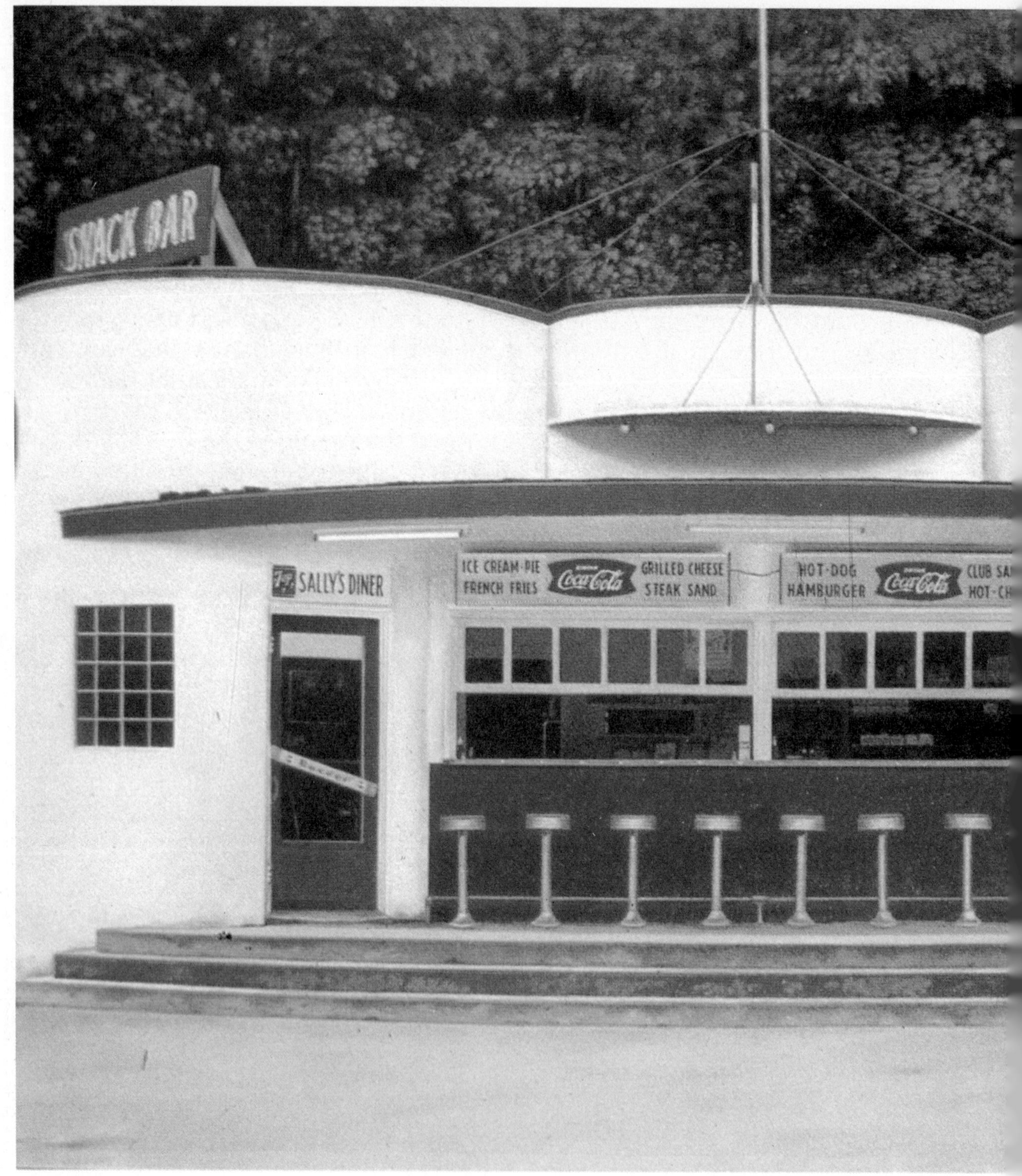
SNACK BAR
SALLY'S DINER
ICE CREAM·PIE
FRENCH FRIES
Coca-Cola
GRILLED CHEESE
STEAK SAND.
HOT-DOG
HAMBURGER
Coca-Cola

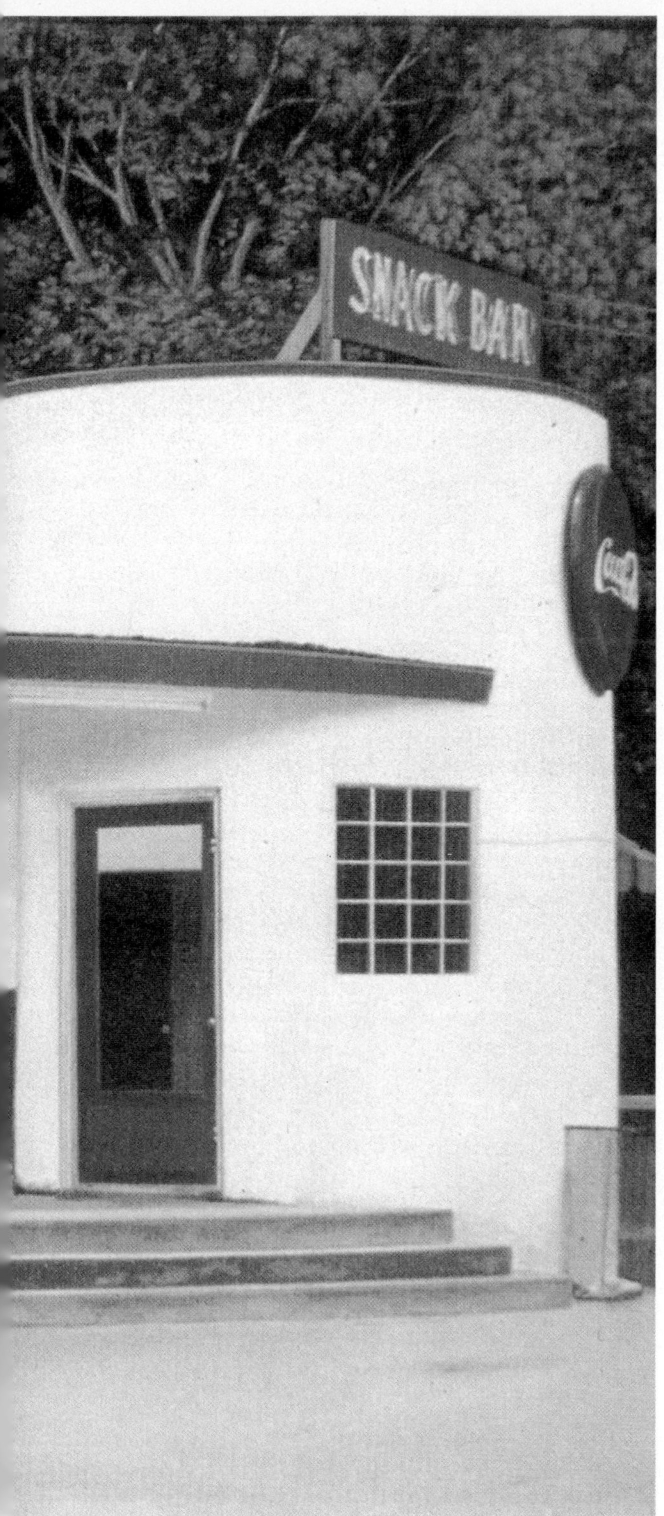

8 Nutrition

The recent surge of interest in nutrition has created numerous self-styled "experts" in the field—all too often, their only credentials being that they eat three meals a day. Nutritional advances since World War II have opened doors to vast stores of knowledge. Unfortunately, much of this knowledge has never reached or is not well understood by the public, and a great deal of it has become clouded by misinformation.

Nutrition is the science of food, its use within the body, and its relationship to good health. It includes the study of the major food components—protein, carbohydrates, fat, vitamins, minerals, and water—and the fifty specific nutrients of which they are composed.

Nutrition is vital to the good health of all people of all ages. When you eat, you are doing much more than simply filling an empty stomach. The eating process ultimately feeds all the cells of the body as it makes material for bones, skin, hair, muscles, hormones, and enzymes, and provides the fuel for efficient operation. Too little food or too much—or worse, too much low-nutrient food—tends to lead to a condition of general debilitation. Irritability increases, mental alertness decreases, susceptibility to disease becomes greater. School teachers have known for many years that well-nourished children usually have fewer learning problems. Such disorders as diabetes and obesity are known to be associated with poor nutritional habits; evidence is now accumulating that dietary factors may be causally related to coronary heart disease, stroke, diabetes, and certain forms of cancer.

But food is to be enjoyed, too. Food left untouched on the plate has no nutritional value. Thus, not only must meals be nutritionally *balanced,* they must also include a *variety* of foods—both to relieve a tired palate and to ensure a full assortment of the many nutrients needed by the body. Personal likes and dislikes must be taken into account. Food must be served attractively and consumed under pleasant conditions.

Because nutrition is a *science,* there is no room for fad and whimsy. Pursuit of purported "magical properties" of certain foods makes no sense at all. Scientists have long known that there is no one perfect food. The "magic" lies in learning how to put together many kinds of food in an enjoyable way that will result in glowing good health.

THE BASIC FOOD COMPONENTS

All foods are composed of chemical compounds. During the process of digestion, these complex compounds are broken down into simpler ones, which then reassemble themselves into other kinds of chemicals that can be directly utilized by the body. Each basic food component—that is, each basic group of chemicals—will be considered separately.

Protein

Protein is made up of twenty-three different amino acids, the "building blocks" of the body. Each of these acids is composed in structurally different ways of carbon, hydrogen, oxygen, nitrogen, and sulfur. Of these twenty-three amino acids, eight are considered *essential.* That is, they cannot be synthesized by the body (as can all of the others) but must be consumed directly.

All the essential amino acids must be present at the same time in order for them to form protein. Since free amino acids cannot be stored in the body, this means that the eight essential acids should be consumed at approximately the same time—preferably at the same meal—if they are to be utilized efficiently.

When all eight of the essential amino acids are present in one food—namely, in those of animal origin (meat, eggs, dairy products)—this is known as *complete* protein. Protein of plant origin (vegetables and grains) is almost invariably *incomplete* protein. However, plant proteins can be combined, either with each other in specific combinations or with animal protein, to form complete protein. Examples include cereal and milk, macaroni and cheese, rice and beans, or—for those fond of Mexican food—refried beans wrapped in tortillas (which are corn-based).

More recent foods on the high-protein scene are "meat substitutes"—vegetable protein that is processed and flavored to provide the taste and protein content of real meat. These products offer a valuable and inexpensive contribution to the diet.

Protein is essential for growth and repair of the body. It is necessary for construction of muscle, hair, teeth, nails, bones, nerve cells, hemoglobin, and enzymes. Proteins are also found in the nuclei of the cells and are responsible for the transmission of hereditary characteristics. (Specifically, these last proteins are known as RNA, or ribonucleic acid, and DNA, or deoxyribonucleic acid.)

It should be apparent that adequate protein must be consumed each day. The average American, however, tends to take in far more than is needed: the Recommended Daily Allowance is 65 grams; average daily consumption is 106 grams. The excess is converted to glucose, which is then either burned as energy or stored as fat—a very expensive source of calories for such usage. Too much protein can also elevate urea levels in the blood.

Protein deficiency *is* a problem in severely deprived areas of the United States, as well as in Indochina, the Middle East, much of Africa, and parts of South America. Extreme deficiency results in *kwashiorkor,* a condition that mainly affects children and causes slow growth, severe mental retardation, bloated stomachs, apathy, and pigment changes (its victims assuming a somewhat purplish appearance).

It should be obvious that the low-protein "fad" diets (to be discussed in Chapter 9) can only have detrimental results. While the dieter is not likely to end up with symptoms of kwashiorkor, even minor protein deficiencies over a period of time will cause fatigue and irritability; antibody production is reduced; the victim becomes more susceptible to infection and recovers more slowly from disease; and wounds and burns heal more slowly. Continued deficiency may eventually lead to anemia and liver disorders.

Carbohydrates

Carbohydrates include both *sugars* (straight chains of carbon "rings") and *starches* (branched chains of carbon rings). (Cellulose is also a carbohydrate, but since it is a nonnutrient, it will not be considered here.) These compounds are less complex than the proteins, being composed only of carbon, hydrogen, and oxygen (no nitrogen or sulfur). They contribute approximately 50 percent of the body's energy needs and are its most economical energy source. Carbohydrates are burned more efficiently than either proteins or fats.

Both starches, which are actually long chains of simple-sugar units, and the sugars we normally eat are broken down in digestion into simple sugars, which are then further converted by the liver into the simplest sugar, *glucose.* Glucose, a single carbon ring, is the only sugar that can be directly utilized by the body for supplying energy.

Some glucose remains stored in the liver and muscles as *glycogen,* ready for immediate release into the bloodstream should blood sugar levels fall too low. Glycogen has the ability to bind large quantities of water. When glycogen stores are depleted, three or four pounds of water are lost along with it—sometimes giving the false impression of quick weight loss. However, as soon as eating is resumed, the lost pounds reappear.

Excess glucose—that which is neither burned as energy nor stored as glycogen—is changed to substances known as *triglycerides* (three fatty acids attached to a glycerol molecule), which are stored in fat tissue as fatty acids.

The most common type of sugar we eat is *sucrose,* which is composed of the two simple sugars glucose and fructose. Refined table sugar is pure sucrose. Fructose by itself is most commonly found as the sweetener in fruits. Lactose is a sugar present in milk and certain milk products.

In addition to fulfilling energy requirements, carbohydrates are also necessary for efficient fat metabolism. If sugar and starch intake is less than 125 grams per day, fat oxidation is incomplete, resulting in the formation of ketone bodies and eventual acidosis when the concentration of these waste products in the blood reaches a critical level, disrupting normal metabolism. Most nutritionists recommend a minimum of 100 grams of carbohydrates per day as necessary for optimal energy levels. Again referring to the popular fad diets, it can be seen why low-carbohydrate versions are ill-advised. Low energy levels result in weakness, lightheadedness, and fatigue.

Recently, sugar has been suggested as the culprit in a variety of diseases and health disorders. But the relationship between sugar consumption and a given disorder is not always simple or direct. For example, in itself, the consumption of sugar does not cause obesity; it is the total number of calories consumed in excess of what is needed that makes a person fat. Sugar has 4 Calories per gram, like all other carbohydrates. The catch is that in candy, pie, cake, and other foods sweetened with sugar, calories tend to be highly concentrated. Excessive use of sugar adds unwanted pounds, but it harbors no unique property that results in obesity when consumed as part of a moderate, balanced diet. Nor does hypoglycemia, or low blood sugar, come from the use of sugar. Actually, hypoglycemia is an extremely rare condition caused by a malfunctioning of the pancreas.

The relationship between sugar consumption and diabetes is more complex. Several animal studies have shown that all the symptoms of diabetes can be produced by feeding the animals high levels of sucrose. Recent research suggests, however, that for 90 percent of the adult population, sugar is not a cause of diabetes, though high sugar intake will aggravate this disease. On the other hand, sugar is a health hazard for the remaining 10 percent of the population who are carbohydrate sensitive. In such persons—15 million of them in the United States—sucrose in the diet results in a large permanent increase in blood triglycer-

FOCUS

Food Fads

In just the last few years, almost everyone from schoolchildren to grandparents has suddenly started "talking" nutrition. Turn on a TV or radio talk show and you're very apt to see an expert—some bona fide, others mostly self-proclaimed—advising millions on what they should or shouldn't eat. TV commercials aimed at children show animated vitamins and minerals and proteins building strong bodies. Almost every month, book publishers bring out yet another miracle diet or shortcut to nutrition.

Now while all this has had the positive effect of making Americans increasingly aware that nutrition is important, the boom has some definite drawbacks, and even dangers. Food fads have become a big business, and with so many conflicting claims, it's understandable that many many people are very confused about just what is—and what is not—good nutrition. Let's try to clear the picture.

First, let me point out that although a good diet permits us to avoid deficiency diseases like rickets or scurvy, and to forestall some of the great killers of our time, like heart disease, even the best nutrition will not keep us young forever, shed weight without effort, avoid all fatigue, headaches, and minor miseries of life. Nor can diet prevent such diseases as arthritis, multiple sclerosis, or muscular dystrophy. And here's where the faddist steps in, a merchant of hope, unhampered by any of the exacting requirements of science, ready with imaginative interpretations of any fact, and with promises to cure or prevent any disease that medicine cannot deal with.

These merchants of hope have been with us since antiquity, with their various potions, philters, and recipes. Our current renewal of interest in nutrition has produced a massive increase in faddist books, bizarre vitamin preparations, and miraculous "nutritional supplements." While the Food and Drug Administration is trying to prevent over-the-counter sales of downright dangerous dosages of vitamins—such as massive amounts of A and D—it is powerless to act against fraudulent books and articles, which enjoy the constitutional guarantee of free speech. Hence, I would like to at least try to warn the public about some of today's fads. Here are ten general rules to help you spot the fad or faddist.

1. Beware of any magic substance that will solve all your problems. Today's big sellers are megavitamins. (One would think that the health-buff's repugnance for chemicals and pills and the "back to nature" view of faddists would militate against their advocating them, but I guess chemicals and pills are fine if they're sold by your friends.) Prolonged ingestion of very large doses of certain fat-soluble vitamins, like A and D, is known to be poisonous. Excessive amounts of D cause calcification and arrest growth, while large amounts of A cause generalized bleeding and bone fragility. The effects of excessive dosages of vitamin E over a long period are unknown, though after a few days, extreme fatigue has been repeatedly observed in some individuals. Large doses of vitamin C over a long period can cause a burning feeling during urination, and, in susceptible individuals, it can lead to small kidney stones. Large amounts of niacin can cause a flushing of the face. The long-term effects of taking other B vitamins are unknown. It may be that they are simply excreted as waste, but we're not sure.
2. A faddist will promise to prevent or cure diseases that doctors generally recognize as incurable. Curiously, the faddists appeal to the paranoid notion that organized medicine is a gigantic conspiracy aimed at withholding "cures" from the people. Of course, any idea that physicians don't care about cures for common diseases, or that they refuse to recognize that they "work," is farcical.
3. Faddists will promise easy solutions (which may defy the laws of nature) to difficult problems. For example, they assure you it's possible to lose weight without worrying about your food intake, because "calories don't count." All you need to do is follow their crash diet, be it steak and martinis or low carbohydrates and high water or whatever, and you will emerge thin as a rail.
4. Faddists recognize only one problem at a time. If you want to lose weight, they will "help" you and damn the consequences to your health. For instance, a recent study at the Peter Bent Brigham Hospital in Boston shows that very low carbohydrate diets (even with plenty of water!) elevate blood cholesterol.

5. Faddists operate on the principle that there's only one factor in the development of complex diseases. Now we are quite certain that a whole range of risk factors contribute to the development of hardening of the arteries, including high blood pressure, overweight, high cholesterol levels, lack of exercise, and cigarette smoking.
6. Faddists lay great stress on blood sugar as an indication of health and mental sanity. They will tell you low blood sugar is the cause of fatigue, depression, and a host of other problems, but they do not tell you that a physician can measure blood sugar and advise you on any problems he may find. Indeed, the idea is that if you are tired, depressed, and so forth, it must be that you have a low blood sugar and you must treat it, according to Mr. X or Miss Y, with such and such a diet. However, your fatigue could be from diabetes, cancer, hepatitis, pernicious anemia or iron-deficiency anemia, or a host of other conditions that a physician—and only a physician—can diagnose.
7. Faddists operate on the basis that if one is good, 100 must be 100 times better. The fact is, one may indeed be good, but 100 can—and often does—kill. This illustrates the principle that "there are no toxic substances, there are only toxic concentrations," meaning that anything, at too high a level, can be poison.
8. Faddists insist that all supermarket foods are "devitalized," because they are deficient in trace minerals, among other things. They also insist these foods are poisonous because they are grown on chemical fertilizers, covered with pesticides, injected with hormones, and overprocessed. The implication is that unless you consume only health-store foods, you, too, will be devitalized. There are so many fallacies in this assertion that it would take a book to answer it, but here are a few thoughts. First, without modern chemical fertilizers, millions in the world would die of hunger. As for trace minerals, widespread deficiencies stop plant growth rather than produce "deficient plants" (exceptions are fluoride and iodide, which are not required by plants). Applying manure instead of "chemical" fertilizer does not restore, say, iodine to soil. In fact, the animals develop goiter, too. The answer is to add iodine to the fertilizer—and iodize salt (or fluoridate water)—to contribute the missing minerals.
9. The faddist would like you to believe all additives are bad. Just look at how ridiculous this is. Take salt for example. It is a chemical, and it is also added to foods. Many additives obviously have marked advantages, whereas some undoubtedly present a risk. The choice is not always easy. Consider the case of nitrites. They inhibit the growth of the organism causing botulism, a deadly disease. They also dye preserved meat pink, instead of an unappetizing brown. On the other hand, they present a special risk to babies and a theoretical, but still unproved, risk of cancer in adults. So nitrites have been removed from baby meats, which are canned so that the risk of botulism is nil. Their use for purely cosmetic purposes of dyeing meat pink has been largely abandoned. But they have been retained where they serve an antibotulism function, and the quest for substitutes goes on.
10. The faddists would have you believe that anything which is "natural" is good. They ignore the fact that the most powerful of all cancer-producing substances, aflatoxin, is manufactured by molds and is perfectly natural. (It grows in peanuts, cereals, and is even found in milk.) So are the toxins of mushrooms or such poisons as strychnine. Natural, unpasteurized milk exposes you to the risk of bovine tuberculosis, uncooked meat to a host of diseases, including trichinosis, taenia infestation, and salmonellosis, to name but a few. "Natural" vitamins have the same arrangement of atoms as those made in a lab, and all atoms are natural.

By all means, then, let us avoid overprocessed foods, and empty calories such as sugar, but don't believe that everything is automatically good for you because it is labeled "natural."

Source: Reprinted from Jean Mayer, "The Cruel Hoax of Food Fads," *Family Health* (June 1974).

ides. This increase is associated with diabetes as well as heart disease.

Recently, a few researchers have suggested sugar (i.e., sucrose) as a causative factor in coronary heart disease; however, this view has not found general support in the scientific literature. But for carbohydrate-sensitive people, sucrose intake significantly increases the risk of heart disease.

The connection between sugar intake and tooth decay seems to be definitely established. Studies of human beings and animals now confirm that sugar is a major cause of *tooth decay* (dental caries). Even so, there is no one-to-one correlation between a person's sugar intake and the number of cavities that develop.

The bacteria usually present in our mouths feed on sugar in two different ways. They use it to create a thick, sticky substance that clings to the surfaces of the teeth and speeds up the accumulation of *plaque,* a composite of debris on the surface of the teeth. Bacterial activity also produces several acids which, when held against the surfaces of the teeth by plaque, attack the teeth with varying measures of success.

Although it is true that some of us are more disposed to develop cavities than others, the kind of sugar we consume has a lot to do with who gets the cavities. Sugar that sticks to the teeth for a long period of time, such as taffy, seems to do the most damage. There is also evidence that sugar taken with meals or consumed with a liquid does less harm than a comparable amount of sugar taken as a snack. Apparently at mealtime the other foods and liquids keep at least some of the sugar from clinging to the teeth surfaces. The National Academy of Sciences suggests rinsing (or better still, brushing) the teeth after eating sweet foods and maintains that if this is done regularly, moderate amounts of sugar should not cause a problem.

Fat

Fat has become an unpopular word recently—yet fat compounds, too, are essential to good health. Besides serving as another energy source, fats—also known as *lipids*—impart flavor and juiciness to many of the foods we eat. Because they move more slowly through the digestive tract, fats also contribute satiety value—that is, the feeling of being "full" after a meal. Fats perform the additional functions of insulating the body, protecting vital organs from mechanical shock, serving as a transport medium for the four fat-soluble vitamins (A, D, E, and K), and contributing to hormone synthesis and the clotting mechanism. As with carbohydrates, unused fats are stored as fatty acids and drawn on by the body as needed for energy. Stored fats are the greatest nutritional reservoir in the body.

Fats, like carbohydrates, are composed of carbon, hydrogen, and oxygen, but with proportionately less oxygen. Basically fats are chains of carbon atoms, some with hydrogen atoms attached. There are different kinds of fat, each with its unique structure. A molecule of *saturated* fat, as the name implies, is complete and has no space for additional material. A molecule of *monounsaturated* fat has room for two more hydrogen atoms, and *polyunsaturated* fat has room for more than one additional hydrogen atom. *Hydrogenated* fats are unsaturated fats to which the missing hydrogen atoms have been added to make them more saturated—a process used in converting liquid vegetable shortenings, for instance, to a more solid form.

Cholesterol, an organic waxy compound, is a lipid of great physiological importance—and is one of the nonessential nutrients. Most of the cholesterol found in the body is synthesized by the body itself in the liver and not taken in through foods. The interest in cholesterol focuses on the established relationship between blood levels of cholesterol and one's risk of heart disease. What is still not fully established, however, is what role *dietary* cholesterol (in the form of eggs, for example) plays in the development of heart disease, and how dietary intake of cholesterol affects blood levels of that chemical.

At present, it is known that saturated fats—found in meat, whole milk, cream, butter, and a few vegetable oils (coconut and palm)—tend to raise blood cholesterol levels by serving as the starting material from which cholesterol can be synthesized in the body. On the other hand, polyunsaturated fats are of vegetable origin—soya, corn, sunflower, cottonseed oils, and others—and these tend to lower blood cholesterol by replacing some of the saturated fats. Monounsaturated fats, such as olive oil, also tend to lower blood cholesterol in the same way, but to a lesser degree than do the polyunsaturated fats.

Except in severely deprived areas of the United States, few Americans have difficulty in consuming sufficient amounts of fat. In general, the opposite is true, with the average percentage of daily calories hovering between 40 and 50 percent fat. Most persons would be far better off if fat was kept between 30 and 35 percent of daily calories. This is easily accomplished by using leaner cuts of fat-trimmed meat; frequent substitution of chicken and fish for high-fat beef, lamb, and pork; and increased use of vegetables and fruits.

Vitamins

Vitamins, along with minerals, are often referred to as "micronutrients." They are required in only trace amounts, yet are indispensable in triggering vital bodily functions. Vitamins do not form new compounds in the way that proteins, carbohydrates, and fats do. Rather, they act as co-enzymes in helping other chemical reactions to take place. For example, calcium cannot become part of the bone structure without the presence of vitamin D.

Vitamins are subdivided into two major groups. The *water-soluble* vitamins, C and the B complex, are easily excreted from the body when consumed in excessive amounts. The real danger of excess vitamin consumption lies in the *fat-soluble* vitamins, A, D, E, and K. These cannot be excreted but rather are stored (as the name implies) in the fatty tissues, where they may build to toxic levels.

For this reason, a word should be said about the dangers of overdosing with vitamin supplements. A number of deaths and cases of unnecessary surgery have been recorded as directly traceable to excessive amounts of one or another fat-soluble vitamin. The hazards of "megadosing" have led the Food and Drug Administration to restrict the amount of vitamin D that may be added to any product, since it is now known that excessive vitamin D causes release of too much calcium, which may result in tissue damage. Between $300 and $500 million is spent annually on unnecessary vitamin supplements. Unless one has a medically diagnosed vitamin deficiency, this money would be far better spent in purchasing nutrients in the form of food.

Minerals

Minerals are inorganic elements needed daily to help form tissues and various chemical substances in the body. They assist in nerve transmission and muscle contraction, and help regulate fluid levels and the acid/base balance of the body.

Iron *Iron* is one of the body's most important nutrients, essential for hemoglobin production in the red blood cells, yet it is also the most frequently deficient in the diet. Only about 10 percent of the average iron intake can actually be used because it cannot be absorbed from the gut—a particular problem for women of childbearing age, who regularly lose considerable amounts of iron through the menstrual process. A woman's iron requirement is almost twice that of a man, and this is the one nutrient that frequently requires supplementation. Such supplements, however, should be recommended only by a physician.

Salt (Sodium Chloride)

Simple table salt (sodium chloride), although a necessary part of the human diet, may bring about problems if it is consumed in substantial quantities. Numerous studies have demonstrated that excessive salt intake can interfere with growth and raise blood pressure, and there is a known association between salt and congestive heart failure, certain types of kidney diseases, and toxemia during pregnancy.

Furthermore, salt may be habit-forming. Apparently human beings have a preference for salt, consuming it in excess of actual need. Sodium appetite seems to be acquired; many believe it develops largely as a result of dietary usage during childhood and early adulthood. Today many doctors and nutritionists recommend reduced use of salt from infancy in order to prevent the salt habit from developing. The major manufacturers of baby food now add to their products only the barest minimum (if any) for accentuating natural flavors.

It is clear that in many hypertensive patients a low-sodium diet reduces blood pressure. In fact, many researchers identify high salt consumption as a cause of *essential hypertension,* or high blood pressure, in human beings; this has already been shown to be true of laboratory animals. According to one view, certain people inherit a susceptibility to this disease, which is triggered by a high-salt diet.

For adults, reducing salt intake is not an easy matter, even if they refrain from adding table salt to their meals. There is some sodium in almost every processed food sold in our supermarkets. Sodium is found not only in such foods as peanuts, pickles, bacon, and potato chips but in items as diverse as corn flakes, canned tuna, candy bars, and instant puddings. It shouldn't be too surprising, therefore, that according to some researchers, Americans consume far more salt than they need.

Water

Water is perhaps the most important of all food components, and second only to air as a necessary substance for the maintenance of life. While the body can survive for long periods without food, four days is the maximum time it can exist without water.

The functions of water are many. It is the medium for transporting nutrients to all the cells of the body, where it then removes cellular waste products to be excreted through the kidneys. Water also acts as a medium for the many chemical reactions of digestion. It is the body's temperature regulator, conducting heat efficiently and cooling the body by evaporation through the skin (perspiration) and lungs. Water is also a component of the breathing process itself. Additionally, it serves as a cushioning device to protect vital organs, and as a lubricant for the joints and central nervous system. Finally, water and some of the chemicals it carries are responsible for bodily structure, maintaining the shape of the cells by equalizing density and pressure between intracellular and extracellular fluids. As much as 80 percent of the body weight may be water, although the average is closer to 60 percent. (A fat person has proportionately less water and more fat in the body than does a thin person.)

An average of two to two-and-a-half liters of water (slightly more than two quarts) per day is the recommended daily intake. Of course, not all of this has to be consumed as plain water; most other nonalcoholic liquids serve as well. Generally speaking, only about 50 percent of the body's water requirement comes directly from liquids; another 25 to 50 percent is from food, and the rest is an end product of metabolism.

It may come as a surprise that the food we eat contains so much water. But most fruits, for instance, contain close to 90 percent water; a "solid" banana contains 75 percent. Lettuce is 95 percent water. Even bread, normally thought of as a somewhat dry food, contains an average of 35 percent water.

The actual amount of water required by the body each day depends on a number of factors —environment, amount of physical activity, season of the year, and type of food ingested. A salty meal or snack raises the sodium content of the body fluids and creates a strain on the kidneys (which under extreme conditions may cease to function). This increased concentration of salts immediately sends out a call for more water to dilute the fluids to their normal state. High-protein foods and alcoholic beverages have a similar effect in tending to overconcentrate bodily fluids. It should be apparent, then, why so many fad-reducing diets are hazardous. Those that tamper with water consumption in any way, such as the "high-protein" diets, can interfere with the body's proper functioning—or worse (see Chapter 9).

Fiber

Fiber, including cellulose and other compounds, is another nonnutritive substance. Also known as "roughage" or "bulk," these compounds are actually a form of carbohydrate but are indigestible by human beings. Common examples of fiber are the bran of cereals, the skin of fruits, and the connective tissue of meat.

Fiber functions as a necessary aid in the digestive process. In the large intestine (the colon) it has the ability to bind with large amounts of water other waste products, forming an easily passed, soft, large stool. Adequate amounts of fiber in the diet result in stools that are increased in both volume and frequency. This, in turn, relieves a certain amount of pressure in the colon, helping to prevent diverticulosis, a physiological problem in which the large intestinal wall weakens and balloons out. The presence of fiber also provides a medium for the growth of certain bacteria that help the body synthesize nutrients such as vitamin K.

More recent studies have tried to demonstrate that increased fiber in the diet will result in lowered risk of colon cancer. But until further research offers more definite proof of the effects of high-fiber diets on the body, most nutritionists recommend moderate amounts consumed as part of a balanced diet. Constipation may indicate a need for slightly increased fiber intake; an ulcer or similar condition may require reduced fiber intake. But otherwise, whole-grain breads and cereals and fresh fruits and vegetables should provide sufficient fiber for the average person. Bran or other such supplements are unnecessary in most circumstances.

Calories

Calories are not nutrients either. They indicate the potential energy value of each food or food component. Energy expenditure—the amount required for every activity or bodily process—is also expressed in Calories. For example, an average-sized apple contains about 100 Calories. A twenty-minute walk will burn up just about as many Calories. (A wedge of apple pie, however, requires one to one-and-a-half hours to "walk off.")

A *calorie* is a measure of heat energy. Specifically, a calorie (small "c") is the amount of heat (or energy) needed to raise one gram of water one degree Celsius. Food energy, however, is actually measured in *kilocalories,* or Calories (capital "C"). A kilocalorie is 1,000 times larger than a calorie and is also referred to as a "large Calorie." Protein and carbohydrate each contain 4 Calories per gram; fat contains 9 Calories per gram. (Thus, one would consume more than twice as many calories in a teaspoon of butter as in a teaspoon of sugar.) Vitamins, minerals, and water contain no calories; fiber, being indigestible to human beings, supplies no calories to the human body.

The number of calories required for optimal health varies considerably among different individuals, depending on age, sex, weight, size, and physical activity. This subject will be covered more thoroughly in Chapter 9.

A BALANCED DIET

Since foods vary so much in their combinations of both nutrients and calories, how is one able to achieve a "balanced" diet each day? There are complicated ways to perform all the necessary calculations, but few people have the time or interest. The simplest device for planning adequate nutrition on a daily basis is through use of the Basic Four Food Groups.

With careful planning, the Basic Four may provide all of the Recommended Dietary Allowances (RDAs) as established by the National Academy of Sciences/National Research Council (see Table 8.1). The RDAs, which are reviewed for possible revision every five years, are estimates of the optimal quantity of each nutrient required. They are estimated values based on those persons with the highest physiological requirements. Thus, when all the recommended allowances are followed, one can be assured of meeting all of one's daily nutritional needs.

The Basic Four

The Basic Four provide a very practical framework for meal planning and form a reliable guide to adequate intake of all the essential nutrients. Sugar, refined fats, and oils are not included since they mainly provide calories and are rarely lacking in the American diet. Briefly, the four groups are:

Meat Group This group includes meats, poultry, fish, eggs, and legumes such as dried beans, peas, and nuts—all good sources of protein. In addition, these foods supply vitamins of the B complex such as thiamine, riboflavin, niacin, B_6, and B_{12}, and the mineral

Table 8.1 Nutrient Requirements: Recommended Daily Dietary Allowances of Vitamins and Minerals

			Water-Soluble Vitamins						Minerals					
	Ages	*Ascorbic Acid (mg)*	*Folacin (µg)*	*Niacin (mg)*	*Riboflavin (mg)*	*Thiamin (mg)*	*Vitamin B_6 (mg)*	*Vitamin B_{12} (µg)*	*Calcium (mg)*	*Phosphorus (mg)*	*Iodine (µg)*	*Iron (mg)*	*Magnesium (mg)*	*Zinc (mg)*
Infants	0.0–0.5	35	50	5	0.4	0.3	0.3	0.3	360	240	35	10	60	3
	0.5–1.0	35	50	8	0.6	0.5	0.4	0.3	540	400	45	15	70	5
Children	1–3	40	100	9	0.8	0.7	0.6	1.0	800	800	60	15	150	10
	4–6	40	200	12	1.1	0.9	0.9	1.5	800	800	80	10	200	10
	7–10	40	300	16	1.2	1.2	1.2	2.0	800	800	110	10	250	10
Males	11–14	45	400	18	1.5	1.4	1.6	3.0	1,200	1,200	130	18	350	15
	15–18	45	400	20	1.8	1.5	1.8	3.0	1,200	1,200	150	18	400	15
	19–22	45	400	20	1.8	1.5	2.0	3.0	800	800	140	10	350	15
	23–50	45	400	18	1.6	1.4	2.0	3.0	800	800	130	10	350	15
	51+	45	400	16	1.5	1.2	2.0	3.0	800	800	110	10	350	15
Females	11–14	45	400	16	1.3	1.2	1.6	3.0	1,200	1,200	115	18	300	15
	15–18	45	400	14	1.4	1.1	2.0	3.0	1,200	1,200	115	18	300	15
	19–22	45	400	14	1.4	1.1	2.0	3.0	800	800	100	18	300	15
	23–50	45	400	13	1.2	1.0	2.0	3.0	800	800	100	18	300	15
	51+	45	400	12	1.1	1.0	2.0	3.0	800	800	80	10	300	15
	Pregnant	60	800	+2	+0.3	+0.3	2.5	4.0	1,200	1,200	125	18+*	450	20
	Lactating	80	600	+4	+0.5	+0.3	2.5	4.0	1,200	1,200	150	10	450	25

*This increased requirement cannot be met by ordinary diets; therefore, the use of supplemental iron is recommended.
Source: Theodore P. Labuza, *Food and Your Well Being* (St. Paul, Mn.: West Publishing, 1977).

iron. Approximately six ounces a day, about two servings, are recommended.

Milk and Milk Products These foods supply more calcium per serving than any other. Indeed, it is difficult to meet the daily calcium requirement without the use of milk or cheese. Foods from this group are also valuable sources of protein, many of the B vitamins (especially riboflavin), vitamin A (if the milk is whole milk), and vitamin D if it has been added to the milk, as it should be. Skim milk, dry skim milk powder, or low-fat milk are good solutions for the weight-conscious, who seem particularly disposed to omitting milk from the daily eating pattern. When using such products, labels should be carefully checked to be certain that vitamins A and D have been added, since these two vitamins are removed from whole milk along with the butterfat.

Two servings (two glasses) a day are generally recommended for adults, two to four servings for children, and four servings for teenagers and nursing mothers. One cup of yogurt may substitute for one glass of milk.

Fruits and Vegetables Foods in this group supply 100 percent of the vitamin C requirement, 60 percent of vitamin A, other vitamins and minerals, and much of the body's fiber requirement. Four servings daily are suggested here, of which one should be a vitamin-C-rich food (citrus, tomato, and cantaloupe, among others). At least every other day, a dark green or deep yellow vegetable should be included for vitamin A. Fruits and vegetables also add texture, color, and variety to the diet.

Breads and Cereals (Whole Grain or Enriched) Foods from this group (including macaroni,

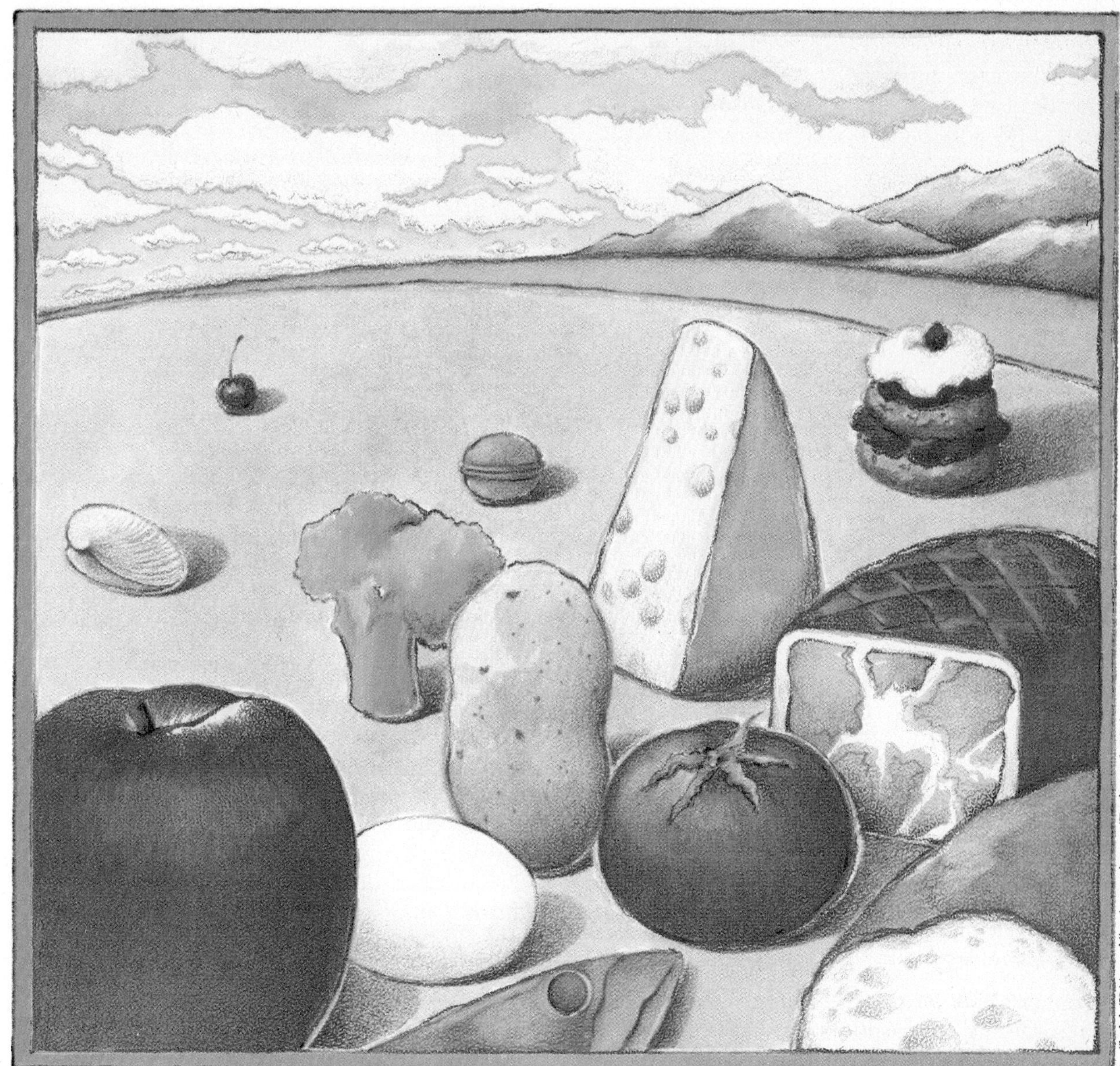

Infield/D'Astolfo Associates/Deborah Volpati and Bill Schmidt

Figure 8.1 To a great degree, food is a matter of personal preference; everyone has certain likes and dislikes for no explainable reason. But the Basic Four provide a practical framework for planning meals and form a reliable guide to an adequate intake of all essential nutrients.

spaghetti, noodles, rice, and similar products) are valuable sources of carbohydrate, thiamine, riboflavin, niacin, and iron. In fact, it is difficult to obtain a sufficient quantity of thiamine and iron (particularly for females) if this group is excluded from the diet. Although four servings a day are recommended, far too many people eat less than this because they view these foods as fattening. In the quibble for calories, it scarcely seems logical to avoid eating bread at 65 or 70 Calories per slice (approximately one ounce) and then eat extra meat at 75 to 90 Calories per ounce.

White bread outsells whole-grain bread by roughly five to one. Enrichment laws enacted in about two-thirds of the states (and followed voluntarily in the others) require that the important B vitamins and iron, partially removed when flour is milled, be replaced to levels equivalent to those in whole wheat flour or bread. This makes concern about overprocessing unnecessary.

Serving sizes will—and should—vary according to individual calorie requirements. For instance, a male tends to be larger, with more bone and muscle, than a female, and other things being equal, would require more calories. Yet in reality a 125-pound female who is physically active throughout the day is likely to need more calories than her 160-pound husband, who spends most of his daytime hours sitting at a desk. Individual calorie requirements will be covered more thoroughly in Chapter 9.

Many of the foods we eat belong to more than one food group. Pizza with sausage, for instance, represents all four groups and is actually a fairly balanced meal if supplemented with milk. Other foods—fats, sugars, spreads, dressings, and condiments, for instance—do not belong to any group. This does not mean that they should be eliminated from the diet; they are enjoyable complements to any meal. But their use should be kept in perspective. If calorie intake must be cut, these are the items that should be sacrificed; those from the Basic Four should be left intact.

Food Labeling

In the past few years, the federal government has gradually increased its regulations governing food labeling. Since 1973, nutrition labeling has been required for any food that has been enriched or fortified, or which makes a specific nutritional claim. (*Enrichment* refers to the process in which specific nutrients lost in processing—thiamine, niacin, riboflavin, and iron—have been restored to the equivalent levels in the natural product, such as whole-grain breads or cereals; *fortification* refers to the addition of one or more nutrients not originally present in that food). Information to be included is sevenfold: serving size; servings per container; and the per-serving amount of calories, protein, carbohydrates, fat, and the percentage of U.S. Recommended Dietary Allowances for certain essential nutrients—protein, vitamins A and D, thiamine, riboflavin, niacin, calcium, and iron. If the quantity of an essential nutrient present in a serving of the food is below 2 percent of the U.S. RDA, an * is placed next to the vitamin or mineral. Even where it is not required, many foods now carry this information voluntarily.

Conversely, there are other statements that are expressly prohibited from appearing on any food label. No type of false or misleading claim may be made for a product or any ingredient in the product; for example, a manufacturer cannot allege that the product will prevent or cure any illness, or that a "natural" vitamin is in any way superior to a synthetic one (since it is not). In 1978, additional legislation was passed governing use of the term "low calorie." Such products must now indeed be low calorie—not more than 40 Calories per serving. "Reduced calorie" foods must have at least one-third fewer calories than other comparable foods.

Hopefully, labeling regulations will continue to advance. Contrary to the opinion of many, food manufacturers also benefit from labeling —the reason so many of them now attempt to aid the consumer by including information voluntarily. Satisfied shoppers are more likely to continue buying a manufacturer's product.

None of this information is helpful, however, if it is not used. Reading labels is a good habit.

Additives and Preservatives

Virtually all processed foods contain additives, which are, for the most part, synthetically produced. They range from *nutrients,* which replace or boost vitamins and minerals, to *bleaches, antioxidants,* and *preservatives,* which prevent or delay spoilage. *Emulsifiers, stabilizers,* and *thickeners* are additives that improve texture, uniformity, or consistency. *Acidulants* control tartness and sourness, whereas *sequestrants* keep products from appearing cloudy. The moisture in such foods as marshmallows and shredded coconut is preserved by *humectants.* There are *firming agents* to keep processed fruits and vegetables from softening, and *curing agents* such as nitrites to preserve and sometimes control food color—especially in meats. And of course, many foods now contain a variety of chemical *coloring* and *flavoring agents.*

In an industry as competitive as the production and distribution of food, attractiveness, taste, and economy are all essential. Both additives and preservatives can contribute to all three qualities. Representatives of the food industry claim that without their use, there would be considerably less total food and variety available. And without preservatives, many foods would be much more expensive because of the enormous spoilage. Moreover, foodborne diseases such as botulism and salmonella would be a constant danger. So safety is a very important consideration.

But what about nutrition? There have been claims that some additives and processing may preserve and even extend health beyond the limits possible with unprocessed or natural foods. For example, certain chemical antioxidants used as preservatives have shown some evidence of slowing down aging in laboratory animals.

Fairly strict laws and policies regulate the food industry. Manufacturers must test food additives, and the Food and Drug Administration (FDA) must examine them and conduct premarket testing. Any chemical that is regarded as a health hazard cannot be added to food. The Delaney Clause, a special section of current food-additives legislation, specifies that no chemical, no matter how small the amount, can be added to food if it causes cancer in human beings or animals.

However, some additives now in use are not as safe as was formerly believed. For example, nitrites, which are widely used to preserve processed meats and enhance the color of the product, are now known to convert to nitrosomines under certain high-heat cooking conditions and in the human body. Nitrosomines are powerful carcinogens. And Red Dye II, one of the most widely used food coloring agents, was also found to be carcinogenic in laboratory test animals.

Legislation concerning color additives specifies that the FDA decide on the colors permitted. By law, proof of safety was required within two-and-a-half years after a color was used, with extensions for safety studies being granted for the completion of those studies "as soon as reasonably practicable." The proof-of-safety deadline expired in 1962, and since that time the FDA has allowed most color additives to be used in foods without completion of the necessary safety studies. Yet most are coal-tar colors; they are members of a suspect chemical family already implicated in studies of several long-term illnesses, including cancer.

These issues are complicated because many of the scientists who test for the effects of food additives are employed directly by the food industry or work for organizations funded by that industry. It seems likely, then, that some conflict-of-interest situations do arise.

Controversy over the safety and benefits of food additives and preservatives will continue, but it seems unlikely that the days of natural foods will ever return, except among small groups who grow their own food. Instead, suspect additives will eventually be replaced by safer ones, and the elaboration of processed food will continue; it may even accelerate. World population pressures, together with increased urbanization, which separates populations geographically from the places in which food is grown, make preserved and processed food more and more important.

For individuals and groups willing to take the time and make the special effort necessary to avoid food additives, there are other options. They may arrange their lives and their environments so that only unprocessed foods are consumed. Many who have chosen this alternative claim improved health as well as a sense of self-discipline.

SPECIAL NUTRITIONAL NEEDS

Children and Teen-agers

Children have essentially the same nutritional requirements as adults, but in smaller amounts. Pound for pound, however, an infant actually consumes more food than an adult. As youngsters approach the teen years, the RDA amounts increase proportionately, and energy (i.e., calories) needs jump considerably to keep up with rapidly growing bodies and the usual high activity levels of most teen-agers.

Teen-agers, especially females, often require extra dietary attention. This seems to be a time when sudden concerns about weight send many of them on a diet, in which they skip important foods such as milk and bread. Iron needs are increasing sharply due to the onset of menstruation. Nutrients frequently deficient among teen-agers include iron, calcium, and vitamins A and C, and care should be taken to see that these are regularly present in the teen diet. While a hamburger, french fries, and a cola drink may make up an occasional enjoyable and nutritious lunch, they do not provide a balanced diet when eaten every day.

As growing independence emerges in the teen-ager, continuing good eating patterns presents something of a challenge to parents. But next to the first three years of life, the years from thirteen to twenty—as child becomes adult—are the most critical of one's life. The requirements for all of this accelerated growth must come from food in the form of regular, balanced, and varied meals.

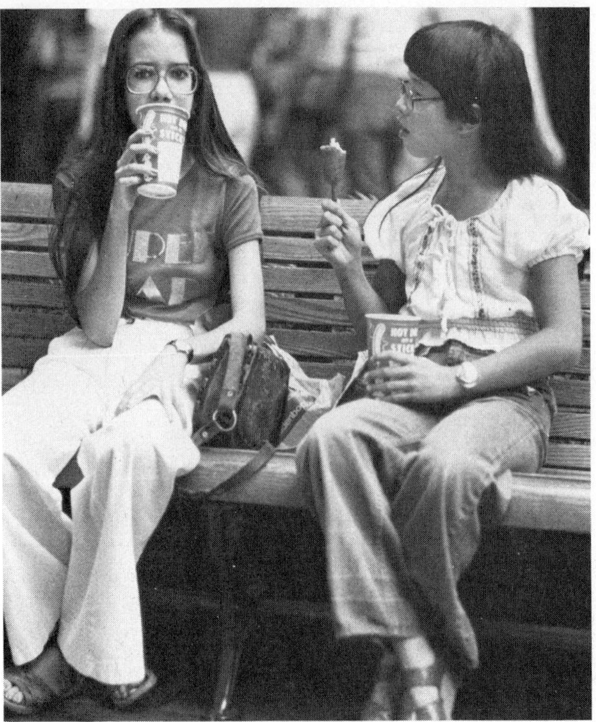

Figure 8.2 Although the nutritional needs of adolescents are considerable, many teen-agers eat poorly balanced meals, which can cause iron and vitamin deficiencies.

Pregnancy

Contrary to a once popular opinion, a pregnant woman does not require significantly more calories than when she is not pregnant. According to the National Academy of Sciences, a typical woman 5 feet 5 inches tall, normally weighing about 128 pounds, requires approximately 2,100 Calories a day when she is not pregnant or one to two months pregnant; 2,400 when three or more months pregnant; and 2,600 to 2,800 when breast-feeding. The 2,400 Calories and increased nutrients can be obtained daily from two to four glasses of skim or low-fat milk; two servings of meat, chicken, or fish; one egg; four servings of fruits and vegetables; and four servings of breads and cereals. All of this should total up to a weight gain of twenty-two to twenty-seven pounds during the entire pregnancy, most of it during the fifth to ninth months.

Admittedly, this leaves little room in the diet for "extras" like salad dressings and rich desserts. Nevertheless, it is imperative for both mother and baby that these guidelines be adhered to as closely as possible. Too many unwanted pounds can complicate delivery and lead to a sometimes depressingly difficult reducing diet postpartum. Still worse are the aftereffects of eating too little, or at least too little of the correct foods. The idea that a baby is a parasite and will take whatever it needs from its mother is strictly a myth. It may get enough calories, but without proper eating habits, the unborn baby will not get enough vital nutrients for proper growth and development. Specifically, the brain is frequently affected, resulting in such conditions as mental retardation, cerebral palsy, and respiratory distress syndrome (RDS), among others. In 1963 the Department of Health, Education, and Welfare reported that almost one million pregnant women were suffering some degree of malnutrition, almost all of it preventable.

Teen-age pregnancies present particular difficulties, both nutritional and otherwise—especially when the teen-ager has been indulging in poor eating habits for a number of years.

Demands of pregnancy coincident with the demands of adolescence can prove detrimental to both mother and baby, and require careful obstetrical care.

The Pill

Women who use contraceptive pills should take extra care to see that their nutritional intake is adequate. The Pill affects certain metabolic processes, and while the need for a few nutrients is actually lowered, other nutrient needs are increased slightly—specifically, vitamins B_6, B_{12}, and folacin. None of these is difficult to consume in sufficient amounts in a reasonably balanced diet.

Estrogen, the major substance in contraceptive pills, is a very powerful hormone, and much is still to be learned of the varying effects it may have. For instance, there is now limited evidence that estrogen increases the rate of ascorbic acid (vitamin C) breakdown, thus increasing the dietary need for that vitamin. While vitamin supplements are not necessary, the "balanced diet" concept cannot be overstressed. A variety of foods eaten in moderation should avert any dietary difficulties.

The Later Years

Life-style changes in later years often create many nutritional problems for the elderly, including weight problems, digestive malfunctions, and varying degrees of malnourishment. Thus, for example, after age twenty-five, indications are that the average American's calorie needs decrease by about 5 percent every ten years—due in part to a slowing of the metabolic processes but also influenced a great deal by the amount of physical exercise one gets.

One of the major problems of the elderly is appetite: loneliness and inactivity can affect it in either direction, thereby causing either underweight or obesity. Intake of vitamins A and C is often inadequate and should be carefully regulated. Calcium levels, too, tend to fall too low in the elderly, contributing to osteoporosis (brittleness of the bones), a condition especially common among older women.

Senior citizens require a balanced diet, like persons of any other age; they just need a little less of it.

NUTRITION AND DISEASE

Chronic nutritional diseases can be roughly divided into two categories—those associated with undernutrition and those associated with "overnutrition" (diabetes, heart disease, cancer, and others). Additionally, there are the simple deficiency diseases, most of which are easily correctable.

Undernutrition

The United States is one of the most affluent countries in the world. After the food stamp program was introduced in the 1960s to augment other forms of government health assistance, it was generally assumed that for the first time in history every American would have enough to eat. Tragically, this is not the case.

What is not understood by most urban dwellers is that certain rural areas of the United States have remained virtually untouched by any type of technology or social reforms. These people barely subsist on too little food, and with no hope of even approaching the principles of variety and balance in their meals. Food stamps are inaccessible, as are medical and dental care.

Such areas include less than 10 percent of the population, but in a country as large as the United States, this is a great number of people. Surely a nation bent on improving the health of underdeveloped countries should also seek new means of reaching and feeding its own destitute populations.

Shockingly, another 10 percent of the U.S. population is also malnourished—and these persons are from the upper income brackets. Greater purchasing power and a rapid living pace seem to encourage poor eating habits. Breakfast is often skipped; other meals are hastily snatched and frequently replaced by low-nutrient, high-calorie snack foods. At least one well-known nutritionist has seriously suggested fortification of the catsup and mustard used in fast food chains!

Overnutrition

The problems of overnutrition are many and varied. Almost without exception, it is not the

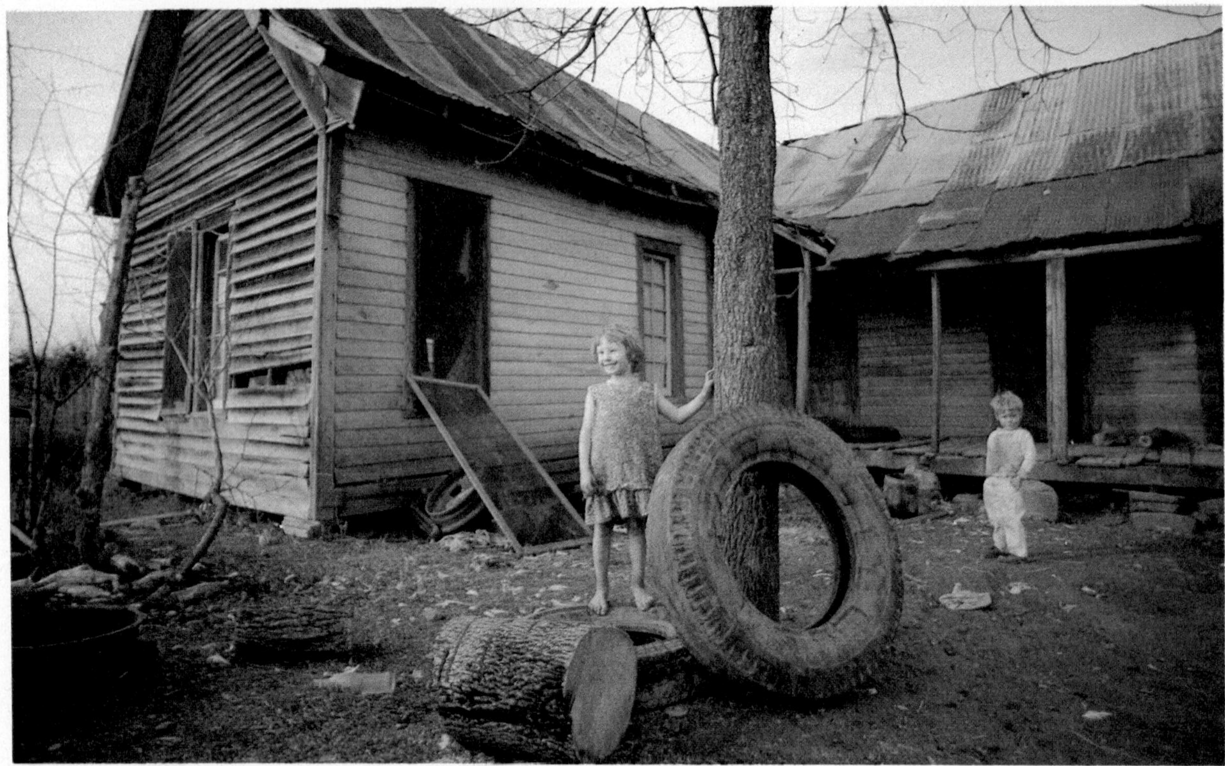

Figure 8.3 Unfortunately, undernutrition still exists in America, especially in areas of rural poverty where people have too little to eat and food stamps are not readily available.

elements of overnutrition per se that create difficulties. Rather, overconsumption of high-calorie fatty or sweet foods leads to obesity—and obesity, in turn, can precipitate or worsen many other conditions.

For example, studies during the past few years have indicated that there is a close association between heart disease and consumption of cholesterol and saturated fat. On careful examination of the data, it becomes apparent that the relationship is not really one of simple cause and effect. What happens is that too much cholesterol and saturated fat in the diet tend to make an individual overweight. Probably the individual also gets too little exercise. There is no doubt that these factors can then contribute to a greater risk of atherosclerosis and coronary heart disease—particularly when combined with other known risk factors, such as cigarette smoking, heredity, and stress. Stroke, too, may be diet related in that an attack is usually preceded by some form of atherosclerosis.

Studies have shown that the risk of heart attack in middle-aged men who are 30 percent or more over their normal weight is double that for middle-aged men still at normal weight. The same studies found that the risk of heart disease is four times greater in persons with high blood pressure (hypertension) than in those with normal blood pressure—and it is known that extra pounds increase the risk of elevated blood pressure by two to three times. The obese often consume more than average amounts of salt, another cause of hypertension.

Similarly, recent research indicates that certain forms of cancer (chiefly, cancer of the colon, breast, and prostate) may be associated with diets high in calories and fat. Currently there is not enough evidence to confirm the precise role played by these substances.

Diabetes is another disease far more prevalent among the obese. That segment of the population that is 30 percent overweight has three times more diabetes than those of normal weight. There is also some evidence that excessive protein consumption may be involved because insulin production is affected by the amino acid leucine. Most doctors today believe that weight control will reduce the risk of diabetes, or at least delay its onset, among those genetically predisposed.

Simple Diet Deficiencies

Except in certain rare hereditary conditions in which one's biological processes may be imperfect (such as pernicious anemia, in which the body cannot manufacture vitamin B_{12}), there is no longer any excuse for simple deficiency diseases in this country. The one possible exception is iron deficiency, which is easily corrected, as discussed in the section "Minerals."

Other vitamin deficiencies do exist, but these are primarily direct results of self-imposed assaults on the body. In alcoholics, for instance, lack of thiamine can ultimately cause death if the deficiency is not corrected in time. New research indicates that smoking destroys some of the body's vitamin C, and therefore a higher intake is needed by those who smoke. Low-carbohydrate fad diets lead to severe losses of both sodium and potassium from the body. Potassium deficiency can cause irregularities of the heart that may be fatal in extreme cases—a possible factor in the deaths associated with such diets.

Moderation—in all aspects of health—is the first requirement for good nutrition.

SUMMARY

1. Nutrition, the science of food, involves its use within the body and its relationship to good health. Eating feeds body cells and fuels the body's efficient operation.
2. Foods are composed of chemical compounds. During digestion, these are broken down into simpler ones, which are reassembled into chemicals that can be directly used.
3. The basic food components are protein, carbohydrates, fats, vitamins, minerals, water, and fiber.
4. Protein is vital for the growth as well as the repair of the body. Meat, eggs, and dairy products are foods that have complete protein. Protein of plant origin (vegetables and grains) is almost always incomplete. To form complete protein, plant proteins can be combined with each other or with specific combinations of animal protein.
5. Carbohydrates include both sugars and starches. They contribute about 50 percent of the body's energy needs and are its most economical energy source. They are also required for fat metabolism.
6. Fats provide a source of energy, impart flavor to many foods, and insulate parts of the body. Stored fats are the greatest nutritional reservoir in the body.
7. Vitamins, indispensable in triggering vital bodily functions, act as co-enzymes and are required only in trace amounts. Minerals help form tissues and various chemical substances in the body.
8. Water is one of the most important of all food components. Fiber, a nonnutritive substance, is necessary to the digestion.
9. The simplest way to plan a balanced diet on a daily basis is to select adequate amounts of food from each of the Basic Four Food Groups.
10. The Basic Four Groups are: (a) the meat group, which includes poultry, fish, eggs, and legumes such as dried beans, peas, and nuts; (b) milk and milk products; (c) fruits and vegetables; and (d) breads and cereals (whole-grain or enriched).
11. Additives and preservatives contribute to the attractiveness, taste, and economy of processed food. They also prevent certain food-borne diseases. In spite of fairly strict laws regulating the food industry, the safety of a number of these chemical substances is questioned by some scientists.
12. Among those who have special nutritional needs are infants and teen-agers, pregnant women, women who use contraceptive pills, and elderly people.
13. Chronic nutritional diseases are of two basic kinds: those associated with undernutrition and those linked with overnutrition (heart disease, cancer, diabetes, and gallstones).

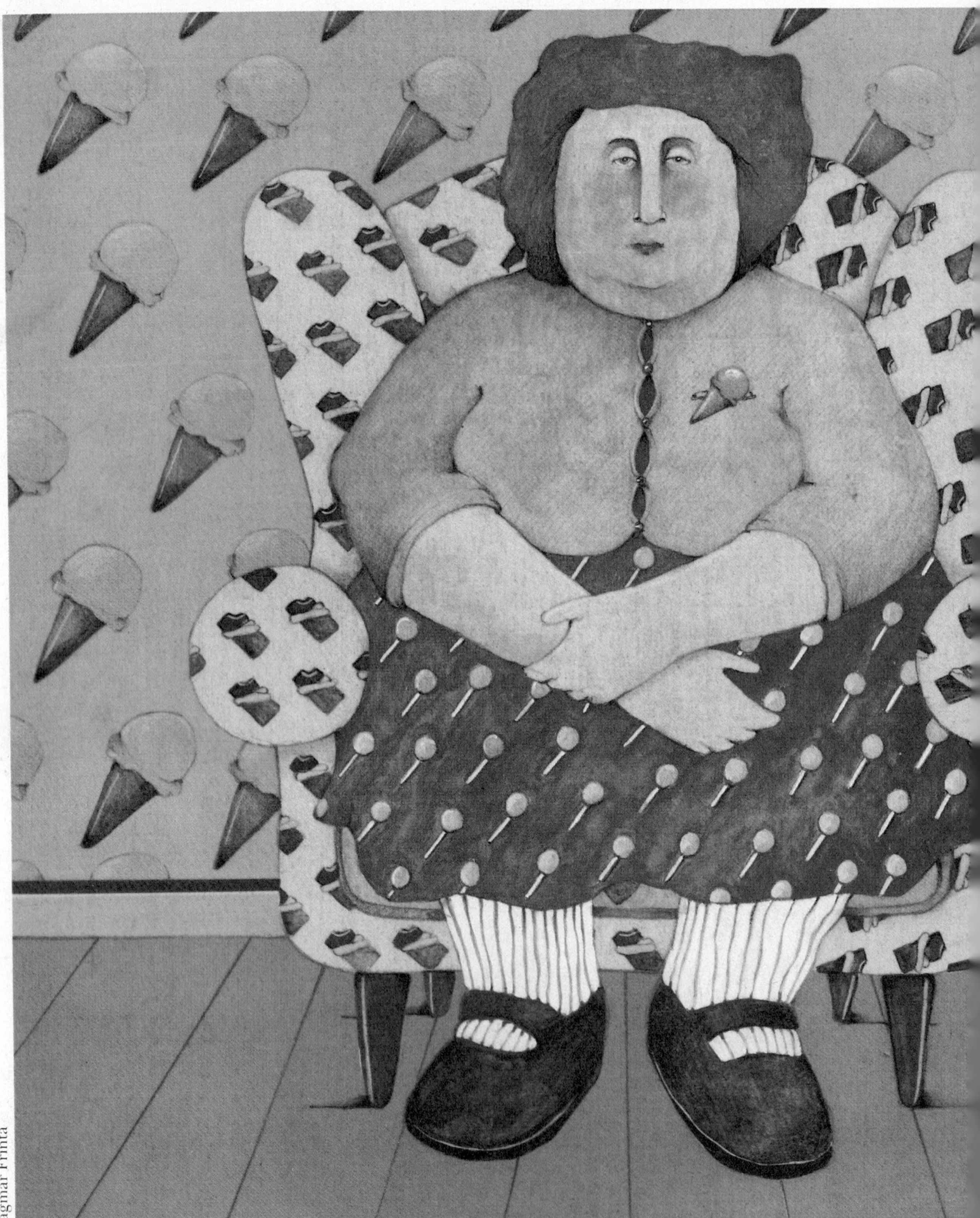

Dagmar Frinta

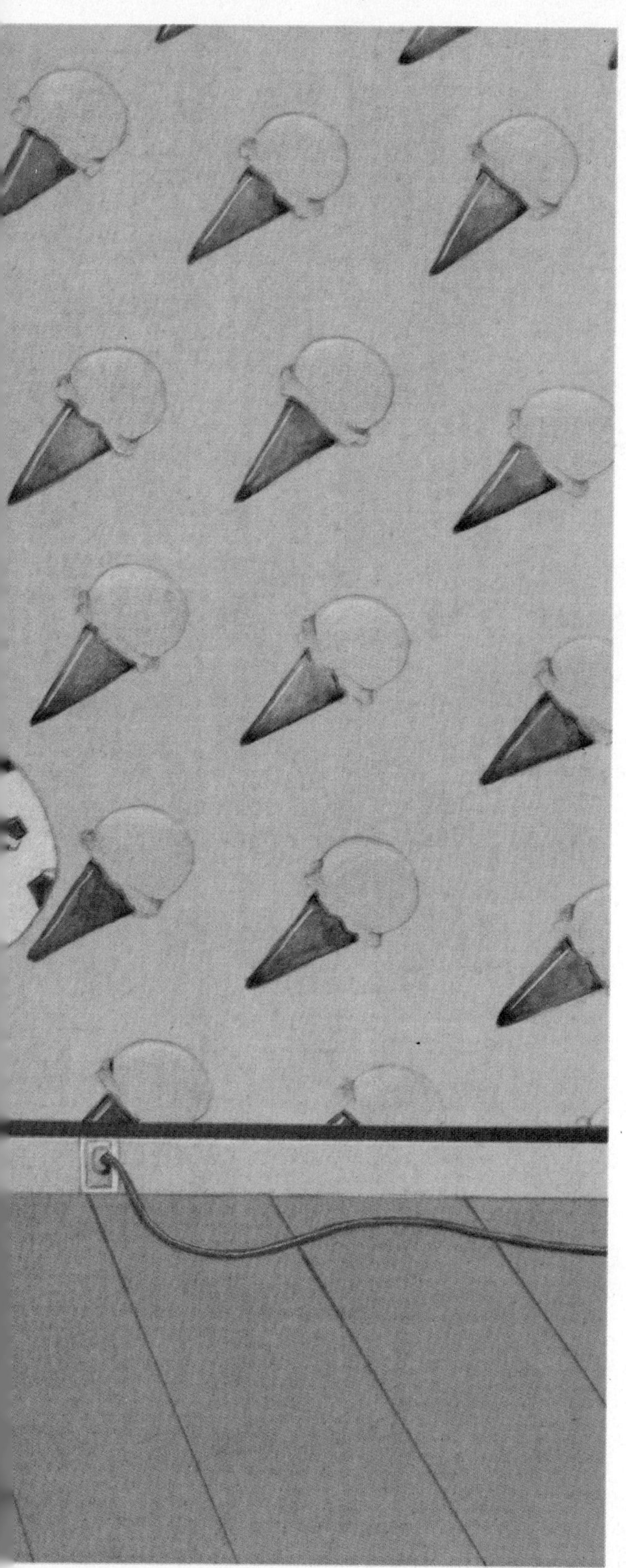

9 Weight Management

Overweight seems to be an American preoccupation. Every year or two, a new book hawks yet another lose-weight-quick fad diet. Supermarkets stock shelves of "diet foods." Commercial weight control groups have sprung up in most major cities, and hucksters are constantly promoting new reducing schemes and gimmicks. Fortunes are made in the weight control business; as one entrepreneur has said, "There's a lot of fat and fear of fat out there to be harvested."

Most of this interest in weight control is motivated by concern for appearance, a desire to have an attractive figure. Overweight can be both a social and an emotional problem in a culture that almost worships slimness. Yet there are also important health reasons for controlling one's weight; overweight is a pathological condition that is associated with a number of serious, disabling, and life-threatening diseases. Experts consider overweight a major health problem in the United States—and one that is still growing. According to a National Center for Health Statistics 1974 survey, both men and women in most age and height categories are heavier than they were in the early 1960s.

This chapter will discuss the differences between overweight and obesity, the causes of overweight, who should control one's weight and why, and the available methods of losing weight.

OVERWEIGHT AND OBESITY

How much should you weigh? Recommendations for desirable weights are usually based on tables published by life insurance companies (see Table 9.1). To compile these tables, the companies have gathered statistics on the average weights of men and women of different heights and body types. Then, since many of these people are overweight, the companies have adjusted the statistics downward to arrive at desirable weights. These tables thus are not absolute but merely approximate guides to healthy weights.

You will note that to use Table 9.1, you need to judge your body frame. To determine this scientifically, a researcher would measure the widths of the shoulder and pelvic girdles and the diameters of the bones at the ankles, knees, wrists, and elbows. You can estimate this, however, by comparing your wrist size with those of other people of your own height and sex.

Generally, if your weight varies less than 10 percent—either more or less—from the weight recommended for your sex, height, and body frame, it is of no health significance. A weight 10 to 20 percent above the table is usually considered *overweight;* 20 to 30 percent above the table may be considered obese; and weight that is 30 percent or more above the recommended value almost always indicates obesity.

In 1971–1972, the Health and Nutrition Examination Survey collected data on the prevalence of obesity among adult Americans. Women had a higher prevalence of obesity than did men, the survey found; 18.9 percent of white women between the ages of twenty and forty-four were obese compared to 16 percent of white men. Black women showed a higher percentage (29.2 percent) of obesity than did white women, while black men had a lower percentage (10 percent) than white men.

Table 9.1 Desirable Weights for Men and Women*

Group	Height (with shoes on)	Small Frame	Medium Frame	Large Frame
Men (one-inch heels)	5′ 2″	112–120	118–129	126–141
	5′ 3″	115–123	121–133	129–144
	5′ 4″	118–126	124–136	132–148
	5′ 5″	121–129	127–139	135–152
	5′ 6″	124–133	130–143	138–156
	5′ 7″	128–137	134–147	142–161
	5′ 8″	132–141	138–152	147–166
	5′ 9″	136–145	142–156	151–170
	5′10″	140–150	146–160	155–174
	5′11″	144–154	150–165	159–179
	6′ 0″	148–158	154–170	164–184
	6′ 1″	152–162	158–175	168–189
	6′ 2″	156–167	162–180	173–194
	6′ 3″	160–171	167–185	178–199
	6′ 4″	164–175	172–190	182–204
Women† (two-inch heels)	4′10″	92–98	96–107	104–119
	4′11″	94–101	98–110	106–122
	5′ 0″	96–104	101–113	109–125
	5′ 1″	99–107	104–116	112–128
	5′ 2″	102–110	107–119	115–131
	5′ 3″	105–113	110–122	118–134
	5′ 4″	108–116	113–126	121–138
	5′ 5″	111–119	116–130	125–142
	5′ 6″	114–123	120–135	129–146
	5′ 7″	118–127	124–139	133–150
	5′ 8″	122–131	128–143	137–154
	5′ 9″	126–135	132–147	141–158
	5′10″	130–140	136–151	145–163
	5′11″	134–144	140–155	149–168
	6′ 0″	138–148	144–159	153–173

*Weight in pounds according to frame (in indoor clothing).
†For women between eighteen and twenty-five, subtract one pound for each year under twenty-five.
Source: Metropolitan Life Insurance Company, 1959.

Body Composition

There is a distinction, however, between *overweight* and *obesity. Overweight* is weight in excess of the average. *Obesity* is a higher than average proportion of fat tissue in the body.

Our bodies are largely made up of lean or nonfat tissues: muscle, bone, cartilage, connective tissue, skin, nerves, and the internal organs. In average young men, about 15 percent of body weight is fat tissue; in highly trained athletes, it can drop to less than 8 percent. In average young women, about 25 percent of body weight is fat; in women athletes, it can drop to below 14 percent. The higher percentage of fat in women is due to an additional layer of fat in female skin plus fat deposits in the breasts, hips, thighs, and lower abdomen.

Fat tissue includes both *essential fat* (that

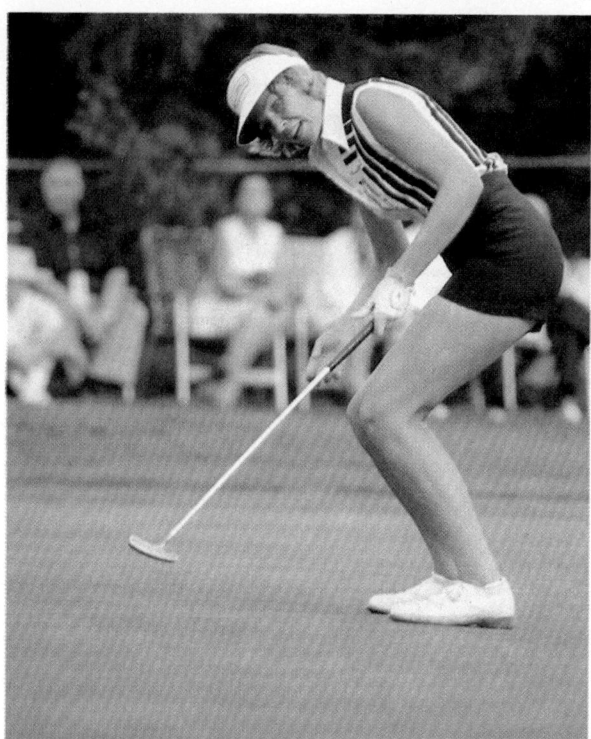

Figure 9.1 The average woman has a higher percentage of fat (usually about one-fourth of her body weight) than does the average man. However, athletic training greatly reduces body fat and increases muscle weight.

which is necessary for normal physiological functioning) and *excess fat.* In men, essential fat is 2 to 4 percent of total body weight. In women, it is 6 to 8 percent.

Since lean tissue is heavier than fat tissue, people can be overweight—in the sense of weighing more than average—without being obese. This is often true of football linemen and serious body builders, who may weigh 20 percent above the weights recommended by the tables because of heavy muscle mass—yet have little fat tissue. Conversely, extremely sedentary people can be obese without being overweight; they may have a lot of fat tissue but little muscle mass.

The effects of these variations in body composition on health are not known. However, it is likely that having excess fat is a greater health risk than simply being overweight.

Assessing Body Fat

How can you tell the proportion of fat tissue in your body? One do-it-yourself method is the *mirror test,* which we all use from time to time: simply looking at yourself nude in a full-length mirror. "If you *look* fat," says nutritionist Jean Mayer, "you probably *are* fat." The mirror test, however, is not objective; studies show that most women make significant errors in judging their own proportion of fat tissue.

A more objective do-it-yourself method is the *pinch test.* With your thumb and forefinger, grasp a fold of skin at your waistline two to three inches to either side of the navel. If the thickness of the skin fold is more than an inch, you are probably fat. Another fairly good method for men is the *abdominal circumference test.* If the circumference of your abdomen exceeds the circumference of your chest, you are probably obese.

Scientists have many more precise methods of assessing a person's actual proportion of lean and fat tissue. In the *densimetric method,* a person is weighed first in air and then while totally submerged in water, to find out his or her specific gravity or overall density relative to water. From this—since lean tissue is heavier than water, while fat tissue is lighter than water—scientists can calculate, using appropriate formulas, the total amount of fat tissue in the body.

Another fairly accurate method is by *anthropometric measurements.* Scientists measure skin fold thicknesses at many different places on the body, circumferences of the trunk, chest, and abdomen, and the diameters of the wrists and ankles. From these data, they can compute the proportion of fat.

CAUSES OF OVERWEIGHT

The direct cause of overweight is straightforward. If we consume more food energy—that is, eat more calories—than our bodies can use up, the excess calories are inevitably stored in our bodies in the form of fat. For every excess 3,500 calories, we gain one pound of fat. The question is, why do so many of us so often eat more calories than we can use? Unfortunately, the fundamental causes of overweight are not well understood.

In laboratory animals, researchers are able to induce overweight in a variety of ways. By inbreeding, they have been able to prove the existence of several "obesity genes" in rats and mice. Scientists can also produce obesity in animals by injuring the appetite regulatory mechanism in the hypothalamus, by manipulating hormone levels, by overfeeding, and by restricting physical activity. Researchers believe that in humans, too, there are probably many different types of obesity with many different causes. And in any one overweight person, many different factors probably contribute to the obesity.

Overweight clearly tends to run in families. If one parent in a family is overweight, 40 percent of the children are also overweight. If both parents are obese, then 80 percent of their children are also obese. Conversely, among children who are overweight, 75 percent have at least one obese parent. Such familial tendencies, however, could be caused by either heredity or environment. While family members do share genes, they also share eating and exercise habits.

Studies of identical twins have shown that *both heredity and environment* are involved in the development of obesity. The existence of a genetic component is demonstrated by the fact that identical twins (who have the same genes) are more similar to each other in weight than are fraternal twins (who have different genes). The existence of an environmental component is shown by the fact that identical twins who are separated and raised in different families differ more in weight than do identical twins raised in the same family.

In humans, researchers have thus far identified only a few, extremely rare, specific obesity genes. They believe that the genetic component in human obesity is probably determined by many genes, and that what is inherited is probably a tendency toward overweight.

In the 1970s, scientists uncovered another intriguing clue about the causes of overweight when they discovered that there are two different types of obesity distinguishable by the fat cells themselves. Some overweight people, it turns out, have a higher than normal *number* of fat cells, sometimes as many as two or three times the normal number. Other overweight people have a normal number of fat cells but are obese because their fat cells are *larger* than normal.

When the people with an excess number of fat cells do manage to lose weight, they never lose these fat cells; the cells simply shrink in size. This type of obesity with excess fat cells usually begins early in life, in childhood or at puberty, and it seems to be far more difficult to overcome than obesity that begins in adulthood. Some 80 percent of overweight children become overweight adults, and approximately 25 percent of overweight adults can trace their obesity back to their childhood. Some evidence suggests that overfeeding during childhood or even infancy may contribute to this excess number of fat cells. Parents who press second helpings on children, exhort them to clean their plates, or reward or comfort them with food may thus be contributing to an overweight problem later in their lives.

In the second type of obesity, many people find themselves victims of "creeping overweight" as they grow older. For many women, weight gained during pregnancy (but there is no need to gain fat during pregnancy) becomes difficult to shed. From age twenty on, basal metabolism slows at the rate of 3 to 5 percent per decade. At age sixty, then, you need perhaps 20 percent fewer calories than you need at age twenty. At the same time, people are likely to eat and drink more as they partake of the "good life." It doesn't take very many extra calories to add up over the years. A mere fifty calories a day over and above what you need will, after ten years, result in a fifty-pound weight gain.

All of us, whether overweight or normal weight, are conditioned to turn to food for many *psychological reasons* over and above our physiological need for fuel. We may be tempted to eat a snack simply because we pass a tempting food stand or see a mouth-watering commercial on television. We may have learned to associate eating with the pleasure of reading or listening to music. We center holidays and other social occasions on lavish meals. We show our love for our families and

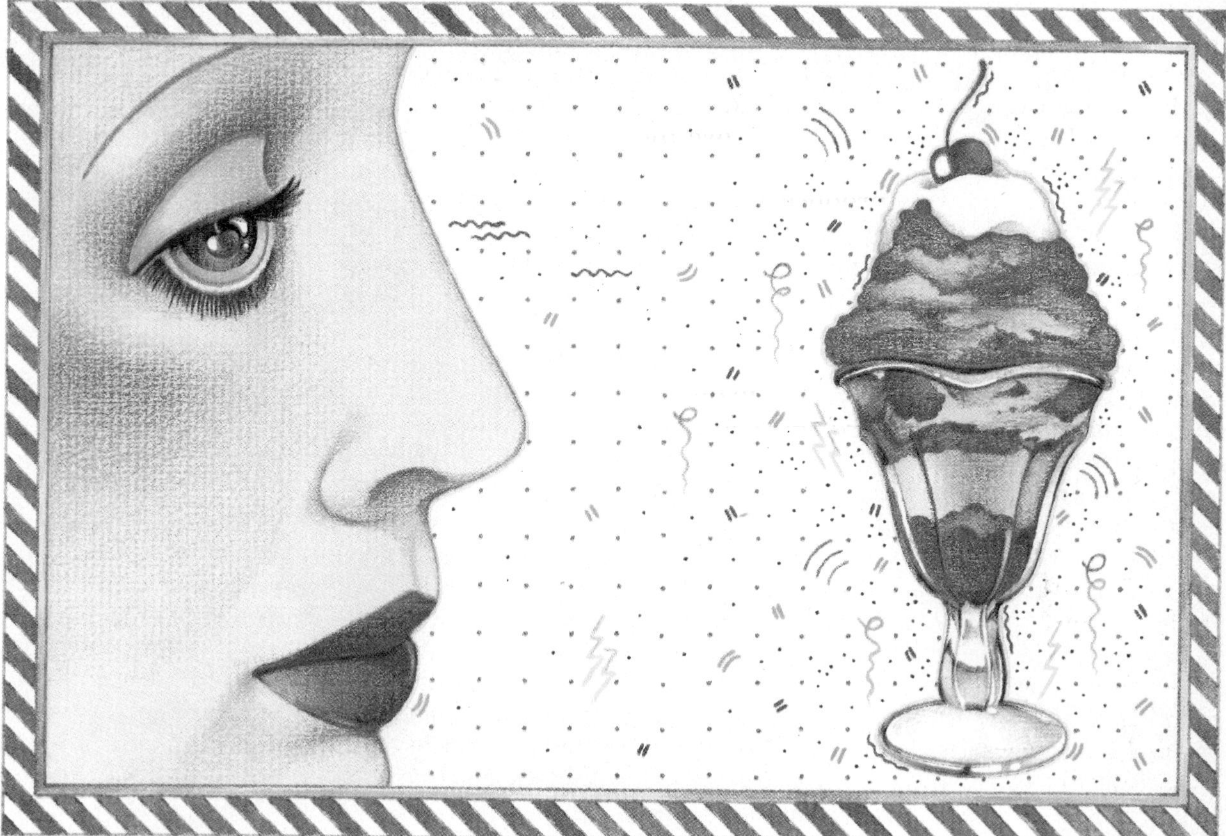

Figure 9.2 Regardless of what we weigh, most of us turn to food for psychological reasons—visual appeal, for instance—that have no relation to our physiological needs.

friends by preparing special foods for them. And we often turn to food for emotional reasons because we are bored, anxious, lonely, depressed, or under stress.

Some recent research, performed in the last decade, suggests that overweight people may be more responsive to such external, nonphysiological cues than are people of normal weight. In experiments conducted by Stanley Schachter, overweights responded more than normals to the taste of food; overweights ate more of food that tasted good. And when researchers manipulated the clock so that people thought it was dinner time when it was not, the normals were not affected but the overweight people ate much more.

Lack of exercise is also associated with overweight. Motion picture studies of obese and nonobese children on school playgrounds and adults in factories showed that the obese exercised much less, both in amount and intensity. Lack of exercise is also probably a factor in the "creeping overweight" of adulthood. To a large extent, we have become a sedentary nation, with all manner of automatic and remote-control gadgets to do our bidding. People who do remain physically active experience much less reduction in their basal metabolism as they age and also gain less weight.

Some research by Dr. Theodore Van Itallie of the Obesity Research Center at St. Luke's Hospital in New York City suggests that *speed of eating* may be related to overeating. People who eat quickly may eat too much because their appetite regulatory mechanism does not have time to signal them that they have had enough. In time, such rapid eating may even switch off the normal regulatory mechanism. Other evidence suggests that *heavy eating late in the day* is more likely to result in overweight in some people.

Other research at St. Luke's has implicated *"junk food" habits* as a possible contributor to overweight. Animals that were fed only highly sugared, low-fiber foods thereafter rejected wholesome standard diets and ate much more of the junk food because it requires more of such food to satisfy hunger. Frequent snacking on high-calorie, low-nutrient foods is habituating. Commercial advertising of such foods and their ready availability in candy counters, vending machines, and fast-food restaurants could be an important cause of the overweight problem.

WHY REDUCE?

While the most obvious reason for losing weight is appearance, there are also important health reasons for reducing. Overweight is associated with a number of major diseases, including several leading causes of death.

The risk of *heart disease* is greatly increased among the obese. People who are 30 percent or more overweight are twice as likely to develop coronary heart disease and have heart attacks as people of normal weight. The excess weight chronically strains both the heart and the blood vessels. Overweight people also tend to have higher levels of blood fats and higher blood pressure and to exercise less—all of which are risk factors for heart disease. Epidemiological studies suggest that overweight is responsible for perhaps 25 percent of all heart disease deaths—or more than 150,000 deaths a year—in the United States.

The risk of developing *hypertension* (high blood pressure) is much greater for people who are overweight. In addition to being a risk factor for heart disease, high blood pressure also increases the likelihood of stroke and kidney disease. In some people with hypertension, losing weight can dramatically reduce their blood pressure, sometimes to the point where they no longer need to take medication for it.

Overweight is also a very significant factor in the development of *diabetes,* a serious metabolic disease affecting millions of Americans. Diabetes involves a derangement of the action of insulin, a hormone produced by specialized cells in the pancreas. The body thus does not use sugar properly, and it builds up in the blood and urine. Diabetes can lead to blindness, heart attack, stroke, and atherosclerosis and is a major cause of death.

Overweight people have twice the incidence of diabetes as people of normal weight, and the more obese they are, the more likely they are to develop the disease. In very obese people, the incidence can be ten times greater than average. The disease is also far more severe in overweight people. Again, losing weight can often dramatically help control the disease.

Overweight may also contribute to certain forms of *cancer.* There is some evidence that overweight women have a higher incidence of cancers of the pancreas, gall bladder, breast, and uterus. In one study, women who had been obese since adolescence had a 75 percent greater incidence of endometrial cancer (cancer of the uterine lining).

Obesity is also associated with kidney disease, gall bladder disease, menstrual disorders, and complications of pregnancy. It overburdens the bones and joints and is associated with certain forms of arthritis and the rupture of intervertebral discs. It interferes with proper functioning of the lungs; in extreme cases, reduced oxygen intake can even threaten brain function.

People who are overweight also suffer definite social, emotional, and vocational disadvantages. Studies suggest that seriously obese high-school seniors have less of a chance of being admitted to college. Many employers avoid hiring the overweight. Sometimes (particularly when the job involves dealing with the public) it is because of the unattractive appearance of the obese. Some other employers, unfortunately, associate fatness with laziness and assume that obesity is a sign of a physical or psychological condition that might interfere with the person's work performance. Many people have a deep-seated prejudice—however unfounded—that the obese are weak, sick, or otherwise disturbed. The obese are thus often shunned socially.

Finally, obesity can be damaging to one's self-esteem. There is no way to measure the effect of never looking really fashionable or well dressed, of failing to qualify for sports and other competitive activities, or of being unappealing to members of the opposite sex.

SUCCESSFUL WEIGHT REDUCTION

Since the direct cause of overweight is eating more calories than our bodies are able to use up, the *only* way we can lose weight is to change our calorie balance so that we consume *fewer* calories than we use. There are two ways to achieve this *negative calorie balance,* as it is called. One is to reduce the number of calories we eat. The other is to increase the number of calories we burn by increasing our activity level. The most successful weight reduction programs combine both approaches.

The cure for overweight is thus simple in principle but—as so many of us know—extremely difficult in practice. The long-term success rate for weight reduction programs is so poor—one in ten at best—that one could consider obesity a chronic disease. Yet many overweight people can and do succeed in reducing.

Long-term weight control requires *permanent changes in both eating and exercise habits.* Crash programs may work in the short run, but they rarely succeed in the long run. Even the idea of dieting to lose weight is a fallacy, because it implies an abnormal eating pattern—and also implies that at some time in the future, one will revert to one's old eating habits.

Most overweight people are experts at losing weight; they have done it many times. They are also experts at gaining weight back again in a "yo-yo" pattern. Nutritionist Jean Mayer calls this the "rhythm method of girth control."

Overweight people must literally relearn how to eat. It is important to learn new eating habits that involve the foods commonly served in homes and restaurants. This does not mean that you cannot change the dishes served in your own home, but you are unlikely to succeed at controlling your weight if you rely heavily on unusual foods. You cannot expect the world around you to gear its habits to your need to lose weight.

Planning a Weight Control Program

To increase your chances of success, it is a good idea to begin by setting specific goals for the amount of weight you want to lose and the rate at which you want to lose it. Then you can work out a program for achieving these goals.

It is important that your goals not be unreasonable. If you have the illusion that you will instantly achieve a model's figure or physique, you are setting yourself up for failure. If, however, you view every pound lost as a small victory, you are more likely to continue your program.

It is not wise to lose weight faster than a pound or two a week unless you are under a doctor's supervision. Thus, if you are thirty pounds overweight, it would be reasonable to aim toward shedding that thirty pounds gradually over the course of a year.

Once you have set your weight-loss goal, the next step is to figure out how many calories you should eat each day in order to achieve that goal. First, use the Calorie Calculator and Activity Level Guide shown in Figure 9.3 to determine the number of calories you now need to eat to maintain your present weight. An eighteen-year-old man, for example, who stands 5 feet 9 inches tall, weighs 180 pounds, and is a student who has a part-time job in the library will need approximately 3,100 calories each day to remain at his present weight.

Let's say his goal is to bring his weight down to 160 pounds by losing 20 pounds over a period of twenty weeks—that is, losing weight at the rate of 1 pound each week. Since one pound of fat equals 3,500 calories, to lose one pound of fat in a week, you need to eat 3,500 calories fewer than you use each week, or 500 fewer calories each day. The student therefore could achieve his goal by eating 2,600 calories a day (3,100 minus 500 calories). If he wanted to lose weight at a rate of two pounds a week, he would need a calorie deficit of 1,000 calories each day, or a 2,100-calorie-a-day diet.

When you are on a low-calorie diet, it is par-

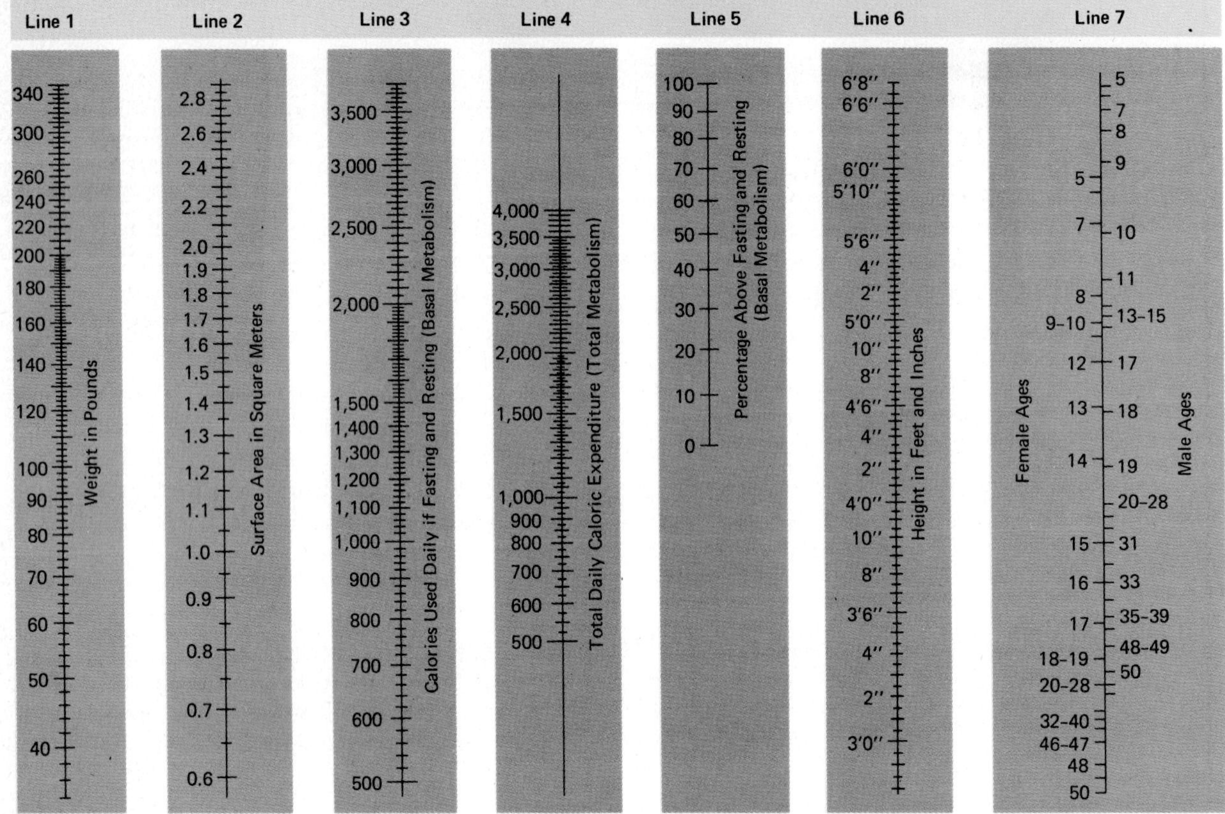

Figure 9.3 The calorie calculator and activity level guide. To determine the number of calories needed to maintain your present weight, follow these instructions:

1. Using a pin as a marker, locate your present weight on line 1.
2. Setting the edge of a ruler against the pin, swing the other end of the ruler to your height, located on line 6.
3. Remove the pin from line 1, and now place it at the point where the ruler crosses line 2.
4. Keeping the edge of the ruler firmly against the pin on line 2, swing its right-hand edge to your sex and age on line 7, using the age of your nearest birthday for the purpose.
5. Remove the pin, and place it where the ruler crosses line 3. This will give you the calories used daily (in twenty-four hours) if you are resting and fasting.
6. To the basal calories thus determined, add the percentage above fasting and resting for your usual type of daily activity, using the following guidelines:
   Add 40 percent if you are a nonworking student whose physical activity is limited to walking to and from classes.
   Add 50 percent if you are involved in physical activity (such as clerical or library work) that includes about two hours of walking or standing daily.
   Add 60 percent if you participate in limited physical exercise (such as disco dancing) or intramural sports of a moderate nature.
   Add 70 percent if your work involves heavy physical activity (such as construction work) or if you participate in a regular, daily exercise program (such as intercollegiate team sports).
   Add 80 to 100 percent if you are engaged in strenuous physical work or participate in intercollegiate sports that have a high rate of calorie expenditure (i.e., basketball, track, and so on).
7. Leaving the pin in line 3, swing the edge of the ruler to the right to the proper percentage on line 5. Where the ruler crosses line 4, you will find the number of calories necessary to maintain you at your present weight if you maintain your present activity level.

ticularly important that you select a diet that is normally balanced among proteins, carbohydrates, and fats, and that includes adequate supplies of vitamins and minerals.

Your actual loss of fat weight on a low-calorie diet can sometimes be obscured by the fact that you can gain or lose water weight quite independently. (There are no calories in water.) Since our bodies are 72 percent water, changes in water content can cause quick and dramatic changes in weight. Indeed, any quick weight loss or gain must be due to water loss or retention because muscle and fat cannot change rapidly. Most quick-weight-loss diets—those that cause losses of more than two pounds a week—rely on such early and dramatic loss of water. On the other hand, some people tend to retain water at the beginning of a reducing diet, so that even though they have a calorie deficit of 500 or 1,000 calories a day, they may not lose as much as a pound a week. These people often become discouraged and drop their diet. If they persevere, however, they do eventually eliminate this extra water and may lose several pounds literally overnight.

You can also lose weight fairly quickly by burning calories stored in muscles and other protein tissue. This can happen on a diet that does not provide sufficient protein. Since a pound of protein contains less than half the calories in a pound of fat, if you are losing weight (other than water weight) faster than one pound for every 3,500-calorie deficit, you are probably losing protein. This kind of diet is very dangerous, because it can damage the heart and other vital internal organs (which are made of protein).

If you are losing weight more slowly than one pound for every 3,500-calorie deficit, you are probably losing fat. Long-term, controlled studies of weight loss have shown that when people lose weight rapidly at the beginning of a diet, this early loss is more likely to be water and protein. Slower weight loss, later on, is more likely to be fat.

The Need for Exercise

In addition to decreasing the number of calories you eat, the other method of achieving negative calorie balance (as mentioned previously) is to increase your activity level. This is an extremely important factor in reducing. It is often easier to exercise more than to eat less, and the most successful reducing plans employ both low-calorie diets and programs of increased exercise.

Many people have the mistaken idea that exercise is of little value in weight reduction. It is true that you need to walk thirty miles, for instance, to burn off the 3,500 calories in a pound of fat. However, if you walk only one additional mile each day—365 extra miles a year—without increasing your calorie intake, you would lose twelve pounds over the course of the year. Furthermore, people who exercise regularly are actually inclined to eat less than sedentary people.

An exercise program for weight control should take the following factors into account:

1. The regularity and frequency of exercise are more important than the kind of exercise.
2. You should schedule a kind of exercise and a time of day for it so that it becomes a routine part of your daily regimen.
3. The kind of exercise you choose should fit your life style and should also be something you enjoy for its own sake.
4. Continuous, rhythmic exercise lasting thirty minutes or more tends to burn the most calories with the least distress. Such exercises as walking, jogging, swimming, and bicycling are the best for both weight control and physical fitness (see Chapter 10).
5. Inactive people over the age of thirty-five should not begin any strenuous exercise program without a complete medical checkup that includes an exercise stress test (see Chapter 10).

Behavior Modification

The most successful method discovered to date for long-term weight control is a process called *behavior modification.* Behavior modification is often employed by professionally led reducing groups, but it is also a process that, to a certain extent, you can do yourself.

Once you have calculated the number of calories you need to eat each day to achieve your weight-loss goals, the next step is to find out what your eating patterns are. What are the cues and circumstances that prompt you to overeat?

To become consciously aware of your eating habits, *write them down.* Behavior therapists often recommend that you keep a detailed written diary of your eating behavior for several days or a week—writing down each meal and snack; the time of beginning and ending it;

Table 9.2 Amount of Exercise Required to Burn Off a Given Number of Calories

Food	Calories	Minutes of Activity				
		Walking	Bicycling	Swimming	Running	Reclining
Apple, large	101	19	12	9	5	78
Bacon, 2 strips	96	18	12	9	5	74
Banana, small	88	17	11	8	4	68
Beans, green, 1 cup	27	5	3	2	1	21
Beer, 1 glass	114	22	14	10	6	88
Bread and butter	78	15	10	7	4	60
Cake, 2 layer, 1/12	356	68	43	32	18	274
Carbonated beverage, 1 glass	106	20	13	9	5	82
Carrot, raw	42	8	5	4	2	32
Cereal, dry, ½ cup with milk, sugar	200	38	24	18	10	154
Cheese, cottage, 1 tbs.	27	5	3	2	1	21
Cheese, cheddar, 1 oz.	111	21	14	10	6	85
Chicken, fried, ½ breast	232	45	28	21	12	178
Chicken, TV dinner	542	104	66	48	28	417
Cookie, plain	15	3	2	1	1	12
Cookie, chocolate chip	51	10	6	5	3	39
Doughnut	151	29	18	13	8	116
Egg, fried	110	21	13	10	6	85
Egg, boiled	77	15	9	7	4	59
French dressing, 1 tbs.	59	11	7	5	3	45
Halibut steak, ¼ lb.	205	39	25	18	11	158
Ham, 2 slices	167	32	20	15	9	128
Hamburger sandwich	350	67	43	31	18	269
Ice cream, 1/6 qt.	193	37	24	17	10	148
Ice cream soda	255	49	31	23	13	196
Ice milk, 1/6 qt.	144	28	18	13	7	111
Mayonnaise, 1 tbs.	92	18	11	8	5	71
Milk, 1 glass	166	32	20	15	9	128
Milk, skim, 1 glass	81	16	10	7	4	62
Milk shake	421	81	51	38	22	324
Orange, medium	68	13	8	6	4	52
Orange juice, 1 glass	120	23	15	11	6	92
Pancake with syrup	124	24	15	11	6	95
Peach, medium	46	9	6	4	2	35
Peas, green, ½ cup	56	11	7	5	3	43
Pie, apple, 1/6	377	73	46	34	19	290
Pizza, cheese, ⅛	180	35	22	16	9	138
Pork chop, loin	314	60	38	28	16	242
Potato chips, 1 serving	108	21	13	10	6	83
Sherbet, 1/6 qt.	177	34	22	16	9	136
Shrimp, French fried	180	35	22	16	9	138
Spaghetti, 1 serving	396	76	48	35	20	305
Steak, T-bone	235	45	29	21	12	181
Strawberry shortcake	400	77	49	36	21	308
Tuna-salad sandwich	278	53	34	25	14	214

Source: Adapted from F. Konishi, "Food Energy Equivalents of Various Activities," *Journal of the American Dietetic Association,* 46 (1965), p. 186.

the place (including what room of your home); whether you are sitting, standing, or lying down; whether you are alone or with other people; any associated activity, such as reading or watching television or talking; your mood; how hungry you were just before eating; the foods you eat; and an estimate of the calories. The therapists also recommend keeping a daily record of your activities, including a record of your exercise periods.

From these records, you should be able to identify the situations that prompt your maladaptive eating behavior. Do you overeat when you catch a whiff or sight of some tempting but high-calorie goodie? Or when you are feeling bored or tense or lonely? You may discover, for instance, that you are ingesting unneeded calories during a morning coffee-and-doughnut break with fellow workers on your job.

Once you have discovered the cues that prompt your overeating, you consciously and deliberately devise ways to change your eating and activity habits by removing, avoiding, substituting, or ignoring these cues. If you have developed the habit of having a drink and a snack while watching television before dinner, for instance, you might, for a week or two, take a walk instead or do exercises while watching the news or move the television to another room. Some people make a point of never associating eating with any other pleasant or relaxing activity, such as reading or watching television or listening to music. Others make themselves follow a rule that they will eat only when seated at a table that is properly set with tablecloth or place mat, napkin, dishes, and flatware. This rule tends to cut down on snacking, since it is inconvenient to set the table just for a snack.

You should also devise some system for rewarding yourself for even small successes. One system is to award yourself tokens or points each time you are able to change a problem behavior; when you have accumulated enough tokens or points, treat yourself to something you want. Your primary reward, however, should be your satisfaction at being able to change your habits and improve your control of your weight.

Some other tips for a successful weight control program are the following:

1. Eat a good breakfast every day, including a complete protein, in order to raise your level of blood sugar after sleep and keep it up throughout the morning.
2. Eat meals at about the same time each day and do not skip meals.
3. Keep portions small and do not take second helpings.
4. Keep portions of high-calorie, low-nutrient foods (such as desserts) especially small.
5. Two or three snacks a day are all right, but they should be small portions of high-nutrient foods such as fruits, dry cereals, or raw vegetables.
6. Eat slowly and savor each bite. You will be satisfied with less total food if you chew it well and do not rush through your meal.
7. You should have specific places, both at home and at work or school, where you do nothing but eat.
8. Never eat because you are anxious or depressed or feel unloved or unappreciated. For emotional outlets, turn to such nonfood activities as social relationships, creative activity, academic pursuits, or sports.
9. Avoid celebrating special occasions, accomplishments, or relationships with food. Instead, treat yourself and others to rewards that do not involve eating. Occasional celebrations involving food are all right if you indulge in them rarely and keep your portions small.

From time to time, you undoubtedly will break your resolve. You may find yourself gobbling chocolate cake directly from the refrigerator. Do not berate yourself unduly; this happens to everyone. The next day, simply return to your planned program of dieting and exercise.

Ultimately, of course, you will want to develop new eating and exercise habits that maintain your desired weight without any such special attention. However, since your old habits probably developed over a period of many years, forming new habits may take months or even years. You need to be patient with yourself and persevere.

One important caution: you should not judge your adequacy or inadequacy as a person by your success or failure at weight control. You should think well of yourself regardless of your weight. Weight control should simply be something you add to your life, not a measure of your worth.

OTHER METHODS OF WEIGHT CONTROL

Some of the methods of weight control are sound and effective. Others, however, are completely ineffective, and still others are downright dangerous.

FOCUS

A Diet to End All Diets

A glassful of orange- or cherry-flavored liquid made from beef hides, tendons, or bones hardly sounds like a tempting beverage, but some weight-conscious Americans will do anything, it seems, to shed excess pounds. The problem is that get-thin-quick schemes can be fatal. A case in point: a few years ago the U.S. Food and Drug Administration (FDA) began receiving reports of the sudden deaths of women who were on faddish low-calorie liquid-protein diets. A typical one was the aptly named *Last Chance Diet.* Women using it ate no food. In a practice known as "modified fasting," they took their nourishment solely from a protein drink made from beef hides, supplemented by vitamins and potassium. To see if there was a common factor in the reported deaths, the Center for Disease Control (CDC) studied the cases of fifteen women who had died while on the Last Chance Diet. The women in question ranged in age from twenty-three to fifty-one, had lost an average of eighty-three pounds after staying on the diet for between two and eight months, and had had no medical problems other than obesity (defined as at least 20 percent overweight). Most of these women, in addition, had been dieting under a doctor's supervision. Autopsies revealed that all fifteen women had died of cardiac arrhythmia, or severe heartbeat irregularity. In all fifteen, researchers also found signs of damage in the middle layer of the heart wall.

What do these findings mean? The theory behind the liquid-protein diets is that consumption of protein alone will induce the body to burn up fat, but not muscle tissue, minerals, or other materials that make up human "lean body mass." Many of these protein products claim to be nutritionally complete, providing all the essential amino acids that the body needs in order to build proteins. As the sole source of nourishment, however, many of these diets supply only about 300 to 500 calories per day —not nearly enough, nutritionists believe, to maintain good health. What's more, FDA tests have shown that the protein supplied by the Last Chance Diet and others is actually of such low quality as to be unusable. Under these circumstances, a dieter's body eventually turns to a more readily available source of protein, namely, itself. The indication, then, is that while the women in the CDC study were on the liquid-protein diet, their insufficiently nourished bodies cannibalized protein from their own lean body tissues. FDA tests on obese rates duplicated the pattern. After a month of feeding on amounts of liquid protein comparable to what the women had taken, 95 percent of the rats in the experiment were dead—suddenly—of cardiac arrhythmia. Of the eleven survivors, all were male.

By the end of 1978, the FDA had learned of more than sixty deaths associated with very low-calorie protein diets, and had received reports of more than 100 other people who complained that the use of protein diet products caused a wide variety of ailments ranging from nausea and diarrhea to irritability, decreased sex drive, and hair loss. Although it was still unclear why women using these diets were so much more prone than men to die of heartbeat irregularity, an FDA panel of medical experts concluded that for both sexes, protein products in low-calorie diets should be used only under the careful supervision of trained medical personnel. At the same time, the FDA issued a regulation requiring the use of warning labels on very low-calorie protein diet products. The agency has also strongly suggested that these diets be avoided by the following groups of people: anyone taking prescription drugs; the elderly; individuals with kidney, liver, or heart disease, or high blood pressure; and pregnant or nursing mothers.

In fact, the FDA has concluded that, for anyone whose goal is to lose twenty-five pounds or less, low-calorie protein diets are unnecessarily hard on the body's vital functions. And since there is little evidence that these diets are more effective than any other methods of weight reduction, they appear to be unnecessarily risky as well.

Fad Diets

Fad diets are often promoted by books with catchy titles—*Diet Revolution, Quick Weight Loss, Live Longer Diet, No Aging Diet, Save Your Life Diet, Zen Macrobiotic Diet, Last Chance Diet*—that are ballyhooed by news stories, advertisements, magazine articles, and authors' appearances on television talk shows.

DOC... COULD THE QUICK-INCHES-OFF DIET DO ANYTHING FOR ME BY TONIGHT?
INCHES I MAY BE LOSING. POUNDS I AIN'T.
I'M NOT ON A STARVATION DIET. I'M FASTING... JUST LIKE GHANDI!
YOU LOOK TERRIFIC - HOW DID YOU DO IT?
I WENT ON A GRAPEFRUIT DIET. MY TONGUE SHRIVELED UP AND I COULDN'T EAT FOR A MONTH.

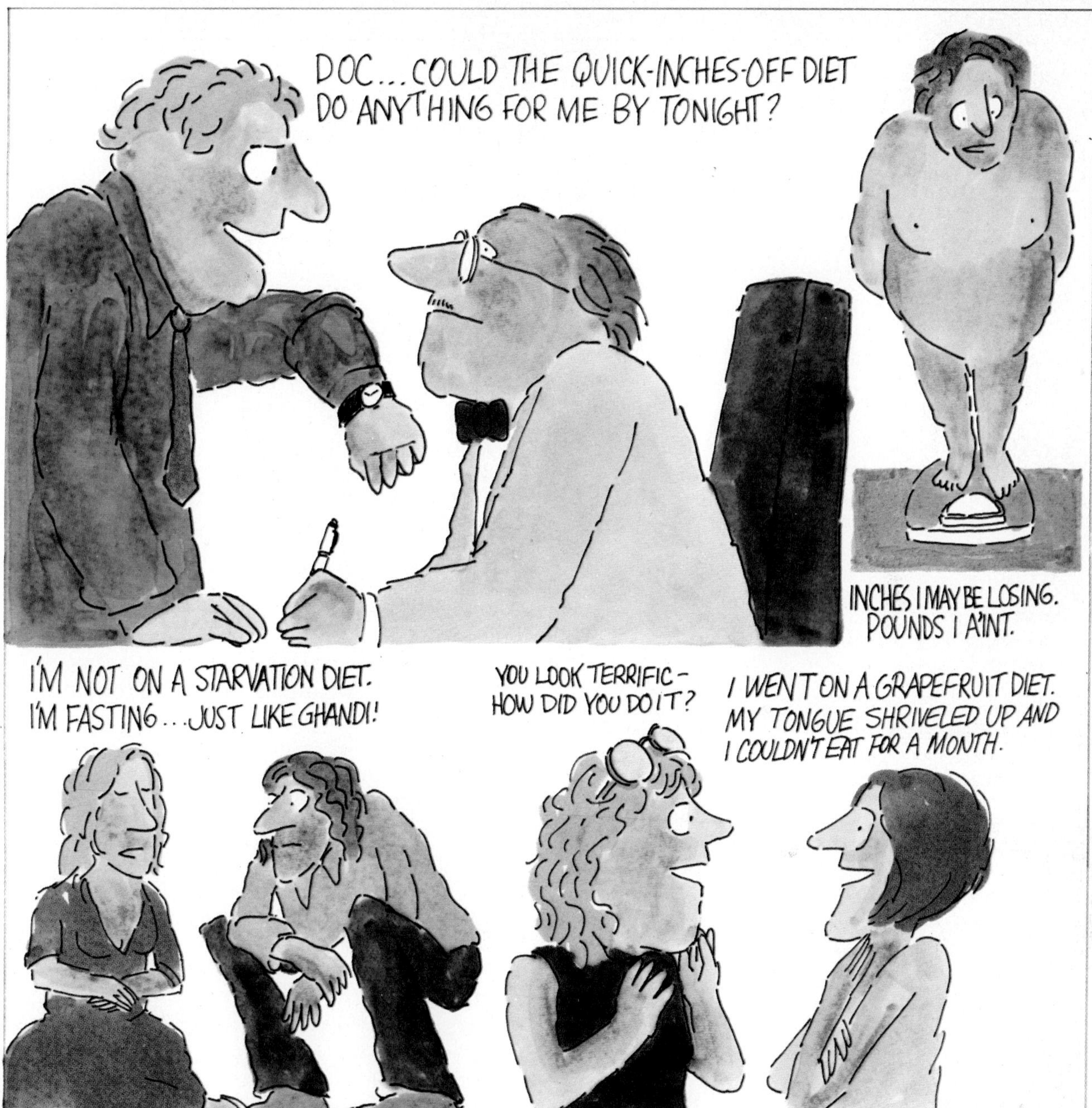

Figure 9.4 There are a number of potentially hazardous diets that rise and fall in popularity from year to year. For example, high-protein, low-carbohydrate diets, such as the *Air Force Diet* and the *Doctor's Quick Weight-Loss Diet,* are dangerously low in necessary carbohydrates, causing excessive protein breakdown and other undesirable metabolic responses. In addition, these diets bring about water loss rather than weight loss and are usually high in fat, which may contribute to atherosclerosis. High-carbohydrate, low-protein diets (such as rice diets) do not supply adequate nutrition, save little in calories, and may cause the dieter to lose protein from his or her body, thus weakening it. Long stays on liquid or formula diets cause such side effects as constipation, diarrhea, nausea, and cramps, because of the lack of bulk (see the Focus box).

These entrepreneurs have offered up virtually every conceivable means of juggling food intake. Many fad diets are wildly unbalanced. They may be high fat and low carbohydrate, or high protein (and fat) plus plenty of water, or low protein and fat and high carbohydrate.

One fad diet, for instance, claims that by eating foods rich in nucleic acids, you can make the cells in your body grow young again. This is nonsense. The fact is that your digestive system breaks down nucleic acids into pieces just as it does other foods.

Many fad diets work in the short run but few, if any, produce long-term weight loss. Some of the more radical diets can cause serious illness and even death. Tragically, a number of young Americans have literally starved themselves to death on the *Zen Macrobiotic Diet.* This diet (which has no connection with Zen Buddhism) is actually a series of diets, each more restrictive than the last. And in 1977, the Food and Drug Administration launched an investigation of thirty-six deaths associated with liquid-protein diets (see the Focus box). While most people can tolerate fad diets for a while without any apparent ill effects, such diets are riskiest for people who have a preexisting health problem.

Sweating

Sweating in steam baths, hot tubs, and plastic exercise suits continues to be a popular means of reducing weight. Water weight can be lost quickly (five to ten pounds in a few hours) through profuse sweating, but this is dangerous. It can cause dehydration and electrolyte imbalance and trigger a variety of illnesses, including kidney, liver, and heart problems and even life-threatening shock. Nor is sweating effective for losing fat. You simply gain the water weight back again the next time you drink a glass of water or other liquid.

Fat Clinics and Health Spas

Physicians and medical clinics that specialize in weight control are often called "fat clinics" or "fat doctors." Some of them offer good programs that include helping people to change their habits. Many, however, use a variety of dubious techniques. One program, for instance, uses a diet of only 500 calories a day plus daily injections of HCG (human chorionic gonadotropin). There is little evidence that HCG, a hormone produced during pregnancy, is useful in weight reduction, but a daily injection of anything would have a psychological effect that might help people stick to such a severely restricted diet. Another popular program controls your food intake by selling you prepackaged (and expensive) diet foods. Other "pill doctors" prescribe elaborate schedules of drugs—vitamins, minerals, diuretics, laxatives, and psychotropic drugs—to supply nutrients, reduce fluid retention, and keep you feeling good on an extremely low-calorie diet. These programs—many of which can be very expensive—can produce dramatic, short-term weight losses, but there is no documentation that they work in the long run.

Health spas or "fat farms" offer live-in programs that involve dieting, exercise, massage, and other forms of pampering. Virtually no research, however, has been published on the long-term effectiveness of such programs. Many wealthy people, however, find that the personal attention and luxurious surroundings make stays at such spas very pleasant.

People often lose ten pounds or more in a week's stay, but this is very misleading. Almost all this weight loss is water loss. Some spas use drugs, diuretic and laxative foods, and steam baths and saunas to achieve this quick loss. In some people, however, as explained previously, such rapid water loss can be dangerous. Live-in programs are not likely to be successful in the long run, because their artificial environments do not reinforce behavioral changes within one's own normal living environment. For a few people, a live-in program may help initiate changes in habits that they continue at home, but it is unlikely that you can learn all the changes needed for permanent weight control in a week or two away from home.

A LIFETIME GOAL

Whether your problem is overweight or underweight, the best way to gain control over it, in the long run, is not by spurts of crash or fad dieting but by making permanent changes in your patterns of eating and exercising—in short, by modifying your life style.

SUMMARY

1. If you weigh more than 10 percent above the weight recommended by life insurance tables for your sex, height, and body frame, you are probably overweight. While overweight is weight in excess of the average, obesity is a higher than average proportion of fat tissue in the body.
2. Methods for assessing obesity include the mirror test, pinch test, abdominal circumference test, densimetry, and anthropometric measurements.
3. The direct cause of overweight is eating more calories than we use up. While the fundamental causes are poorly understood, among the factors that seem to be involved are genetics, environment, psychological conditioning, and lack of exercise.
4. Overweight is associated with heart disease, hypertension, diabetes, and other diseases. It also carries social, emotional, and vocational disadvantages.
5. The only way to lose weight is by consuming fewer calories than we use. This can be accomplished by decreasing caloric intake and/or by increasing activity level. The most successful weight reduction programs combine both approaches.
6. To identify the circumstances in which you tend to overeat, keep a written record of your eating behavior for several days. Then you can consciously modify maladaptive eating habits.
7. Other methods of weight control include fad diets, sweating, fat clinics, and health spas. Some of these are sound and effective; others are ineffective or downright dangerous.

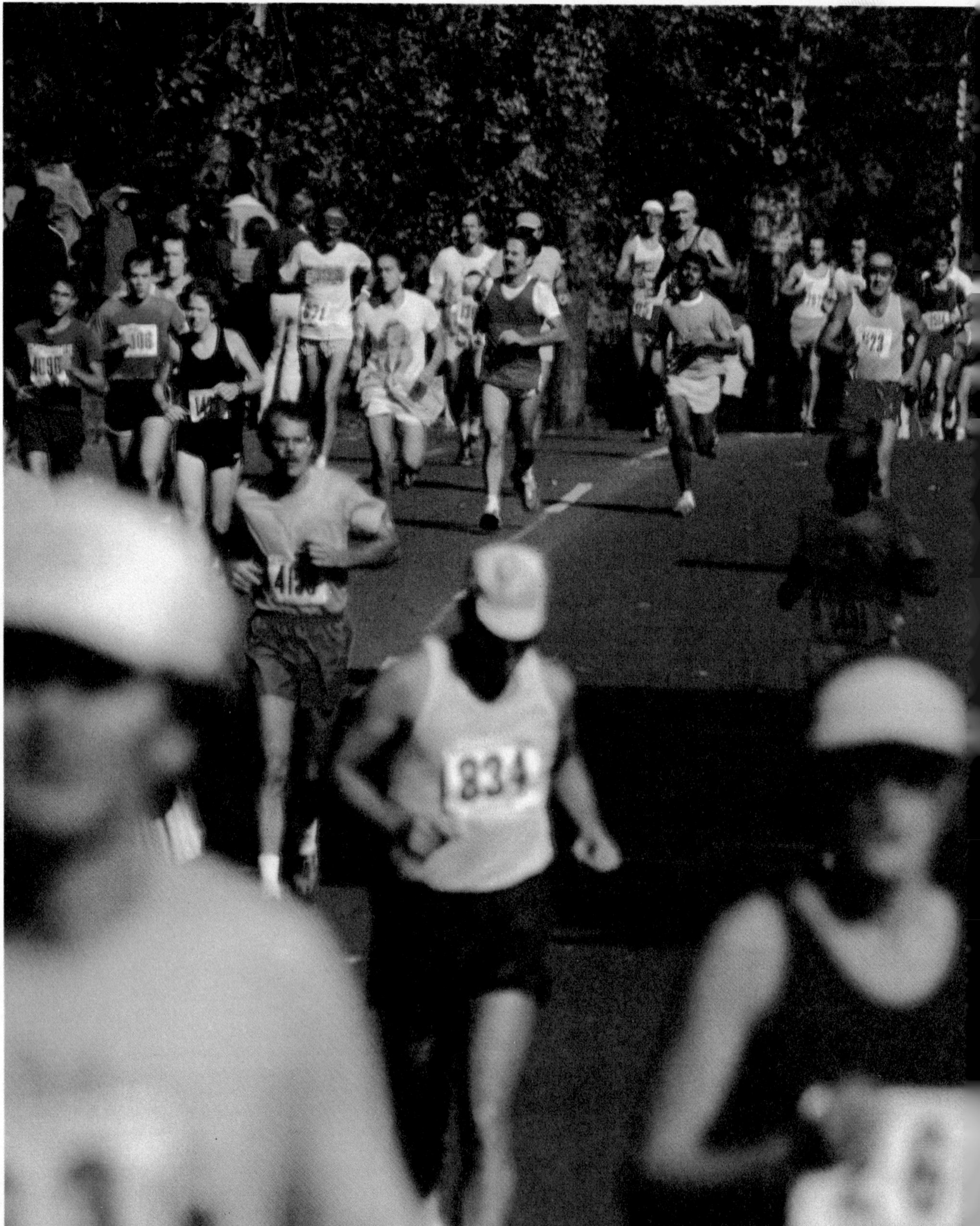
834

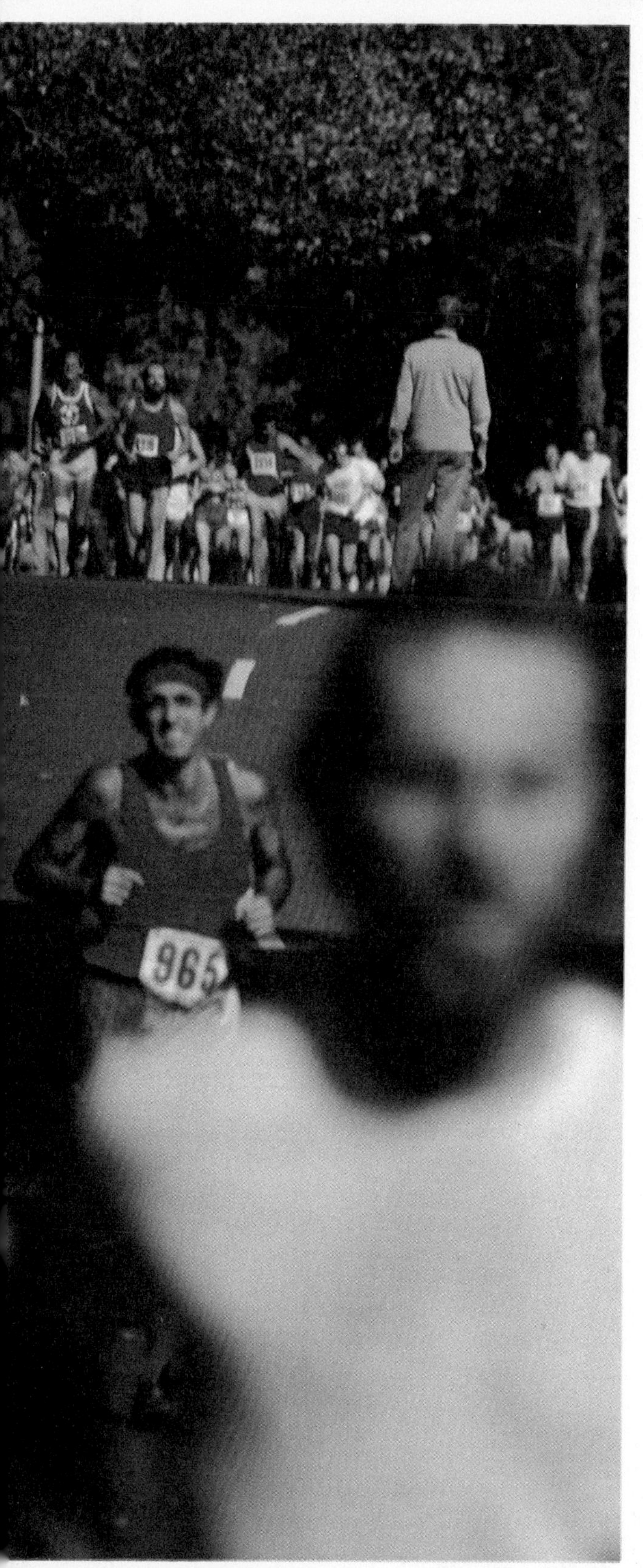

10 Physical Fitness

Americans who only a few years ago were leading sedentary lives are now exercising for both recreation and health. Today, it is fashionable —not eccentric—to be seen around town in warm-up suits or tennis togs. It is no longer unusual to come across joggers almost anywhere at any time. A vast industry has sprung up to provide sports clothes, footwear, and other gear for all this new physical activity. Exercise and fitness are definitely *in.* This phenomenon appears to be both permanent and still growing. It may well be the most important, health-promoting shift in the American life style in this century.

THE ROLE OF FITNESS

Some of this new physical activity is channeled into organized or competitive sports requiring a specific number of players or special equipment (a boat, skis) or locale (court). But more importantly, much of the new activity is aimed instead at exercise training of the individual, with the goal of improving the physical fitness of one's own body. Such fitness is important for both physical and mental health.

Exercise training is obviously vital to the athlete, who needs optimal physical conditioning in order to perform at his or her best in competition. Most of us are thrilled when we watch record-breaking performances. Top athletes demonstrate how much the human species can achieve, just as do the most accomplished artists, musicians, and scientists. Such champion athletes are driven from both within and without and must devote grueling hours—even years—to their training. While many of us admire this dedication, few of us share the need or the inclination to put in the time and effort necessary for such preeminence. Still, the champion and the harried student or businessperson share the same basic anatomy and physiology, the same need for physical fitness, and the same capacity to respond to exercise training.

Until relatively recently in human history, people were unable to survive without well-honed physical skills needed to find food and shelter and to escape danger. Today, however, our technology and social philosophy have so changed the physical requirements for survival that even some severely handicapped people can lead productive lives. Nevertheless, there is imprinted upon our bodies a need to move —a fundamental need that modern sedentary life may even intensify. During the times of starvation and deprivation, our efficient fat-storage mechanism may have helped assure survival. But in these times of overnutrition and underactivity, this same mechanism conspires against health and survival. Thus physical fitness is relative to the times and the circumstances. There is an appropriate level of physical activity for each individual. At the minimum, this activity should be of the kind, intensity, and frequency sufficient to keep a person fit for the world he or she lives in.

Physical fitness is more a means than an end in itself. It enables a person to use physical abilities to maximize his or her emotional, intellectual, and social attributes and achieve "total fitness." You do not have to be a dedicated athlete to achieve this kind of fitness. With a personal commitment to a physically active life style, virtually any man or woman can be fit; the key is motivation. You can only achieve fitness if you actively work toward it. The tragedy is that many people simply accept physical deterioration and early aging. There are better alternatives. Understanding of fitness and action based on that understanding are essential—especially in urban communities, where there is often more reinforcement for sedentary living than for physically active living.

THE ELEMENTS OF FITNESS

Physical fitness mainly involves the development of three elements: strength, suppleness, and stamina.

Strength is the basic muscular force required for movement. Strength is normally developed by overcoming resistance, which can be supplied by the parts of the body itself; by the whole body when lifting, pulling, walking, or climbing; by another person's body, as in football or wrestling; or by inanimate objects such as grocery bags, trash cans, books, or barbells.

The quickest and most direct means of improving strength is through weight training, a form of *isotonic* exercise. Calisthenics, such as push-ups, sit-ups, and pull-ups, are also useful isotonic exercises. Isotonic exercises develop strength through repeated rhythmic movements. *Isometric* exercises, on the other hand, produce static muscular contractions that result from pushing or pulling against a stationary object such as a tension bar. Isometric exercises may also improve strength. However, isotonic exercise, which involves movement, is generally preferred because it does not inhibit blood flow or raise blood pressure to the same extent that isometric exercise does. Moreover, weight training seems to bring about greater strength achievement over a wider range of movement than isometrics, which tend to have an effect that is limited to specific angles of application.

Suppleness, or flexibility, is the quality of muscles, bones, tendons, and ligaments that permits full range of movement in a joint. One may be supple in some joints but not others. There may even be large differences in suppleness between the same joints on opposite sides of the body. Many people, for instance, have a greater range of movement in one shoulder than the other. One's ability to move one's limbs and joints through their full range is maintained by periodic bending and stretching exercises. Immobilization or restricted movement of a limb or joint often leads to reduced suppleness and may give rise to postural or orthopedic problems.

Stamina, or endurance, is the quality that enables an individual to mobilize energy to sustain movements over an extended period of

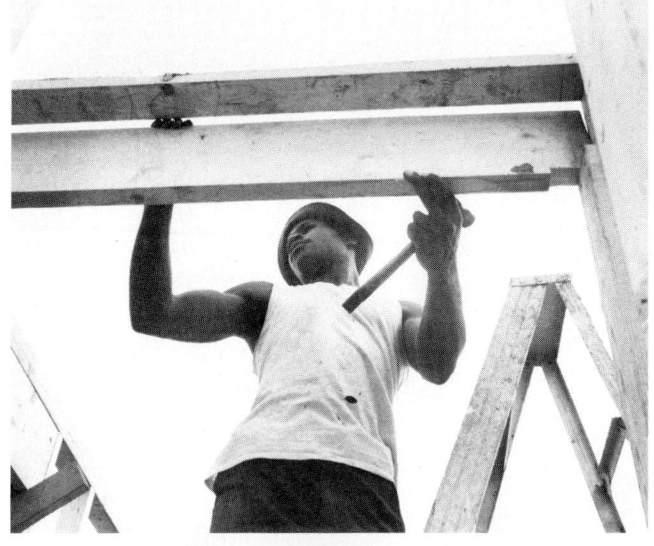

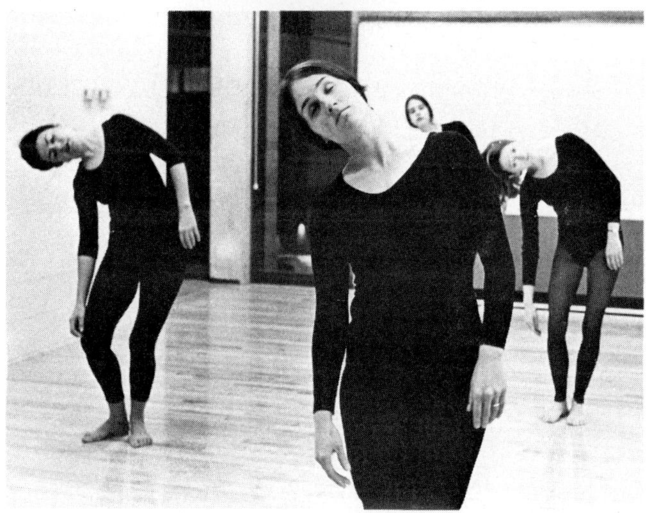

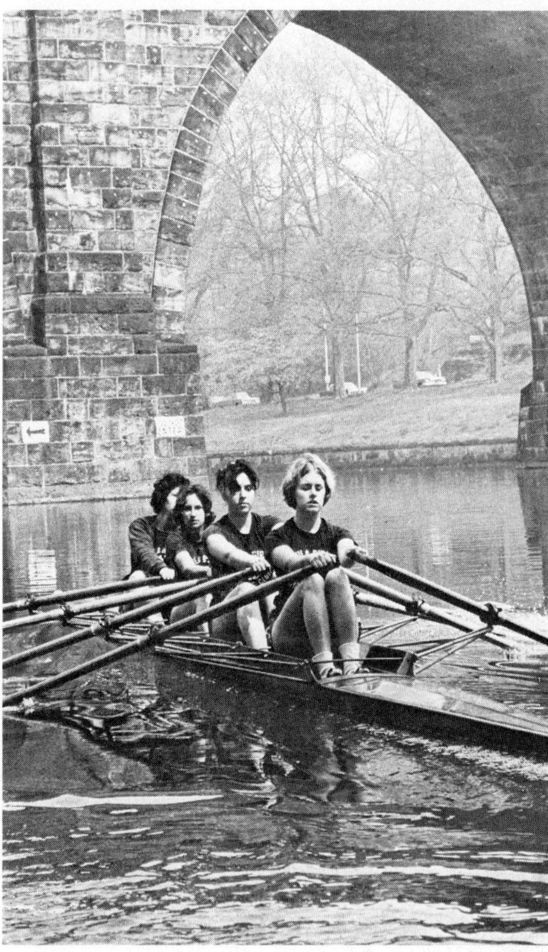

Figure 10.1 The three main components of fitness: *(Top left)* strength, for lifting or carrying; *(Bottom left)* suppleness, for reaching and bending; and *(Right)* stamina, for climbing stairs and walking long distances.

time. As will be discussed later in this chapter, stamina is largely a matter of developing an adequate oxygen-transport system. Stamina is normally achieved by sustained exercise of the whole body, involving the large muscles and putting the major joints through a wide range of motion. Whole-body exercise includes running, bicycling, swimming, and cross-country skiing. Weight training may also help to build stamina, when relatively light weights are used with more repetitions.

The fitness elements cannot be developed or maintained unless the specific exercise experience is reasonably intense and frequent. People who lead sedentary lives offer a marked contrast to those whose life styles provide activity of the kind, intensity, and frequency that are necessary for the development and maintenance of strength, suppleness, and stamina. Some of the easily identifiable effects of training are summarized in Figure 10.2

Compared with an untrained person, the trained individual is essentially leaner, stronger for his or her body size, has an enhanced circulatory and energy-mobilization capacity, and recovers more quickly after exercise. Endurance training also helps to develop cardiovascular fitness, which may be a defense

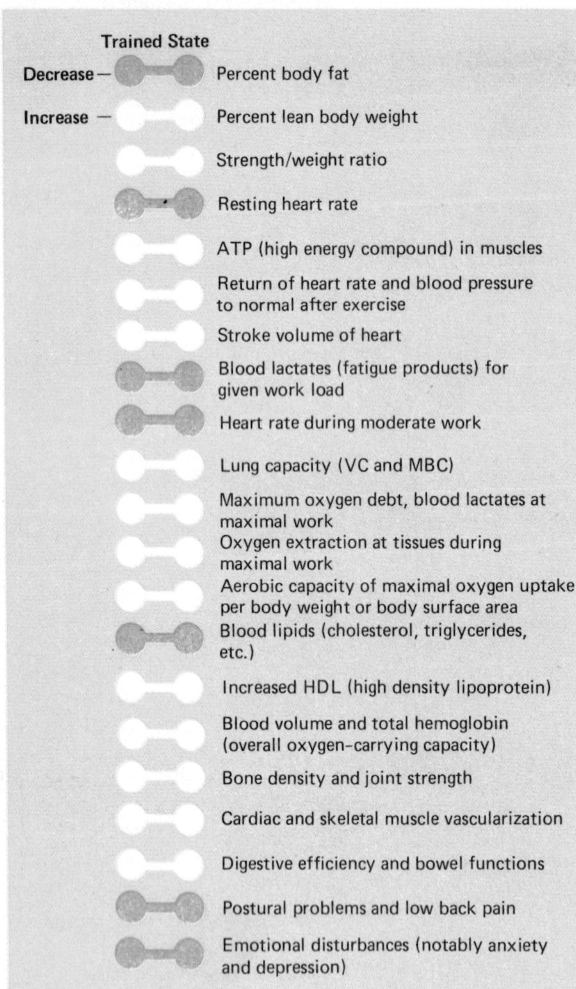

Figure 10.2 A summary of the physiological effects of training.

against heart and blood-vessel diseases (see Chapter 16). The untrained individual often exhibits the physical characteristics associated with early aging. Physiological middle age for the unfit may arrive before they are chronologically twenty-one years old. At the other end of the fitness spectrum, there are vigorous "youngsters" chronologically in their sixties and beyond. There is evidence to indicate that training postpones physiological aging in adulthood and enhances strength and stamina in old age. However, a declining suppleness may be one infirmity shared by the fit and unfit senior citizen, because deterioration of joints does not appear to be reversible.

EXERCISE AND HEALTH

For centuries, human beings have been vaguely aware that exercise and fitness are important to their well-being. Not until recently, however, has science begun to document the nature and extent of the relationship between exercise and health. Studies comparing the cardiovascular systems and heart-disease experiences of sedentary and active workers in specific occupations have shown that the more active workers have less disease and lower death rates than their sedentary counterparts. If persons are compared on the basis of exertion, the least active tend to have the greatest degenerative disease and death rates, with quality of health and life span increasing in direct proportion to increased physical activity.

Fascinated by this kind of evidence, two American physicians, Wilhelm Raab and Hans Kraus, reviewed the many studies on the subject, added some research of their own, and in 1961 published a book, *Hypokinetic Disease,* which cataloged a wide variety of human disorders that occur more often among sedentary people than among the physically active. "Hypokinetic" pertains to insufficient movement; these disorders are specifically linked with or complicated by too little exercise. Some of the hypokinetic disorders identified were chronic fatigue, shortness of breath, overweight, digestive upsets, headache, backache, anxiety states, muscular weakness and atrophy, musculoskeletal (muscle, bone, joint, ligament, tendon) pain and injuries, high blood pressure, atherosclerosis, coronary artery disease, and generalized, accelerated, degenerative aging.

What is the connection between lack of exercise and each of these disorders? Exercise provides greater physical reserves and improves body structure and functioning. The health-promoting effects of exercise are dynamic in that the various positive effects interact with and reinforce each other. The total impact on health, therefore, is greater than the sum of the separate effects.

FOCUS

The Running Mania

Jogging and running have become more than a sport, more than a passing fad; they have evolved into almost a national mania. The President's Council on Physical Fitness and Sports estimates that 6.5 million Americans jog, a third of them once or twice a week. Young men and women go out on jogging dates. Middle-aged executives in running shoes and shorts, jogging at lunchtime, are now a common sight on city streets. An eighty-five-year-old Santa Monica grandmother has competed in half-mile and one-mile races. Some doctors suggest jogging as physical therapy for people who have had heart attacks. Even the nation's dogs have caught on and no longer bother to bark or wag their tails.

Some of the most serious and dedicated joggers eventually evolve into marathoners. A marathon is a grueling race of 26 miles, 385 yards, named after the ancient Greek city of Marathon. In 490 B.C., so the story goes, a long-distance runner ran the 26-odd miles from Marathon to Athens to bring the news of a Greek victory in battle over the Persians. The most famous modern marathon is run in Boston; each year in mid-April several thousand men and women run a tortuous course from Hopkinton, Massachusetts, into downtown Boston. In recent years, New York City has also staged a marathon that begins on Staten Island and snakes through all five boroughs of the city before ending up in Central Park. The New York marathon even draws handicapped entrants who "run" the course in wheelchairs.

Beyond the marathoners are a breed of runners who call themselves "ultramarathoners." One of the classic ultramarathons is a fifty-mile race from London to Brighton, on the English Channel. A number of ultramarathoners have run across the United States from Los Angeles to New York, or vice versa. The record set in 1977 for this 3,000-mile distance was 53 days and 7 minutes.

Why have jogging and running become so popular? For ordinary joggers, at least, it is an easy and inexpensive sport to take up. It does not require elaborate personal equipment (only a good pair of running shoes), a long series of lessons, membership in an athletic club, a long drive to the beach or the mountains, or the necessity of finding partners or teammates. One can simply go out and *do* it, with a minimum of fuss. But beyond this, an increasing number of Americans are discovering that it both feels good and makes sense to take good care of the only body any of us will ever inhabit.

Released Tension

Exercise may provide the movement activity to physiologically express and release tension that accumulates when one is under stress. Primitive human beings survived, in part, through their "fight or flight" reactions; when danger threatened, the body reacted by releasing adrenaline into the bloodstream. This hormone sharpened and quickened physical responses. In modern life, environmental stress is still a very real part of human experience, though dangers seldom threaten one's life. Still, the body reacts in the same fashion as it did when threatened by wild beasts.

Primitive human beings were required to move, to work, to "exercise" in order to survive. Modern urban people under stress are often required to sit still and appear relaxed and calm, thereby inhibiting natural expression. Accordingly, the hormone-induced tense state is not resolved in activity. Unresolved stress is persistently accompanied by constricted arterioles, high blood pressure, and increased heart rate. Such unremitting stress is thought to contribute to a variety of degenerative effects, particularly in relation to the digestive and cardiovascular systems. Deliberate and appropriate exercise, then, enables modern people to release psychological tension and achieve physical relaxation.

Thaddeus Kostrubala, a San Diego psychiatrist, has recently discovered that stamina training—jogging at three-fourths of one's maximum capacity (determined by a medical stress test) for one hour or more three times a week—not only improves physical fitness but also produces psychological benefits such as relieving depression and anxiety. Some long-distance runners have even reported feelings of euphoria—a so-called "runner's high"—and a trancelike state after an hour or more of running. There is now some evidence that such experiences may be due to the release of certain chemical neurotransmitters in the brain, which trigger altered states of consciousness similar to those induced by drugs. This natural chemical response of the brain may be responsible for the almost religious zeal with which so many people are becoming committed to running.

Another southern California psychiatrist, William Glasser of Los Angeles, has introduced the phrase "positive addiction" for this state of mind described by runners, other athletes, and also by people who mediate or perform some other repetitive activity for a specified period of time each day. Some runners have told him, Dr. Glasser says, that when they don't run they sometimes have actual withdrawal symptoms.

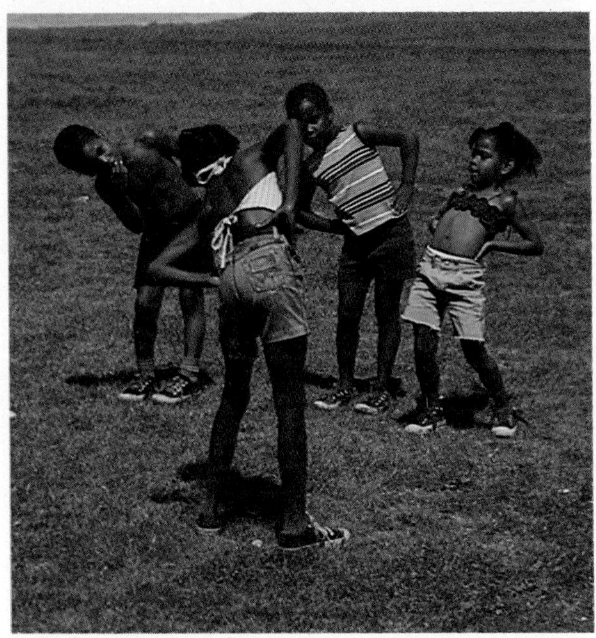

Figure 10.3 A group of children exercising. Physical activity during the developing years helps to strengthen muscles, bones, and organs and will have a lasting positive effect during later years.

Strength and Resistance

Appropriate exercise and fitness have maintenance values for a number of tissues and so survival value for the whole organism. Untrained muscles grow smaller and weaker than trained muscles. When a broken arm is immobilized in a cast for several weeks, *atrophy* begins to take place; the muscles waste away, and the bones and joints deteriorate with inactivity. Astronauts' muscles grow weak and deteriorate rapidly in weightless environments unless they exercise artificially. Such exercise compensates for the absence of the minimal exercise involved in maintaining posture and simple movement against gravity. Sedentary people suffer the same kind of atrophy, weakness, and resulting vulnerability to injury.

Support of Developmental Growth

Children require exercise for normal growth and development. Although sedentary youngsters may survive, their muscles, bones, nervous systems, hearts, and lungs, and the functions dependent on these organs, are impaired by insufficient movement. Exercise is necessary for fitness at any age, but if restrictions are imposed on it during the developmental years from birth to age twenty, a child may become permanently handicapped. The handicap may become seriously apparent only at middle age, however. Deprived of the benefits of physical fitness in the developmental years, the middle-aged man or woman frequently suffers from a variety of hypokinetic disorders, such as those mentioned above. Medical treatment may provide some relief when these disorders strike, but it is sad to realize that they could have been prevented or postponed by fitness in childhood and continued fitness through life.

HOW FIT IS "FIT ENOUGH"?

What generalizations are justified in view of the broad range of individual goals and abilities? Ultimately, one decides this issue for oneself, taking into account one's own perceptions, understanding, and life style. However, health science research, observations of physicians, and experiences in physical education have evolved some criteria that may be useful in making this decision.

Fit enough to maintain orthopedic integrity—that is, to enjoy active living with minimal risk of orthopedic injury or disability—is one aspect of the "how fit" question. Men and women should be strong and supple enough and have the skills to work and play with ease and without risk of muscle or joint injury. This type of fitness is relevant to such diverse activities as lifting babies and trash cans, pushing vacuum cleaners and lawn mowers, swimming a half mile or playing three hard sets of tennis.

But why not just do what one has to and wants to, and let one's fitness grow and adapt accordingly? For one thing, the body adapts to the specific demands placed on it and no more. In youth, this adaptation works fairly well because of the natural resiliency of the young organism. A younger person who "overlifts" or "overexerts" may develop a few sore muscles or become fatigued but quickly recovers. Natural resiliency diminishes with age, however. If one does nothing more strenuous than lift babies or push lawn mowers, the body adapts to those limits, and even slight exertion beyond the normal may produce injury or fatigue. Therefore, controlled extra training beyond the routine minimal daily demands is needed to maintain a safety margin for those inevitable times when an additional demand is imposed.

To develop and maintain strength and suppleness in adults, calisthenic activity is most useful. Bending and stretching exercises (all body parts in all directions and to the limit without inordinate strain), bent-knee sit-ups, leg half-squats, and a wide variety of additional controlled no-strain movements are among the best exercises to maintain orthopedic adequacy. Once these minimal levels of muscular fitness are achieved, one might add exercises such as push-ups and pull-ups, or use weights, pulleys, or springs if one's exercise goals go beyond minimal orthopedic safety.

Fit enough to protect against heart attack is often cited as a criterion. There is, of course, no absolute protection against heart attack, but the development of stamina (cardiovascular-respiratory endurance) appears to be one way

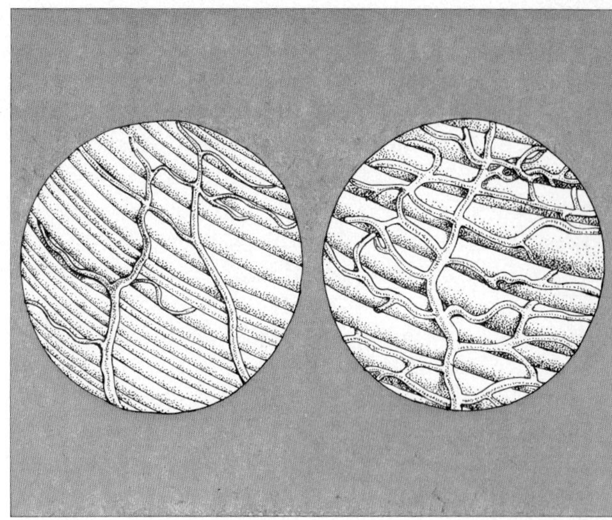

Figure 10.4 Capillarization. On the left is a drawing of an untrained muscle with relatively few capillaries. On the right is trained muscle with thicker fibers and increased number of capillaries.

to reduce some of the risk factors for coronary artery disease (see Chapter 16).

Stamina training (to be described in detail later) involves continuous rhythmic cardiovascular-respiratory overload, lasting from eight minutes to an hour or longer depending on the individual's level of fitness and fitness goals. The body responds to the demands imposed by this training by adapting; that is, it rebuilds itself in order to accommodate future training demands with less or no stress. In time, the muscles involved develop an increased vascularization, and the increased size of the capillary network offers more available routes for oxygen transport by the blood. The ability of the hemoglobin in the red blood cells to carry oxygen is also improved.

In the coronary system of a fit person the circulation serving the heart may provide valuable protection—increased blood flow—against a fatal heart attack. If a clot or spasm blocks a coronary vessel and causes a heart attack, there is the possibility that the richer blood flow promoted by stamina training will compensate for a blocked vessel. Accordingly, damage is likely to be slighter and recovery quicker.

With training, the heart becomes stronger and more efficient. An increased amount of blood is pumped on each beat, with a more complete emptying of the heart, even though the heart will not increase much in size. Cardiac output at resting is not affected because the resting heart rate becomes slower. Whereas the normal adult resting pulse rate is around seventy beats per minute, and eighty to ninety beats is not unusual in untrained individuals, the stamina-trained adult usually has resting pulse rates of fifty-five to sixty beats per minute. Consequently, the heart beats thousands of times less per day, which appears to be beneficial in reducing the wear and tear on heart valves and blood vessels.

Stamina training stresses other body systems, thereby stressing the body as a whole, and in this way also contributes to the welfare of the heart. Exercise burns calories, which contributes to weight control. In typical adult training programs occurring three days per week, partially trained participants expending energy at about 400 calories per session may undergo a weight reduction of about seventeen pounds per year as a concomitant benefit of stamina training. Rhythmic, relaxing stamina exercises tend to release muscle tension through motor expression of emotions and to reduce stress stimuli and their unnecessary burden on the heart. Finally, the entire respiratory sytsem is employed in adapting to training. Typically, the lungs increase the amount of air inspired and expired at one time (vital capacity) and the maximum amount of air taken in over a period of time (maximum breathing capacity). Together, the adaptive effects of stamina training build and maintain the complex oxygen-transport system and thus protect against heart attack.

WHAT EXERCISE AND HOW MUCH?

Exactly how much and what kind of exercise is needed for fitness? Although precise answers to this question depend on individual variations in development, prior fitness, and particular goals sought, useful guidelines have been provided by fitness research and health professionals.

Because strength, suppleness, and stamina and the supporting structures and functions diminish not only with disuse but also at an accelerating rate with age, it is important to continue to move in ways that maintain these capabilities. Resiliency and resistance to injury tend to diminish with age; therefore, exercise of an easy, flowing, rhythmic nature is indicated, rather than movement demanding quick bursts of strength, speed, or violent effort. Calisthenics should fully stretch the muscles and joints as gently as possible instead of requiring powerful, forced stress. Sports and endurance activities in adulthood should be accompanied by a preliminary calisthenic routine to maintain reserve strength and suppleness and to avoid potential injury.

Stamina training is the most vital form of adult exercise. When properly conducted so as to be individually appropriate, such training is well within the capabilities of all normal adults regardless of age. The major concept of stamina training has been termed "aerobics" by Kenneth H. Cooper, a physician who conducted major research projects in adult fitness for the United States Air Force. *Aerobic* means "with oxygen," or, in this sense, extended exercise in which the oxygen demands of the body are being met by a sufficient delivery. Some examples of aerobic exercise are vigorous walking, longer-distance running and jogging, jumping rope, bicycling, swimming, and cross-country skiing. Exercise in which the demand exceeds the supply and produces "oxygen debt" is termed *anaerobic.* An example of an anaerobic exercise is sprinting a quarter-mile: one goes so fast that one can get only part of the oxygen one needs during the sprint itself; one has to make up the oxygen debt afterward.

When an activity is especially energy demanding (as in sprinting), the amount of available oxygen is not sufficient. In these instances, some additional energy is available anaerobically—that is, without oxygen. It is obtained by the splitting of sugar (glucose) and the production of lactic acid in the absence of adequate oxygen. This mechanism is a limited one that brings about the fatigue that everyone has felt at one time or another through overex-

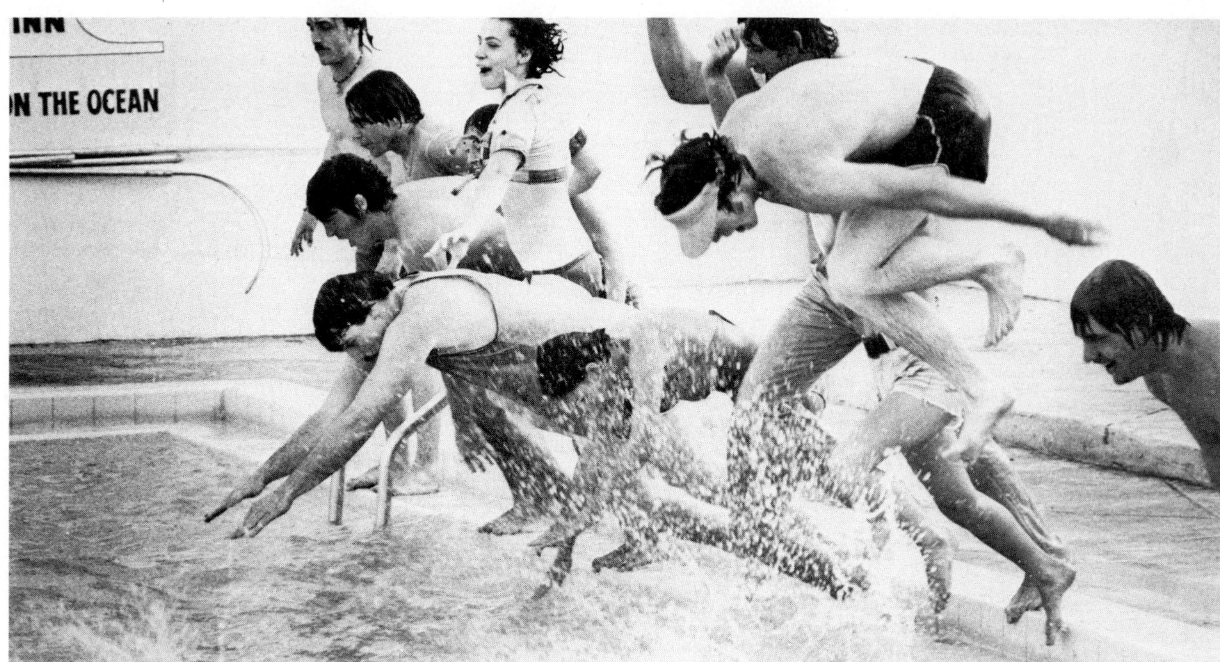

Figure 10.5 Swimming is an aerobic exercise that can be used to increase stamina and to improve both cardiovascular and respiratory efficiency.

ertion. The greater one's aerobic capacity, the more intense the activity that can be supported before anaerobic processes are called upon to supply energy needs.

Cooper's studies and others have shown that controlled aerobic exercise of sufficient duration and intensity is more comfortable, less hazardous, and produces better results than anaerobic spurts. The minimum duration of aerobic exercise for a "training effect" is about eight minutes. Less exercise than that produces little or no improvement; more leads to greater and faster improvement.

The optimum duration for aerobic exercise training has not yet been established, but for normal individuals interested in their general fitness, fifteen to thirty minutes appears to be sufficient. Progress is slow with less than fifteen minutes of exercise, and more than one hour yields diminishing returns.

How frequent should aerobic workouts be? Cooper, building on the findings of other exercise physiologists, determined that the positive adaptive effects of an aerobic workout last about two days, after which "detraining" begins. Ideally, then, intervals between workouts should not exceed two days. Daily workouts result in the greatest progress, but four days per week appears to be a more realistic frequency in busy life styles.

PLANNING FOR FITNESS

When it comes to exercise, Americans tend to do either too much or too little. A parent will play football all afternoon with the children and then get no exercise for the rest of the week. What is essential for lifetime fitness is continuous, regular exercise combining calisthenic effects with stamina training. It requires physical activity several times a week. Such a program is not compatible with sporadic exercise, fitness fads, and the like. Some words of caution are in order.

1	Precede your cardiovascular exercise period with at least ten minutes of "warmup" exercises.
2	Start slowly and progress gradually.
3	It is better to exercise before a meal than right after a meal. After eating allow at least two hours before the exercise program.
4	Ideally, exercise should be done in the temperature range of 40° to 85°F., with humidity less than 60 percent. Rubber or plastic suits are not recommended.
5	Allow sufficient time (at least ten minutes) to "cool down" after exercise before taking a hot shower. This may be accomplished by slow walking at the temperature at which the exercise was performed.
6	Avoid sitting or standing still immediately after exercise. Keep moving slowly to "cool down." This prevents fainting.
7	Do not exercise when not feeling "up to par." Return to a lower level of effort following illness.
8	Aching joints and muscles are a sign of inadequate conditioning—too fast a pace too soon. Musculoskeletal pains commonly occur in the first two weeks, but normally disappear shortly thereafter. Should symptoms persist, a reevaluation is in order. Using proper shoes and socks and taking it easy at the beginning will help you avoid many foot and leg problems. Overweight individuals should be especially careful.
9	Abstain from any alcoholic beverages for at least four to five hours prior to exercising, and minimize use at other times.
10	Never end your exercise period with a sprint.
11	Discontinue your exercise and check with your physician should any of the following conditions develop during or following exercise: a. Pain in the chest, teeth, jaw, neck, or arm. b. Significant difficulty in breathing. c. Light-headedness or fainting. d. Irregular heart rate persisting during exercise and recovery period. e. Disabling musculoskeletal discomfort or swelling of joints. f. Excess fatigue as indicated by constant lethargy, malaise ("indefinite discomfort"), or an uncoordinated gait with weakness after exercise. g. Unexplained weight loss. h. Persistent nausea or vomiting after exercise.

Figure 10.6 Precautions for cardiovascular exercise.

A Few Cautions

One should try to avoid *overexertion.* It does not contribute to overall fitness, because activity is reduced while one is recovering. Injuries may also result either from a mishap because of fatigue or from overworking bones, joints, or muscles. If one begins exercise training gradually and is satisfied with steady though slow progress achievable with the previously outlined principles, the likelihood of overexertion is minimized. Mistakes, however, are possible, and the following signs of overexertion should be watched for:

1. Pulse rate not recovered to 120 beats per minute or lower within two minutes of stopping exercise.
2. Subjective feeling of fatigue not passed within ten minutes of stopping workout. (Proper workout should leave one relaxed, refreshed, and pleasantly tired rather than deeply fatigued.)
3. Lingering fatigue and difficulty in sleeping.
4. Fatigue the day following a workout.
5. Chest pains, which should be evaluated immediately by a doctor.

Any combination of these signs calls for reexamination of one's fitness program and a reduction in strenuousness.

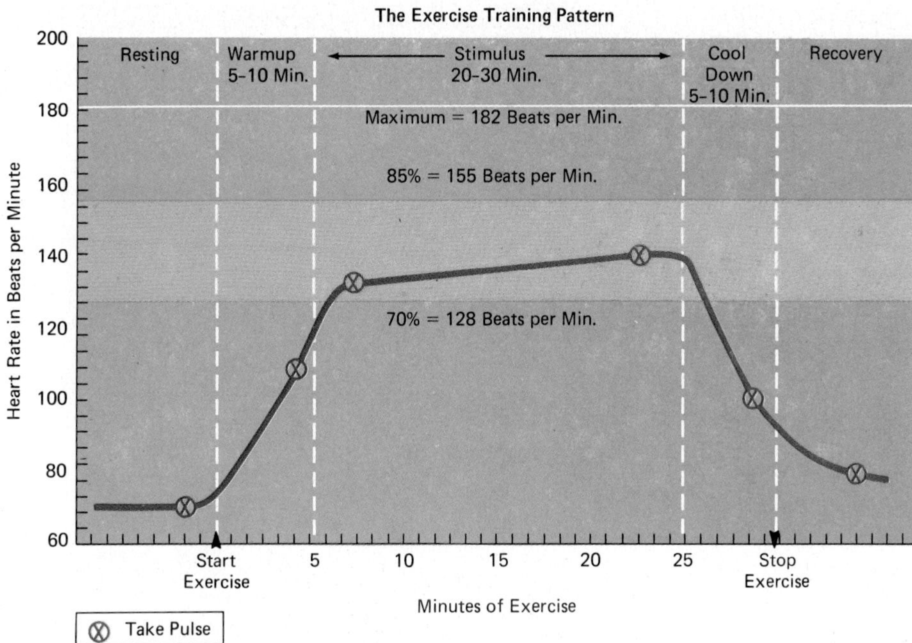

Figure 10.7 A typical aerobic training session. The person should feel as if he or she is working hard but within comfortable limits. For example, overexertion is less likely if you can carry on a conversation while running.

Recent research points out that, while regular, rigorous exercise is beneficial to many people, it can be dangerous to others. In the District of Columbia, for example, three men—a congressman, an economist, and an aerospace engineer—died in a single week while jogging. Many sports medicine specialists are urging people to exercise—*but* in moderation. People who jog to excess are liable to suffer "overuse" injuries such as "runner's knee," stress fractures, and inflammations of the bones, joints, and tendons.

Strenuous exercise may also be harmful to tense, competitive Type A personalities (see Chapter 16). Exercise, instead of relaxing these people, often has precisely the opposite effect—aggravation of tension. Their determination to run that extra yard or lift that extra ten pounds can actually add to their stress load and *increase* the likelihood of a heart attack.

In light of these findings, *medical clearance* for beginning a fitness program is wise, especially for the inactive or those over thirty-five. A number of medical conditions are aggravated by physical exertion and should be ruled out by a medical examination and an exercise stress test before an endurance program begins. It is a good idea to plan one's tentative fitness program and present it for approval to a physician who is aware of one's physical condition and past medical history.

Recreational sports require performance that is difficult to control. Hence, sports are not as useful for maintaining fitness as a combination of calisthenics and endurance training. Few sports provide the continuous, rhythmic, controlled overload and range of movement called for. Competition is always an invitation to overexertion. Also, most active sports have certain requirements that do not provide regular or frequent enough activity; one has to have a court, for example, or a team for many games.

And particularly as one gets older, competitive sports are not to be recommended as the best form of exercise. Since one's joints can tolerate less stress, one should avoid sports involving violent body contact and sharp stops and starts and instead pursue activities involving more continuous, rhythmic motion. Sports do, however, supplement a controlled fitness program. The "fit" person is likely to enjoy many extra years of sports competence.

Fitness *gadgets and devices* may be useful but certainly are not essential. Weights, springs, and other devices for increasing resistance help build strength beyond minimal levels, but they have little use in developing endurance. Exercise bicycles and treadmills provide endurance training, but jogging in place is just as helpful. It is to be expected that a consumer-oriented culture would develop consumer products to facilitate fitness even though, obviously, fitness needs can be adequately met without them.

Fitness fads are rampant, and most are harmful at worst and inadequate at best. Isometrics, which create muscle tension without movement, may build some strength, especially in weak individuals, but they do not maintain or improve joint flexibility or maintain endurance. Food-for-fitness fads come and go, but the only way to achieve and maintain physical fitness is through appropriate exercise and eating a balanced diet. Seconds-per-day "miracle programs" are widely advertised, but none will work because fitness training requires more time than a few seconds to produce physiological effects. Some may actually be harmful to weak, untrained muscles. Spot-reducing exercises are useless because one cannot tailor the loss or redistribution of body fat through exercise. Fat distribution is primarily genetically determined, so exercise has little effect.

Establishing a Fitness Program

An ideal program of exercise for physical fitness is, obviously, one that incorporates all the principles presented here, that is consistent with each individual's goals, and that is realistic in terms of individual and environmental limitations. There is virtually an infinite variety of exercise options that can be adjusted

HOW TO Develop a Daily Fitness Program

Have you been putting off exercising because you feel self-conscious about being out of shape? Have you been making excuses about not having the time or money to buy sporting equipment or to join a health club? Here is a program of daily exercise that you can follow by yourself, quickly and inexpensively.

To increase flexibility fitness:

1. Do ten to fifteen minutes of stretching exercises. Do not bounce—just hold the stretched position for several seconds. Gradually work up to holding each stretch for thirty to sixty seconds. Use this exercise to increase the flexibility of those areas of your body that are tight.

To increase strength fitness:

1. Each day, do several sit-ups with bent knees, or any way that you can. Breathe normally during this exercise, and do not strain to do more than you are able.
2. Keeping your lower body on the floor, do several push-ups in any comfortable way. Again, breathe normally, and do not strain yourself.

To increase the efficiency of heart and lungs:

1. Start your aerobic activity by walking. Gradually over many days and weeks increase the amount and speed of walking until you are able to walk for one hour briskly without stopping. Your walking activity should not cause your heartbeat to exceed 75 percent of your maximal heart rate (for example, at age twenty, not more than 165 beats per minute). You should, therefore, not be out of breath or unable to talk during this activity.
2. Always start your aerobic activity by warming up for five to ten minutes at a slower rate (for example, at 60 percent or less of your maximal heart rate). At the end of your activity, it is important that you "cool down" in the same way. *Do not* end your exercising with a sprint.
3. After you are able to take a daily brisk walk for an hour, you may substitute other aerobic activities (such as bicycling, running, swimming, or jumping rope) for your daily hour of exercise. *Remember* to warm up beforehand, not to exceed a level of 75 percent of maximal heart rate during the activity, and to cool down afterward.

to one's needs and desires. In terms of total health benefits to be derived, however, a program should include some form of controlled, continuous, rhythmic exercise, such as jogging, swimming, or bicycling, that will raise the heart rate. But one's exercise program need not be complex or elaborate (see the How To box).

If one has been sedentary for a period of months or years, the prospect of engaging in this kind of exercise and incorporating it into one's permanent life style may seem ominous and impossible. Yet those who have tried it have been amazed at how quickly they adapt and become enthusiastically habituated to regular exercise.

Exercise and Aging

A fitness program can confer lifelong benefits. Over the past twenty years evidence has accumulated that proper exercise slows down many of the degenerative changes associated with age. A person who stays physically fit can arrive at age sixty-five with the strength, suppleness, and stamina typical of a person thirty years younger who has not exercised. A San Diego study that followed a group of men in an adult fitness program over a ten-year period demonstrated that these men were able to maintain the same high level of fitness throughout this period—a period in which sedentary men usually experience sharp declines in their fitness. Another study, at the University of Southern California, showed that many older people, even people over seventy, can still improve their fitness through proper exercise.

Virtually all of the favorable physiological effects of training listed above continue to occur at all ages. In addition, exercise can diminish or reverse the loss of calcium from bone (which commonly happens in older people, particularly in women) and thereby reduce the risk of fractures. Likewise, by maintaining muscle and joint strength and suppleness, ex-

Figure 10.8 Caring for your health and physical fitness will pay off in a variety of ways as you grow older. These older people continue to enjoy participation in football, bicycling and other sports—one of the benefits of having kept their bodies in top condition.

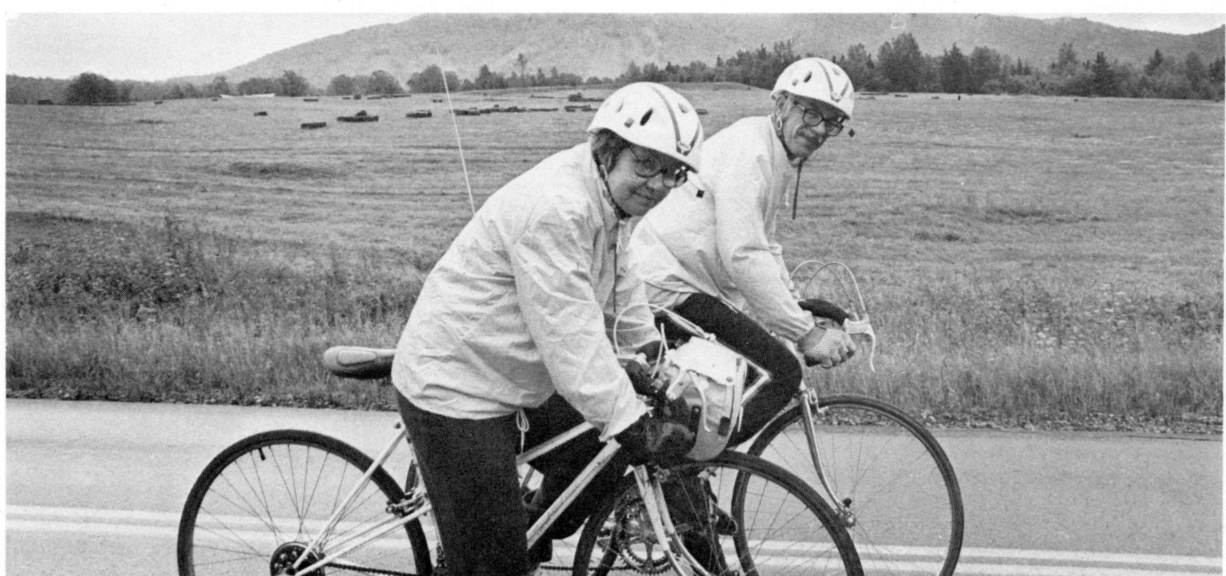

ercise can lead to less orthopedic injury and pain in later life. In osteoarthritis (degenerative joint disease), pain in the joints may be inevitable, but exercise can prevent or resolve much of the related disability. The most important effect of stamina training, of course, is on the cardiovascular and respiratory systems. This effect probably helps prevent heart attacks and improves chances of recovery should a heart attack occur.

How should one's patterns of exercise change with age? Within a wide range of individual differences, from about the age of twenty-five on, exercise should become less sporadic and violent and more and more of a continuous, rhythmic nature. Good sixty-year-old tennis players play quite differently from good twenty-five-year-old players. Older players perform less violently but maintain an easy rhythm that gets maximum results with the least risk of injury. Ideal forms of exercise for older people include walking, jogging, swimming, and bicycling. The latter two are less stressful orthopedically. If older adults prefer more violent exercise and sports, it is important that they warm up carefully, with gentle bending and stretching, and gradually increase the intensity of exercise in order to prepare the body for strenuous activity with minimum risk of injury. Even so, the older athlete is still more subject to muscle, tendon, joint, and bone injury.

A LIFETIME NEED

Functional fitness that provides adequate strength, suppleness, and stamina for living is gained and maintained by appropriate exercise. Moreover, physical recreation may help resolve the stresses of contemporary life. Thus the learning of physical skills and the development of a lifelong commitment to exercise may be a primary requisite for health for people living in modern industrialized societies. It is not a matter of choosing between exercise and other activities, as those who say that they have "no time for exercise" contend. Instead, exercise increases one's capacity both to carry out and to enjoy those other activities. Its benefits are twofold. First, if physical fitness adds years to life (and there is strong evidence that it does), then the time invested is repaid with interest. Second, because fitness maintains capacities at a high level, one realizes health benefits immediately.

Despite the current exercise and fitness revolution, America's urban and suburban life styles still exert tremendous pressures toward sedentary living. However, physical activity is available to those who understand the advantages of exercise and believe in its importance. Physical fitness is not a temporary or intermittent need but continuous throughout life. Its substantial benefits are enjoyed most by people who incorporate appropriate exercise into their life styles.

SUMMARY

1. Physical fitness is important not only for athletes but for everyone, for both physical and mental health.
2. Physical fitness involves the development of three elements: strength (the muscular force required for movement); suppleness (flexibility); and stamina (endurance).
3. If people are compared on the basis of their physical activity, the least active tend to have the greatest degenerative disease and death rates, with quality of life and life span increasing in direct proportion to increased physical activity.
4. How fit is "fit enough"? One should be strong and supple enough to work and play without risk of muscle or joint injury. Calisthenic activity is most useful in maintaining orthopedic adequacy. One should also be fit enough to protect against heart attack. The development of stamina (cardiovascular-respiratory endurance) appears to be one way to reduce the risk factors for coronary artery disease.
5. Aerobic exercise is extended exercise in which the oxygen needs of the body are being met continually by sufficient oxygen delivery. In anaerobic exercise, the oxygen demand exceeds the supply, and the body goes into "oxygen debt." Sprinting is an anaerobic exercise. Running, jogging, jumping rope, and swimming are aerobic exercises.
6. In planning a fitness program, one should get medical clearance and avoid overexertion.

Most competitive sports are not as useful for maintaining fitness as calisthenics and endurance training. Most fitness gadgets and devices are not essential, and most fitness fads are useless.

7. A fitness program can confer lifelong benefits. While exercise capacity does diminish with age, virtually all of the favorable physiological effects of traiing continue to occur at all ages.

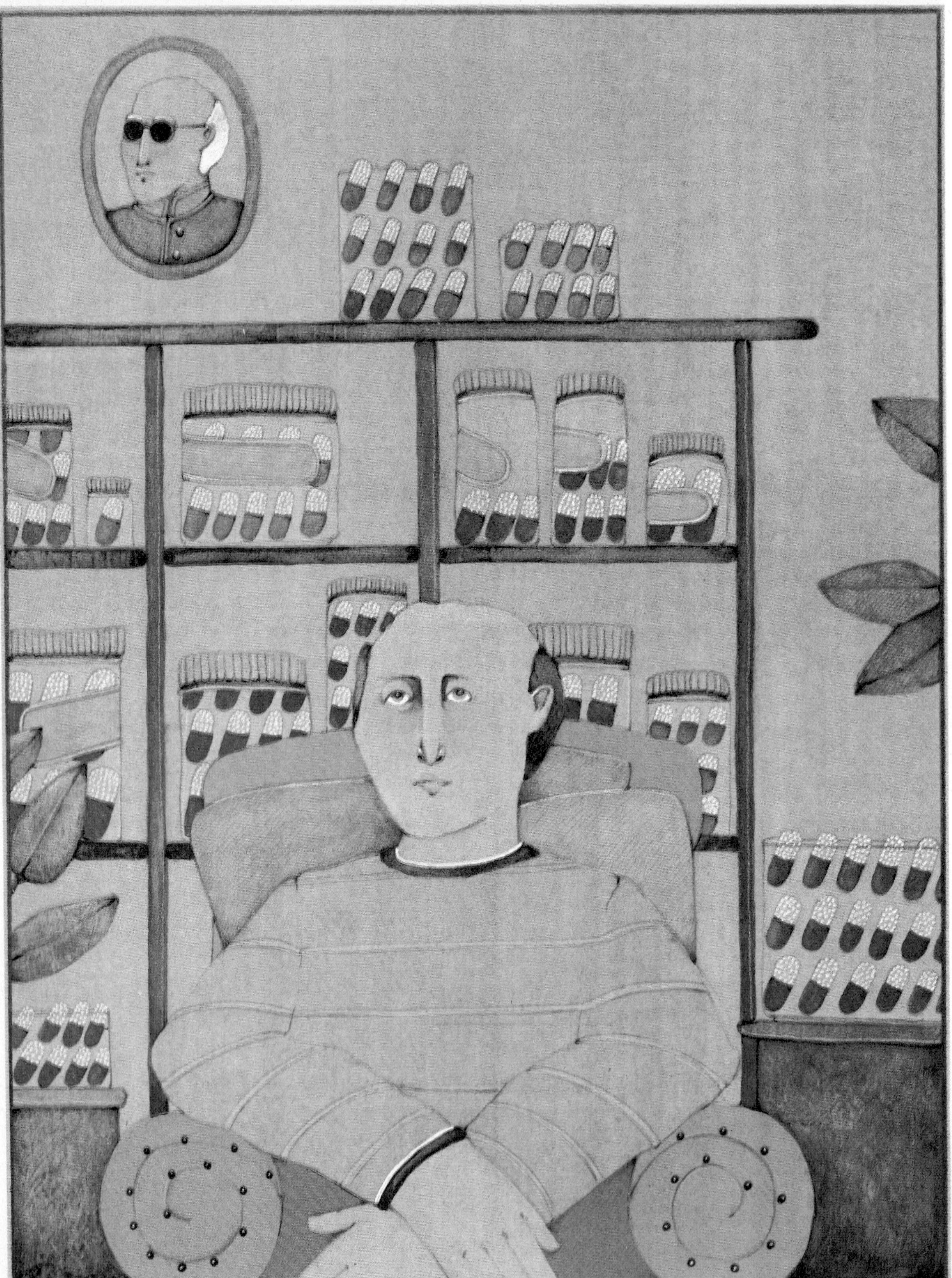

Dagmar Frinta

IV SUBSTANCE USE AND ABUSE

When we read about ancient history we learn that, even then, people throughout the world used many of the same drugs for healing, escape, and pleasure that we use today. But although drug use seems to date back as far as human history, in this century the number of available drugs has proliferated beyond the imagination of even the most fanciful cave dweller.

Not only do we have available vast numbers of over-the-counter and prescription drugs to cure physical ailments, but we also have access to an incredible range of *psychoactive drugs,* which chemically alter our behavior. Abuse of the psychoactive drugs has become a critical health problem among people of all ages in recent years, and these substances have become the center of medical, legal, and moral controversies. Part IV studies the nature of drugs and the roles they play in our lives.

Chapter 11 provides an overview of the world of drugs—defining drug abuse, outlining the stages of drug dependence and drug-using behavior, and examining the use, effects, and potential for abuse of the major psychoactive drugs. It also contains guidelines for the safe use of over-the-counter and prescription drugs, which many people abuse, too.

Chapter 12 focuses on this country's most widely abused drug—alcohol. And Chapter 13 is a study of cigarette smoking—perhaps the most graphic example of a drug habit that can have disastrous long-term effects on overall health.

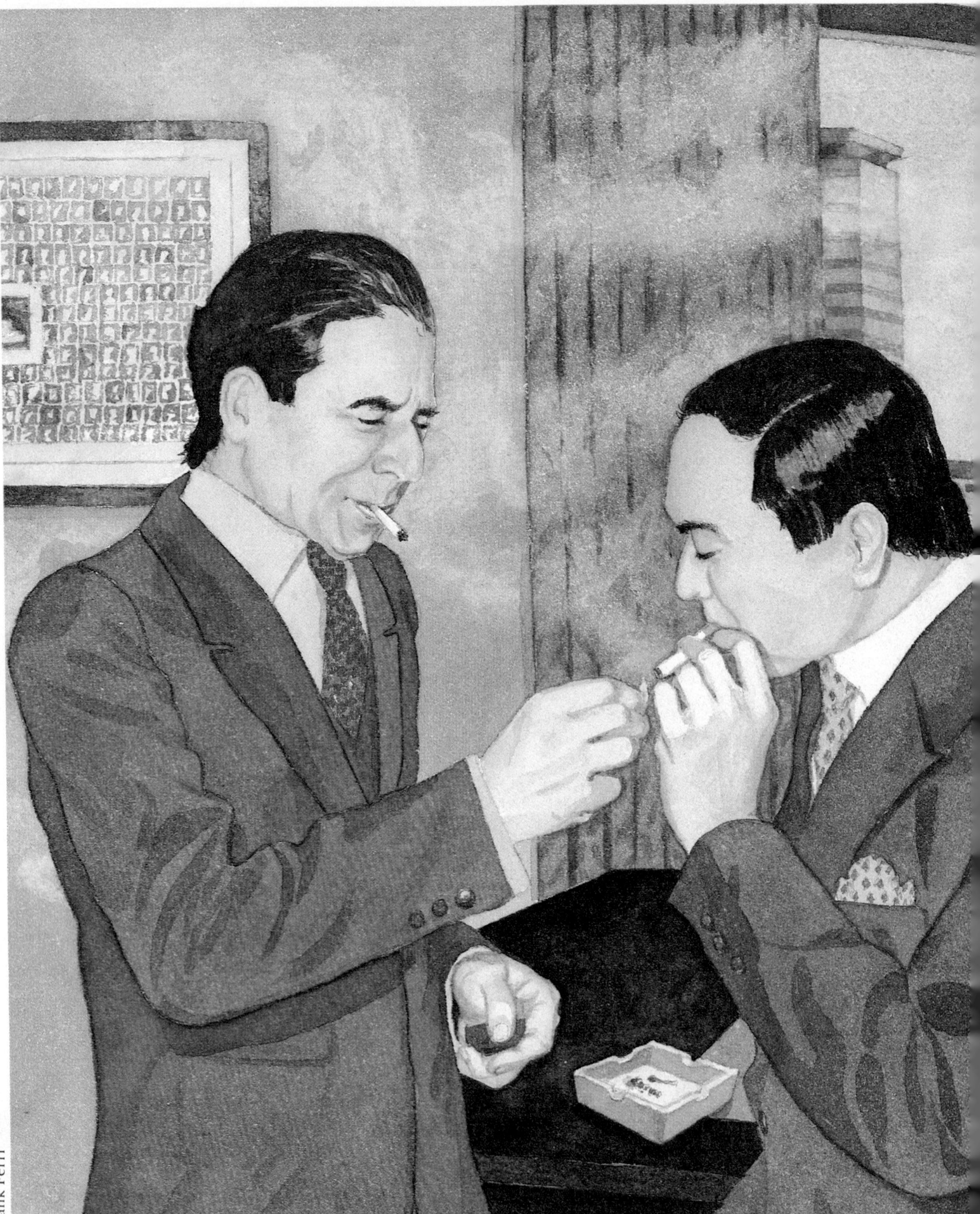

Frank Ferri

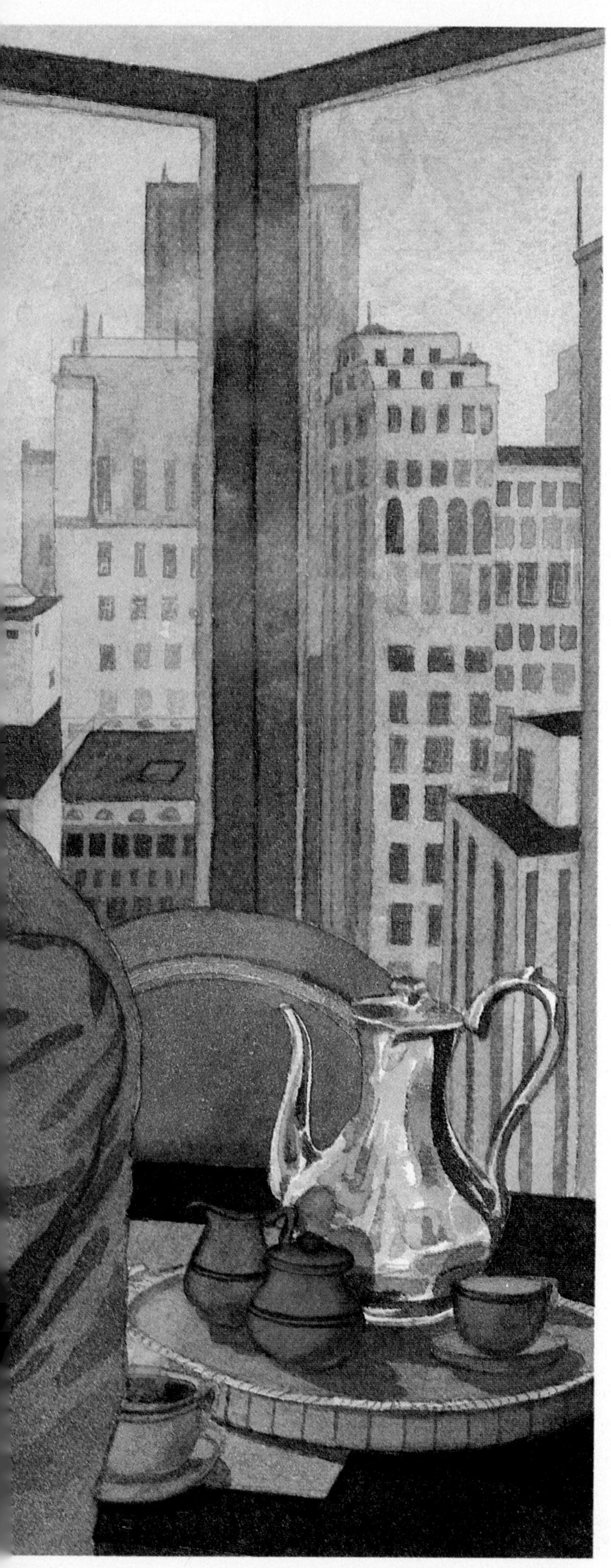

11 Drugs and Drug Use

America today has been called the most drug-oriented society in history. There is no question that we are drug-saturated, with an enormous variety of chemical substances available both legally and illegally. Drugs are a part of almost every medical treatment, and they help lubricate our social occasions. People use drugs freely to give themselves a lift, to help themselves relax, to feel better or not so bad, out of habit, or just because it is the thing to do. Americans are continuously barraged by advertisements touting different brands of alcohol or tobacco, aspirin, cold remedy, or other drugs. Not only do these ads sell products, they also sell the idea that drugs can provide immediate solutions to human problems.

This barrage is not all exaggeration, of course. Drugs do save lives and improve human health by curing diseases, helping to limit the size of families, and controlling mental illness. Cigarettes do satisfy the smoker, and alcohol does ease tensions. Barbiturates may bring the restful oblivion of sleep; opiates ease pain; and the minor tranquilizers reduce anxiety. Caffeine, cocaine, and the amphetamines give psychological and physiological boosts, and other drugs produce highly pleasurable feelings of euphoria or well-being. Drugs are easy to take, and their effects are often immediate. It is no mystery, then, why so many people believe that "relief is just a swallow away" or why chemical means of escaping and coping are—and will continue to be—so popular. However, people are often inclined to carry a good thing too far and abuse these substances, ignoring or failing to prevent and control their destructive aspects.

The question is not whether people will use drugs. The evidence is that virtually everyone does and will. The real issues are who will use what drugs, for what purposes, with what benefits and risks, and with what short- and long-term consequences. The challenge is to develop those drug-using practices that maximize the constructive uses of these substances while minimizing their destructive aspects.

What exactly are drugs? What constitutes drug abuse? Why do some people become abusers of drugs while others do not? What are the major psychoactive drugs and how widely are they abused? Are the over-the-counter drugs that are sold in drugstores and supermarkets really safe? What should a patient know about prescription drugs before taking them? These are some of the questions that will be discussed in this chapter.

WHAT IS A DRUG?

A *drug* is a chemical substance that alters structure or function in a human organism. Thus, aspirin, antibiotics, antihistamines, and antacids, as well as the mind-altering or *psychoactive* drugs, are included in this definition. In medicine, a drug is any chemical compound administered to help in the prevention, diagnosis, or treatment of disease.

A sizable fraction of all drugs acts directly on the brain and central nervous system. Because of their chemical nature, they either facilitate or impede the normal transmission of impulses from nerve cell to nerve cell within the brain or nervous system. Modifications in nerve transmissions are perceived by the individual as an alteration of awareness or mood. Drugs that create such perceptions are called psychoactive drugs. The major psychoactive drugs include alcohol, nicotine, caffeine, the barbiturates, major tranquilizers (antipsychotics), minor tranquilizers (antianxiety drugs), antidepressants, amphetamines, cocaine, marijuana, opiates (opium, morphine, heroin), and the psychedelic-hallucinogens (LSD, mescaline, PCP).

Over-the-counter (OTC) drugs are used for temporary relief from minor health problems. Common OTC drugs include aspirin, antacids, antihistamines, and laxatives. Specific information about the effects and abuses of psychoactive and OTC drugs is provided later in this chapter. Knowing the available facts may help you to decide what role these substances should or should not play in your own life. (Alcohol is discussed in Chapter 12, nicotine in Chapter 13.) Prescription drugs, which can cure some illnesses, include the antibiotics (see Chapter 14); guidelines for using them intelligently are explained in this chapter as well.

WHAT IS DRUG ABUSE?

Some drug experts make a distinction between misuse and abuse. To *misuse* a drug is to use it in ways or amounts that are not medically indicated, according to one definition. A wide spectrum of substances can thus be misused, ranging from agents with profound effects on the brain to caffeine, headache remedies, and antibiotics. A common kind of drug misuse in the United States is the excessive consumption of nonprescription, over-the-counter (OTC) drugs, a topic that we will discuss below. However, this concept of misuse—all nonmedically indicated drug use—would include *all* use of alcohol and nicotine. It is thus not a very helpful definition.

Drug abuse can also be a confusing term, because two distinct concepts enter into its definition. From one standpoint, to abuse a drug is to use it to an extent that produces a measurable impairment of psychological or physiological functioning. From another standpoint, the difference between drug use and drug abuse depends on how a particular society at a particular time views a certain drug. What is considered normal as opposed to pathological use thus varies from drug to drug, from dosage to dosage, from situation to situation, from culture to culture—and even among the subcultures of a given society.

In Western society, for instance, a chronic alcoholic is considered a drug abuser—yet the three-martini lunch or occasional drunkenness is acceptable in many circles. Likewise, the use of barbiturates as prescription sleeping pills is sanctioned, but taking the same dosage in a

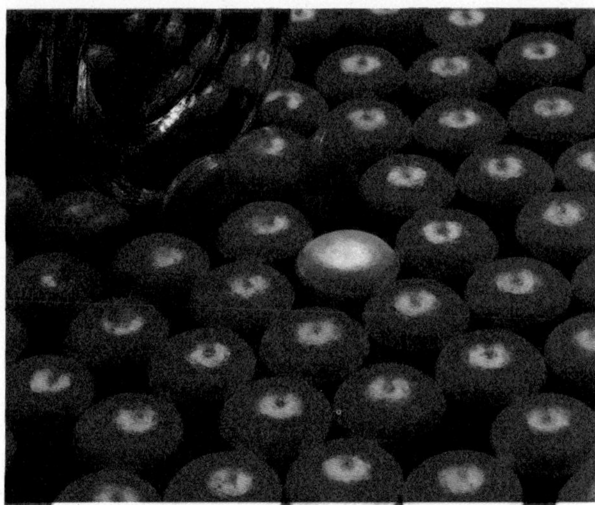

Figure 11.1 How a society defines drug abuse depends on the times and the circumstances under which the drug is taken.

social situation to induce euphoria is considered abuse. Using a medically prescribed opiate (such as morphine) to relieve depression or tension (rather than pain) is considered flagrant drug abuse. Yet many opiate users in the United States are people being treated legally for terminal cancer or other chronic, severe pain or are people who were formerly dependent on heroin and are now on methadone maintenance. Few would consider these people abusers.

What constitutes drug abuse also varies with the times and circumstances. In the early 1960s, when the use of LSD was limited to small numbers of intellectuals and research workers, American society tolerated LSD use (perhaps because they heard little about it) as a research tool for investigating certain aspects of mental processes. When in the mid-1960s, however, the use of the drug spread beyond the laboratory and became widespread among high-school and college students, use of LSD became equated with abuse. Within a short period of time, the manufacture, sale, or possession of LSD was not only condemned but became a crime.

Another common definition of drug abuse is an *unlawful* use of a drug. By this definition, any use of alcohol or nicotine by people under eighteen or twenty-one (depending on the state) would be considered abuse, and alcohol would be the most extensively used illegal drug. To avoid these problems inherent in the social and legal definitions of drug abuse, we will use the following definition: *drug abuse is an amount, frequency, or pattern of use that impairs normal functioning.*

HAZARDS AND COSTS OF DRUG USE AND ABUSE

It is hard to measure the risks of drug taking objectively or to balance them against potential benefits. Nevertheless, the risks can be measured in a number of ways. Economically, for instance, one can calculate not only the dollar cost of the drugs themselves but also that of the legal penalties involved in their use. The cost of drug taking can also be measured in terms of time—time lost from school or work while in the drugged state or recovery from it, or time spent in hospitals or jails. Even more significantly, the hazards of overdoses or long-term heavy use can also be counted in terms of addiction, mental disorder, disability, impaired functioning, injury to others, crime, and even death.

Psychologically, the risks of drug use can be evaluated subjectively in terms of decreased autonomy and freedom, decreased alertness and self-control, and loss of goals. Biologically, the costs of drug use can be evaluated in terms of their physiological effect on the human body. These biological effects are influenced by a number of variables.

The Physiological Variables

Pharmacology is the study of drugs and their effects. It is an exceedingly complex science, and the physiological reasons why and how most drugs act as they do are still not fully understood. Clear, objective knowledge of the biological risks associated with the use of any specific substance is therefore difficult to determine. It is known, however, that individuals vary enormously in their inherent response to different drugs. A number of the pharmacological factors involved in this variation are known

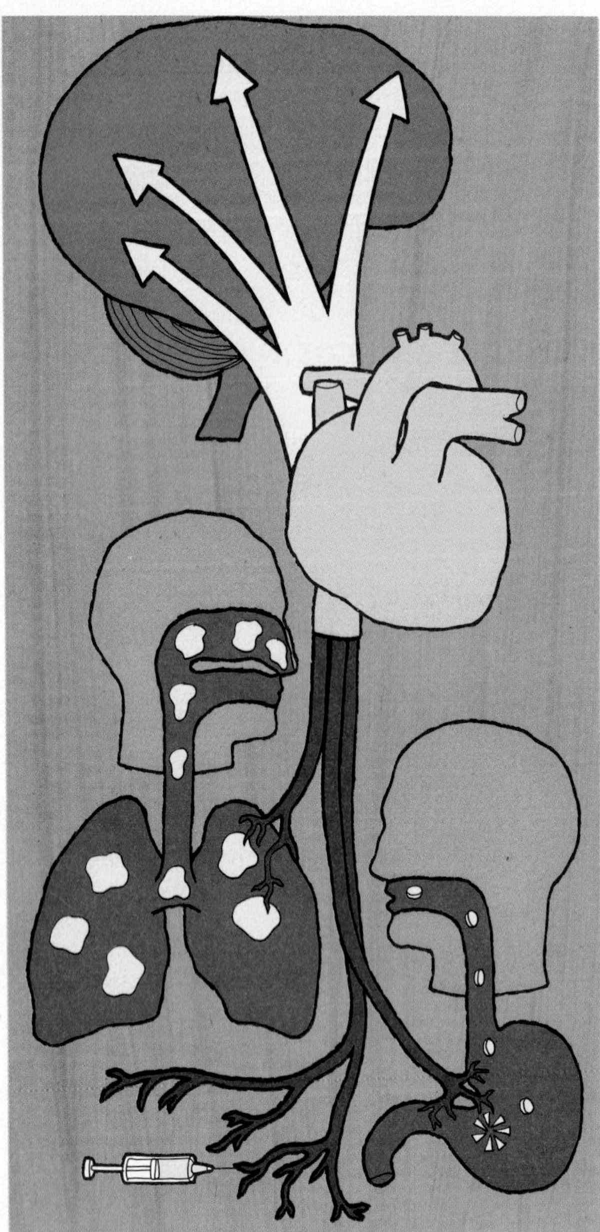

Figure 11.2 Drugs reach the brain by several routes—via the digestive tract if ingested, the respiratory system if inhaled, or the bloodstream directly if injected.

and are useful in considering one's own use of drugs.

One of the most important variables is *dosage.* Theoretically, any drug is safe at some small dosage, and any drug can be *toxic* (harmful or poisonous) at some higher dosage. As Jean Mayer has said, "There are no toxic substances, only toxic concentrations." One alcoholic drink is mildly relaxing; two or three may produce euphoria and impair sensory and motor performance; while the equivalent of ten to twenty drinks ingested over a short period of time can depress the nervous system, stop breathing, and cause death. Dosage is a function not only of the actual amount of the drug taken but also of body size, metabolism, the routes by which the drug is administered and excreted, and the individual's inborn sensitivity. Generally, the larger the person, the higher the dose that will be required to produce a given effect. Drugs inhaled or injected into a vein produce greater and more immediate responses than the same drugs taken by mouth or injected into a muscle. And some individuals may be considerably more or less sensitive than average to a given dose. These factors affect dosages of all drugs, whether used medically or recreationally.

Potency varies enormously from drug to drug and also affects dosages. At the same dosage, some drugs are much more powerful than others. Only 0.2 milligram of LSD is required to

Figure 11.3 Potency of drugs in the same category, such as the sedative-hypnotics, can vary greatly. Thiopental is a common anesthetic, but the small difference between an effective dose and a lethal one makes it a very dangerous drug in the hands of anyone but a medical expert. On the other hand, Valium, when taken alone, is considered relatively safe; only an enormous dose could cause death.

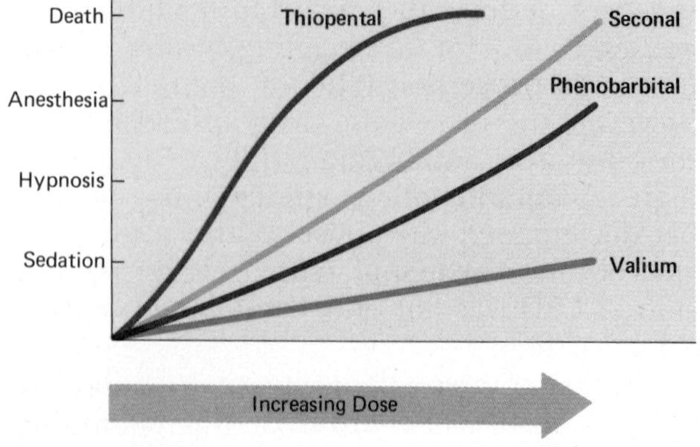

produce the same effects as 2 milligrams of psilocybin or 200 milligrams of mescaline.

Another important factor is a drug's *solubility*. Drugs that are water-soluble generally cannot reach the central nervous system because they are blocked by the so-called blood-brain barrier. (One exception is alcohol, which, although water-soluble, passes the blood-brain barrier because of the small size of its molecules.) Lipid-soluble (fat-soluble) drugs, on the other hand, are able to reach the central nervous system because they penetrate cell walls, which are largely fat. Most psychoactive drugs are highly lipid-soluble. This also means that they remain in the body longer. They must be metabolized and broken down into water-soluble compounds before they can be excreted by the kidneys. Some barbiturates require several days to be metabolized completely, as does the active chemical in marijuana, THC.

The specific *site* within the body where a drug acts—that is, the specific location where it, because of its chemical nature, alters functioning—is also a critical factor. Psychoactive drugs, for example, do not change what brain cells actually do. They merely stimulate or depress normal nerve transmission; they alter a potential that is always present. For example, LSD is believed to produce its wild hallucinatory experiences by blocking the inhibition of certain sensory areas of the brain, thereby allowing a flood of nonintegrated signals and perceptions.

Transient physiological variations also affect an individual's response to a drug. Variations in the functioning of internal organs, particularly the liver, can alter the effect of a drug. Fatigue or stress can also change a person's response. Women's ability to metabolize alcohol varies with the phase of their menstrual cycle; a given amount on the twenty-eighth day of the cycle will produce a higher blood level of alcohol than the same amount on the first day of the cycle. And the presence of other drugs in the system can boost, inhibit, or otherwise alter one's reaction to some drugs. (See the discussion below on drug interactions.)

The *setting* and one's own *set* also powerfully influence a drug's effect. Set refers to what one has learned to expect from a drug, and psychoactive drugs tend to deliver what one expects. It is not known whether this is more psychological or physiological. The social setting also conditions the perceived effects of psychoactive drugs. An individual is likely to react quite differently to three drinks at a sedate dinner party with the boss than to the same three drinks at a sporting event with a friend.

Drug Toxicity and Interactions

There are no absolutely safe drugs; all drugs—whether psychoactive, prescription, or over-the-counter—have side effects and are potentially poisonous. Any drug can be harmful in large enough doses, in impure forms, and in combination with other drugs. Some 30,000 people die each year from adverse reactions to drugs. (This number does not include deaths associated with the use of alcohol or tobacco.) There are also more than 284,000 hospital emergency room visits a year related to drugs. In addition to these acute toxic reactions, drugs can also cause long-term side effects, ranging from fetal malformations to cancer.

A growing problem in the United States is adverse reactions caused by interactions between two or more different drugs, taken either simultaneously or sequentially. This is especially significant considering the trend toward multisubstance abuse by American men and women of all ages and social classes. (See the Focus box.) When two drugs are taken at the same time, they sometimes will interact *synergistically*. That is, the sum of their combined action can be more (or less) than the sum of their separate actions. One plus one may equal not two but four, five, or even ten. A classic example of drug synergism is the common combination of alcohol plus barbiturates. A less-than-lethal amount of alcohol plus a less-than-lethal dose of barbiturates can add up to a more-than-lethal dose as a combination. Alcohol can also affect the action of other drugs, sometimes in unpredictable ways. It may reduce the effectiveness of anticonvulsant drugs and some antidiabetic drugs. On the other hand, it can increase the tendency of aspirin to cause stomach or intestinal bleeding.

Table 11.1 The Hazards of Combining Alcohol with Other Drugs

Avoid Combining with	Possible Effects	Possible Results
Amphetamines		Loss of alertness, coordination skills, and judgment
Antihistamines	Increases the central nervous system depression of alcohol	Drowsiness, respiratory depression, loss of consciousness in severe cases
Barbiturates	Increases the effects of both alcohol and barbiturates	Drowsiness, respiratory depression, coma, and death from large doses
Codeine	Increases the effect of codeine	Respiratory depression, dizziness, drowsiness
Fumes from carbon tetrachloride and lacquer thinner		Liver and kidney failure, death
Insulin	Increases, by as much as 21 percent, the rate of metabolism of alcohol in the diabetic	Normal doses of insulin insufficient to control diabetes, diabetic shock and coma
Oral antidiabetics (Diabinese, Dymelor, Orinase)	Increases the effect of alcohol due to a buildup of acetaldehyde	Drowsiness, possible severe nausea and vomiting

STAGES OF DRUG DEPENDENCE

In addition to the risks of acute toxicity or wasting money, another risk of drug use is that of developing dependence on the drug. There are several escalating levels of drug dependence.

Habituation

Drug users may reach a state in which they feel compelled to continue the use of a drug in order to maintain the state of well-being it produces. At this point, the user is said to be *psychologically dependent* on the drug or *habituated* to it. When deprived of the drug, the habituated person becomes restless, irritable, or anxious. Unlike the physically dependent drug user (who will be discussed later), however, the person whose dependence is only psychological does not suffer any physical withdrawal symptoms.

Under this definition, millions of Americans are habituated to their spouses, to television, and to hobbies, as well as to a wide variety of drugs, including caffeine and tobacco, alcohol and amphetamines. Whether or not such psychological dependence is a problem can be determined only on an individual basis, using the definition of drug abuse cited earlier.

Tolerance

One characteristic of chronic drug use is that the user often develops *tolerance* to the drug. This means that the body becomes adapted to the drug and requires ever-increasing doses to achieve the same responses that smaller doses formerly elicited. Thus the first time a person drinks alcohol, half a glass of wine or liquor might make him or her drunk, while later, half a bottle or more might be required to produce the same effect.

Tolerance may also mean that a user can take larger and larger doses without suffering acute overdose effects. A long-time heroin user, for example, can tolerate dosages that would kill a new or moderate user. Tolerance also imposes a heavy financial burden on the user of an expensive drug.

FOCUS

Multisubstance Abuse

The growing problem of multisubstance abuse was brought to public attention early in 1978 when outspoken former First Lady Betty Ford checked into the Alcohol and Drug Rehabilitation Center at the Long Beach (California) Naval Hospital for treatment. For years, Mrs. Ford had suffered from flareups of arthritis and from pain due to a pinched nerve in her neck. "I am not only addicted to the medication I have been taking for my arthritis, but also to alcohol," she admitted in a public statement. "Over a period of time, I got to the point where I was overmedicating myself." One of her sons, Steve, added that his sixty-year-old mother was "fighting a very, very rough battle" against the effects of alcoholism and of Valium, a minor tranquilizer, the most frequently prescribed drug in the United States, which is sometimes used as a muscle relaxant.

Mrs. Ford's candid and gallant admission emphasized the growing tendency for Americans to use not just one but two or more drugs at the same time. This is sometimes called "polydrug use." This trend toward the use of multiple drugs is evident in both medical practice and the nonmedical use of drugs. A study in a Baltimore hospital showed that hospitalized patients received, on the average, eight to eleven different drugs during their stay there. And according to the National Institute on Drug Abuse, the *majority* of drug users take more than one legal or illegal drug. Mrs. Ford's mixture of drugs and alcohol is one of the most common combinations. Nearly 48,000 people a year are admitted to hospital emergency rooms suffering from reactions caused by combining alcohol with other drugs; this combination causes 2,500 deaths a year. Another classic combination is that of amphetamines and barbiturates. Some people take amphetamines in the morning in order to "get going" and feel alert and energetic enough for their day's activities. Then, in the evening, they find that they need barbiturates in order to calm down and go to sleep. These make them feel drowsy and sluggish the next morning—so they take amphetamines again. Such a cycle of "uppers" and "downers" tends to be self-perpetuating and extremely difficult to break.

Mrs. Ford's hospitalization for dual drug dependence also focused attention on the large numbers of women who take prescription psychoactive drugs. Almost twice as many women as men take such drugs. About 42 percent of American women (32 million) have taken tranquilizers, compared to only 27 percent of men (19 million). The same is true for both sedatives (16 million women, compared to 12 million men) and stimulants (12 million women, compared to 5 million men). Another startling fact: while the median age of white men and black men and women who die from drug-related causes is twenty-eight, the median age of white women who die from drugs is forty-three.

Physical Dependence

Physical dependence involves actual changes in the user's physiological state.* The body now requires frequent administration of the drug in order to avoid an extremely painful condition known as the withdrawal syndrome. Both tolerance and withdrawal symptoms always accompany physical dependence.

The *withdrawal syndrome* is a temporary physical illness that occurs when someone who is physically dependent on a drug either no longer receives it at all or receives much less than the amount to which the body has become tolerant. The delirium tremens (DTs) of an alcoholic is a withdrawal syndrome. The alcoholic may suffer convulsions, hallucinations, nausea and vomiting, tremors (the shakes), and even death.

For a dependent person, drug use pervades his or her life and activity. Although almost anything can produce psychological dependence (habituation), physical dependence is most likely with the depressants (alcohol and opiates) and the sedatives (barbiturates, Quaalude, Doriden, Miltown).

*Although *addiction* may be the more familiar term for physical dependence, it will not be used here due to its extremely negative connotations.

PATTERNS OF DRUG-USING BEHAVIOR

In 1973, the National Commission on Marijuana and Drug Abuse attempted to correlate various patterns of drug use with their underlying motivations. The commission was able to identify five more or less progressive patterns of drug use: (1) experimental use; (2) social or recreational use; (3) circumstantial or situational use; (4) intensified use; and (5) compulsive use.

By far the largest group of people who have ever used drugs (other than alcohol, tobacco, caffeine, and medicines) are strictly *experimental users.* They are motivated primarily by curiosity and by a desire to experience new feelings or moods. This experimentation is usually part of a social activity. An example of experimental use is smoking marijuana, for the first time, at a party. Such use does not usually result in any long-term or permanent impairment, although some drugs or high dosages can have serious adverse effects, including fatal reactions. Experimental drug use is not risk-free, but the risks are ordinarily low.

Social or recreational use occurs in social settings in which the participants wish to share with others an experience they perceive as acceptable and pleasurable. Examples would be serving wine at a dinner party or cocaine use among a small group of friends. Compared to experimental use, social-recreational use is more patterned, more planned, and a more regular component of social events. Recreational use is socially motivated. It usually does not escalate in frequency or get out of control, nor is it sustained by any significant degree of dependence. Most drinkers are recreational users of alcohol. As with experimental use, the risks of recreational use, either to the individual or to society, are usually low. For some drugs, however, such as heroin, alcohol, and Quaalude, recreational use can quickly escalate to destructive dependence.

The vast majority of drug users fall into the above two categories. While their drug use is often disapproved of by others and may sometimes be unlawful, it usually does not adversely affect their lives. Studies by a New York psychologist have documented that students who use drugs experimentally or recreationally are virtually indistinguishable—emotionally or intellectually—from their non-drug-using classmates.

In *circumstantial or situational use,* the user perceives a need for chemical help in accomplishing a task or coping with a situation. Such use tends to be regular, but limited to a specific circumstance. Some examples of situational users are students who use stimulants to stay awake while studying for exams, truckers who rely upon drugs to extend their endurance, athletes who use them to improve their performance, and people who go on alcoholic binges when they feel under unbearable stress. The immediate physiological and behavioral effects of such use, especially in higher doses, carry greater risks both to the individual and to society than does experimental or recreational use. The long-term risks are also higher. One is more likely to escalate to more intensive drug use or fail to develop other means of coping with situations.

Intensified use is repeated (usually daily), long-term self-medication with high dosages of one or more drugs in an attempt to get relief from a persistent problem or to maintain a desired level of performance perceived as impossible without drugs. Some examples are the unfulfilled housewife who consumes tranquilizers to reduce anxiety and the pressured executive who gains relief through heavy drinking. While most such intensive drug users remain stable both socially and economically, this use pattern has strong components of dependence. The individual's autonomy and control over such use may be constantly in jeopardy.

Compulsive use is the pattern in which the individual has largely lost control of his or her drug use, having "progressed" to levels of psychological or physiological dependence beyond the will to discontinue without experiencing great discomfort. Heavy drug use is central and dominant in the lives of compulsive users. Their individual and social functioning are therefore seriously impaired. Such profound dependence can be wholly psychological, as in the case of drugs such as marijuana and cocaine, or it can be both psychological and physiological, as with drugs such as barbiturates, alcohol, and the opiates. With these

HOW TO Recognize a Drug Problem

Are you afraid that a friend or relative may have a drug problem? How can you be certain?

Drug use, especially in the early stages, is hard to identify. But don't play detective; you'll do better just to ask the person about his or her experiments with drugs. Open communication will make both of you more comfortable.

If, however, your friend or relative has become *dependent* on a drug, communication may prove more difficult: drug abusers generally do everything possible to conceal their habit. Don't jump to hasty conclusions: you could falsely accuse a completely innocent person. Tablets or capsules, for example, may be legitimate prescriptions, and unusual behavior may be totally unrelated to drug abuse. However, there are some signs that commonly point to a drug abuse problem:

1. Changes in attendance at school or work.
2. Changes in normal work habits, efficiency, or other capabilities.
3. Poor physical appearance, including inattention to dress and personal hygiene.
4. Wearing sunglasses constantly and at inappropriate times (indoors or at night, for example) to hide dilated or constricted pupils or bloodshot eyes, and to compensate for the eye's diminished ability to adjust to sunlight.
5. Unusual attempts to cover the arms in order to hide needle marks.
6. Association with known drug abusers.
7. Stealing items that can readily be sold for cash in order to support a drug habit.

Source: National Institute on Drug Abuse, *Drug Abuse Prevention* (Washington, D.C.: U.S. Department of Health, Education, and Welfare, 1978); Drug Enforcement Administration, *Drug Abuse and Misuse* (Washington, D.C.: U.S. Department of Justice, 1978).

drugs, an added motivation to continue drug use is the desire to avoid painful withdrawal symptoms. Some examples of compulsive users are pack-a-day smokers, physicians dependent on morphine, "skid row" alcoholics, heroin-dependent "street junkies," the cocaine-dependent "snow nose," the marijuana "pothead," and the multisubstance abuser. Compulsive drug use poses the highest risks, both to the individual and to public health and safety. Compulsive drug users are responsible for an awesome amount of crime, illness, suffering, and human and economic waste.

CAUSES OF DRUG USE AND ABUSE

Although the availability of drugs, individual curiosity, and even chance all play a role in determining who will and who will not use or abuse drugs, other factors are also important. Different people will respond differently to their first exposure to the same amount of the same drug, and they will also take different lines of action with respect to their subsequent use of that or other drugs. To account for these individual differences, experts have explored two main areas that might influence use and abuse of various drugs: *psychological* factors and *sociological* factors.

There is no agreement among psychologists and sociologists as to which of these factors is more important. Most drug experts believe that sociological factors are usually of greater significance in determining drug *use,* while psychological factors are usually the major forces contributing to drug *abuse.*

Psychological Factors

According to drug authority Joel Fort, "The most important determinant of the drug effect is the personality and character structure of the person consuming the drug, including mood, attitude and expectations . . . what comes out of the mind-altering experience primarily depends upon what you are as a person." The effect experienced when taking the drug is, in turn, one of the many determinants involved in the *motivation* toward continuing to use it.

Motivation for taking drugs can vary from a simple desire for pleasure or euphoria, relaxation, or socialization to a need to escape from reality to a search for meaning, identity, or new ideas and perceptions. In trying to untangle the complex, underlying motivational factors that influence a particular drug user to become a drug abuser, behavioral scientists have come up with a number of theories, none of which is completely satisfactory.

Some researchers feel that people who abuse drugs have an underlying emotional immaturity or inadequacy that seems to be relieved by taking drugs. These investigators contend that the emotional disorder ultimately would become apparent to some degree whether or not drugs were abused. (This theory has largely replaced an older school of thought which held that all drug abusers are morally weak or sinful people who simply overindulge themselves.) It does not follow, however, that all people who have emotional disorders become drug abusers or vice versa. Other psychological and social factors also play a role, as do the availability of alternatives to drug use and the individual's motivation to use these alternatives. A person who is so psychologically constituted that he or she can cope with the frustrations and disappointments of living is unlikely to come to depend on drugs for assistance. (We are not speaking of cases where a person has become dependent on a drug after legitimate medical use of it—for example, dependence on morphine prescribed to relieve the pain of an injury.)

It may be that specific types of emotional disturbances determine, at least in part, what drugs will be abused. It seems conceivable that people suffering from anxiety, depression, or delusions might seek out those drugs that would most effectively counteract these particular maladies. However, attempts to classify opiate, alcohol, and amphetamine abusers into distinct psychological categories have so far not been particularly successful, nor have efforts to construct psychological "profiles" of alcoholics or opiate abusers. Part of the difficulty lies in the present inability to define the "predependent" personality.

For example, anxiety can be viewed as an expression of an unresolved conflict between drives and inhibitions. Alcohol (as well as barbiturates) is thought to decrease anxiety by reducing inhibitions, and alcoholics are said to relieve these conflicts by acting out their drives, such as aggression, dependence, and sexuality. On the other hand, opiate abusers may achieve similar relief from anxiety by reducing drives instead of inhibitions. They are viewed as more passive, avoiding rather than seeking aggression.

In summary, the most popular psychological theory today about the causes of drug abuse is that most abusers have psychological disturbances that are both profound and extensive. This theory holds for most drugs, whether opiate, barbiturate, alcohol, or amphetamine. Whether or not these psychological disturbances existed before the drug abuse and, in fact, led directly to it is not yet established. It is also possible that compulsive, long-term use of drugs so exaggerates preexisting emotional disorders that a previously undetectable disorder might become severe and pronounced.

Sociological Factors

In the United States, social and cultural factors are perhaps the most significant in promoting drug use and abuse. The fact that people use any drug at all is culturally determined. A growing body of thought contends that life style contributes even more than psychological make-up in determining who will and who will not take and abuse specific drugs. Life style is, by and large, a product of cultural environment. More specifically, our drug-oriented society influences who uses what drugs in many ways: by the psychological pressures it exerts on its members, by selecting or restricting the socioeconomic or subcultural group one can associate with, and by providing exposure to drugs.

Children are exposed, as they grow up, to the example of adults using drugs freely. Children get their cues to appropriate behavior by observing, emulating, and modeling themselves after the adults in their world. To a large extent, then, young people who use or abuse drugs are merely doing in their own way what they see the important adults in their lives do, at home and in school, in films and on television.

Individuals are also constantly exposed to information and discussion about drugs in newspapers, magazines, and television programs. Exposure to drug advertising also subtly conditions the individual to seek and accept drugs as ways to solve a variety of problems.

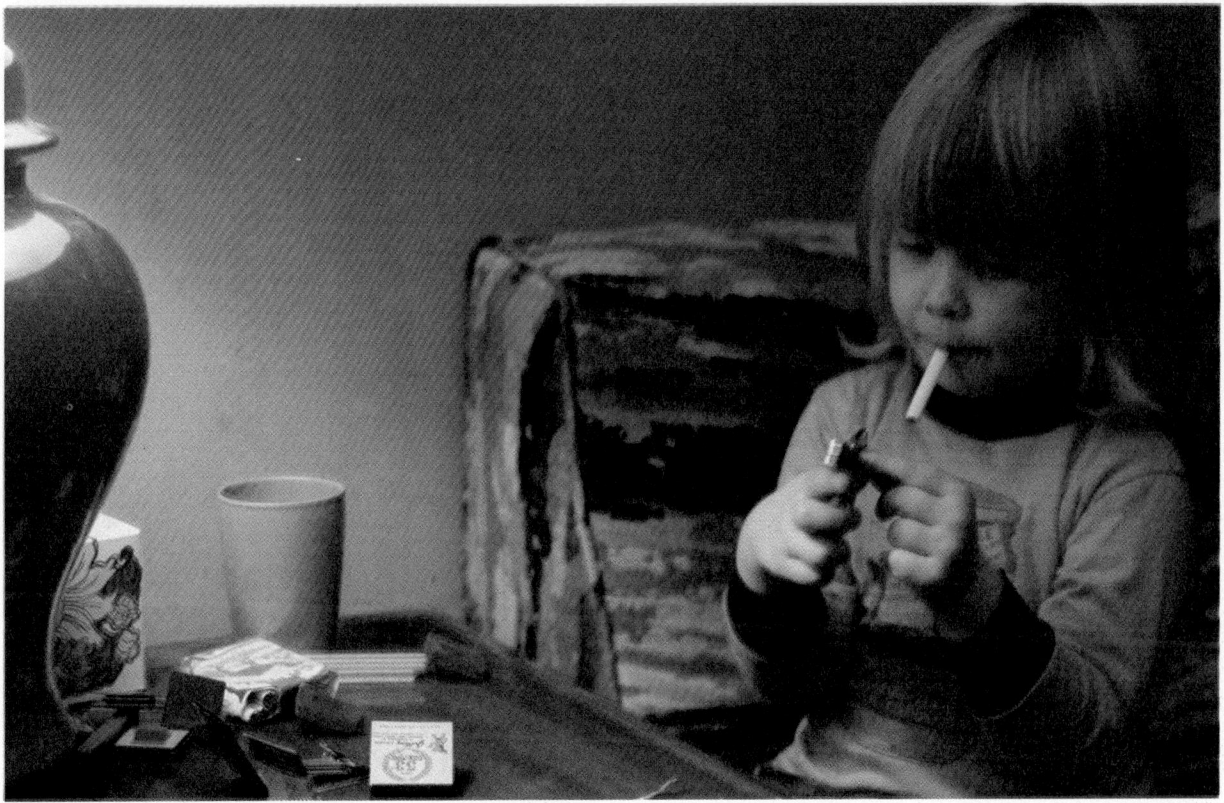

Figure 11.4 When young people use or abuse drugs, they are often trying to imitate the important adults in their lives.

"Want to be sexy, youthful, and happy? Drink ______." "Tired? Take ______." "Tense and nervous? Take ______." "Got a cold? Take ______." It is no surprise, then, that millions of Americans feel that there is a pill, drink, or cigarette for every problem.

The pharmaceutical industry and physicians must also assume a share of the responsibility for drug abuse. Pharmaceutical companies spend more than $4,000 a year per physician on drug advertising. Physicians themselves are trained in a tradition of "pharmacological magic." A Chicago study showed that the writing of a drug prescription is an almost invariable part of a visit to a physician, a ritual performed by the doctor and expected by the patient. The prescription, the study found, was often unnecessary medically. Its apparent purpose was to terminate the patient's visit. There is no doubt that both patients and physicians too readily adopt chemical means for resolving problems.

There are also powerful economic and political forces contributing to the widespread use of drugs. Despite the fact that the Public Health Service considers cigarette smoking the nation's largest single preventable cause of disability and death, another branch of the federal government feels obligated to pay millions of dollars to farmers each year in subsidies to support the price of tobacco. And the use of unlawful drugs is powerfully impelled by the astronomical profits that importers, dealers, and middlemen can make in the black market.

Why People Use Drugs Drug use can be a *way into* specific experiential or social groups. In their desire to belong, many people succumb to *peer-group pressures*— the need to do what "everyone else" is doing. In order to be ac-

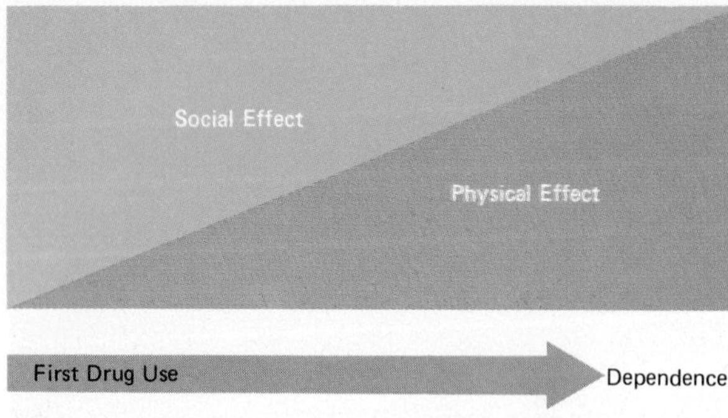

Figure 11.5 The first use of a drug is usually experimental—the result of peer pressure or other social forces. As use continues and dependence increases, the person becomes more and more involved with the physical effects of the drug and less and less concerned with its social aspect.

cepted into a group, an individual is often drawn to experimenting with whatever the group-sanctioned drug is, whether it be alcohol, tobacco, barbiturates, narcotics, amphetamines, cocaine, or Quaalude, even if otherwise he or she might have no particular interest in the substance. Peer-group pressure is a major factor in the drug use of the young couple at a cocktail party. One of the tragic problems of such experimentation is that toxic or even lethal overdoses of drugs can result from ignorance, carelessness, impurities, or fraud. Furthermore, experimenting with drugs is a gamble that *can* lead to abuse or destructive behavior. And for those who have not yet learned who or what they are, the need to use the drug over and over again to maintain their identity with the group may become even more important than the effects of the drug itself.

People also use drugs as a *way of coping* with their life situation, its pressures, disappointments, and the inability to see a way to become upwardly mobile. And, most of all, people use drugs because of their usually *pleasurable effects.*

The 1977 National Survey on Drug Abuse documented that the use of unlawful drugs in the United States today is very much an age-related phenomenon. While the majority (60 percent) of young adults between the ages of eighteen and twenty-six have used marijuana, only 28 percent of those between the ages of twelve and seventeen have used it and only 15 percent of adults over twenty-five. While the use of the stronger unlawful drugs is much less widespread, the same tendency holds true: they are used significantly more by people between the ages of eighteen and twenty-five than by those either younger or older. Apparently as people finish school, start their professional careers, and assume the responsibilities of marriage and family, they tend to taper off their use of these drugs.

Many experts believe that these sociological factors, interacting with emotional problems, play the major role in drug abuse. Thus, depending on the drug, anyone can get "hooked." Any solution to today's many drug problems must take into account these social roots.

THE PSYCHOACTIVE DRUGS

The psychoactive drugs comprise a great variety of substances with one common property—the ability to alter consciousness or mood. These drugs are widely used and abused; they are most often taken for relief from psychological and social problems or for pleasure and recreation. The common psychoactive drugs can be divided into six major categories: (1) depressants, (2) major tranquilizers, (3) antidepressants and lithium, (4) stimulants, (5) psychedelic-hallucinogens, and (6) cannabis (marijuana).

DEPRESSANTS

Depressants are drugs that slow down or reduce the activity of the central nervous system, particularly the brain. Among the most commonly used depressants are alcohol; the sedative-hypnotics; the opiates (including heroin and morphine); methaqualone (Quaalude, Sopor); volatile chemicals such as gasoline or toluene (glue); and the drugs used in medicine to produce general anesthesia (such as ether and nitrous oxide, or laughing gas). In small doses, these depressants produce sedation or sleep. In larger doses, they can produce coma and death.

Alcohol, which is the most widely used of all these central-nervous-system depressants, will be discussed separately in Chapter 12. Throughout this chapter, however, the reader should also keep in mind the fact that alcohol, too, is a drug and one of the most commonly abused mind-altering substances.

Sedative-Hypnotics A sedative is an agent that calms or relaxes a person. The word *hypnotic,* when used in reference to a drug, means an agent that induces sleep. The difference between sedative action and hypnotic action is merely a matter of degree. The same drug in smaller doses can act as a sedative, while in larger doses it acts as a hypnotic. As a group, the sedative-hypnotics are the most widely used depressants after alcohol.

The sedative-hypnotics can be divided into three major categories. One group is the *barbiturates,* which are synthetic drugs. In the United States, pentobarbital (Nembutal), secobarbital (Seconal), and amobarbital (Amytal) are the most commonly used and abused barbiturates. While the barbiturates are similar chemically and pharmacologically, they differ in their speed and duration of action.

A second major group of sedative-hypnotics is the *benzodiazepines,* a class that includes the widely prescribed drugs Valium and Librium. These are also called *minor tranquilizers,* a term that also includes another pharmacological category typified by meprobamate (Miltown). The third major group of sedative-hypnotics consists of a number of drugs that are unrelated chemically: paraldehyde, chloral hydrate, methaqualone (Quaalude, Sopor), and glutethimide (Doriden). Most nonbarbiturate sedative-hypnotics have come into widespread use only in the last two decades. Generally, these drugs affect the central nervous system in much the same way as the barbiturates and alcohol, and have similar side effects, disadvantages, and dangers to the barbiturates.

The sedative-hypnotics reduce anxiety and may cause slurring of speech, loss of muscular coordination, and eventually drowsiness or sleep. As with alcohol, there is great variation in the severity of these effects and the amount of impairment of cognitive functioning, depending on the individual and the particular tasks he or she is performing. Moderate doses rapidly produce drowsiness in most people, but when these drugs are taken for altering awareness or social reasons, the individual can become tolerant of heavy doses and keep awake.

In medicine, the barbiturates and other sedative-hypnotics are widely used for treating insomnia, controlling epileptic seizures, producing daytime sedation, and allaying anxiety. They are also used to modify the effects of other drugs such as stimulants or painkillers. Sedative-hypnotics are usually taken in the form of pills, but they sometimes are injected. Doses of about 50 milligrams several times a day usually have a sedative effect.

It is believed that abuse of sedative-hypnotics, particularly the barbiturates, exceeds that of opiates. The patterns of sedative-hypnotics abuse range from infrequent sprees aimed at gross intoxication to prolonged, compulsive daily use of large quantities, where the abuser is preoccupied with securing and maintaining adequate supplies. The original contact with the drug may be either through a prescription or an illicit-drug subculture. In a medical patient, abuse may develop gradually. It may begin with prolonged use for insomnia and progress to larger and larger doses each night, plus a few capsules at particularly stressful times during the day. Eventually, the drug may become a major focus of the user's life.

If the user keeps daily consumption of barbiturates at or below 400 milligrams, there will probably be no physical dependence. However, a variety of side effects may occur, including hangovers, nausea, headaches, dizziness, and drowsiness, and the user may be subject to accidents.

Daily use of 500 milligrams or more of barbiturates (or equivalent doses of other sedative-hypnotics) usually produces classical physical dependence. Such abuse can rapidly develop tolerance for up to fifteen times the usual dose. Without the drug, the abuser suffers acute withdrawal symptoms. These symptoms begin with nervousness, trembling, and weakness. If untreated, the person can suffer epileptic-like seizures, a toxic psychosis with delusions and hallucinations, and loses of consciousness. The most severe symptoms of untreated withdrawal last about four days and can be fatal.

The barbiturate abuser, like the severe alcoholic, often becomes mentally confused; frequently is obstinate, irritable, and abusive; and is usually unable to function adequately in daily activities. This behavior is in marked contrast to that of the opiate abuser, who usually remains passive and is able to function moderately well.

According to the Public Health Service, barbiturates and other sedative-hypnotics account for over 15 percent of drugs involved in visits to hospital emergency rooms, and are implicated in nearly 20 percent of all drug-related deaths. Barbiturate overdose accounts for more than 3,000 known deaths a year. It is also the most frequent method of suicide among American women. Many accidental deaths result from the combined use of alcohol and barbiturates, neither of which would have been fatal by itself. Unfortunately, the treatment of barbiturate abusers is still in a primitive state.

By contrast, the benzodiazepines carry a much lower risk of morbidity and mortality. Diazepan (Valium) has become the most widely used prescription drug in the United States. Between May 1976 and April 1977, according to the National Institute on Drug Abuse, physicians wrote more than 57 million Valium prescriptions for more than 3 billion pills. In the same period, there were also more than 15 million prescriptions written for Librium and early 10 million for meprobamate. Valium—primarily when used in combination with alcohol or other drugs—led to an estimated 54,400 visits to hospital emergency rooms, more than any other single drug. Yet these minor tranquilizers were involved in far fewer deaths proportionally than the barbiturates: there were 3 Valium-related deaths per 10 million pills, compared to 73 deaths per 10 million pills for Nembutal and 119 deaths per 10 million pills for Seconal, both of which are barbiturates.

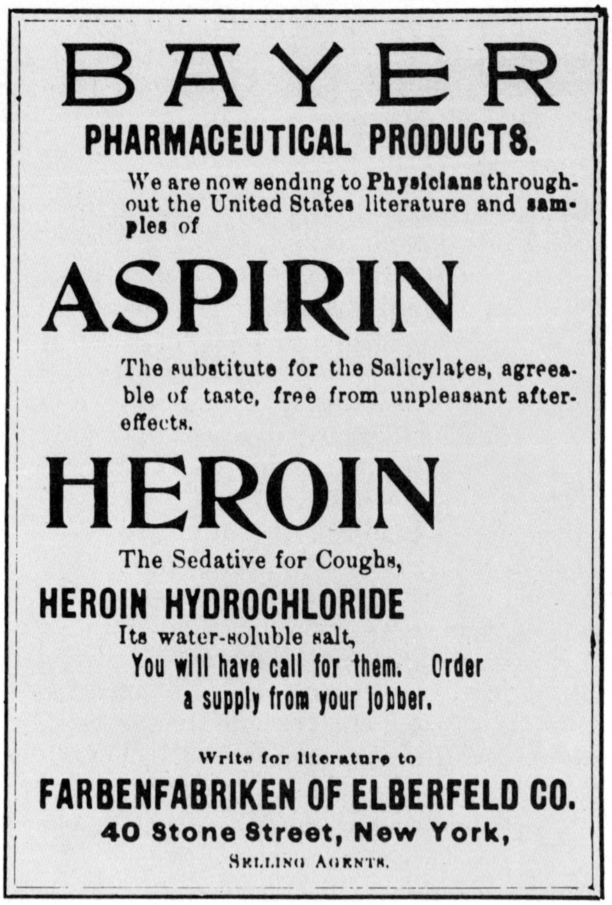

Opiates The central-nervous-system depressants known as the *opiate alkaloids* include opium, morphine, heroin, and codeine. Together with the synthetic drugs Demerol and methadone, these are classified as *opiates* (formerly called narcotics) and are widely used both in medicine and illicitly. The opiates can be taken in a variety of ways: opium is swallowed or smoked; morphine is injected; heroin is commonly injected or sniffed; and methadone is either swallowed or injected.

Figure 11.6 Opiates were active ingredients in many patent medicines sold around the turn of the century. They were peddled as cures for an endless variety of ailments, ranging from arthritis to impotence.

Opium is a juice derived from the opium poppy. Its active ingredient is *morphine,* which is widely used for medical purposes. *Heroin* is derived from morphine. Although it is used for medical purposes in England and a few other developed countries, it is barred from medical use in the United States and is the most popular of the illicitly used opiates. Pure heroin is about two and one-half times more potent, weight for weight, than morphine. Street heroin, however, averages only 3 to 5 percent pure. Medically used morphine preparations are therefore far more potent than street heroin.

The opiates have a high potential for tolerance and dependence. The usual starting dose of heroin is 3 milligrams. Tolerance, however, can increase a user's needed dose to 1,000 milligrams within several months. Heroin dependence thus can become a very expensive habit, costing a hundred dollars a day or more.

The opiates initially relieve tension and anxiety, decrease physical drive, and produce drowsiness. Some users experience a sense of well-being or euphoria, but others—particularly if they are not anxious or in pain—experience distinct unpleasantness. In medicine, the opiates are used to reduce pain, control diarrhea, and suppress coughs.

The opiates have more potential for dependence than either alcohol or the sedative-hypnotics. Nevertheless, only a minority of people exposed to opiates, either medically or on the black market, continue to use them to the point where they become dependent.

According to the National Institute on Drug Abuse, there are about 1,700 deaths a year in the United States due to heroin and morphine (compared to about 2,500 from alcohol). Some of these deaths are accidents due to variations in the strength of street drugs and also in individual tolerance. Others are suicides or murders by overdose. Still others are due not to the effect of the drugs themselves but to complications—such as hepatitis or endocarditis (inflammation of the membrane lining the heart)—caused by unsterile injections.

Although the symptoms of withdrawal from heroin or morphine are less severe than those from alcohol or the barbiturates, they can be excruciating to the addict. About four to six hours after the last dose, runny eyes and nose, yawning, and perspiring appear. As these symptoms increase in intensity, addicts also suffer intestinal pains and diarrhea, nausea, and vomiting. Heart rate and blood pressure increase. Their skin breaks into goose pimples; their muscles and bones ache severely; and they feel weak and depressed. These symptoms reach a peak in twenty-four hours and are usually over within forty-eight hours.

When opiate abuse occurs, both short-term treatment and long-term rehabilitation are necessary to overcome the effects of the drugs and permit abusers to lead normal lives. In the United States, treatment for heroin dependence has been almost nonexistent. It has often involved "cold turkey" withdrawal in jails, extended medical and psychiatric care in hospitals or clinics, or confinement in public health facilities. More recently, self-help groups (such as Daytop), which are based on the principles of Alcoholics Anonymous, have tried to provide a more intensive and supportive environment for rehabilitation.

One of the most active programs to help heroin abusers involves the use of the drug *methadone.* Methadone is an inexpensive, long-acting synthetic opiate that can be taken by mouth. It has been used as a painkiller in both Europe and the United States since World War II. In 1964, Dr. Vincent Dole and Dr. Marie Nyswander of Rockefeller University found that they could keep abusers off heroin by slowly building up a daily maintenance level of methadone, which blocked the withdrawal effects of heroin without interfering with its euphoric effect, but had little euphoric effect itself. Since then, methadone treatment clinics have been opened in many cities, with the largest and most ambitious programs in New York City and Washington, D.C.

In these programs, heroin abusers come once a day to drink a dose of methadone in a cup of orange juice. Within weeks, they have lost their craving for heroin. In most maintenance programs, they then continue indefinitely to take 60 to 120 milligrams of methadone daily. Urinalysis is done regularly to detect any use of heroin, other opiates, amphetamines, or barbiturates.

In theory, the ex-heroin abusers are able to stop the criminal activity that supported their expensive habit, and—while on methadone—can live an essentially normal life, going to school or working. The cost for treatment is much less than the cost of keeping the person in prison.

From the start, however, methadone treatment has been controversial, and it has not proved to be a panacea for the heroin abuse problem. Methadone in itself can cause dependence, and critics point out that the treatment simply substitutes one opiate for another. In fact, a black market in methadone has developed. While a daily moderate dose of the drug does not seem to impair functioning in any way, overdose can cause death, particularly when combined with other depressants, such as alcohol, heroin, or barbiturates. In 1976, Drs. Dole and Nyswander themselves reported that while thousands of former heroin abusers have been rehabilitated, "The great majority of heroin addicts in our cities remain on the streets, and programs have lost their ability to attract them to treatment."

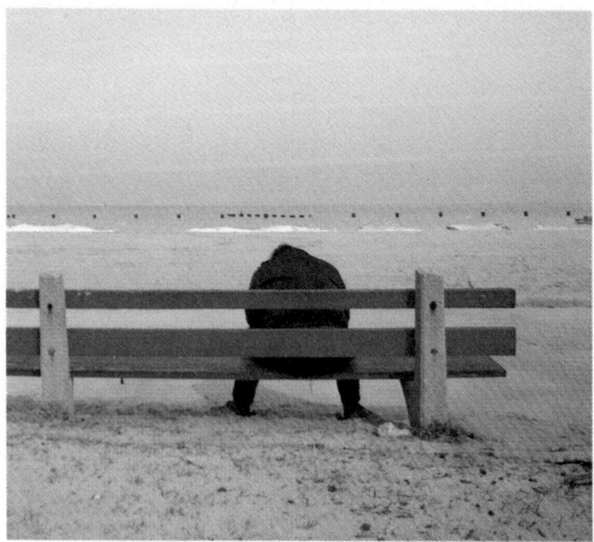

Figure 11.7 Depression—the most common emotional disorder—can be treated by drugs such as the tricyclics, which elevate mood and increase activity and drive.

Major Tranquilizers

The term *tranquilizer* is very misleading, because it is applied to two totally separate categories of drugs with different uses and side effects. One category is the so-called "minor tranquilizers," discussed above in the *Sedative-Hypnotics* section. These minor tranquilizers, which include the benzodiazepines (Valium and Librium) and meprobamate (Miltown), are more accurately called *antianxiety drugs.*

The other category is the *major tranquilizers,* which are more accurately called the *antipsychotic drugs.* These include several pharmacological classes: the phenothiazines (Thorazine, Mellaril), the butyrophenones (Haldol), and the thioxanthenes. These drugs are used to treat serious psychiatric illnesses, particularly schizophrenia, the most prevalent psychotic condition, in which people may lose contact with reality and experience delusions and hallucinations. Hundreds of thousands of psychiatric patients take these drugs on a long-term basis, often for years at a time. The phenothiazines increase a person's sensitivity to alcohol, and all the antipsychotic drugs may produce some neurological side effects. However, these drugs do not produce dependence and are rarely abused.

Antidepressants and Lithium

A number of important medical advances have recently been made in developing drugs that act directly on *affective* disorders in mood. The *antidepressants,* or mood elevators, are used to treat people with depression, the commonest emotional disorder. These drugs include the monoamine oxidase (MAO) inhibitors and the tricyclics (imipramine). The MAO inhibitors have a number of dangerous side effects and have been largely replaced by the less toxic tricyclics. In certain individuals, these drugs elevate mood and increase activity and drive. These effects do not appear immediately, but only after the person has taken the drug for many weeks. The antidepressants seem to be more effective in treating individuals with severe depression unmixed with such other components as anxiety, hostility, and hyperactivity.

According to current theory, a person's moods are influenced by the activity of certain biochemical substances—called *neurotransmitters*—that carry impulses from nerve cell to nerve cell in particular parts of the brain involved in the emotions. If there is too little neurotransmitter activity, the nerve impulses travel sluggishly and the person feels depressed. The antidepressant drugs are believed to alleviate depression by increasing the available supply and activity of these key neurotransmitters.

Lithium is one of the newest drugs for the treatment of mood disorders. It is effective in improving patients with mania, a condition characterized by exaggerated euphoria, hyperactivity, and excessive self-confidence. Lithium is also useful in treating manic-depression, a less common form of depression in which a person swings from manic "highs" to extreme "lows."

Stimulants

The most commonly used central-nervous-system stimulants are caffeine, nicotine, amphetamines, and cocaine. Nicotine will be covered in Chapter 13. The discussion here will focus on caffeine, amphetamines, and cocaine as representative of this group of drugs.

Caffeine *Caffeine* is the main active ingredient in coffee, tea, cocoa, cola drinks, and over-the-counter preparations for overcoming fatigue (No-Doz, for example). Although caffeine is a potent CNS stimulant, the low doses normally consumed produce only mild effects. Because the drug is so readily available and inexpensive, and because of its social acceptability and relative harmlessness, caffeine is the psychoactive drug most widely used by Americans of all ages.

The dose of caffeine in a single cup of coffee or tea relieves drowsiness and muscle fatigue, stimulates thinking, and promotes more sustained physical and intellectual activity. The nicotine in one cigarette is roughly comparable in effect to that of the caffeine in one cup of coffee. The amount of nicotine normally consumed thus also acts as a mild stimulant. Both caffeine and nicotine produce tolerance and habituation.

Caffeine abuse can occur when people consume excessive amounts of caffeine-containing beverages: six or more cups of coffee or bottles of cola a day. The physical symptoms of such caffeine overconsumption include restlessness, irritability, insomnia, and aggravation of peptic ulcer and high blood pressure.

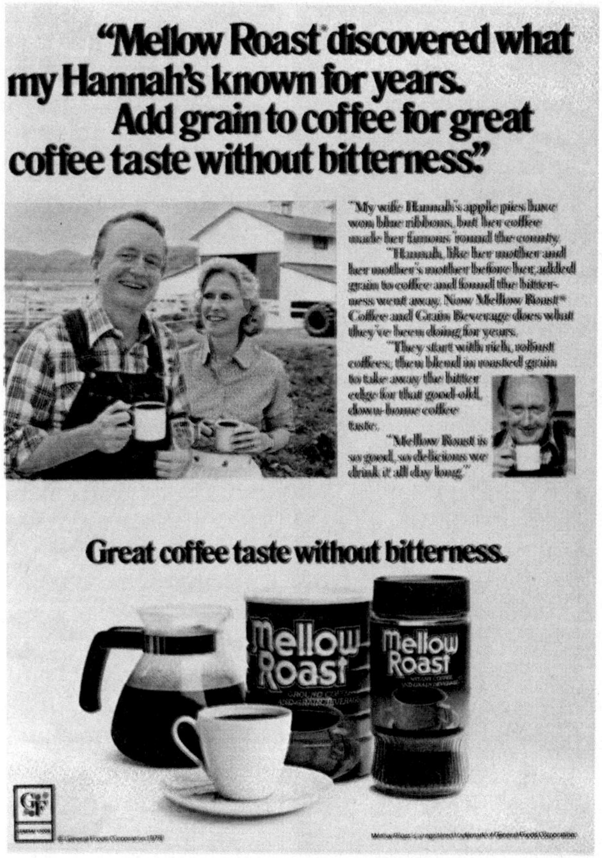

Figure 11.8 The wide popularity of coffee, tea, cocoa, and cola drinks makes caffeine the most commonly used psychoactive drug in the United States.

Amphetamines The amphetamines ("uppers") are a group of synthetic drugs that include Benzedrine ("bennies"), Methedrine (methamphetamine or "speed"), Preludin (phenmetrazine), and Dexedrine ("dexies"). In low to moderate doses, amphetamines usually produce a sense of increased energy and alertness; an elevation of mood; anxiety and irritability; and a decrease in both fatigue and appetite. In medicine, amphetamines have been used as diet pills, although they are ineffective as an appetite suppressant for more than a few weeks. They can sometimes improve performance in activities requiring extreme physical effort and endurance, such as military combat or athletics, by shortening physical reaction time and improving motor coordination. However, their improvement of performance is limited and they are dangerous when thus used because they increase both heart rate and blood pressure.

One nonmedical pattern of amphetamine use is the taking of low doses, in the form of pills, for limited periods of time by students cramming for exams, tired politicians and executives, and long-distance truck drivers. However, the material learned while under the influence of amphetamines can often be recalled only while on amphetamines. And using amphetamines to stay awake while driving is risky because the drug's effects often wear off abruptly. The user may quickly become drowsy and even fall asleep.

Amphetamines are much more abused than caffeine. Tolerance develops in a relatively short time, and the user must gradually increase the dose to achieve the initial effects. Prolonged use or large doses are nearly always followed by depression and fatigue; side effects can include insomnia, headaches, dizziness, agitation, confusion, and delirium. For some individuals, a pattern of prolonged use may ultimately lead to a paranoid psychosis, involving delusions, hallucinations, unfounded suspicions, and hostility.

Intravenous injection of large doses of amphetamines rapidly leads to abuse. Individuals may have a *run,* during which they inject the drug every few hours for a period of several days. During this time, they may eat little and remain awake continuously. Immediately after each injection, they experience a pleasurable feeling called a *flash* or *rush,* and for several hours they feel invigorated and perhaps euphoric. When they begin to feel uneasy and irritable, they take another injection. A run ends when users run out of the drug or become too disorganized or paranoid to continue. They then may sleep for twelve to eighteen hours or longer. Afterward, most users are lethargic and some are depressed. Taking amphetamines again relieves the lethargy and depression, and the cycle begins anew.

Although no withdrawal symptoms per se follow amphetamine abuse, there is usually some physical discomfort—such as prolonged sleeplessness and irregular eating—associated with abrupt cessation of high doses. Intravenous use may cause death due to burst blood vessels or stroke, as well as to infections (hepatitis, endocarditis) from unsterile needles.

Chronic amphetamine use can gradually erode personal, social, and work relationships until the user can focus on nothing but procuring and using the drug. This progressive elimination of formerly meaningful activities closely resembles the classical dependence syndrome of the opiates.

People who go on runs frequently try a variety of depressants to counteract the discomfort they feel afterward. They often find that barbiturates or heroin not only help them come down but also produce pleasurable feelings of their own. With time, heroin use can become more frequent.

Cocaine The stimulant *cocaine* ("coke") is a drug extracted from the leaves of the South American coca bush. Cocaine's effects and abuses are similar to those of the amphetamines, but it has not been used as extensively in the United States because it is not as readily available and is extremely expensive.

In medicine, cocaine is used as a local anesthetic. It numbs tissue and constricts the blood vessels, and is primarily employed in surgery on the membranes lining the nose and throat.

Recreationally, a powdery form of the drug known as "snow" is usually sniffed or "snorted" through the nose. Abusers, upon developing tolerance, often switch to intravenous injections, sometimes combining cocaine with heroin.

The "high" from cocaine—the feeling of well-being, increased energy, and sociability—is more intense than that from the amphetamines but does not last as long. Repeated cocaine inhalation irritates the mucous membranes lining the nose, and chronic users typically have nasal congestion or a runny nose. Prolonged use can also cause deterioration of the septum (the wall between the nostrils). Cocaine produces particularly strong psychological dependence or habituation. Chronic users may experience restlessness, anxiety, and irritability. Some people develop a characteristic cocaine psychosis, which may include tactile hallucinations of "bugs" crawling on the skin. Cocaine can kill, although uncommonly, as a result of seizures, respiratory arrest, and coma.

In the past, such eminent personalities as Sigmund Freud have been cocaine users. In recent years, the drug reportedly has become extremely fashionable among rock musicians, movie stars, and other celebrities. Its cost can

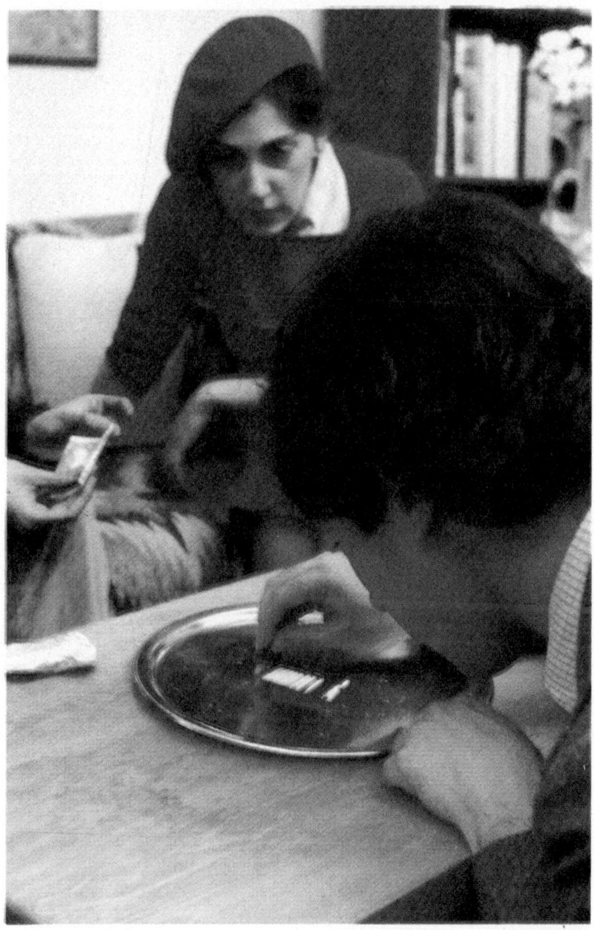

Figure 11.9 Cocaine has become very fashionable recently, and more and more young people are trying it.

run to more than twenty dollars for a fifteen-minute "high." It is possible that this expense itself (it has been called "the champagne of drugs"), plus elaborate cocaine-taking rituals, are strongly reinforcing elements in some social circles. Despite the cost, the 1977 National Survey on Drug Abuse found that about 20 percent of young adults between the ages of eighteen and twenty-five have tried cocaine, and more than half of them know people who have used the drug. This was a marked increase from 1972, when only 10 percent had used it. In most states, however, illegal dispensing and possession of cocaine are prosecuted as severely as is that of heroin. The legal risks of cocaine use, therefore, are particularly serious.

Psychedelic-Hallucinogens

This is actually a grab-bag category, which includes a variety of drugs also called *psychotomimetics* or *psychotogenics.* This group includes lysergic acid diethylamide (LSD), phenylethylamine derivatives (peyote, mescaline), the indole derivatives (psilocybin, DMT), and phencyclidine (PCP, Sernyl).

There is no sharp line separating these substances from other classes of psychoactive drugs. Under certain conditions or at high doses, a variety of other drugs (including alcohol) can also induce illusions, hallucinations, delusions, paranoia, and similar alternations of mood and behavior. The features that usually distinguish the LSD-type drugs from other classes are their greater likelihood of producing these effects and the greater intensity and duration of the experience.

Although marked tolerance can develop with frequent use, these drugs cause little compulsive drug-seeking behavior and no physical dependence. Mescaline, LSD, and psilocybin have a cross-tolerance to each other and are generally similar in their effects. They may therefore exert their effects through a common, although unknown, mechanism. Since LSD is the best known and understood of these drugs, it will be discussed as a representative example.

LSD The ingestion of even one-millionth of an ounce of LSD or "acid" will produce noticeable effects in most people. An average dose of 150 to 250 micrograms produces slight dizziness, weakness, dilation of the pupils, and particularly such perceptual alterations as intense visual experience, distorted time sense, heightened auditory acuity, and *synesthesia*—the blending of two senses so that the person "hears" colors or "sees" sounds. Psychological symptoms include the flooding of consciousness with numerous thoughts in new combinations, rapid changes in mood, and a feeling that one's body is distorted. These effects usually occur in sequence. Physical changes come first, then the perceptual alterations, and finally the psychic changes. There is considerable overlap, however, among the three phases.

As with other drugs, the sort of experience one will have with LSD, particularly with average doses, is determined in large part by the purity of the drug, the setting, the user's personality and mood, and what he or she expects of the drug.

There is a disturbing incidence of abuses resulting from LSD and related drugs. Severe panic reactions ("bad trips") sometimes occur. Both occasional and chronic users can experience acute, short-term psychotic reactions and *flashbacks.* Flashbacks are brief, sudden, unexpected perceptual distortions and bizarre thoughts—similar to those experienced while on an LSD trip—that can occur months or years after the pharmacological effects of the drug have worn off. In some people, LSD can precipitate serious depression, paranoid behavior, or chronic psychoses. Fatal accidents and suicides have also resulted from the use of LSD.

Other Psychedelic-Hallucinogens Although LSD is representative of the psychedelics, the use and effects of related drugs do vary in many ways. Again, it must be emphasized that these effects (especially with moderate doses) largely depend upon factors such as the setting and the expectations of the individual.

Phencyclidine (PCP, Sernyl, Angel Dust) is a very dangerous and perplexing drug, which has become increasingly available and popular in recent years. It was originally developed for medical use, but was discarded because of its unpredictable, adverse side effects. Its wide availability is due to the fact that it can be readily made from common chemicals in makeshift laboratories. In small doses (1 to 5 milligrams), PCP produces a floating feeling of euphoria and an overall numbness, together with mild loss of inhibitions. In larger doses (5 to 15 milligrams), it commonly produces body distortions, reduced perception of pain, impairment of thought and speech, disorientation of time and place, restlessness, or quiet withdrawal. At 10 milligrams or more, PCP may induce behavior mimicking psychoses, including catatonia or paranoid schizophrenia. People under the influence of PCP may become seriously agitated and combative; they may be very difficult to control; and they may behave in ways that are dangerous to themselves and others. Not all PCP experiences produce these effects, but the fact that reactions to it are so unpredictable—from person to person or from time to time in the same person—makes PCP an exceedingly hazardous drug.

Mescaline, in the form of peyote buttons, is the ceremonial drug of the (Indian) Native American Church. It is also popular with drug users who value "natural" drugs and shun synthetic drugs such as LSD. Mescaline, however, can also be produced synthetically.

Psilocybin, which comes from the Mexican mushroom psilocybe, has less intense effects than LSD and is probably the safest of the psychedelics. Dimethyltryptamine (DMT), diethyltryptamine (DET), and dimethoxymethylamphetamine (DOM or STP) are similar to LSD in many ways. DMT and DET produce effects more quickly, and STP induces longer trips.

Cannabis (Marijuana)

Marijuana and hashish are the main active drug preparations derived from the hemp plant *Cannabis sativa,* which is grown around the world. In average doses (such as the amount inhaled from smoking one or two joints), marijuana acts somewhat like a sedative-hypnotic, somewhat like alcohol, and somewhat like a stimulant, as well as having some unique properties of its own. *Hashish* is a concentrated resin made from the plant leaves. It is thus more potent than crude marijuana.

The active ingredient in marijuana and hashish is a chemical called tetrahydrocannabinol (THC). The amount of THC in a given preparation determines its potency. THC has recently been produced synthetically, but it is difficult to make and thus too expensive to be widely available either for research or unlawful use.

Marijuana has become an extremely popular drug among young adults, and more and more adolescents are using it as well. In 1977 the National Institute on Drug Abuse reported that three out of five Americans between the

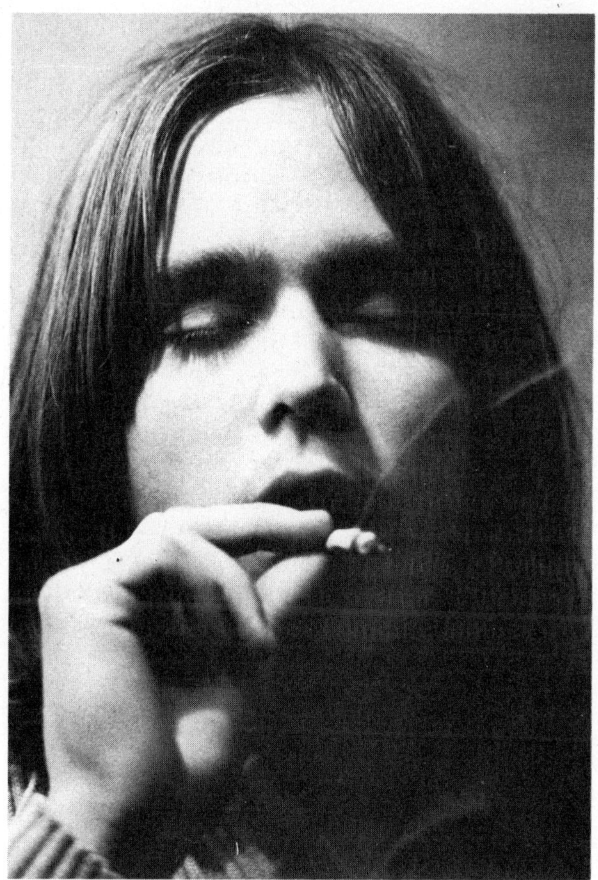

Figure 11.10 The effects of marijuana vary from person to person, depending largely on the user's expectations and past experience with the drug.

ages of eighteen and twenty-five had tried marijuana; one in four were current users. Among high-school seniors, one in eleven used marijuana on a daily basis. Between 1976 and 1977, the number of twelve- to seventeen-year-olds who used marijuana increased by 25 percent.

Short-Term Effects In moderate doses, a common effect of marijuana is the alteration of sounds, colors, and other sensory phenomena. There is wide variation in these perceptual changes, and marked differences between individuals in their awareness and interpretation of them. These differences are significantly influenced by the user's expectations and previous experience with the drug. The chronic user may get a "high" from low-potency marijuana, while the neophyte may feel nothing from the same dose.

As with other drugs, the effects of cannabis on mood and personality also vary. Initially, there may be a slight apprehension, then a pleasant lassitude interspersed with euphoria. Later, the sedative effects of the drug predominate and often produce sleep. The acute physical effects of marijuana are minimal. They include an increase in heart rate and also dilation of blood vessels in the eye (causing characteristic reddened eyes).

With higher doses of marijuana, the behavioral effects are determined more by the drug properties per se than by psychosocial factors. With these higher doses (and occasionally with low doses in susceptible individuals), the changes described above may be markedly exaggerated. Subtle alterations of sensory input become gross distortions, the user may feel inundated by myriad sensory cues from the environment, and he or she may be unable to think clearly. Such effects on thought processes lead some users, especially neophytes, to think they are losing control over their minds. The user's mood changes from the usual relaxation and tranquility to a state of anxiety and panic.

Long-Term Effects The long-term effects of cannabis consumption are still being researched. It is difficult to evaluate the relative role of other factors—such as poor nutrition, use of other drugs, and socioeconomic conditions—in producing changes in chronic cannabis users. Nevertheless, scientists predict that long-term heavy use will produce, in some susceptible individuals, an impairment of certain cognitive functions, such as short-term memory and the ability to sustain attention. A few vulnerable long-term users of excessive amounts of marijuana are likely to show persistent changes in mood and sensory abilities. Although cannabis does not produce physical dependence, a small percentage of chronic users may increasingly center their lives on the drug, gradually withdrawing from other activities that were once meaningful to them.

According to the National Institute on Drug Abuse's 1977 report, researchers have identified several high-risk groups that may be es-

VIEWPOINT

Is Marijuana Safe?

With millions of Americans getting high on marijuana these days, scientists have begun to study the long-term physical and psychological effects of marijuana smoking. Because this is such a new area of research, findings pave often been contradictory or inconclusive.

In a classic study of marijuana smokers, Zinberg and Weil found that marijuana has few serious damaging physical effects and that it is a relatively harmless intoxicant. The physical changes they observed include a moderate increase in heart rate and reddening of the whites of the eyes. They found no effect on blood-sugar levels, pupil size, and respiratory rate. Zinberg and Weil point out that although the long-term effects of marijuana smoking are not yet known, these relatively mild short-term findings make serious, long-term damage unlikely. Some researchers are worried, however, about the irritating effect marijuana has on the lungs, which may result in chronic respiratory disorders. Others believe heavy use of marijuana may cause chromosome breakage or abnormalities, but more research is still needed to confirm or deny this connection.

Researchers have an even more mixed view of the psychological effects of marijuana smoking. Even though most believe that there is no simple cause-and-effect relationship between marijuana smoking and psychological dependence, they point to other serious psychological effects that may result from regular smoking.

Studies have shown that marijuana smokers have experienced visual and auditory hallucinations, distortion of visual perception, depression or overexcitement, shift of time orientation from past or future to present, and paranoid delusions of persecution or grandeur. Smokers may also have trouble remembering what was said and have gaps in their stream of thought. Teen-agers who smoke marijuana may be more prone than adults to these psychological problems. Driving while under the influence of marijuana may also be dangerous in some cases.

Basically, evidence indicates that marijuana has much less noticeable effects than alcohol. "As a result it seems possible to ignore the effects of marijuana on consciousness, to adapt to them, and to control them to a significant degree."

Source: Norman E. Zinberg and Andrew T. Weil, "The Effects of Marijuana on Human Beings," *The New York Times Magazine*, March 8, 1969, pp. 376–381. Deena D. Dell and Judith A. Snyder, "Marijuana: Pro and Con," *American Journal of Nursing* (April 1977), pp. 630–635.

pecially susceptible to adverse effects from marijuana. These include young people under the age of eighteen, who are at a critical stage of physical and psychological development; people with heart or lung impairments; and those with a history of serious psychological problems.

Possible Medical Uses In recent years, investigators have been paying increasing attention to several possible medical applications of marijuana—or, more likely, purified THC. Some researchers are studying its effectiveness in relieving the nausea and vomiting associated with chemotherapy for cancer. Others are testing it on glaucoma, an eye disease in which the pressure inside the eyeball is increased. Marijuana may be helpful in reducing this pressure in some patients. These medical studies are mostly preliminary, but since January 1979, physicians may legally prescribe marijuana as a medication.

Over-the-Counter Drugs

There is a vast assortment of drugs that can be purchased legally, at drugstores and supermarkets, without a doctor's prescription—the so-called proprietary or over-the-counter (OTC) drugs. These include everything from mouthwashes to antacids, antiperspirants to cough medicines, cold remedies to deodorant soaps. The OTC drugs are big business; there are hundreds of thousands of them on the market, and Americans spend between $3 and $4 billion a year on them. Since 1972, the Food and Drug Administration has been conducting a massive review of the safety and effectiveness of these OTC drugs. The scorecard so far is mixed. Some of the drugs (aspirin) are useful and effective; some (laxatives) are widely misused; and others (daytime sedatives) are often unnecessary. All, however, must be used with discretion. For one physician's recommendations as to what your medicine cabinet should contain, see Table 11.2.

These OTC drugs are intended only for use in treating temporary, minor aches and illnesses. The trouble with such self-medication is that it depends upon self-diagnosis—and one may or may not be right about the need for

Table 11.2 Your Home Pharmacy (Store all medications out of the reach of children.)

Ailment	Medication
Allergy	Antihistamines
	Nose drops and sprays
Colds and coughs	Cold tablets/cough syrups
Constipation	Milk of magnesia, bulk laxatives
Dental problems (preventive)	Sodium fluoride
Diarrhea	*Kaopectate, paragoric
Eye irritations	Eye drops and artificial tears
Hemorrhoids	Hemorrhoid preparations
Pain and fever (in children)	*Aspirin, acetaminophen
	†Liquid acetaminophen, aspirin, rectal suppositories
Poisoning (to induce vomiting)	†Syrup of ipecac
Skin problems	
Dry skin	Moisturizing creams and lotions
Fungus	Antifungal preparations
Sunburn (preventive)	Sunscreen agents
Sprains	*Elastic bandages
Stomach, upset	*Nonabsorbable antacid
Warts	Wart remover
Wounds (minor)	*Adhesive tape, bandages
(antiseptic)	*Hydrogen peroxide, iodine
(soaking agent)	*Sodium bicarbonate
Vitamin deficiency	§Vitamin preparations

*Starred items are basic and should be included in every medicine cabinet.
†Daggered items are musts in homes with small children.
§Not routinely recommended. True vitamin deficiency is rare.
Source: From Donald M. Vickery and James F. Fries, *Take Care of Yourself: A Consumer's Guide to Medical Care* (Reading, Mass.: Addison-Wesley, 1978), p. 44.

the medication. The threat to health and even life posed by use of these medications without sufficient information is significant. With all these drugs, you should carefully read what the labels say about dosages and warnings. Some of the OTC drugs you are most likely to use include the following.

Aspirin and Acetaminophen

Probably the most widely used of all drugs, aspirin is marketed both alone and in combination with other drugs. It is often the only significant ingredient in many cold and pain remedies. In 1977, the FDA review panel found aspirin both safe and effective for the temporary relief of minor aches and pains and for reducing fever and body-joint inflammation. Aspirin does not cure the underlying disorders; it merely relieves these symptoms.

Aspirin does have drawbacks. It is the leading cause of poisoning deaths among children under five. It can also upset the stomach, cause ulcers to flare up, interfere with blood clotting, or cause ringing in the ears.

Since all aspirin has the same effect, it makes sense to buy the cheapest brand. Do not buy a large economy size if you do not use aspirin much; the average shelf life of aspirin is only three years. If the pills smell vinegary when you open the bottle, the aspirin has begun to deteriorate and you should discard it.

Acetaminophen, which is sold under several brand names, is also safe and effective for reducing fever and temporarily relieving minor aches and pains. According to the FDA, however, there is no basis for claims that it is safer than aspirin. Acetaminophen can cause liver damage and also disturb the action of the kidneys.

Antacids

Antacids neutralize hyperacidity of the stomach; the FDA says they are good for heartburn, sour stomach, and acid indigestion—all conditions related to the effects of stomach acid. While the stomach does normally secrete hydrochloric acid, hyperacidity is relatively rare, and does not cause most minor stomach upsets. These are usually due to overeating or not relaxing while eating. Antacids are valuable, however, in treating peptic ulcers under the supervision of a physician.

Some antacids are absorbed into the body from the gastrointestinal tract. The chief absorbable antacid is sodium bicarbonate, an alkaline substance that is meant to neutralize the excess acid in the stomach. The problem is that the sodium bicarbonate promptly leaves the stomach and passes into the intestinal tract, where it is absorbed into the bloodstream. In large doses, it may disturb the body's acid-base balance. It does not relieve the basic cause of the hyperacidity and it may stimulate the stomach to secrete more acid in a "rebound" effect.

Other types of antacids are not absorbed by the body and thus do not disturb the body's acid-base balance. However, they may cause diarrhea (if they contain magnesium) or constipation (if they contain aluminum). Most nonabsorbable antacids contain both these ingredients to minimize both side effects.

Antacids come in both liquid and tablet form. The liquid form is more effective, because it coats more of the stomach wall. The pills may not do the job unless you chew them thoroughly.

Antihistamines

Antihistamines act, it is believed, by suppressing symptoms caused by the body's release of a substance called histamine, which dilates the capillaries and plays a major role in allergic reactions. Antihistamines thus can temporarily shrink swollen membranes and block such symptoms as a runny nose, sneezing, watery eyes, and itching due to allergies or common colds. However, antihistamines do not affect the release of histamine in the first place; they do not cure the allergy or shorten the course of the cold. They only relieve the discomfort.

The side effects of antihistamines can be severe in some individuals: they can cause drowsiness, dizziness, blurred vision, headaches, nervousness, and nausea. Prolonged use can permanently damage the mucous membranes of the nose, throat, and sinuses, and thus diminish normal body defenses against infection.

Laxatives

The FDA review panel, in 1975, found that "there is widespread misuse of self-prescribed laxatives." Many people take laxatives because they believe—erroneously—that it is harmful not to have a bowel movement every day. Actually, says the FDA, the normal range is from three a day to three a week. When a person does take a laxative, it completely evacuates the bowels; several days thus go by before the bowels return to their normal habits. This often leads people to take more laxatives, in a vicious circle, and develop a laxative habit.

The FDA warns that you should not take a laxative for longer than a week except under the supervision of a physician. Prolonged use can seriously interfere with normal bowel movements, and using them for acute stomach pain, vomiting, and other digestive tract symptoms can threaten your life. It is far better to rely upon proper diet (raw vegetables, fruits, whole-grain foods) and adequate fluid intake to control constipation.

If you do take a laxative, bulk laxatives are recommended because they have no contraindications or side effects. They pass through the digestive tract without being absorbed into the body. They work by drawing water into the stools, forming a thick solution that provides bulk. The other recommended laxative is milk of magnesia, which is mild and works by retaining water in the bowels and thus softening the stools.

Antidiarrhea Preparations

You should use an antidiarrhea drug only in cases of severe diarrhea, and you should try a clear liquid diet first. The FDA review panel, in 1975, judged that only four ingredients are effective against diarrhea: three opium derivatives (opium powder, tincture of opium, and paregoric) and polycarbophil. If diarrhea persists, you should see a physician.

Emetics

Every household with small children should have on hand a bottle of ipecac syrup to induce vomiting in case of accidental poisoning. In most cases of poisoning, you should get the child to vomit and empty the stomach as soon as possible in order to rid the body of the poison. However, if he or she has swallowed a strong acid or alkali or petroleum product, you should not induce the child to vomit, because these substances will do additional damage, destroying tissue or inflaming the lungs, as they come back up. Instead, give the child milk to neutralize the caustic agent. In either case, says the FDA, you should *first* call your doctor, poison control center, or hospital emergency room for advice.

PRESCRIPTION DRUGS

Prescription drugs, which are often stronger than over-the-counter drugs, have more potential for both good and bad. On one hand, prescription drugs can actually cure some diseases, not merely alleviate symptoms, but, on the other hand, they can also cause more serious adverse reactions.

If you do need a prescription, it is important that you tell the doctor if you are already taking any other drugs, because many drugs interact adversely with each other. You should also tell him or her about any food or drug allergies you may have. Some people, for instance, are allergic to penicillin. Before leaving the doctor's office with a prescription, you should know the answers to the following questions.

What is the drug? You should know not only the brand name but also the so-called "generic" name. This reflects its chemical composition, which is more informative than the brand name.

What is the drug supposed to do? All too often doctors gloss over this legitimate question by saying something like "It's to make you feel better." You are entitled to know precisely what effect the drug is expected to have on both your disease and your body.

How should I take the drug? Drugs can come in pills, liquids, or other forms. They can be swallowed, injected, inhaled, applied on the skin or mucous membranes, or taken as suppositories inserted in a body orifice. If you are to take the drug orally, should you take it with or without water or other liquids? Many drugs need to be taken with water to dissolve them or dilute their intensity. Aspirin, for instance, should always be taken with water to avoid stomach upset. On the other hand, tetracycline, a commonly prescribed antibiotic, should not be taken with milk or milk products.

When should I take the drug? Instructions to "take three times a day," for instance, do not tell you whether you should take the drug every eight hours, or whether you can take it with meals. Some drugs should be taken on an empty stomach so that the body absorbs them better. Others should be taken on a full stomach because they may otherwise irritate the stomach lining.

Does taking the drug require any change in diet or activities? In the case of a number of drugs, you should not drink alcohol while you are under prescription. Some other drugs may cause drowsiness or interfere with your coordination, so you should avoid driving, working with dangerous machinery, or other hazardous activities.

How long should I take the drug? Should I refill the prescription? You can stop taking some drugs as soon as the symptoms disappear. With some other drugs, it is necessary to keep taking them long after the symptoms have gone. This is often true of antibiotics: if you stop taking them too soon, the infection is likely to recur.

What if I accidentally miss a dose? With some

drugs that have a cumulative effect, it might lower the level of drug in your body to a point where it does little good—yet it might be dangerous to double up the next dose.

What side effects can I expect? All drugs can cause side effects ranging from the trivial to the serious. You should know whether to expect serious effects and, if so, how they can be treated.

What is the drug likely to cost? This is particularly important if you must take the drug over a long period of time. Sometimes you can save money if your doctor prescribes by generic rather than brand name. And sometimes the price of prescription drugs varies enormously from one pharmacy to another. You may want to shop prices by telephone.

Studies show that many patients never fill the prescriptions their doctors give them, and of those who do, over half make mistakes in taking them. Two common and potentially dangerous mistakes are sharing prescription drugs with other people and not discarding old medications. As with the psychoactive and OTC drugs, excessive, unnecessary, or incorrect use of prescription drugs can have damaging effects. The more you understand about *any* drug you take, the more likely you are to use it correctly and wisely.

SUMMARY

1. A drug is any biologically active substance foreign to the body that is deliberately introduced to affect its functioning. Drugs that act directly on the brain and central nervous system are called psychoactive drugs.
2. Drug abuse is excessive use of any drug that measurably damages health or impairs social or vocational adjustment.
3. Among the factors influencing the effect of any given drug on an individual are its dosage, its potency, its solubility in water or lipids, the site in the body where it acts, the setting in which it is taken, and the individual's own set or expectations.
4. There are no absolutely safe drugs; all drugs have side effects. Some 30,000 people die each year from adverse drug reactions. Drugs can also cause long-term harmful effects. Adverse interactions between two or more different drugs, taken at the same time, are a growing problem.
5. The escalating levels of drug dependence are psychological dependence (habituation), tolerance, and physical dependence. When a physically dependent person does not receive the drug, he or she may suffer withdrawal symptoms.
6. The five progressive patterns of drug use are experimental, social or recreational, circumstantial or situational, intensified, and compulsive use.
7. There is no agreement among experts about the causes of drug use and abuse, but most believe sociological factors are more important in determining drug use, while psycological factors are more important in contributing to drug abuse.
8. Depressants are drugs that slow the activity of the brain. The most widely used depressants (after alcohol) are the sedative-hypnotics, which include the barbiturates, the minor tranquilizers, and a group of chemically unrelated drugs. Barbiturates and other sedative-hypnotics are implicated in nearly 20 percent of all drug-related deaths.
9. The category of depressants known as the opiates includes the opiate alkaloids (opium, morphine, heroin, codeine) and the synthetic drugs Demerol and methadone. The opiates have more addictive potential than either alcohol or the sedative-hypnotics.
10. The major tranquilizers, the antidepressants, and lithium are used in medicine to treat people with schizophrenia, mania, depression, and other serious mental disorders.
11. The major central-nervous-system stimulants are caffeine, nicotine, the amphetamines, and cocaine. Caffeine is the psychoactive drug most widely used by Americans. Cocaine has become increasingly popular in recent years.
12. The psychedelic-hallucinogens include LSD, which produces intense perceptual alterations, and PCP (Angel Dust), which is a particularly dangerous drug because of its unpredictability.
13. The active ingredient in marijuana and hashish is tetrahydrocannabinol (THC). Marijuana acts somewhat like a sedative-hypnotic,

somewhat like alcohol, somewhat like a stimulant, and also has some unique properties of its own.

14. There is a great variety of over-the-counter (OTC) drugs available in drugstores and supermarkets. Common OTC drugs include aspirin, antacids, antihistamines, and laxatives. Some of these drugs have been found to be effective; others are widely misused.

15. If you need a prescription drug, you should ask its generic name, what it is supposed to do, how and when to take it, whether it requires any changes in your diet or activities, and what side effects to expect.

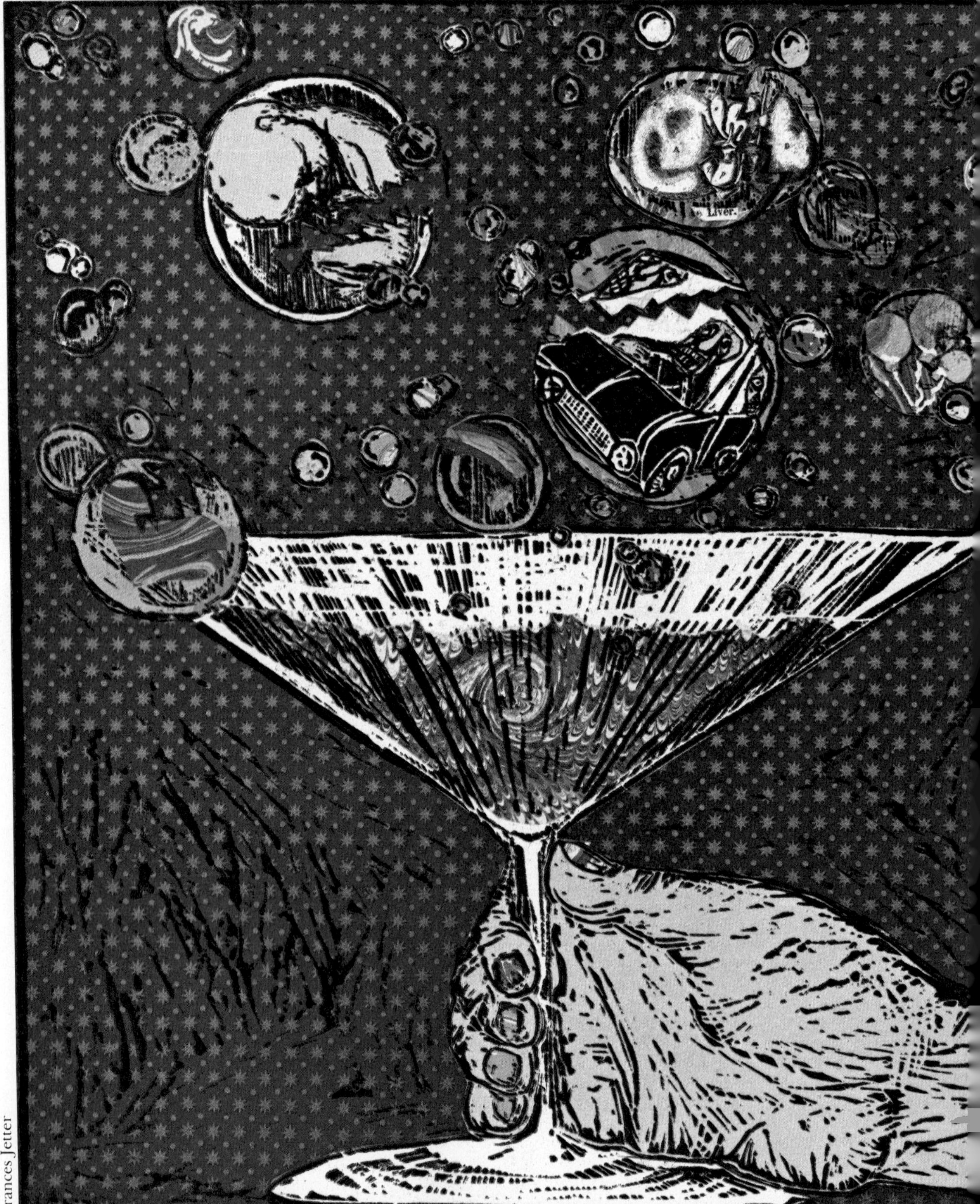

Frances Jetter

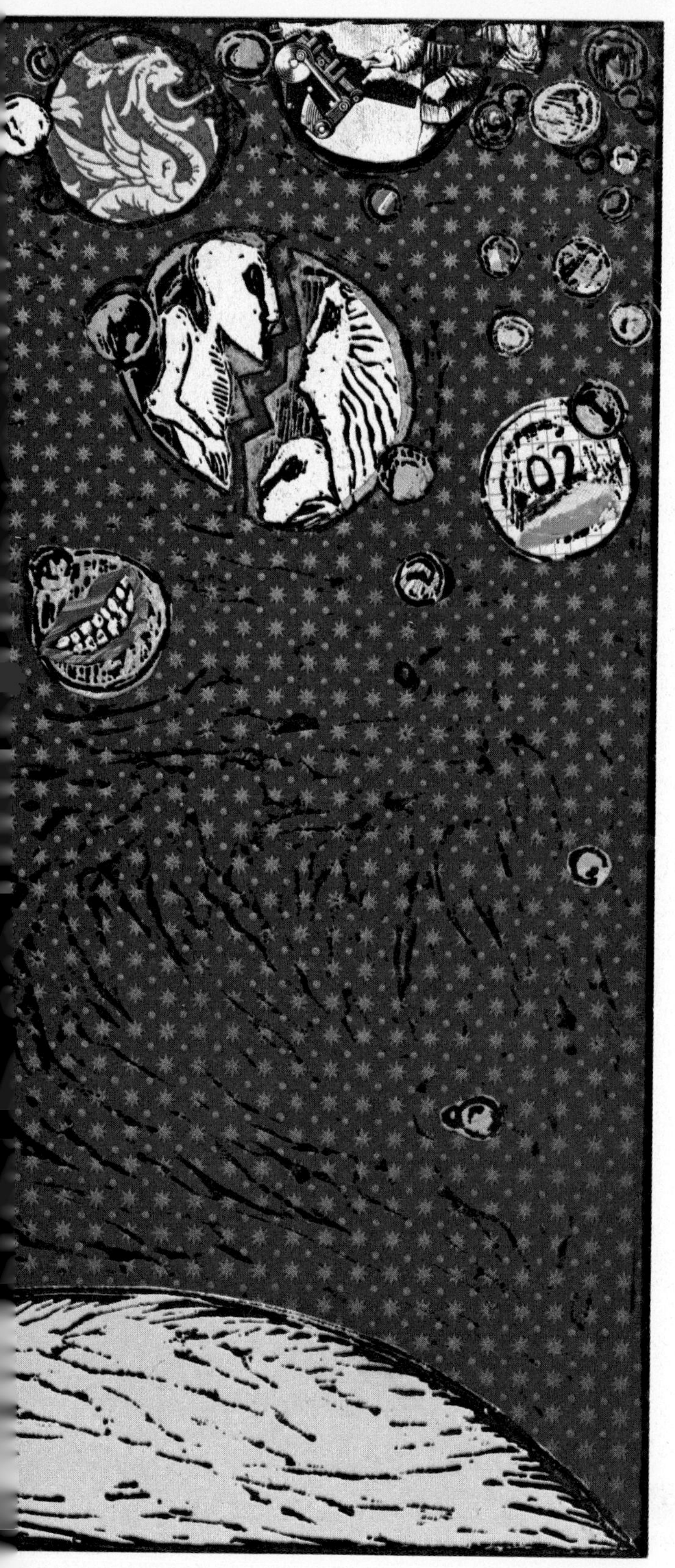

12 Alcohol Use and Abuse

Abuse of alcohol is one of the biggest health and social problems in the United States today. It is estimated that there are more than 15 million persons whose drinking is associated with serious problems, including about 10 million who are alcoholics. More than 50 percent of the fatal accidents and a high proportion of the injuries occurring on the nation's highways involve drivers or pedestrians who have had too much to drink. Alcohol use is often associated with crime, poverty, and other social problems. Alcohol also contributes to physical illness, mental illness, and family conflicts. Why, under these circumstances, do people drink?

When used in moderation, alcohol can reduce anxiety and tension and bring on a feeling of relaxation and well-being. These effects help explain why alcohol has had an accepted place in so many human societies. Nevertheless, few societies have been able to enjoy the benefits of alcohol without the complications inherent in the intoxicating properties of alcohol, a drug that can adversely affect any user temporarily and upon which many drinkers become dependent.

What are the physiological effects of alcohol on the human body? What are its psychological effects? What factors influence a person's response to the effects of alcohol? How does society affect alcohol use? What causes alcoholism? And how can it be treated? These are some of the questions that will be examined in this chapter.

PHYSIOLOGICAL EFFECTS OF ALCOHOL

Alcohol is a systemic drug, carried by the bloodstream to act on the central nervous system with both physiological and psychological consequences. Pharmacologically, alcohol is an anesthetic, a tranquilizer, and a depressant. It may seem at times that it is a stimulant, because it can spark conversation and activity in social settings. In fact, however, alcohol induces such mood changes because it depresses the part of the brain involved in sending out instructions to the body. This results in the most measurable of alcohol's effects—impairment of motor coordination. It is not known precisely how alcohol acts on brain cells to produce these acute effects. Under certain circumstances, even moderate doses of alcohol can also act on the brain to produce confusion and hallucinations.

Moderate amounts of alcohol can also affect the cardiovascular system by increasing the heart rate and dilating blood vessels near the skin. This vasodilation gives the drinker an illusion of feeling warmer, although actually the person is losing heat from the body more rapidly. Alcohol also increases secretion of saliva and stomach acid and is a mild diuretic.

As with other depressant drugs, daily alcohol intoxication produces a state of tolerance and physical dependence. When alcohol is stopped, the person undergoes withdrawal symptoms, the intensity of which reflects the degree to which the person is dependent. In those who are chemically dependent on alcohol, the withdrawal illness or abstinence syndrome can involve severe seizures and hallucinations or delirium tremens (DTs).

The "hangover" that follows a few hours' intoxication is frequently considered a state of mild withdrawal. Its severity is related to both

Table 12.1 Estimated Deaths Related to Alcohol in the United States, 1975

Cause of Death	Number of Deaths	Percent	Estimated Number
Alcohol as a direct cause			
Alcoholism	4,897	100	4,897
Alcoholic psychosis	356	100	356
Cirrhosis	31,623	41–95	12,965–30,042
Total	36,876		18,218–35,295
Alcohol as an indirect cause			
Accidents			
Motor vehicle	45,853	30–50	13,756–22,926
Falls	14,896	44.4	6,614
Fires	6,071	25.9	1,572
Other*	33,026	11.1	3,666
Homicides	21,310	49–70	10,442–14,917
Suicides	27,063	25–37	6,766–10,013
Total	148,219	29–40	42,816–59,708
Overall total	185,095		61,034–95,003

*Includes all accidents not listed above; but excludes accidents incurred in medical and surgical procedures.

Source: Ernest P. Noble, ed., *Third Special Report to the U.S. Congress on Alcohol and Health* (June 1978), p. 13; data from Nancy Day, *Alcohol and Mortality.* Paper prepared for National Institute on Alcohol Abuse and Alcoholism under Contract No. NIA-76-10(P). (January 1977); and National Center for Health Statistics, *Vital Statistics of the United States, 1972,* vol. 2 (Washington, D.C.: U.S. Government Printing Office, 1975).

the amount and duration of the drinking and the mental and physical condition of the individual. One may have a headache, be weak and nervous, feel nauseated and vomit; the heart may beat faster, and one may have difficulty thinking. Unfortunately, there is no cure for a hangover. Neither coffee nor vitamins nor the "hair of the dog" does much good, although aspirin, rest, liquids, and solid food do help. Fortunately, hangovers usually last less than thirty-six hours.

Prolonged heavy use of alcohol often brings a high rate of serious illness. It may bring on temporary or permanent psychotic conditions. Alcohol can irritate the stomach and contribute to gastrointestinal disorders, such as gastritis. Alcoholics frequently suffer from malnutrition and vitamin deficiency, because alcohol, which provides calories and depresses the appetite, does not supply vitamins and essential amino acids. Excessive alcohol intake damages the liver; it increases fat deposits and leads to cirrhosis of the liver, a serious disease in which the liver tissue degenerates. Heavy alcohol use is also associated with cancers of the mouth, pharynx, larynx, and esophagus, especially if the drinker also smokes. Heavy drinkers have significantly shorter life spans.

Alcohol Absorption and Blood Alcohol Level

As a psychoactive drug, alcohol is unique in that its effective dose is much greater than that of most other intoxicants. For example, full effects of LSD are observed upon ingestion of ten-millionths of an ounce, or about three-tenths of a milligram. Barbiturates need roughly 1,000 times larger amounts (about 300 milligrams) than LSD. With alcohol, intoxication follows an ingestion of about 50 to 100 grams (2 to 4 ounces), that is, 200 to 300 times more than barbiturates and almost a million times more than LSD. This difference occurs primarily because most of the alcohol ingested does not reach the brain. The body absorbs alcohol into the bloodstream partly through the lining of the stomach and partly through the small intestine. Once in the blood, between 80 and 90 percent of the alcohol is broken down in the liver and other tissues, eventually to carbon dioxide and water. The rest may circulate through the brain before being eliminated through the kidneys or sweat glands.

The *blood alcohol level*—the concentration of alcohol carried by the blood to the brain—determines how much effect the drug will have on a person's behavior. Whenever the rate at which alcohol is absorbed into the blood is greater than the rate of breakdown and elimination, the excess of unaltered, nonoxidized alcohol is able to reach the brain, where it produces its intoxicating effect.

The body oxidizes alcohol at a fairly constant rate, with variations depending largely on the size of the liver, which in turn is somewhat dependent on body weight. For example, the liver of a person weighing 150 pounds would oxidize about 0.3 ounce of pure alcohol an hour—roughly the alcohol to be found in 0.6 ounce of 50 percent whiskey or 7 ounces of 4 percent beer. A smaller, lighter person, with a correspondingly smaller liver, would have a higher alcohol level in the blood reaching the liver and possibly an even higher level in the blood leaving the liver.

Although there are individual variations, most people will experience little noticeable effect at a concentration of up to .02 percent alcohol in the blood (.02 grams per 100 milliliters of blood, or 2 parts of alcohol per 10,000 parts of blood). Some recognizable sensations will generally occur between the levels of .03 and .05 percent. These sensations may include lightheadedness, a sense of relaxation and well-being, and release of some personal inhibitions, often leading the drinker to say or do things not in that person's normal behavior pattern. By the time the blood concentration reaches .1 percent, there is major depression of sensory and motor functions. The drinker may stagger slightly, fumble objects, and have some trouble saying even familiar words.

If alcohol concentration reaches .2 percent, the drinker will usually be both physically and psychologically incapacitated. At .3 percent the drinker is in a stupor, and concentrations above .4 percent lead to coma. A concentration of .6 or .7 percent would cause suffocation and death. Fortunately, such a high concentration rarely occurs, because most drinkers lose consciousness before they consume that much al-

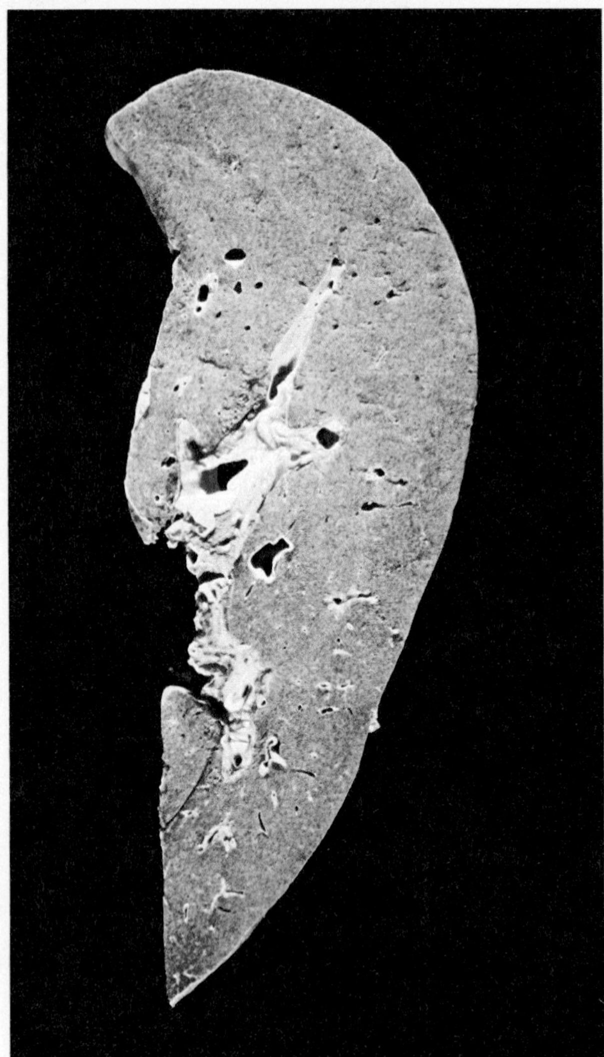

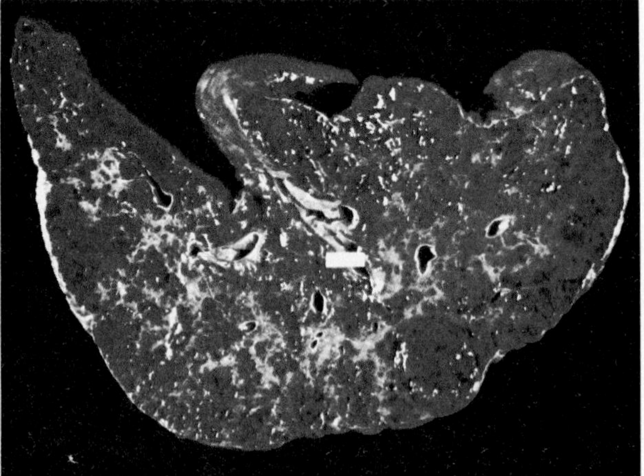

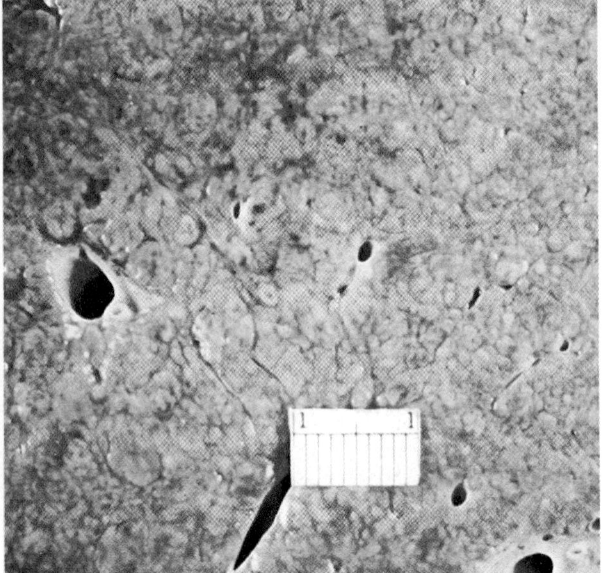

Figure 12.1 *(Left)* A normal human liver. *(Top right)* A cirrhotic liver. Cirrhosis of the liver is characterized by hardening of the liver through the formation of scar tissue. *(Bottom right)* Close-up of a cirrhotic liver. The scar-tissue cells interfere with the liver's functioning capacity. Although the condition is irreversible, its progress can be slowed by discontinuing alcohol consumption and correcting dietary inadequacies.

cohol or because the alcohol irritates the stomach and the drinker vomits before absorption of a fatal dose occurs.

Blood alcohol level depends on the amounts and forms in which alcohol is *consumed,* the rapidity with which it is introduced, or *absorbed,* into the bloodstream, the volume of blood into which it is *diluted,* and the rate at which it is *removed* from the bloodstream. Many factors influence each of those four aspects.

Type of Beverage Alcoholic beverages vary greatly in strength as measured by the concentration of alcohol they contain. Distilled liquor contains a greater percentage of alcohol than beer or wine. One ounce of pure alcohol could be ingested from a 2-ounce shot of 50 percent (100-proof) whiskey, from 5 ounces of reinforced wine, from 10 ounces of natural wine, or from two 12-ounce bottles or cans of beer. The alcohol content of each beverage, then, is

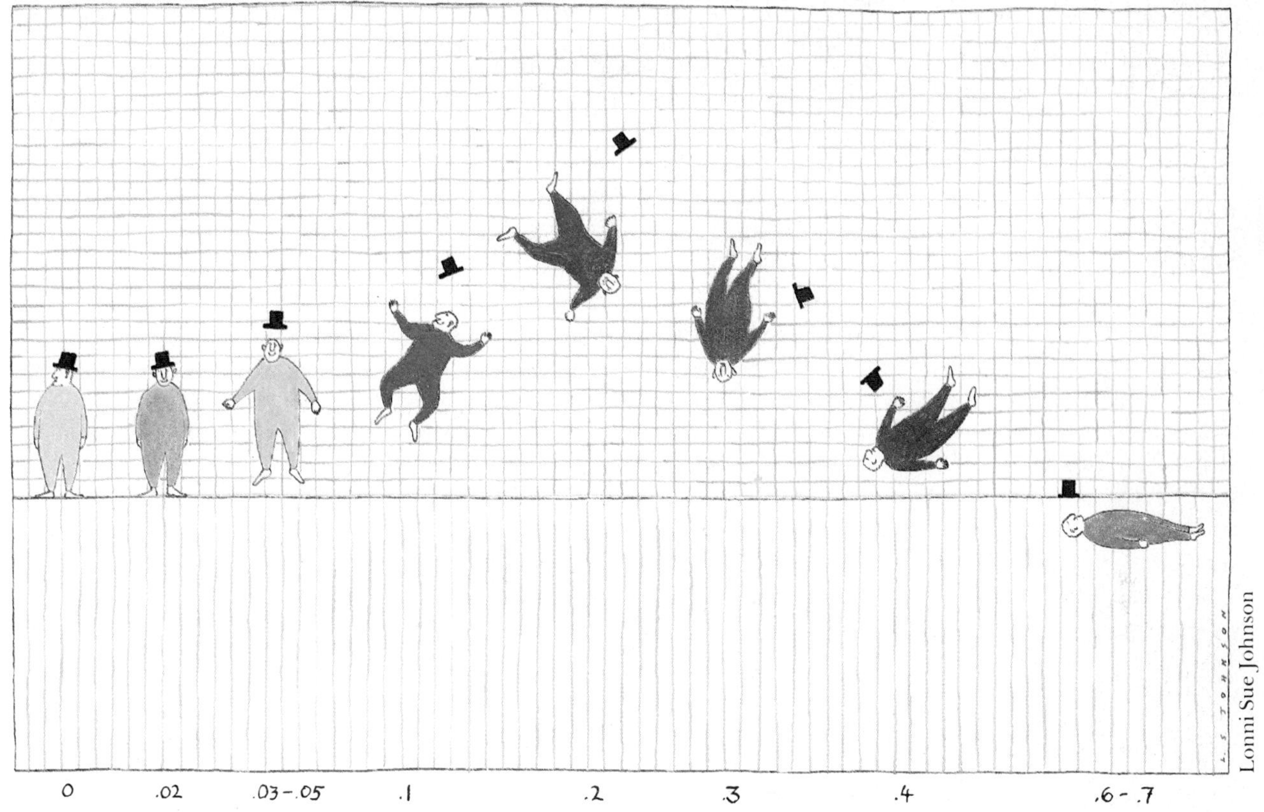

Lonni Sue Johnson

Figure 12.2 Blood alcohol levels and their effects on a drinker's behavioral state.

very important in determining what effect a certain drink will have.

Body Weight The concentration of alcohol in the blood obviously depends on both the amount of alcohol absorbed and the volume of blood into which it is absorbed. Blood volume is related to body weight. If it is assumed that a 200-pound person has roughly twice as much blood as a 100-pound person, all other factors being equal, the heavier person can consume twice as much alcohol for the same final concentration of alcohol in the blood and hence the same effect.

Because women generally weigh far less than most men, most women cannot safely drink as much as most men.

Rate of Consumption For alcohol to reach the brain and affect behavior, it must be consumed and absorbed more rapidly than it is oxidized. Absorption rates depend partly on rate of consumption. An ounce of alcohol in whiskey (2 ounces of liquid) can be downed in an instant, but even the veteran drinker will take at least a few minutes to get down the equivalent amount of alcohol in two bottles of beer. Differences in consumption time become more significant when larger amounts of alcohol (and liquid) are involved. The rate of consumption (but not absorption time) is influenced by custom and by the setting where drinking takes place. For example, on some occasions one sips a drink slowly, but on others one may be urged to chug-a-lug.

Rate of Absorption The rate of absorption is significantly affected by what is in the stomach when one is drinking. When people drink on an empty stomach, there is usually nothing present in the stomach to slow down the absorption process. Therefore, absorption takes place rapidly enough to produce a noticeable effect even from relatively small amounts of alcohol. On the other hand, alcohol that is consumed with food, especially after a large meal, will be absorbed much more slowly. In fact, the half-ounce of alcohol sipped from an after-dinner cordial may well be broken down almost as rapidly as it is absorbed. The same would be true of an after-dinner beer, because people tend to drink almost any liquid more slowly after a meal than before. There is some evidence that beer contains substances that may slow absorption time slightly and that the common carbonated sodas with which whiskey is often mixed may slightly accelerate the absorption process.

Other Biochemical Factors

Additional factors affecting the individual's response to alcohol should be mentioned, although they are perhaps the least understood. In some cases, they may involve permanent or temporary differences in the efficiency of the absorption and/or the breakdown processes. Some people are particularly sensitive to alcohol, and even small amounts produce unpleasant reactions for them. And people with certain diseases (diabetes and epilepsy, for example) should not drink. Such people should not be encouraged or pressured to drink merely for the sake of conformity—nor should anyone else. Many people seem more susceptible to alcohol's effects when they are extremely fatigued or have recently been ill. Such people find they simply cannot drink the way they usually do without experiencing uncomfortable effects.

Alcohol in Pregnancy In the last ten years, researchers have discovered that one condition that seriously influences the amount of alcohol a person should drink is pregnancy. Physicians now realize that even moderate drinking during pregnancy can have extremely harmful effects on the unborn baby. Women who are chronic alcoholics run a substantial risk of giving birth to babies with a pattern of birth defects now called the *fetal alcohol syndrome.* The children are stunted in their growth, may be mentally retarded, and have malformed faces, extremities, and hearts. According to the Public Health Service, a pregnant woman who drinks 3 or more ounces of absolute alcohol (six average drinks) a day definitely risks harm to her baby. It is not yet known whether fewer than six drinks a day also can harm the baby. However, the Public Health Service recommends that pregnant women drink no more than 1 ounce of absolute alcohol a day—that is, no more than two mixed drinks containing an ounce of liquor each, or two 5-ounce glasses of wine, or two 12-ounce cans of beer (see also Chapter 14).

Drug Interaction A serious problem occurs when people drink at the same time that they are taking other drugs. If the actions of two or more drugs are directed to the same body systems, their combined effect is often more powerful than might be expected from adding the independent effects. For example, both alcohol and phenobarbital (a barbiturate) are depressants. The combination of the two, each in doses well below the lethal level, can kill a person. Occasionally there is a lot of publicity about the death of a prominent person who took what would ordinarily be a nonlethal dose of a barbiturate while under the influence of alcohol. Nevertheless, far too little attention is given to the potentially serious outcome of drinking while a person is taking almost any form of medication, including numerous over-the-counter remedies that contain drugs with sedative or depressive properties.

At any given time in the United States, 20 to 30 million people may be using sedative antihistamines for allergies, for colds, or as sleeping aids; 15 million may have prescriptions for tranquilizers or antianxiety drugs. All these people should be warned that the drugs they are using cannot safely be combined with alcohol.

PSYCHOLOGICAL EFFECTS OF ALCOHOL

As with the other mind-altering drugs, the effect on the mind of average doses of alcohol depends mainly on the user's underlying personality and character interacting with the setting and the drug. The psychological effects of alcohol include two distinct but related categories. First, there are the effects on overt behavior, including perception, reaction time, motor tasks and skills, and cognitive processes—learning, remembering, thinking, reasoning, and problem solving. Second, there are the effects on emotional behavior, such as fear, anxiety, tension, hostility, or euphoria.

Numerous studies have demonstrated that alcohol, even in small amounts, has a harmful influence on task performance. The effect of given amounts of alcohol on performance increases with the complexity of the task, its unfamiliarity to the performer, and the inexperience of the performer with drinking. At the same time, however, the person has the illusion of better than normal reactions, perceptions, and discriminatory powers. This false sense of well-being compounds the effect of alcohol by misleading the drinker into believing that it is possible to safely undertake dangerous tasks (such as driving) or to make decisions demanding discriminatory judgment.

There are many psychological factors that may affect the influence of alcohol on any one individual. These include the individual's motives for drinking, the family's orientation and use of alcohol, the person's own previous experiences with it, and the customs and beliefs of the culture about alcohol.

As with all aspects of human behavior, there is, of course, a fundamental relationship between physiological and psychological responses to alcohol. The intensity of a drinker's physiological reactions can be partly influenced by such psychological factors as experience with drinking and expectations, and a physiological factor such as fatigue can affect psychological responses to drinking.

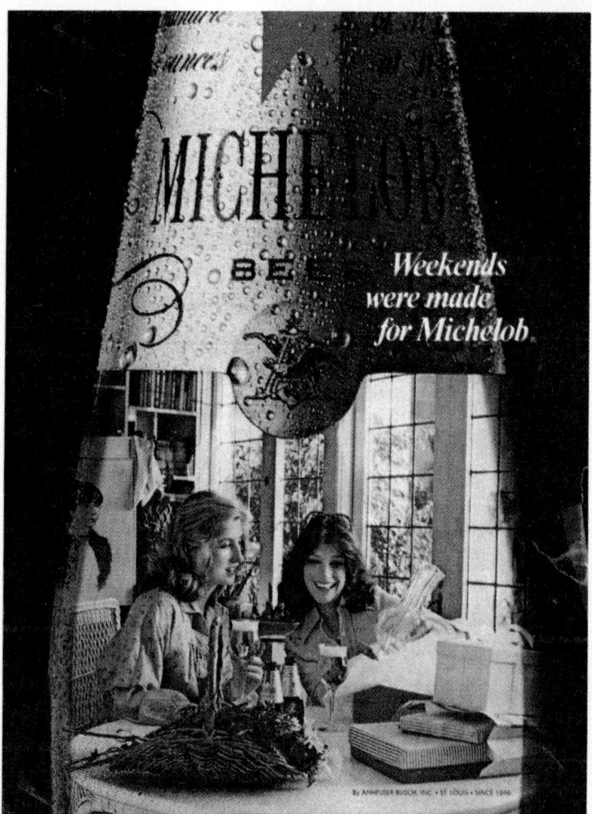

Figure 12.3 Motivation and experience play major roles in determining a person's response to alcohol. If you drink only a few leisurely beers on weekends, you will generally not suffer alcohol's harmful effects.

Motivation

Individuals who are seeking to maximize the effects of alcohol—who drink for the effects that alcohol produces—have learned to adjust their choice of beverage and their speed of consumption to produce the desired effects. On the other hand, those whose drinking is more related to the symbolic meaning of alcohol usually select beverages and circumstances that minimize the intoxicating effects of alcohol. For example, a person who really wants to get drunk, whether to forget problems or to celebrate something, will often choose distilled whiskey and will drink it rather rapidly. Someone else who just wants to be polite at a party may drink wine or beer, or a mixed drink with low alcohol content, or a strong drink but nurse it along slowly.

Role of Experience

Another factor that appears to influence the effect of alcohol on the individual is the amount of prior experience the drinker has had. When all other factors are kept constant, the individual who has had little prior experience with alcohol is likely to display more variable and less pleasant responses than the experienced drinker. This difference may be explained partially by the strangeness of the sensations and a tendency for some people to overreact to various kinds of new experiences. It may also reflect an attempt by drinkers to conform to what they assume their reactions should be.

Some people appear to be more intoxicated than might be warranted by the amount of alcohol they have consumed. Conversely, as people become experienced drinkers, they often learn to compensate for some of the alcohol-induced behavioral responses. They can appear to be more sober than might be expected from their alcohol consumption. These differences are essentially psychological adaptations to the experience of drinking. At the physiological level, people appear to have some capacity for adapting to the irritating properties of alcohol. A novice taking a strong drink for the first time may throw it up—a reaction not too different from that of children who experiment with tobacco. All these differences should not, however, be confused with alcohol-induced *tolerance.*

Tolerance of alcohol, like that of many other psychoactive drugs, is built over a period of drug abuse. Progressively higher amounts of alcohol are "tolerated" with no recognizable signs of depressant action. Even though some heavy drinkers can tolerate much more alcohol than moderate drinkers or nondrinkers, the degree of tolerance to alcohol is modest compared with that of many other psychoactive drugs. For example, persons who are dependent on opiates can develop a tolerance for amounts that are many times greater than what would be lethal for the nondependent user.

Drinking and the Family

For most people, the question of whether to drink or not first comes up within the family, and it is there that one's earliest attitudes toward drinking are formed. Several studies have found that the setting of people's first exposure to alcohol is most often the family and their first drinking companions are most frequently family members. About half of those who drink say that they first tasted or experimented with alcohol by the age of ten. There is also a high correlation between young people and their parents in regard to drinking frequency and the amounts and types of beverages they consume. Within the family, most people also acquire the sense of security or insecurity that may affect the psychological meaning that alcohol has for them and thus their motivation for drinking.

DRINKING IN AMERICAN SOCIETY

Within this century, with the exception of the Prohibition period, a gradual but steady trend toward the use of alcohol by more and more people has been recorded. In a recent study of American drinking practices, it was estimated that 100 million Americans above the age of fifteen, including about eight out of ten adult men and six out of ten adult women, use alcoholic beverages. The vast majority of those who drink appear to use alcohol without noticeable danger or damage to themselves or others except when they drive after drinking, but the drinking habits of at least 15 million people cause distinct problems. This last group includes the estimated 10 million who are alcoholics and others who are often temporarily incapacitated from safely or effectively carrying out their various activities.

Drinking Among Youth

Despite relatively recent concerns about marijuana and other drugs, drinking among young people has been a consistent cause of friction between the generations. In American society, drinking has long been permitted only for adults. Until recently, the sale, purchase, or use of alcoholic beverages to or by persons under the age of twenty-one was illegal in most states. Following the lowering of the voting age from twenty-one to eighteen, many states reduced the legal drinking age to eighteen. There is still a great deal of controversy over this question, however, and Kentucky, which many years ago changed the voting age to eighteen and now considers an eighteen-year-old a legal adult, still prohibits drinking before the age of twenty-one. And some states that

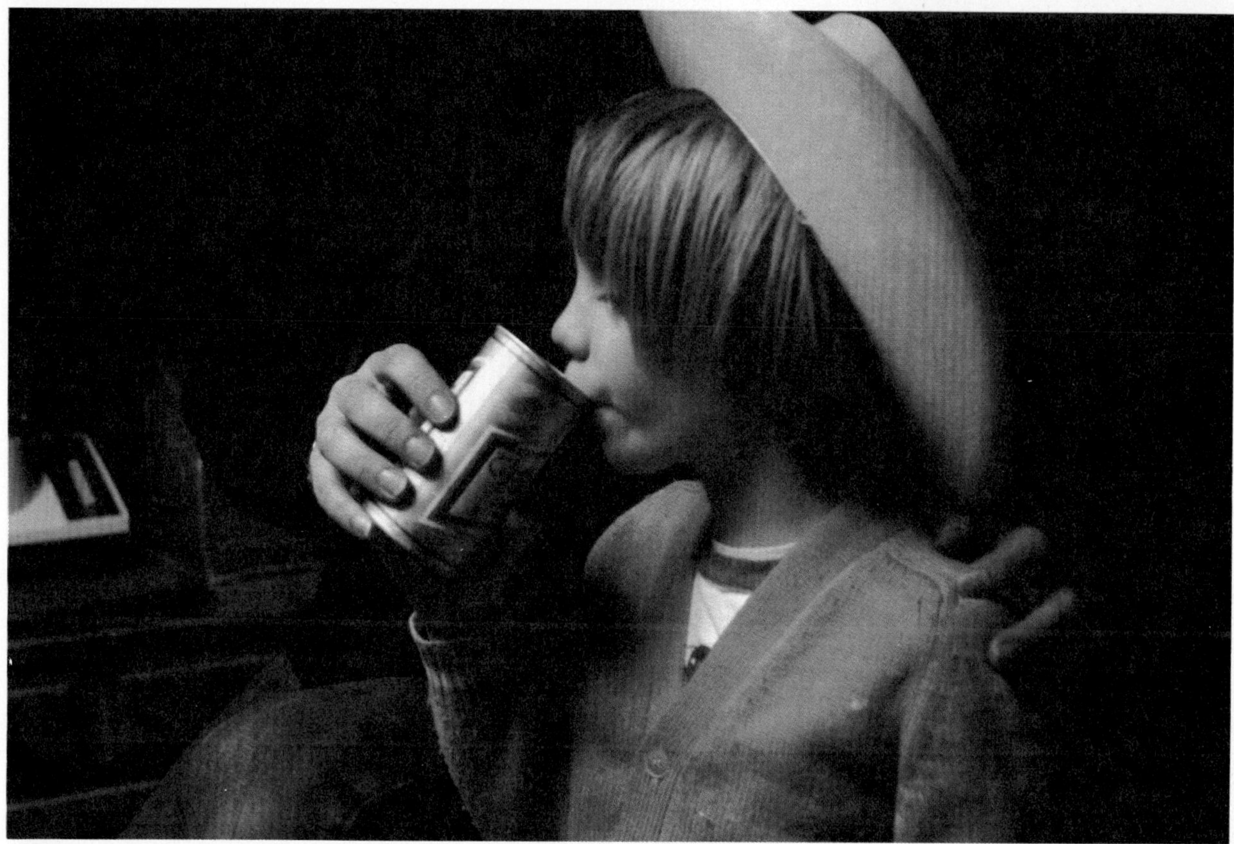

Figure 12.4 The family is the earliest influence on attitudes toward drinking.

lowered the legal drinking age are now considering raising it again.

Adult examples, attitudes, and restrictions have enhanced the attraction of alcohol for young people as a symbol of adult status, of rejected authority, or of "forbidden fruit." As a result, adults seem to have stimulated the kind of drinking that involves risks more than they have controlled it. The same thing has probably also been true of much of the education about alcohol—required by the laws of every state—which, until recently, so insulted the intelligence of students that it appears to have inspired the very behavior it was intended to discourage.

For a few years, concern about alcohol use among youth seemed overshadowed by concern about use of other drugs, notably amphetamines and marijuana. In more recent years, however, young people have been turning to alcohol in increasing numbers. According to the 1977 National Survey on Drug Abuse, 85 percent of young adults between the ages of eighteen and twenty-five and over 50 percent of youths between twelve and seventeen had tried alcoholic beverages at least once. Nearly 70 percent of the young adults and 30 percent of the teen-agers between twelve and seventeen were current users of alcohol (defined as having used it in the month prior to the survey). Since this survey was based on interviews with people living in households—but not places of traditionally high alcohol use, such as military installations and college dormitories—the survey, if anything, may underestimate alcohol use by young people (see the Focus box).

By comparison, marijuana use was well behind alcohol use. Only 60 percent of the eighteen- to twenty-five-year-olds and 20 percent of

FOCUS

Teen-Agers and Drinking

Not only has there been an increase in alcohol consumption by teen-agers in recent years (see the section *Drinking Among Youth*) but young people are also drinking at younger and younger ages. A survey by the National Institute on Alcohol Abuse and Alcoholism (NIAAA) in 1974 discovered that among high-school seniors, 93 percent of the boys and 87 percent of the girls had tried alcohol. Among seventh graders, 63 percent of the boys and 54 percent of the girls had tried it.

Further evidence of the extent of drinking among teen-agers comes from studies done at one suburban school system in San Mateo County, south of San Francisco. In 1973, 40 percent of the senior-class boys and 29 percent of the senior-class girls reported that in the previous year they had drunk some sort of alcoholic beverage fifty or more times. Among the ninth graders (thirteen- and fourteen-year-olds), 23 percent of the boys said that they drank just as often. In each case, these percentages were nearly double what they had been in a 1970 study.

Teen-age drinkers are a cross section of the student body. They

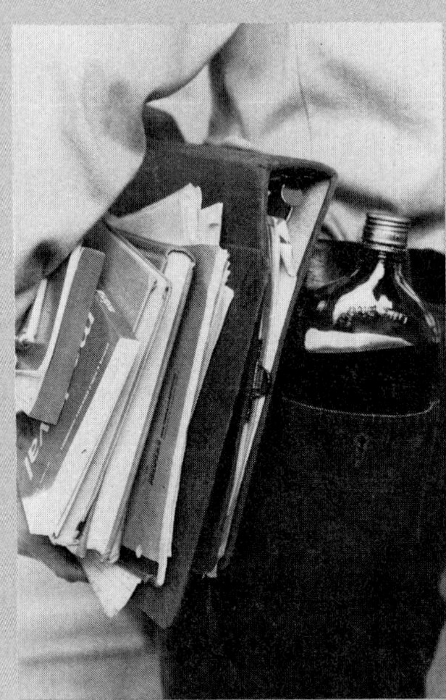

"represent all levels of scholastic achievement and aspiration—53 percent expect to go to college and beyond," according to another survey conducted by the National Highway Safety Traffic Administration in 1974, and "they report the same range of sports and extracurricular activities as the students who are not involved in social drinking."

This widespread teen-age drinking is apparently one factor in the popularity of the new, so-called "pop wines," the fruit-flavored beverages that are too sweet for the tastes of many adults but seem to be a transition drink between soda pop and harder alcoholic beverages for many young people. Beer, however, still remains the number one choice of young drinkers. It contains significantly less alcohol (6.4 percent in most states) than the pop wines (about 9 percent).

Not surprisingly, the rise in drinking among teen-agers has also brought an increase in their drinking problems. The 1974 NIAAA survey found that 23 percent of the students had signs of a potential drinking problem, which the Institute defined as getting drunk four or more times per year. Approximately 5 percent of the students were already problem drinkers, defined as getting "high" or "tight" at least once a week. Arrests of people under age eighteen for drunken driving increased by more than 400 percent between 1960 and 1973. And Alcoholics Anonymous reports that it is getting more and more teen-age members.

the twelve- to seventeen-year-olds had tried marijuana, and about 25 percent of the young adults and 15 percent of the youths were current users.

Intoxication and Society

Whenever a society permits the use of alcohol, some people drink to the point of drunkenness and others drink enough so that their inhibitions against antisocial behavior are weakened. In some societies, intoxication generally occurs only in connection with certain ceremonial events, and provisions are made for protecting drinkers from themselves and society from their drunkenness. In some segments of American society, by contrast, drunkenness is socially reinforced. Adults say (when they are sober) that drunkenness is disgusting—yet they get drunk themselves.

The intoxicated person is euphoric and talkative, lacks inhibitions, and is frequently aggressive. Speech is slurred and movements are uncoordinated so that the person even has difficulty walking. Someone who becomes very drunk may go into a stupor and become unconscious. Although rare, it is possible for a severely intoxicated person to die as a result of depressed respiration and heart action. A large number of accidental deaths and suicides occur following heavy drinking. Most of the deaths from alcohol result from suffocation. Usually the person has vomited while not fully conscious and suffocated on fluid inhaled into the lungs. This is a real danger and one reason a drunk should not be put to bed to "sleep it off."

Most of the hundreds of thousands of persons who are repeatedly arrested, convicted, and jailed for public intoxication, only to be released and then arrested again in a continuing cycle, are problem drinkers. Increasingly, communities are providing centers for detoxification (literally, "depoisoning" or "drying out") and treatment in place of jail terms for some of their chronic publicly intoxicated drinkers.

Drunkenness is by no means confined to the public offender. In fact, most intoxication today occurs in men and women who live with their families, hold jobs, and maintain stable community ties. In the past, these persons were often protected when drunk, unless intoxication occurred so frequently or with such dire consequences that the drinker lost family, job, or both. People who drink excessively are also often impaired by alcohol even when they do not necessarily seem drunk. Their perception of time and space may be altered, their judgment faulty, and their reaction time and thinking slowed—all without obvious signs of drunkenness.

The problems created by people under the influence of alcohol, in public or otherwise, have been compounded as society has become more technological and as more and more jobs and activities require exacting skill and judgment. The more demanding the job, the less satisfactorily workers may be able to perform while under the influence of alcohol or while suffering the aftereffects of intoxication. It is impossible for most people to avoid everyday activities that will be affected by immoderate alcohol use.

The most vivid example is the case of personal transportation. In the days of the horse-drawn vehicle, drunken or alcohol-impaired drivers were rarely a threat to anyone but themselves and their horses. But the automobile and truck are far more dangerous. In 1978, the Secretary of Health, Education, and Welfare reported that the use of alcohol by drivers and pedestrians in the United States is responsible for one-half of all traffic fatalities (about 23,000 deaths) and one-third of all traffic injuries. Drinking also leads to a high proportion of accidents in private aircraft, in the home, and in industry.

ALCOHOLISM

Although intoxication in a privately protected environment may occur occasionally without causing undue harm, any intoxication that coincides with the need to drive, work, or make decisions may lead to serious consequences. When intoxication occurs repeatedly, causing problems of personal health or interfering with psychological or social functioning in the family, job, or community, the person can be considered a problem drinker. Problem drinkers who have developed a physical dependency on alcohol or who have lost their ability to stop drinking once they have started or to refrain from drinking in inappropriate situations are *alcoholics.*

The definition of an alcoholic includes both social and medical concepts. Repeated use of alcohol can lead to psychological dependence —habituation—and to physical dependence. The person dependent upon alcohol is usually so impaired in the ability to function in normal activities that social interactions are considerably restricted; often, however, the losses to the person, the family, and society are great.

Signs of Alcoholism

What are the early warning signs of alcoholism? How can one tell when a friend's drinking

HOW TO

A Guide to Sensible Drinking

People have always enjoyed drinking—it is a pleasant ingredient in many social situations. But too much of a good thing can have nightmarish results, and excessive drinking is no exception. It can cause —and has caused—misery, deterioration, and death.

You can avoid these dire consequences simply by drinking sensibly. You will keep your good judgment on and off the road, you will escape the horror of alcoholism, and, if nothing else, you will save yourself the embarrassment of being drunk.

How do you drink sensibly? First, you need to be aware of what alcohol is and what it can do to you. Then, use your common sense. Here are a few pointers:

1. Restrict your drinking—even on special occasions.
2. Avoid drinking daily or regularly.
3. Keep track of how much you are drinking. Don't exceed your limit.
4. Dilute spirits with soda, water, or juice so the alcohol will be absorbed more slowly.
5. Avoid two-liquor mixes like martinis and manhattans.
6. Never gulp down your drinks.
7. Never drink on an empty stomach.
8. Learn to refuse alcoholic beverages politely but firmly in favor of juice or a soft drink.
9. Avoid bars and cocktail lounges when you are just killing time (at an airport, for example).
10. Delay your first drink at parties or dinners as long as possible.
11. Develop the ability to converse while drinking; this will help you space your drinks.
12. If you are hosting a party and serving alcohol, be sure to offer coffee, soft drinks, and food as well.
13. Plan your transportation so that the driver is never alcohol impaired.
14. Think about your drinking. Is it getting out of hand?
15. If a friend suggests that you have a drinking problem, take it seriously and get help.

Remember: The best thing to mix with alcohol is caution!

Source: Adapted from *The Alcoholic American*, National Association of Blue Shield Plans, 1970.

has become a serious enough problem that he or she should be steered toward a treatment program? (See the section *Treatment* later in this chapter.)

Dr. Morris Chafetz, former Director of the National Institute on Alcohol Abuse and Alcoholism, has listed some of the danger signs of a problem with alcohol: being intoxicated four or more times a year; needing to drink in order to go to work or to school or out socially; driving while intoxicated; sustaining bodily injury needing medical attention as a consequence of intoxication; getting into trouble with the law as a consequence of drinking; doing something under the influence of alcohol that one contends one would never do when sober.

What Causes Alcoholism?

There are no completely satisfactory theories about the causes of various types of problem drinking. Increasingly, simple learning theory is being used to explain it: a person is tense and takes a drink. The drink relieves the tension, thus reinforcing the behavior. The next time the person is in a tense situation, he or she will again take a drink. Researchers have also looked into liver metabolism, the function of the central nervous system, hormonal imbalances, vitamin and nutritional deficiencies, personality disorders, and the role of culture. Most authorities now agree that alcoholism is caused by many interrelated factors, which vary from person to person.

Although the existence of specific biological deficiencies or sensitivities has not been identified, their possible contribution to alcoholism cannot be ruled out. Alcoholism definitely does run in families. This could be due to either environmental reasons or heredity, or to a combination of the two.

A number of psychological traits have been identified in individuals who drink excessively. Alcoholics tend to experience greater psychological discomfort than most other people. They have deep-seated feelings of inadequacy or are often anxious or depressed. Most alcoholics often experience intense psychological or social stress, and drinking provides temporary relief. Yet repeated intoxication invariably causes physical, psychological, or

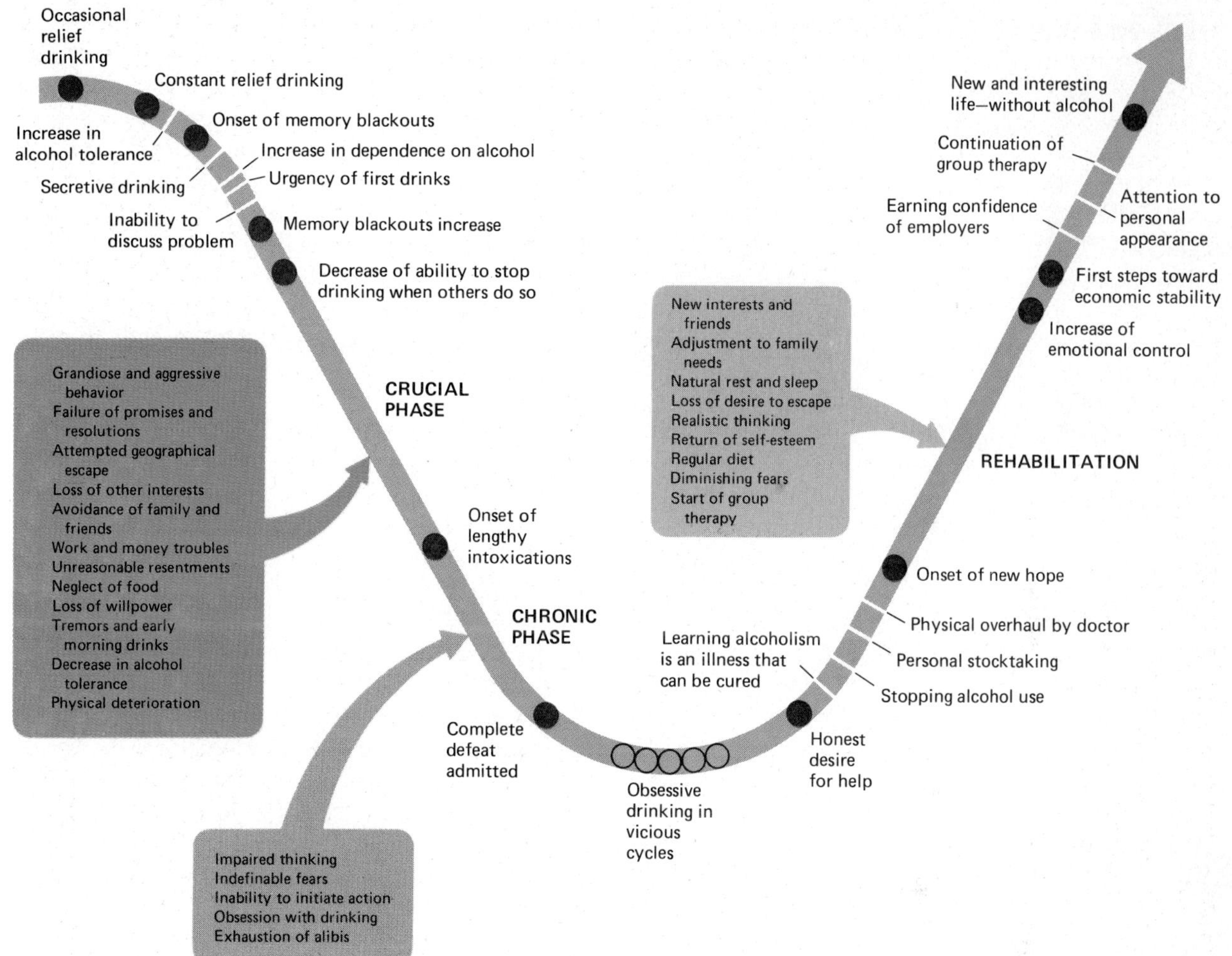

Figure 12.5 The road to alcoholism and recovery. *Source:* Adapted from M.M. Glatt, "Group Therapy in Alcoholism." *The British Journal of Addiction* (January 1958). Copyright © by M.M. Glatt. An improved chart is in M.M. Glatt, *A Guide to Addiction and its Treatment* (Lancaster, England: MTT Medical and Technical Publishing Co.)

social problems that, in the long run, can only increase this stress.

Whatever their pattern of alcohol use, alcoholics are seeking the intoxicating effects of alcohol. Some alcoholics are sober most of the time but go on binges. Others follow regular patterns of drinking, perhaps drinking heavily every night, or only on weekends or holidays. Some, once they start drinking, seem compelled to continue until they reach a peak level of effect. Others try to maintain an alcohol-induced euphoria for as long as possible.

Diagnoses of alcoholism are not precise. Alcoholism has long been a stigma. As long as they are able, the alcoholic and often his or her family and friends may try to deny or conceal the situation, in order to prevent the alcoholic from losing job and respectability.

It is estimated that in the United States, there is one problem drinker for every ten people who use alcohol. Alcoholics are found in all regions of the country, at all educational and income levels, and in all occupations, from highly paid business executives to skid row derelicts, from suburban mothers to blue-collar workers. There are significantly more men than women alcoholics (probably four to one), but the proportion of women alcoholics seems to be rising. The highest incidence of alcoholism was once among middle-aged men, but today it is among men under the age of thirty.

When alcoholism develops early in life, it

often occurs after only two or three years of heavy drinking. When it develops later in life, it usually follows many years, perhaps six to ten, of steady, heavy drinking. Among teenagers, however, for reasons that no one knows, the process is so speeded up that they can become alcoholics after only three or four months of high alcohol consumption.

The prevalence of problem drinking is also related to differences in customary beliefs and patterns of alcohol use. Conditions that favor the rapid absorption of sufficient alcohol to affect behavior are associated with higher rates of intoxication and increased exposure to alcoholism. Such conditions are generally found in societies where most drinking is done on an empty stomach and involves beverages with a high alcohol content in relatively undiluted form. Such conditions tend to prevail at the typical late-afternoon American cocktail party. Not only is the buffering effect of food missing, but also people tend to drink more rapidly when they are not eating.

Treatment

The alcoholic requires support at all levels, ranging from family members to the attending physician. The treatment of alcoholism requires a broad-gauged approach capable of dealing with the physical consequences of prolonged drinking while the alcoholic is helped to change those social and personality factors that have contributed to the alcoholism problem.

Ideally, treatment programs should provide medical, psychological, and social-work resources and should involve the support and participation of the alcoholic's family, employer, and other significant persons. The organization Alcoholics Anonymous (AA) provides important therapy for alcoholics. AA's services are completely free and are based on mutual support and understanding of the problems of alcoholism through personal experience. Contact with AA can be made anywhere in the United States. There is an organization for spouses of alcoholics, Al-Anon, and there is also one known as Alateen, in which teen-age sons and daughters of alcoholics meet to help one another. Many physicians have found that Antabuse (disulfiram), a tablet taken daily that produces a toxic reaction if any alcohol is consumed, can help their alcoholic patients maintain sobriety while receiving other treatment. Group and individual psychotherapy, social-work services, vocational counseling, operant conditioning, and other traditional and innovative approaches are often used in combination with AA and Antabuse. Treatment generally emphasizes full acceptance of the problem drinker as an ill human being who needs long-term specialized outpatient help.

Facing the Problem

Although intoxication, incidental and chronic, has long presented problems for societies, the consequences of intoxication have increased as the demands of a more and more complex society have created roles requiring physical dexterity, mental alertness, and decisive actions. On the one hand, the more complex the society, the more pressures it places on individuals who use alcohol for temporary (and illusory) relief. On the other hand, the more complex the society and demanding its roles, the less tolerance it affords for individuals whose physical and mental functioning are compromised by alcohol. This dilemma is one that contemporary society faces not only with respect to alcohol but with respect to a wide range of other behavior-altering drugs. It presents a challenge to the coming generations to develop intelligent and effective methods of utilizing the benefits of alcohol and other drugs without incurring their liabilities.

SUMMARY

1. Alcohol abuse is a major social and health problem in the United States. There are more than 15 million Americans with serious drinking problems and 10 million alcoholics. Excessive drinking is a factor in more than 50 percent of fatal automobile accidents.

2. Pharmacologically, alcohol is an anesthetic, a tranquilizer, and a depressant. Although at times it seems to be a stimulant, it is

not. It produces mood changes by depressing the part of the brain controlling behavior, judgment, and memory.

3. Prolonged heavy use of alcohol can lead to psychotic conditions, gastrointestinal disorders, malnutrition, cirrhosis of the liver, certain types of cancers, and a shortened life span.

4. The effect of alcohol on a person's behavior is determined by the blood alcohol level. Most people experience little noticeable effect with up to .02 percent of alcohol in the blood. At .1 percent, there is major depression of sensory and motor functions. Concentrations above .4 percent lead to coma.

5. Blood alcohol level depends on the strength of the alcoholic beverage consumed, body weight, the rate of consumption, and the rate of absorption.

6. Women who drink heavily during pregnancy run a risk of giving birth to a child with a pattern of birth defects called the *fetal alcohol syndrome,* in which the baby is stunted in growth, mentally retarded, and has deformities of the face, extremities, and heart. The Public Health Service recommends that pregnant women drink no more than the equivalent of two mixed drinks a day.

7. The psychological effect of drinking is influenced by a person's motivation for drinking, experience, and family, cultural, and ethnic background.

8. In recent years, teen-agers have been drinking alcoholic beverages in increasing numbers. Alcohol use is well ahead of marijuana use.

9. Alcoholics are problem drinkers who have developed a physical dependence on alcohol, or who can no longer stop drinking once they have started or refrain from drinking in inappropriate situations.

10. While the causes of alcoholism are still poorly understood, many alcoholics have been helped by the treatment program provided by Alcoholics Anonymous.

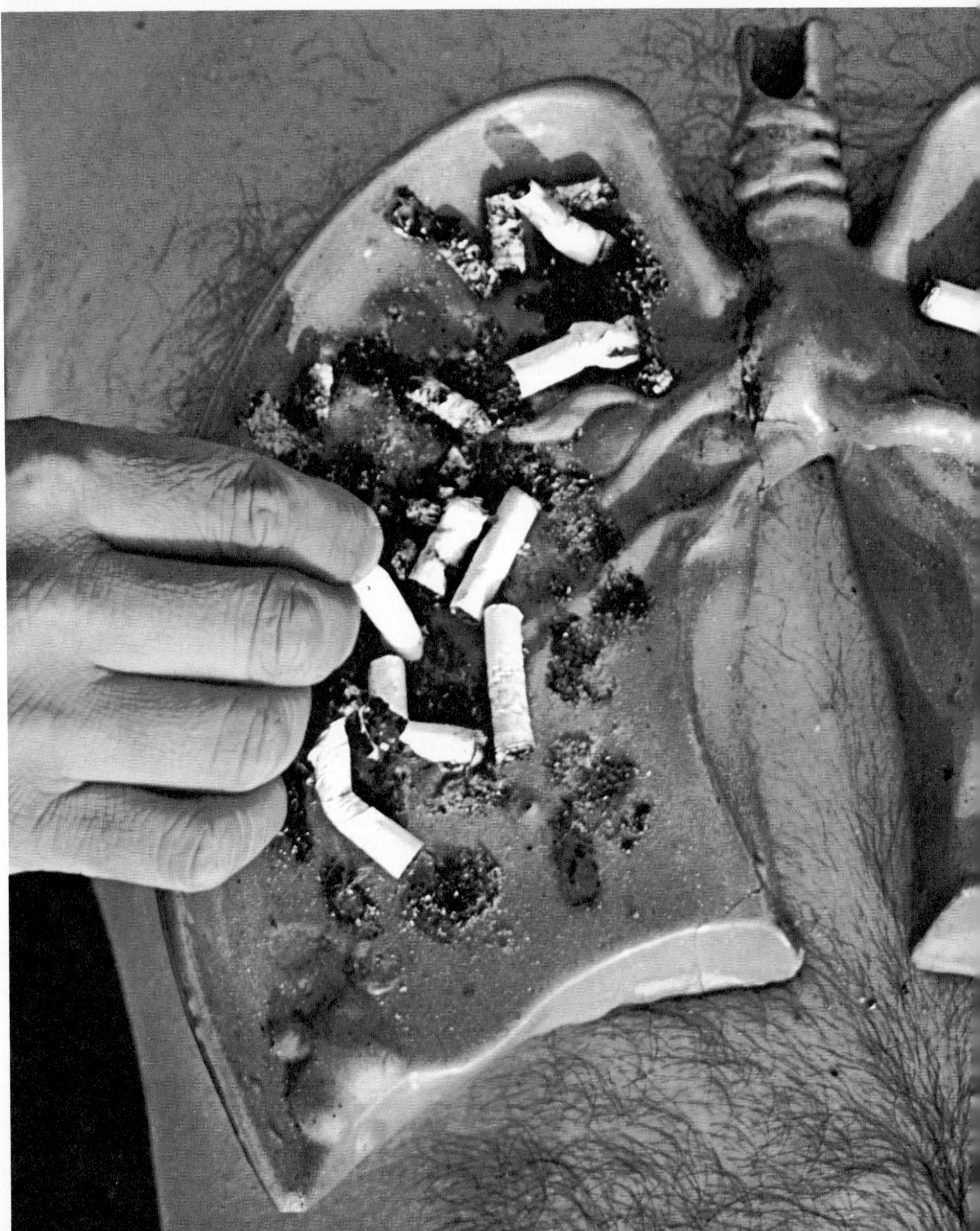

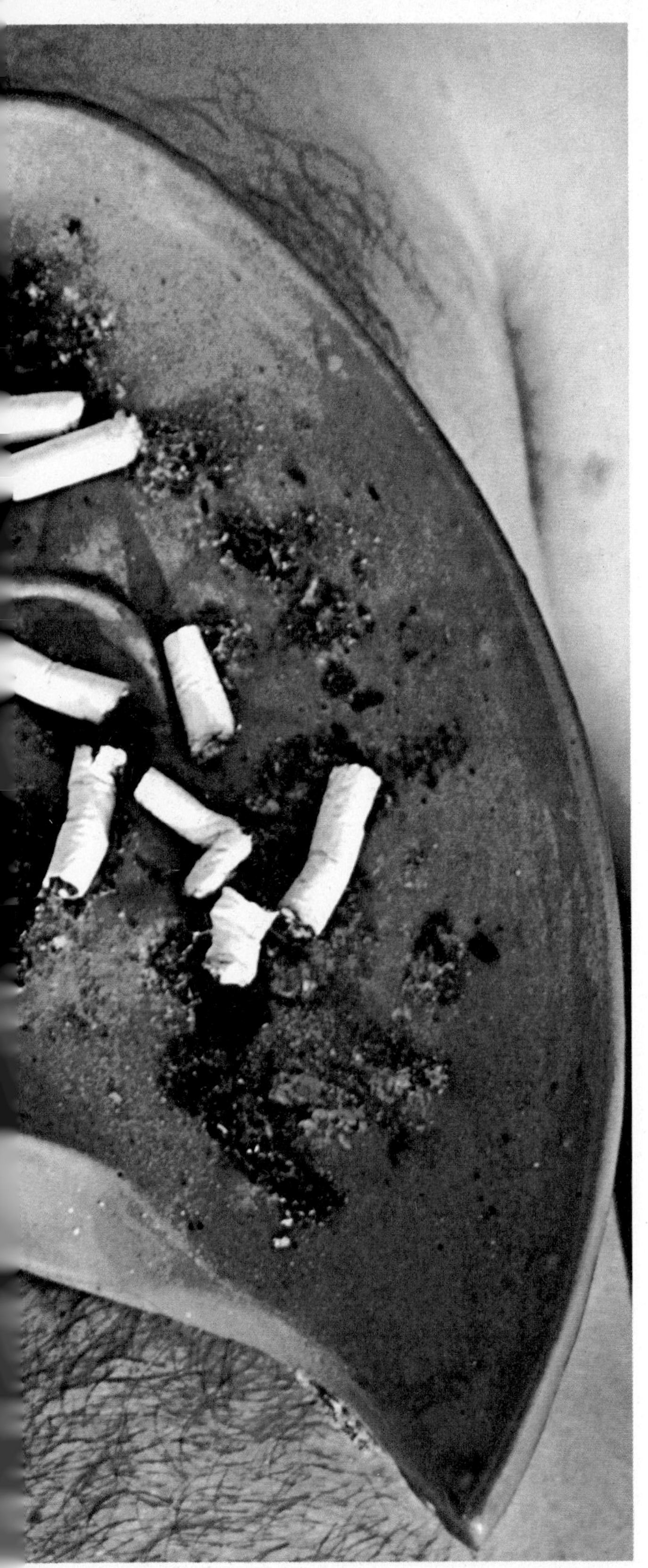

13 Smoking and Health

In 1964 the U.S. Surgeon General presented his committee's report on the health hazards of cigarette smoking. And for the first time, Americans began to realize the gravity of the smoking problem. The committee had considered the results of many investigations, in animals as well as humans, and had evaluated a large number of comprehensive epidemiological studies involving millions of people of all backgrounds in the United States, Canada, and Great Britain. The conclusion, as reported by the Surgeon General, was in no uncertain terms: "Cigarette smoking is a health hazard of sufficient importance in the United States to warrant appropriate remedial action."

Since then, further medical studies have reaffirmed this conclusion again and again. The Public Health Service's 1975 report, *The Health Consequences of Smoking,* states, "Cigarette smoking remains the largest single unnecessary and preventable cause of illness and preventable death." All packages of cigarettes and all cigarette advertising must now, by law, carry the label: "Warning: The Surgeon General has determined that cigarette smoking is dangerous to your health." And in 1979, the Secretary of Health, Education, and Welfare and the Surgeon General jointly released a massive, 1,200-page *Report on Smoking and Health* that reviewed in detail more than 30,000 scientific studies. The new report presented "overwhelming proof" of the link between cigarette smoking and disease and also emphasized that now that women are smoking more, they, too, are suffering the same serious health consequences as men. The HEW Secretary says, "People who smoke are committing slow-motion suicide."

Nevertheless, tens of millions of Americans —exercising their right to a free choice even in matters of their own health—continue to smoke hundreds of billions of cigarettes each year. Yet, there are signs of a turning tide. Nine out of ten smokers say that they would probably stop if there was an easy way. And around the country, nonsmokers are becoming increasingly militant about *their* right to breathe air unpolluted by cigarette smoke.

THE MANUFACTURED EPIDEMIC

About one hundred years ago, cigarettes were homemade and were smoked by a few rugged individualists. But the invention of the cigarette-making machine in 1881 spawned an industry that was turning out 4 billion cigarettes a year at the turn of the century. By the 1920s, yearly cigarette production hit 80 billion. By 1978, smokers were puffing away their lives and polluting the air with the help of some 615 billion cigarettes. In the same seventy years, lung cancer grew from a relatively rare disease to the killer of more than 78,000 Americans in 1977. Bronchitis, emphysema, cancers of the kidney, pancreas, and bladder, and heart disease have also been on the rise, thanks in part to tobacco smoking. In fact, the 1979 Surgeon General's Report concludes that cigarette smoking is responsible for 346,000 deaths *each year!*

Studies in which selected groups of people (physicians, war veterans, industrial workers, and so on) were monitored for as long as ten years have dramatically revealed the body-damaging, life-shortening effects of excessive cigarette smoking. Cigarette smokers have an approximately 70 percent greater overall mortality rate from disease than do nonsmokers, according to the 1979 Surgeon General's Report, and the rate differences depend on how much or how long the subject has been smoking. The mortality rate is also higher for smokers who inhale and for those who start smoking at an early age. The mortality rate for women, which is generally lower than for men, has also increased in proportion to the extent of their smoking. Mortality rates are almost normal for cigar and pipe smokers, although these smokers are more susceptible than are total abstainers to lip and certain other cancers.

The excessive mortality rate observed in cigarette smokers is caused by a variety of diseases, but 80 percent of the increase is tied to lung cancer, bronchitis, emphysema, other respiratory ailments, and heart disease. Lung-cancer incidence is eleven times greater, death from pulmonary diseases six times more frequent, and coronary artery disease almost two times greater than for nonsmoking subjects (see Figure 13.1). Nonsmoking, lifetime members of the Seventh-Day Adventists experience almost no lung cancer, even though their jobs and areas of residence expose them to a wide variety of other environmental pollutants. Conversely, in Iceland, where air pollution is low, a sharp rise in lung cancer followed the large increase in cigarette consumption that took place in the post-World War II years. Thus, the dramatic difference in lung-cancer incidence between smokers and nonsmokers is much more directly related to cigarette smoking than to air pollution. This fact is not surprising, considering the amount of self-contamination to which a smoker is deliberately subjected. Smoke from a typical nonfilter cigarette contains about 5 billion particles per milliliter—50,000 times as many as an equal volume of polluted urban atmosphere.

In addition to this increased mortality, millions of heavy smokers are chronically disabled by emphysema, bronchitis, and other respiratory diseases. Heavy smokers are much more likely to be ill and to miss work more often. For example, according to the National Center for Health Statistics, seventeen- to forty-four-year old smokers lose 50 percent more workdays than nonsmokers in the same age bracket. To this loss of work, time, and wages, one must add the cost of increased medical and hospital bills; according to government figures, smoking adds, each year, between $5 and $7 billion to the nation's total health care costs. This, of course, is a bill that every one of us—whether or not we smoke—helps pay in the form of taxes and insurance premiums. Careless smokers are also responsible for 13 percent of resi-

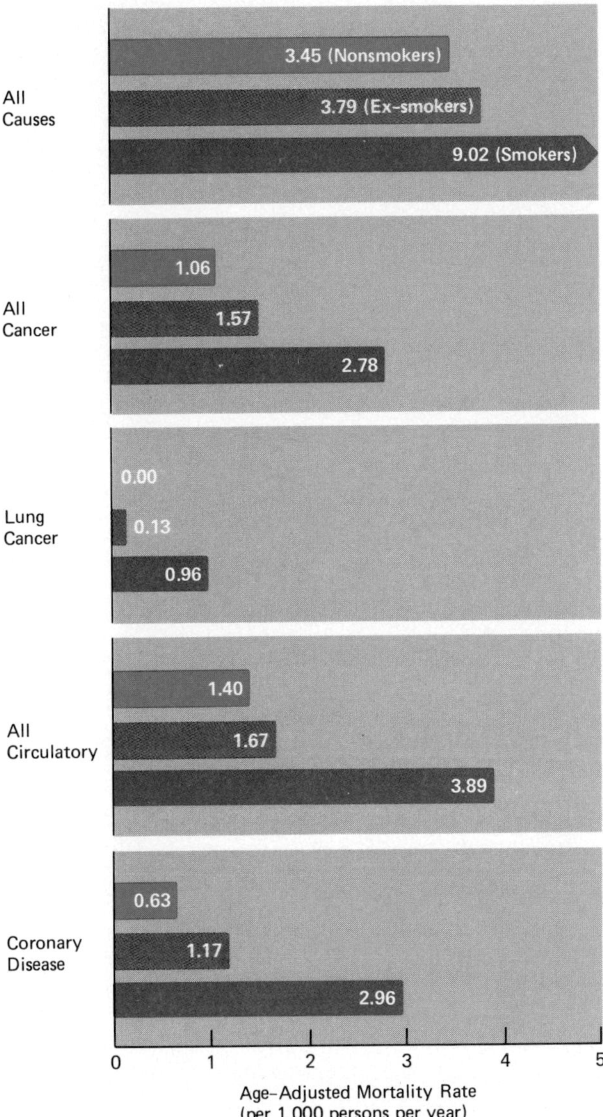

Figure 13.1 Death rates for cigarette smokers, ex-smokers, and nonsmokers by selected diseases.

dential fires, the National Fire Data Center reports, and smoking is the most common cause of deaths (29 percent) and injuries (18 percent) in such fires.

COMPONENTS OF CIGARETTE SMOKE

To help determine what portions of tobacco smoke are responsible for the various diseases associated with cigarette smoking, chemists have meticulously broken down the smoke into its components and then tested the various fractions on laboratory animals. Thus far, they have identified more than 1,200 different toxic chemicals, and the number is still growing. When it burns, the average cigarette produces about one-half gram of smoke, 92 percent in the form of gases (a number of them known to be toxic) and 8 percent as ash, a tar-rich condensate, and a "wet particulate matter" comprising hundreds of different substances.

The tarry condensate can be separated chemically into three parts: acidic, basic, and neutral. In animal tests, the neutral part shows by far the highest *carcinogenic,* or cancer-causing, activity: it contains *benzopyrene,* one of the deadliest carcinogens known, and many other chemicals of the same family. The acidic part of the tarry condensate contains phenol and other materials that are not carcinogens but, some cancer researchers believe, could activate a "dormant" cancer cell to grow and spread.

Nicotine, the "drug" characteristic of tobacco, was found to occur in the basic fraction of tarry condensate. It is not a carcinogen. Rather, it has been linked circumstantially to some of the other smoke-supported diseases.

Nicotine is an agent affecting primarily the nervous system. Like other drugs in this category, it produces habituation and tolerance. It is known that nicotine mimics some of the effects of the neurotransmitter acetylcholine, enhancing transmission between nerve cells when applied in low doses and blocking it at the higher dose range. A number of the body's responses to inhalation of nicotine are viewed as consequences of these effects. For example, nicotine is known to increase the heartbeat fifteen to twenty-five beats per minute while constricting blood vessels in the extremities. Thermograms (heat pictures) taken of smokers' hands and feet dramatically show the decline in temperature in fingers and toes after a cigarette is smoked. Other effects of nicotine are suspected to take place at the level of the smooth muscles regulating the constriction of the bronchioles—an important component of respiratory disorders.

SMOKE AS A DISEASE AGENT

Lung Cancer

When the tarry portion of cigarette smoke is applied to the skin, lungs, and other tissues of mice, rats, or hamsters, the compounds it contains produce cancer in the experimental animals. Recent experiments showed that lung cancer could be produced in dogs made to smoke seven cigarettes a day (through incisions in the trachea) for a period of more than two years. Among dogs that smoked filter cigarettes or half the number of nonfilter cigarettes, some did develop abnormal cell changes in lung tissues that pathologists suspect would eventually lead to cancer. However, the dogs that smoked more of the nonfilter cigarettes showed more of these changes.

One of the most comprehensive studies of the effects of cigarette smoking on human lung tissue was carried out at the Veteran's Administration Hospital in East Orange, New Jersey, where autopsied lung tissue from several thousand individuals was thoroughly examined.

A significant finding was the high incidence of *hyperplasia* among heavy and moderate smokers. In hyperplasia, the *basal cells* that underlie the bronchial lining become irritated and begin to pile up in layers, usually five or more deep. The next most noticeable difference in the respiratory passageways of smokers is the loss of ciliated *columnar cells.* These cells include fine hairlike projections, or cilia, on their surface. The cilia wave back and forth and usually keep harmful materials out of the lungs. Following the loss of the ciliated cells, the remaining cells flatten out and enlarge, taking on the "squamous" structure invariably found in patients with lung cancer.

Most pertinent to lung cancer itself was the appearance of disordered nuclei in the affected lung cells. Cells of this type are seen in *carcinoma in situ,* a localized cancer that may break through to the underlying basal cells, proliferate, and spread throughout the rest of the body. Hyperplasia, the loss of ciliated cells, and the abnormal nuclei were prevalent in patients who died of lung cancer. The researchers also found that among former smokers these three conditions had regressed, suggesting that in the premalignant state, at least, the lung-cancer process may be reversible.

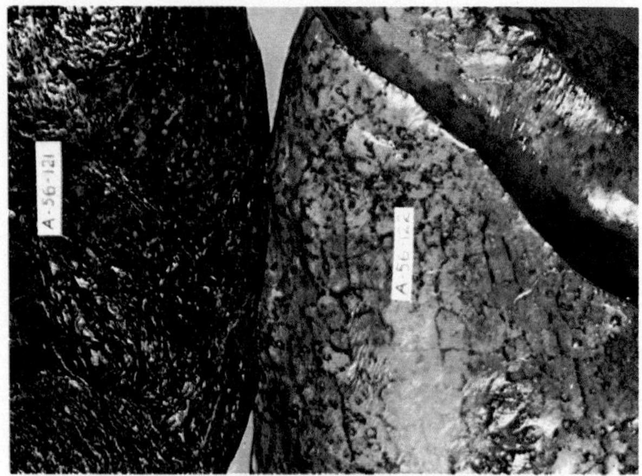

Figure 13.2 A heavily carbon-pigmented lung typical of smokers and coal miners is compared to a normal lung surface. This carbon pigmentation is more frequent in urban and industrialized areas, and it may even appear in the lungs of nonsmokers.

Other Cancers

The death rates for cancers of the mouth, larynx, and esophagus are significantly higher for smokers than for nonsmokers. These cancers affect cigar and pipe smokers as well as cigarette smokers, probably because of the heat and chemicals fed directly into the mouth through the pipe stem or cigar. The lips, tongue, and mucous membranes of cigar and pipe smokers are especially vulnerable to *leukoplakia,* a whitish thickening that is considered to be an early form of cancer.

Together with lung cancer, cancers of the esophagus and trachea have risen sharply since 1935, along with a similar increase in tobacco consumption. Researchers have also linked bladder cancer to cigarette smoking; pack-a-day smokers are twice as likely to die from the condition as are nonsmokers. Toxic materials released while smoking are eliminated through the urine. These are believed to be a prime

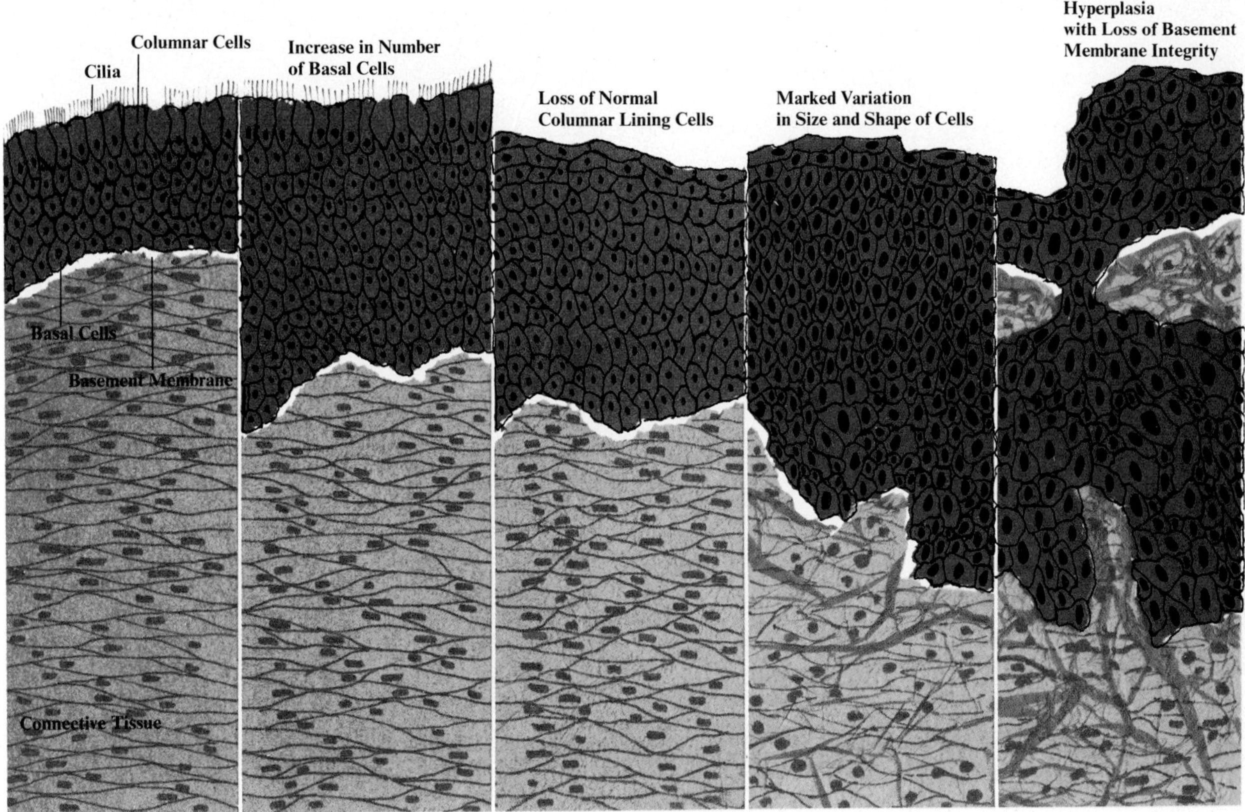

Figure 13.3 The process of hyperplasia. Basal cells that underlie the bronchial lining become irritated and begin to increase in number. This is followed by loss of the ciliated respiratory epithelial cells that function to keep harmful materials out of the lungs. The remaining cells then take on a characteristic "squamous" structure.

factor in bladder cancer. An increased incidence in cancers of the pancreas and kidney may also be the result of excessive smoking.

Heart Disease

Heart attack occurs twice as frequently among cigarette smokers, and sudden death from heart attack occurs three times as frequently in persons who smoke a pack or more a day. In fact, heart attack is the leading cause of excessive deaths suffered by smokers as a group. The risk of heart disease increases in proportion to the number of cigarettes a person smokes and also to the number of years he or she has been smoking.

The physiological processes linking smoking to heart attacks are poorly understood. However, two components of cigarette smoke are implicated: carbon monoxide and nicotine. Carbon monoxide is a colorless, odorless, and poisonous gas that combines with the hemoglobin in red blood cells and reduces the amount of oxygen that reaches body tissues. Nicotine, it is strongly suspected, among other toxic substances, constricts coronary vessels and interferes with nerve signals regulating heartbeat, thereby reducing the supply of oxygen in the heart muscle. It is also probable that nicotine increases the clotting capability of the blood, thereby increasing the likelihood of thrombosis (formation of a blood clot) in coronary vessels. Nicotine also impairs lung function and elevates blood pressure, thus contributing to the chain of events that put unnecessary strain on the heart.

Bronchitis and Emphysema

The familiar hacking cough and large amount of mucus coughed up by cigarette smokers are now known to be the early symptoms of two serious diseases—bronchitis and emphysema, the two most common of the chronic obstructive pulmonary diseases (also known as COPD). These conditions are thought to result when various chemical components of cigarette smoke break down vital tissue in the bronchi or lungs. In bronchitis, the threadlike cilia that normally sweep foreign particles out of the lungs are damaged. The resulting irritation leads to inflammation and narrowing of the bronchial airways, and the affected individual chokes on the excess mucus that is formed. In emphysema, the lungs' tiny air sacs also lose their elasticity and burst. There is trouble in exhaling sufficiently, and used air is trapped in the lungs, giving the person a characteristic "barrel chest" appearance. In both diseases, the person suffers from chronic cough, shortness of breath, and susceptibility to respiratory failure.

WHY START A LIFE UNDER A CLOUD?
Smoking is harmful to your baby's health. Quit for both of you. For help call your American Cancer Society.

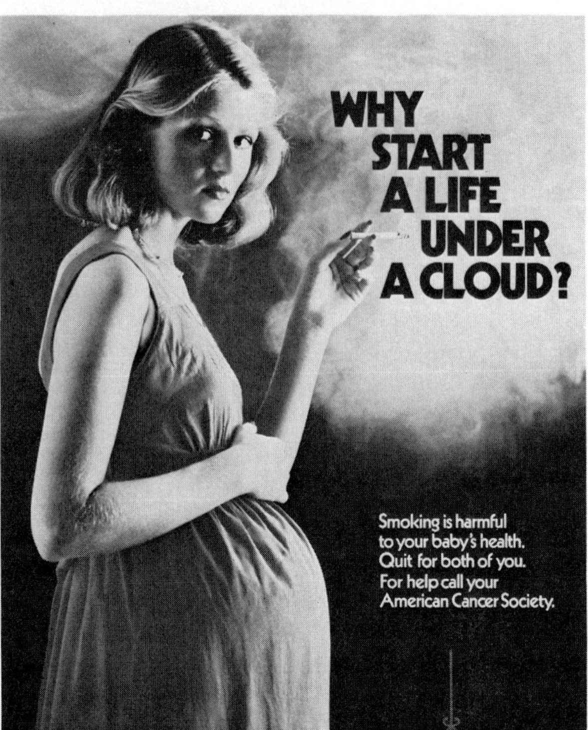

Figure 13.4 A pregnant woman who smokes can cause serious harm to her unborn child.

Smoking and the Pill

In the late 1970s, several different studies showed that cigarette smoking greatly increases the risk of heart attacks, strokes, and other cardiovascular disorders among women who take birth control pills. One California study found that women who both used the pill and smoked were twenty-two times more likely to suffer from certain kinds of strokes than women who did neither. The risks increase with age, according to the Food and Drug Administration, and with heavy smoking (fifteen or more cigarettes a day). Since 1978, the FDA has required that birth control pills be labeled with the warning: "Women who use oral contraceptives should not smoke."

Smoking and Pregnancy

A pregnant woman who smokes can adversely affect her unborn child. Several large studies, involving tens of thousands of pregnancies, reveal that mothers-to-be who smoke have twice as many spontaneous abortions and stillbirths and two to three times as many premature babies as nonsmokers. Furthermore, babies born to women who smoke during pregnancy are on the average nearly one-half pound lighter, according to the 1979 Surgeon General's Report, than babies born to nonsmokers. In one study, researchers calculated that one out of five babies who died would have been saved if their mothers had not been smokers. The precise way in which tobacco smoking affects the fetus is not known. It has been suggested that the oxygen supply to the fetus may be reduced by carbon monoxide (one of the gases in cigarette smoke) poisoning the red blood cells or by nicotine constricting the arteries and reducing the blood flow across the placenta. The Public Health Service says, "Stopping smoking is recommended during pregnancy."

It's Not Too Late to Quit!

Fortunately, some of the damage to the lungs and other parts of the body caused by smoking can be reversed when and if a person does quit. The chances for a longer life span gradually improve as the time off cigarettes increases. According to the 1979 Surgeon General's Report, after ex-smokers have gone fifteen years without smoking, their overall mortality rates approach those of nonsmokers. Similarly, an ex-smoker's chances of dying of lung cancer also gradually decrease the longer he or she is off cigarettes, until after ten to fifteen yeas they too approach those of nonsmokers. And the ex-smoker's risk of a heart attack is also substantially reduced.

People suffering from bronchitis, emphysema, and other chronic lung diseases likewise often experience a significant improvement in their health when they quit smoking. Most cough less and breathe more easily. However, some of the damage to the delicate lung tissue from these diseases is permanent and irreversible. Air sacs destroyed by emphysema never regain their elasticity, and blocked bronchial airways may never reopen.

PROFILE OF THE SMOKER

At the turn of the century, the typical smoker was a middle-class working man who perhaps believed that smoking made him seem more manly. Women who smoked were considered fast, loose, and capable of almost any depravity. The cigarette was considered a "filthy weed" fraught with undertones of impending disaster for the human race.

During the 1920s, men of all professions and backgrounds turned to the cigarette. The flappers joined them; they considered smoking a fashionable mark of sophisticated decadence. It was not until the late 1930s that advertising began to build shining images for cigarettes and the people who smoked them. Smokers were the heroes of the day: fighter pilots, soldiers in the foxhole, tank drivers, doctors, and good-looking nurses.

With television came visual proof that cigarette smokers were the "good guys." The smoker was a tough, handsome cowboy driving a herd of cattle across the Western plains. The "right" cigarette became a sexual lure, attracting bikini-clad beauties off their surfboards into the waiting arms of handsome young men. Another cigarette advertiser conferred a kind of medical certification on smoking, pointing out that more doctors smoked their cigarettes than any other leading brand.

In the 1950s and 1960s, advertising campaigns were aimed heavily at the youth market, particularly college students. Air travelers received complimentary cigarettes with their meals, and children memorized catchy advertising jingles that glorified "good" cigarettes.

As a result of this drum beating, more and more men, women, and children became smokers. By 1964—the year of the Surgeon General's first report—more than one-half of American men and nearly one-third of the women smoked daily, a total of 50 to 60 million smokers. In the age group between twenty-five and thirty-four, nearly 60 percent of the men and 44 percent of the women smoked.

Since then, however—as the health message has gotten across—the percentage of Americans who smoke cigarettes has been declining. According to the 1979 Surgeon General's Report, only 37.5 percent of American men and 29.6 percent of women over the age of seventeen are now smokers.

However, there has been a disturbing upward trend in smoking by two groups of people: adult women and teen-aged girls. Although the percentage of women who smoke has been dropping, the women who do smoke are now smoking more heavily—inhaling more, smoking more cigarettes per day—and also have been smoking for longer periods of time. And as women's smoking habits are shifting more toward those of men, the women are increasingly suffering the same sorts of serious health consequences. Mortality rates from lung cancer are increasing much more rapidly among women than among men; lung-cancer deaths among women have increased fourfold in the last thirty years.

Among teen-aged girls, there has been a dramatic increase in smoking. Since the 1960s, the percentage of girls between the ages of twelve and eighteen who smoke has nearly doubled (to 15.3 percent) and is now nearly

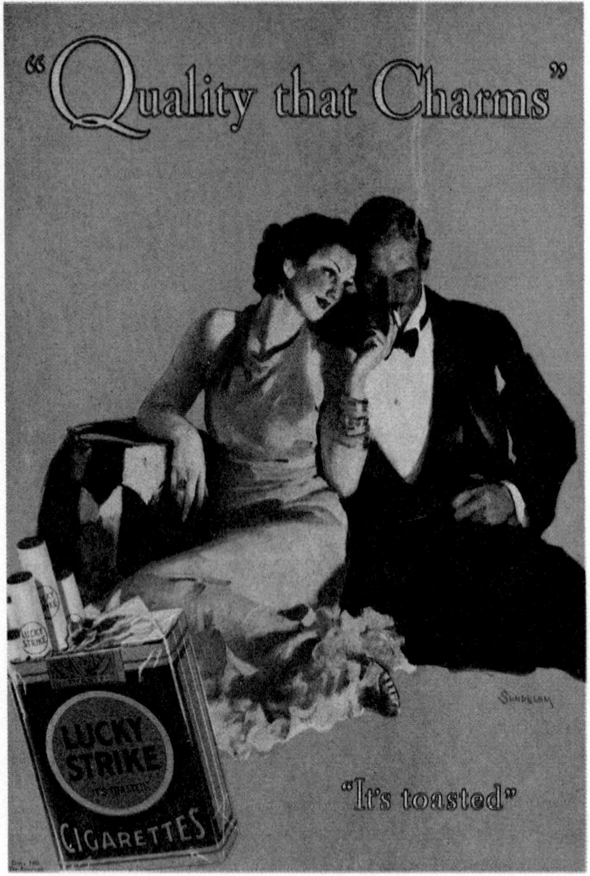

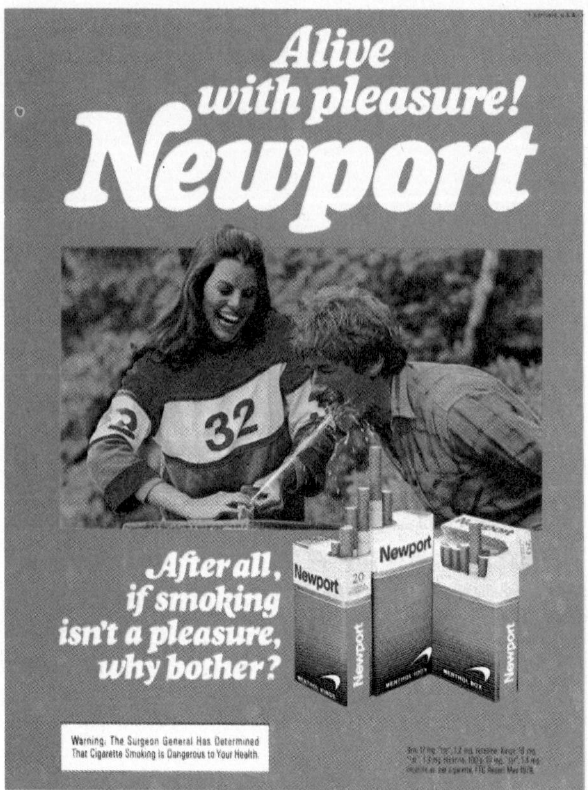

Figure 13.5 In the early 1930s, smoking was considered a mark of sophistication. Today, catchy advertising still lures many people to cigarettes.

the same as that of teen-aged boys (15.8 percent). According to the 1979 Surgeon General's Report, 100,000 American children twelve or under are smokers. In one large West Coast urban area, one out of five children is smoking by the age of twelve.

WHY PEOPLE SMOKE

Social and Psychological Factors

Generally, adolescents begin smoking—and most adults continue smoking—in large part because many other people smoke and because the use of nicotine and other drugs is institutionalized in society. Some 53 million Americans smoking an average of twenty cigarettes a day represent a lot of social reinforcement, as does several hundred million dollars of advertising per year. To smokers, smoking is relaxing and pleasurable; something to do with their hands; a means of communication, role playing, and filling time; a brief "lift"; a comfort; or a sensory pleasure. This pleasure, coupled with the fact that smokers try to cope with many of their interpersonal relationships and emotional problems (tension, gratification of needs, and so on) through smoking, produces a profound psychological dependence.

Some further insight into why people smoke comes from a 1975 American Cancer Society study of teen-aged girl smokers. Generally, these girls were well aware of the health hazards of smoking, but they lived in an environ-

Table 13.1 Cigarette Smoking Among American Teen-Agers, 1965 and 1975

	Current Smokers (in millions)	Total Population	Percent of Smokers
Boys (13–19)			
1965	2.3	12.4	19
1975	3.1	15.0	21
Girls (13–19)			
1965	1.2	12.0	10
1975	2.9	14.5	20
Total (13–19)			
1965	3.5	24.4	14
1975	6.0	29.5	20

Source: U.S. Department of Health, Education, and Welfare, Center for Disease Control, National Clearinghouse for Smoking and Health, Program Research Division, DHEW Publication No. (HSM) 74-8701, 1977.

ment of smokers. Most of their parents (84 percent of the fathers, 64 percent of the mothers) smoked or had smoked; most of their parents (87 percent) knew the teen-agers smoked; and a third of the parents condoned it. The girls' peers—two-thirds of both their male and female friends—also smoked. Half of the girls reported that their schools provided special "smoker" rooms, and 70 percent claimed that their doctors had not warned them about the hazards of smoking. Cigarette smoking among these girls, the study found, also seemed to be associated with rebellion against the adult world.

Pharmacological Factors

While smoking clearly becomes a habit, experts differ as to whether cigarette smoking and nicotine are truly addictive in the sense of producing physical dependence, including withdrawal symptoms when the drug is stopped. (See the discussion of psychological and physical dependence in Chapter 11.)

The peculiar effects of nicotine and the convenience of cigarettes together make smoking an "ideal" drug. The initial effect of nicotine is mildly stimulating—a lift—but the lingering effect is felt as a mild depression, setting up the need for the next cigarette, which can be conveniently carried, lit, and held.

A STUBBORN PROBLEM

Many of the things that can be done to deglamorize smoking, reduce starting, and reinforce quitting have already been initiated—such as the elimination of cigarette advertising from television and radio and the required label warning, "Cigarette smoking is dangerous to your health."

In the United States, things seemed for a while to take a turn for the better. Between 1964 and 1979 some 29 million Americans successfully quit smoking. However, government statistics show that the per capita consumption of cigarettes by Americans over eighteen, while it has declined since 1974, was still nearly 4,000 in 1978. Americans are still among the world's heaviest smokers, says the Department of Health, Education, and Welfare.

The problem is a stubborn one. It's very difficult for a person to kick the habit once nicotine dependence has become established. According to the 1975 survey by the National Clearinghouse for Smoking and Health, nearly two-thirds (61 percent) of current smokers have made at least one serious attempt to stop smoking—and have failed. Curiously, for reasons no one knows, it seems to be more difficult for women than for men to give up smoking. Only one person out of ten is a hard-core smoker totally uninterested in breaking the habit.

The Power of the Tobacco Industry

There are many economic, social, and political forces that make the quick elimination of cigarette smoking unlikely. The 600,000 farm families who produce the 2 billion pounds of tobacco consumed every year experience lung cancer at the same increasing rate as the rest of the population, but will statistics convince them that they should change their occupation? Will a congressman from a tobacco-producing state agitate for the elimination of cigarettes if it means political suicide?

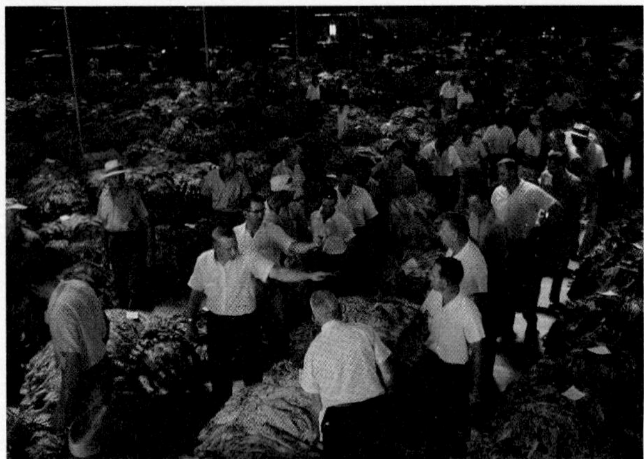

Figure 13.6 A tobacco auction. In spite of the mounting medical evidence against smoking, economic, political, and social forces help to perpetuate it.

The federal government finds itself on both sides of the fence. On one side, it pays out money to underwrite an aggressive anti-tobacco crusade; on the other, it supports tobacco manufacture with agricultural subsidies. And, although it is the U.S. Department of Health, Education, and Welfare that is designated to attack cigarettes, federal agencies—including HEW—benefit from the more than $2.3 billion that the government receives every year from tobacco taxes. Similarly, hard-pressed state and local governments collect their own cigarette tax money, amounting to approximately $3.7 billion a year.

Other major beneficiaries of the tobacco culture are the advertisers who so energetically foster competition between brands; the magazines, newspapers, and billboard owners who prosper through cigarette advertising; the thousands of people who manufacture, ship, and sell cigarettes; and the distributors and vending machine operators who together grossed more than $15.8 billion from cigarettes in 1977.

Pervading this aggregation of pleasure seeking, vested interests, economic pressures, and personal greed is the obstinate insistence of the tobacco industry that there is no link between cigarette smoking and ill health.

KICKING THE HABIT

There are many methods of stopping smoking, ranging from simply quitting "cold turkey"—which some authorities consider the most effective method—to elaborate, highly structured (and sometimes expensive) group programs that may taper off cigarette smoking over a period of many weeks. No one method is right for everyone. As Dr. Daniel Horn, Director of the National Clearinghouse for Smoking and Health, has put it: "There is no program, no matter how weird, that has not helped somebody and there is no program, no matter how good, that has not failed to help many people who tried it."

There are a number of products on the market offered as aids to do-it-yourself quitting programs: books, records and cassettes; over-the-counter tablets; and sets of graduated filters designed to reduce, over a period of weeks, a person's tar and nicotine intake. Since people carry out these programs on their own, the experts find it hard to evaluate their effectiveness.

Some programs involve hypnosis, usually one or more sessions, where a practitioner puts the prospective quitter into a mild trance and then coaches him or her about how to stop. Other programs rely on aversion techniques. They may administer mild electric shocks, or have the person breathe stale cigarette smoke or smoke extremely rapidly, in an effort to associate smoking with an unpleasant experience.

There are a wide variety of group programs and clinics, some sponsored by voluntary health organizations, such as the American Cancer Society, the American Heart Association, and the American Lung Association. Other stop-smoking programs are run as commercial businesses. Group programs usually involve lectures, films, discussions, and practical tips on how to stop. Many use the "buddy system," pairing off participants so that they can bolster each other's resolve. Some of these programs meet regularly over a period of weeks; others are concentrated five-day programs. Some hospitals even offer intensive, twenty-four-hour-a-day, live-in programs.

In considering the cost of a program, one

HOW TO

Kick the Habit—for Good

Have you ever tried to quit smoking? Do you know someone who wants to give it up, but just can't?

It's tough to break the cigarette habit, but 29 million Americans *have* done it. The American Cancer Society has compiled a list of methods that some of these people have used—successfully—to help them quit for good. Here are a few that you can recommend to others—or try yourself:

1. Smoke an *excess* of cigarettes (three or four packs) for a day or two to spoil their taste; then quit. Or quit when you have a cold or the flu, and have no desire for cigarettes.
2. Write down your reasons for not smoking. Read your list often and add new reasons when you can.
3. List a few things you would like to buy. Calculate their cost in terms of packs of cigarettes. Put the money you used to spend daily on cigarettes into a special piggy bank. Then splurge!
4. Bet a friend that you can quit. Bet with your cigarette money.
5. Never buy cigarettes by the carton. Finish one pack before you buy another.
6. Never carry cigarettes, matches, or a lighter.
7. Change brands every week. Your new brand must have less tar and nicotine than the old one.
8. Smoke only during even- or odd-numbered hours.
9. Smoke only half a cigarette. Inhale only every other puff.
10. Say "I don't want to smoke," not "I've quit smoking." If you do have a cigarette, you won't feel that you've broken your resolution.
11. Help someone else to quit.
12. Always ask yourself, "Do I need this cigarette or is this just a reflex?" If you really need the cigarette, go to a mirror and watch yourself light up.
13. If you crave a cigarette, take ten deep breaths. Strike a match while you hold the last breath. Exhale slowly, blowing out the match. Crush the match into an ashtray as if it were a cigarette. Get back to work immediately.
14. After you quit, use your lungs more: increase your activities and exercise moderately.

Source: Adapted from the American Cancer Society (California Division), San Francisco, Cal.

should include the cost of continuing to smoke. A two-pack-a-day smoker can easily spend several hundred dollars a year on cigarettes. Also, the sponsors of the program should be asked what its success rate is after one year. Many people find it easier to give up cigarettes than to stay off of them. Good stop-smoking programs have success rates of 30 to 40 percent at one-year follow-ups.

THE RIGHTS OF NONSMOKERS

The Surgeon General's Reports suggest that tobacco smoke in enclosed indoor areas is an important air pollution problem. Carbon monoxide levels of sidestream smoke (smoke from the burning end) reach 42,000 parts per million. (The Environmental Protection Agency sets 100 parts per million as the maximum clean air standard.) Carbon monoxide levels in smoke-filled rooms can be sufficient to harm the health, says the Public Health Service, of people with chronic bronchopulmonary disease or coronary heart disease.

While most people suffer some discomfort from heavy concentrations of tobacco smoke, people allergic to such smoke suffer the most. About 10 to 15 percent of Americans are allergic to tobacco smoke and suffer reactions ranging from mild eye irritation and upper respiratory congestion to life-threatening asthma attacks.

Increasing numbers of nonsmokers are more militantly demanding their right to breathe air free from tobacco smoke. Many nonsmokers are asking smokers not to light up in certain places. Some have established no-smoking rules in their cars and homes. In 1976, a New Jersey woman who is allergic to tobacco smoke sued her employer, the telephone company, for the right to a smoke-free working place—and the New Jersey Superior Court set a precedent by ordering a ban on smoking in the office she shared with other workers.

Collectively, nonsmokers in many communities have organized groups such as ASH (Action on Smoking and Health) and GASP (Group Against Smokers' Pollution). These groups have succeeded in securing nonsmokers' rights laws that prohibit smoking in certain

No Smoking
Please
smoking is
permitted only in
designated areas.
Minnesota
Clean Indoor Air Act
1975 Legislative Statute

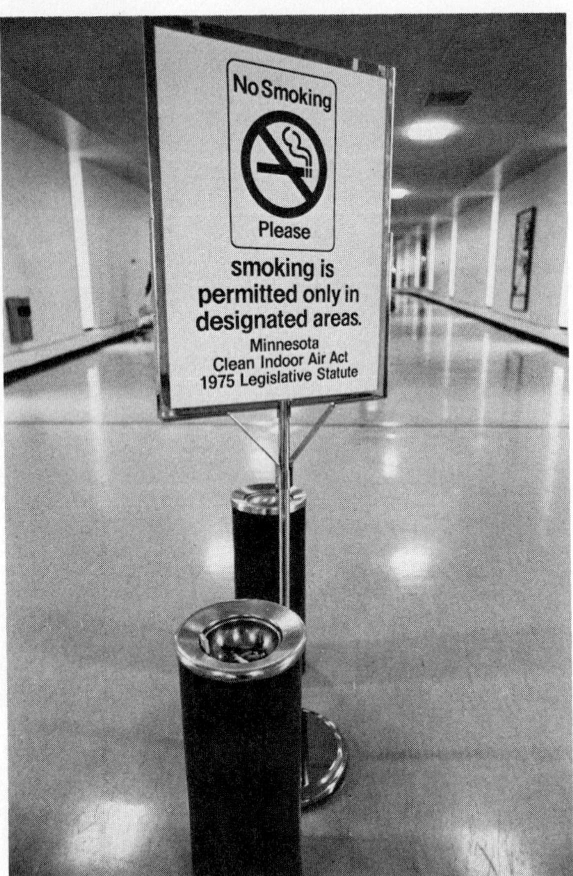

Figure 13.7 The growing militancy of nonsmokers has led to the prohibition of smoking in many public places.

public places—usually those where people have to spend time, such as food markets, public waiting rooms, service lines, and elevators. By 1978, at least twenty-eight states had passed "clean indoor air" laws restricting smoking in public places and certain facilities like hospitals and nursing homes.

Laws are not automatically obeyed, especially when they go counter to established traditions and habits. As substantial numbers of nonsmokers overtly express support for these laws, however, a profound change is taking place not only in public smoking but in the social acceptability of smoking in general. This erosion of public tolerance of smoking may, in the long run, have a greater impact on this deadly and crippling habit than all the scientific and educational efforts combined.

SUMMARY

1. Smoking is hazardous to health. Smokers have a 70 percent greater overall mortality rate from disease than do nonsmokers.
2. More than 1,200 toxic chemicals have been identified in cigarette smoke. The "drug" in tobacco is nicotine, which primarily affects the nervous system. Another component, benzopyrene, is one of the deadliest known carcinogens.
3. Smokers are eleven times more likely than nonsmokers to die from lung cancer. Death rates for cancers of the mouth, larynx, and esophagus are also significantly higher among smokers.
4. Heart attacks occur twice as frequently among cigarette smokers as among nonsmokers, and heart attack is the leading cause of excessive deaths among smokers.
5. Millions of heavy smokers are also chronically disabled by emphysema, bronchitis, and other respiratory diseases.
6. Cigarette smoking greatly increases the risk of heart attacks, strokes, and other cardiovascular disorders among women who take oral contraceptives.
7. A woman who smokes during pregnancy can harm her unborn child. Smoking mothers-to-be are more likely to have spontaneous abortions, stillbirths, and premature babies.
8. After fifteen years off cigarettes, the overall mortality rates and lung-cancer death rates of smokers approach those of nonsmokers.
9. In recent years, the percentage of Americans who smoke has dropped significantly. By 1979 only 37.5 percent of men and 29.6 percent of women smoked. However, there has been a dramatic increase in the number of teen-aged girls who smoke.
10. It is not easy for a person to stop smoking once nicotine dependence is established. Nine out of ten smokers say that they either have tried to quit and failed or would quit if there was an easy way.
11. Some of the methods of stopping smok-

ing include quitting "cold turkey," graduated filters, hypnosis, aversion techniques, and commercial group programs.

12. Carbon monoxide levels in smoke-filled rooms can become high enough to harm the health of nonsmokers. Nonsmokers are becoming increasingly militant about their right to unpolluted air.

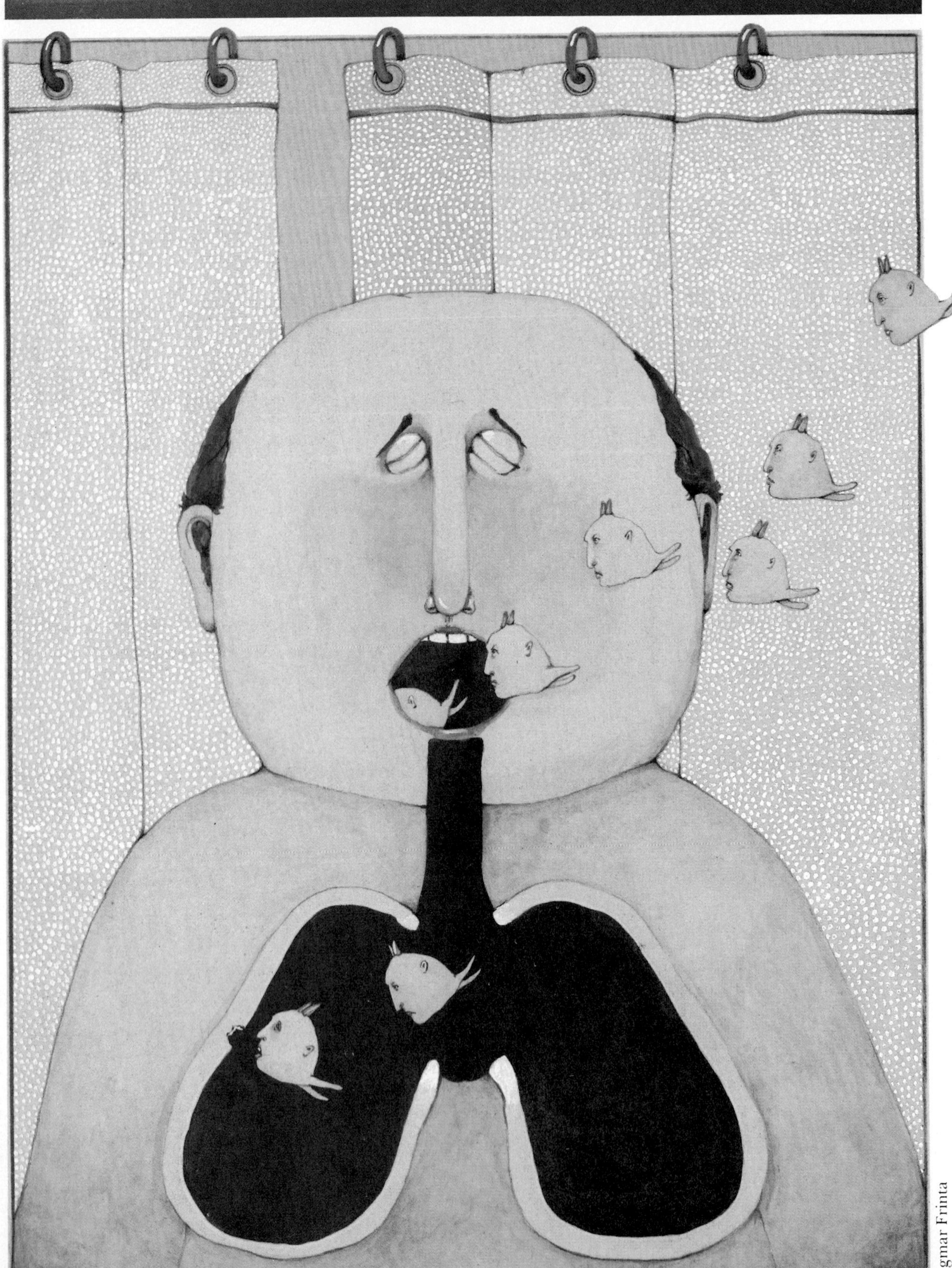

Dagmar Frinta

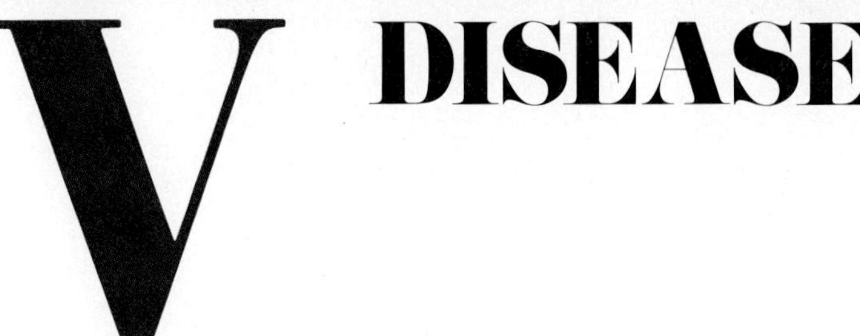

V DISEASE

Disease is a threat that human beings have always had to face. Even as our technology evolved and we grew more and more able to protect ourselves from starvation and other terrors, we were still victimized by a great number of diseases. Then, about a century ago, the picture began to change as, one by one, most of these historically dreaded illnesses were conquered by advances in medical science.

However, the technological progress that brought these diseases—such as tuberculosis, diphtheria, and whooping cough—under control also triggered the increased incidence of other types of afflictions. Until just a few years ago, many Americans thought that they could smoke, overeat, avoid exercise, and endure stress without risk of adverse consequences. We know differently now, but the diseases of life style—notably cancer and cardiovascular diseases—are our major health problems today.

Part V examines the struggle against disease from the highest levels of research and decision making to the personal level—what *you* can do to guard against illness. Chapter 14 discusses the causes and changing patterns of disease, as well as the most common infectious diseases that remain at large. Today's leading killers, cancer and the cardiovascular diseases, are the subjects of Chapters 15 and 16 respectively.

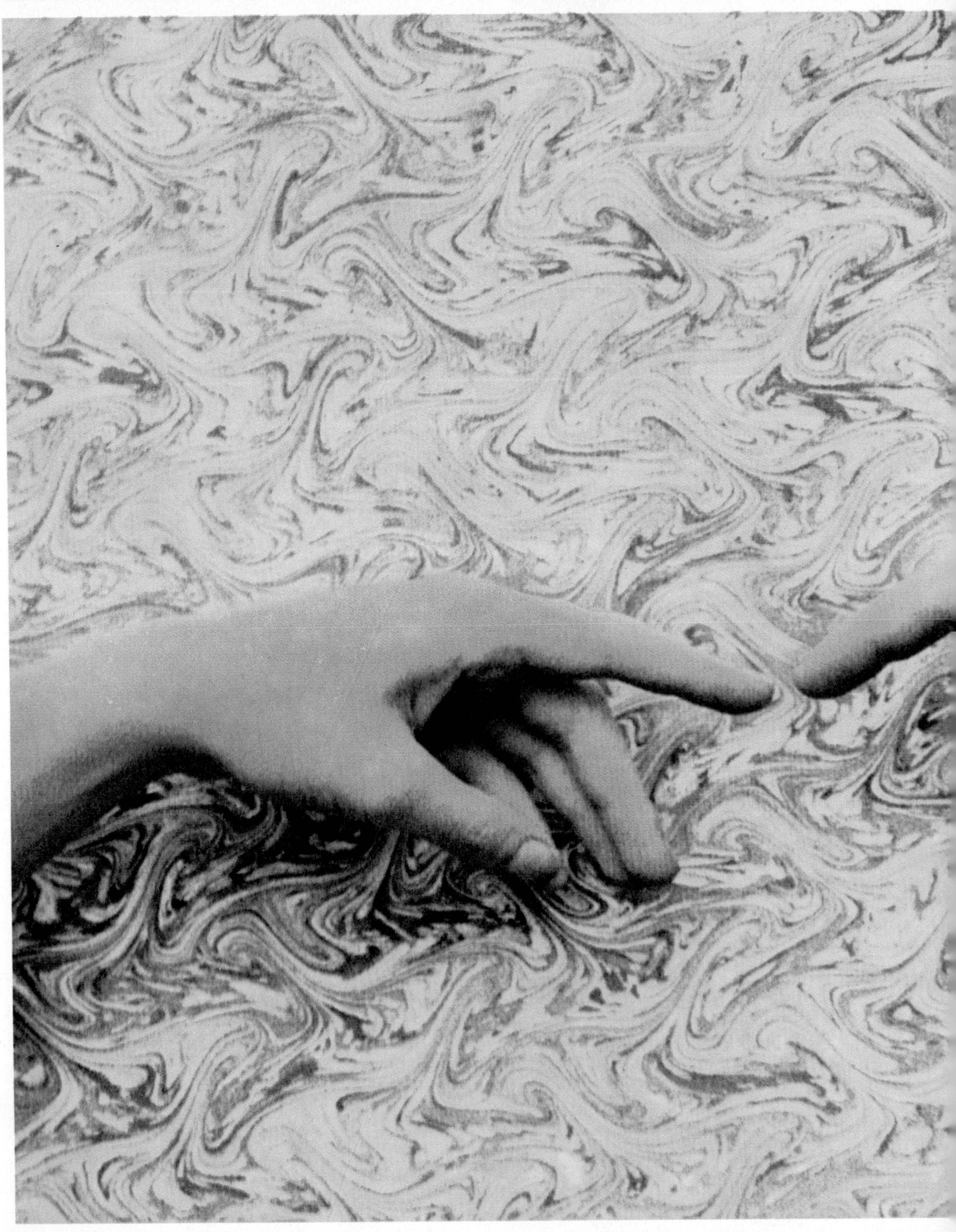

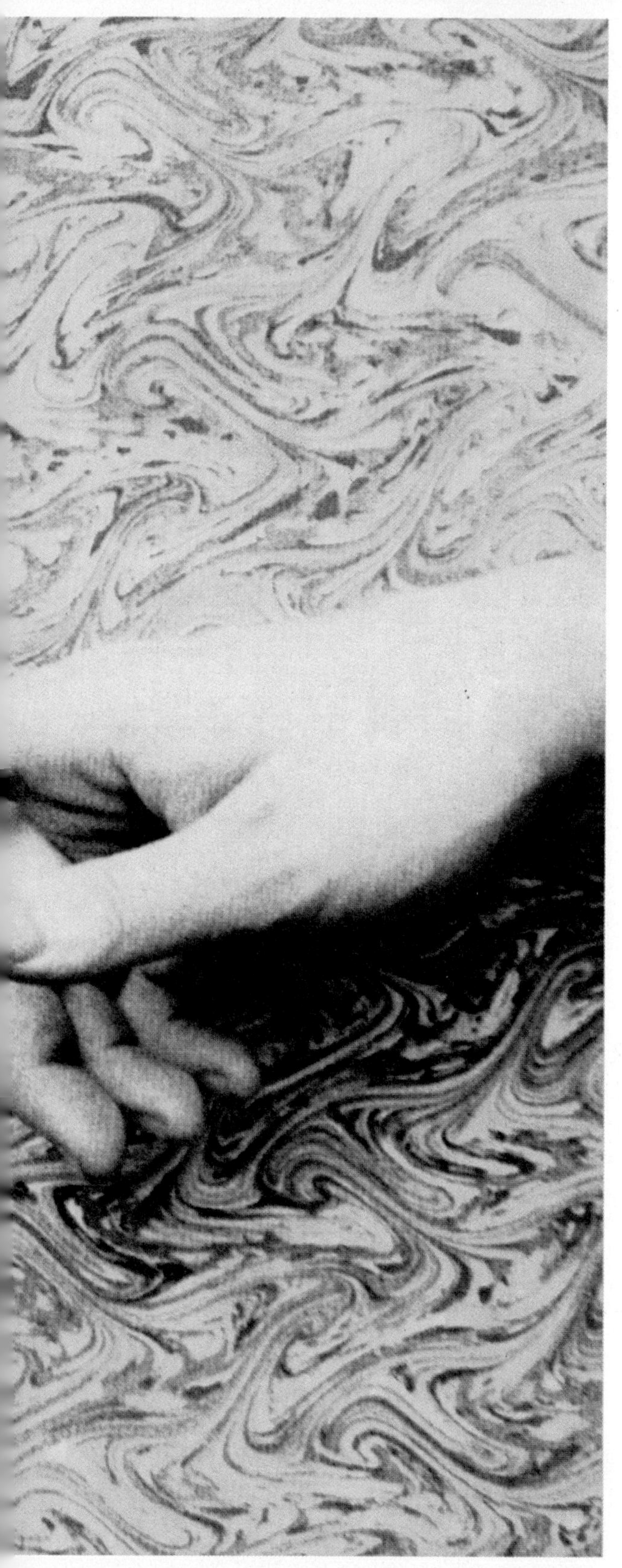

14 Communicable Diseases

People have desired a long and healthy life since prehistoric times. As long ago as 2000 B.C., the Babylonians perceived that good health was not entirely a matter of chance or "the will of the gods." A thousand years later, the Egyptians commonly followed simple sanitary practices by constructing "earth closets" and public drainage pipes, and used numerous pharmacological preparations in treating the ill. Health measures were further elaborated upon by the Jews, whose Mosaic laws are now considered to have comprised the first formal hygienic code.

Unfortunately, this limited development of health knowledge was followed by centuries of little progress. Throughout the Middle Ages, disease and death were generally blamed on the "demons" of superstition or the "punishment" of religion. Cultural and religious practices prohibited autopsies, thereby limiting severely any real study of the human body. Were it not for the practice of *quarantining*—the restriction on leaving or entering a premises if an infectious disease has been diagnosed—epidemics of leprosy, diphtheria, typhoid, and bubonic plague would probably have succeeded totally in what has been called "mankind's nearest approach to complete annihilation."

Perhaps the most devastating example of the result of uncontrolled health measures occurred during the fourteenth century when bubonic plague, or the "Black Death," ravaged Europe. At least one-third of the population died; in England alone, the population fell from 3.8 million in 1348 to 2.1 million in 1374.

The economic, moral, religious, and social effects were enormous.

But the destruction wrought by the plague gradually made people aware that poor sanitation and neglected personal hygiene had provided an optimal environment for the spread of disease. Cities were terribly dirty; vermin and rats thrived in the streets. People bathed infrequently, if at all, and soap was rarely used. In the centuries following the plague, communities worked to improve sanitation, construct hospitals, and reduce crowding.

During the Renaissance, scientific thought began to displace preoccupation with the supernatural. The sixteenth and seventeenth centuries witnessed medical milestones such as Vesalius's studies of anatomy, Anton van Leeuwenhoek's discovery of the microscope, and Marcello Malpighi's study of tissue structure. But comprehensive knowledge of disease causation was still far in the future.

DISEASE ANALYSIS

The systematic study of the distribution and dynamics of disease among populations is known as *epidemiology.* The ultimate goal of the epidemiologist is to *prevent* disease, by studying not only patterns of disease but also patterns of good health. Examination of disease patterns eventually tells us something of its causation; causation usually offers clues to prevention. We now know that malaria, for example, can be controlled by draining swamps and other breeding grounds of the mosquito carrier. Many other such diseases of the past are now almost unheard of in the United States, though this is not necessarily true for the rest of the world. There are still 200 million cases of goiter worldwide, even though we have long known it can be easily prevented by adding sufficient iodine to the diet.

In order to study a disease pattern, epidemiologists must consider the frequency of its occurrence in relation to a number of factors—geographic, ethnic, economic, social, and cultural—as well as fluctuations that occur due to sex, physical environment, and personal habits. Various types of data are utilized: (1) *mortality rates*—the number of deaths occurring in a given population; (2) *morbidity* or *incidence rates*—the number of cases of a disease diagnosed in a given population; (3) *life expectancy* (at the time of birth)—the average number of years one may expect to live; (4) *infant mortality*—the number of infant deaths occurring before age one; (5) *maternal mortality*—the number of pregnancy-related deaths occurring before, during, and after childbirth.

Almost all tables listing the above information are usually expressed on the basis of cases per 100,000 population. For example, as can be seen in Figure 14.7, the heart disease death rate in the United States in 1976 was 339.2 persons per 100,000 persons in the country. The figures are not percentages (which would be per 100 population), but are much lower than that. A mortality rate of 337.2 per 100,000 would indicate that .337 percent of the population died of heart disease in that year. (Note that this figure is a percentage of the total population—not a percentage of total deaths.)

Age is the single most important epidemiological variable. Frequently statistics on death and disease are age-adjusted so that comparisons can be made from year to year. Age-adjusted figures eliminate the effects of an aging population; that is, the adjusted rates assume that the age structures of the populations being compared are the same. For example, it would be inappropriate to compare the general cancer death rate in the United States in 1900 with that in 1978. In 1978, a larger portion of the population was over age sixty; other things being equal, more cancer would occur simply because of the age distribution factor. In adjusting rates, a standard population (say, that of 1940 or 1960) is chosen, and rates are calculated on the basis of that population's age distribution.

Generally speaking, an *epidemic* occurs when a disease affects a larger number of people in one area than it normally would. While this concept is usually thought to involve hundreds of thousands of victims, the term is often used relatively. One case of yellow fever or a few cases of plague in the United States might be considered an epidemic today, simply because those diseases are so rare here. Conversely, thousands of colds on a winter day in New York City would not be considered abnormal.

Diseases that occur normally in a given area and at a relatively consistent level are considered to be *endemic* to that area. Diseases become *pandemic* when they spread beyond their usual geographic confines. Cholera, for example, was endemic to the Celebes Islands of Indonesia but has become pandemic since 1961.

Possible causative agents of disease cannot be studied without also studying the absence of the agents in a comparable selection of people. Those groups *not* exposed to the factor being studied are called *control groups*. By using controls, the effects of factors *not* being tested are eliminated. In studying the possible effects of cigarette smoking on disease, for example, it was necessary to compare the disease rates of cigarette smokers with those of nonsmokers who were similar in every way except their smoking histories.

Detection of causal association is occasionally hampered by the existence of *multifactors*—two or more factors acting together to produce a particular disease condition, although neither by itself will do so. In the past, progress was sometimes delayed for decades as the search continued for a single causative agent. The interplay of multifactors is explained more fully in the following section, *Causes of Disease*.

Once all data have been collected, they must be analyzed and interpreted. The manner in which data are analyzed and put into perspective can lead to widely differing conclusions. No single study should ever be deemed the final word on any subject.

What epidemiologists look for is a pattern of *consistency* in their results. Using the cigarette analogy, when the first epidemiological studies were published in 1950, no firm conclusions were drawn. More work was needed to confirm the results. When, by 1964, dozens of human studies had been finished and the conclusions were unanimous, a verdict could be registered.

The real problem for public health policy makers is the occasional necessity of offering preventive health advice on the basis of incomplete evidence. For example, more than two decades of scientific work have examined the possible effect that a diet rich in cholesterol and fat can have on one's chance of developing heart disease. As of this writing, the interpretation of most public health scientists is that there might be a link between diet and heart disease, although the case is far from proven. But what should be recommended while the issues are being resolved? The decision is difficult, and caution in making recommendations is generally the guideline. Certainly the possible adverse implications of a public health program should be considered along with the possible benefits.

In spite of the difficulties of data collection, and the uncertainties of interpretation and application, epidemiology is useful—if not indispensable—in many ways, particularly in determining disease trends, development of measures for prevention or control, and analysis of disease outbreaks. In the past, such studies usually involved a communicable disease or poisonous agent, but as these problems have gradually come under control, epidemiologists are increasingly concerning themselves with chronic diseases, including cancer, heart disease, and diabetes. Indeed, almost everything we know about the causation of human cancer has been derived from epidemiological observations—specifically, that smokers have higher rates of lung cancer, that fair-skinned individuals exposed to a great deal of sunlight have a higher rate of skin cancer, that daughters of women exposed to the drug DES have a higher rate of a rare type of vaginal cancer, and that children exposed to high-dose radiation have higher rates of thyroid cancer as young adults.

CAUSES OF DISEASE

Disease, or "dis-ease," is defined as the incorrect functioning of an organ, part, structure, or system of the body. Obviously, then, there are many kinds of causes.

"Cause," however, is an inexact term. What we are really talking about is a *causal association*—or, in other words, one's *risk* of developing a disease. As has already been mentioned, while early epidemiological studies dealt primarily with infectious (communicable) diseases such as cholera, the emphasis has now shifted toward study of the noninfectious, or *chronic,* disorders like cancer and coronary heart disease. In both types, however, the ac-

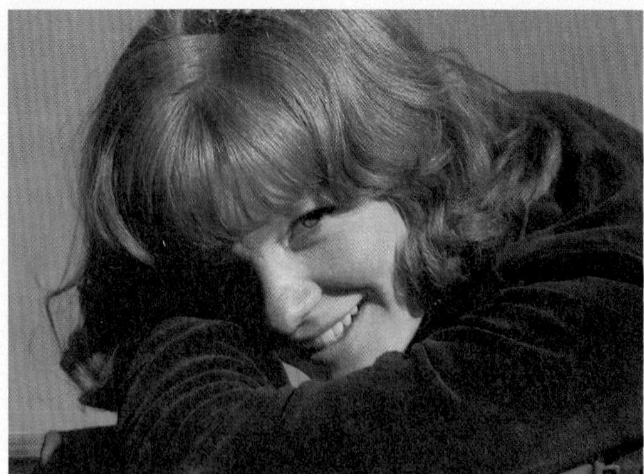

Figure 14.1 Is the possibility of this woman developing skin cancer due to heredity or environment?

tual presence of disease and the establishment of risk are based on three factors: *environment, contact,* and *susceptibility.* Without the presence of all three factors for a specific disorder, the disorder will not occur.

For example, it is necessary for the victim of an infectious disease such as yellow fever (1) to be living within an *environment* that provides a source of the infectious agent and favors its development and transmission, (2) to have come in *contact* with the infectious agent, and (3) to be *susceptible* as a host to the disease. Similarly, coronary heart disease may result from (1) psychosocial and economic *environments* that cause or reinforce behaviors leading to the development of the ailment, (2) *contact* with specific disease-inducing factors (such as elevated blood cholesterol, high blood pressure, smoking, and perhaps poor diet and lack of exercise), and (3) individual *susceptibility* (genetic predisposition, the undermining influence of other diseases, and so forth).

Table 14.1 details some specific causes of disease: heredity, environment, infection, diet, drugs, stress, and degenerative processes. One must keep in mind, however, that the multifactor principle is frequently operative in determining one's risk of disease. That is, often an illness results from not just one disease-causing agent but from a combination of several factors. Thus one individual might develop heart disease as a result of the combination of two or more factors, such as heredity, poor diet, stress, smoking, and lack of exercise. Similarly, some cancers may involve viruses interacting with environmental irritants and stress, or could result from the combination of two high-risk exposures—for example, alcohol and tobacco teaming up to cause cancer of the mouth, or asbestos and cigarette smoking causing lung cancer. Thus, in addition to the specific treatment required for a given disease, it is often crucial to protect the patient against other agents that might take advantage of his or her debilitated condition to impose their own damaging—even lethal—effects.

AGENTS OF INFECTION

Many people fear microorganisms, or microbes, and refer to them as "germs." But not all microbes are harmful. Specialists have estimated that actually only a limited number of the known microbial species are *pathogens*—that is, organisms that regularly cause disease.

Those organisms with which people live most intimately and harmoniously are called resident, or *endogenous,* microbes, meaning that they reside within the human host. These microbes are so small that the billions of them in one body combined would probably not take up much more than one and a quarter measuring cups. Most of them are quite compatible with the health of the human body and in fact may contribute to its welfare—for example, by manufacturing essential vitamins and amino acids in the intestines. However, endogenous microbes cannot be regarded as completely or permanently harmless simply because they are inoffensive under normal circumstances. When these circumstances change, serious disease may result.

Other organisms are *exogenous*—that is, they are not normal residents of the human body. Such organisms will cause disease if they gain a foothold of any kind. But even if they invade, a variety of circumstances determine whether the invasion will lead to disease. The number of organisms present, the health of the individual exposed (including fatigue, resistance, and so on), and even the individual's environment are often involved.

Table 14.1 The Causes of Disease

Agent	Roles	Examples
Heredity	Parents can pass genetic defects to their children. Heredity can predispose people to certain diseases.	Genetic disorders—sickle-cell anemia, PKU, Tay-Sachs disease, hemophilia, cystic fibrosis Genetic predisposition to stomach and skin cancers, schizophrenia
Environment	Environmental conditions such as pollution, socioeconomic factors, and individual life style can damage health.	Bronchitis or asthma aggravated by air pollution Mercury or cadmium poisoning due to water pollution Hearing loss and stress due to noise pollution Undernutrition due to poverty Skin cancer due to overexposure to the sun Various diseases caused or aggravated by drug abuse (see below)
Infection	Infectious agents—usually bacteria or viruses—cause disease by entering and reproducing within a host organism.	Common cold Influenza Tuberculosis Mononucleosis Hepatitis Syphilis Gonorrhea
Diet	Malnutrition (the wrong diet ingredients), undernutrition (insufficient amounts of food), and overeating (consumption of too many calories) can cause or contribute to a variety of health problems.	Vitamin-deficiency diseases—scurvy, pellagra, rickets Heart disease, some cancers, diabetes, and infertility (from overeating)
Drugs	Dependence on drugs—both psychoactive substances and medical preparations—can damage health. Overuse of antibiotics contributes to resistant strains of bacteria. Overuse of drugs can cause harmful side effects. Some drugs have a *synergistic* effect—they can greatly increase the danger from another risk factor.	Lung cancer (from cigarettes) Heart attack (from cigarettes, the Pill) Cirrhosis of the liver (from alcohol)
Stress	Stress can be a contributing factor to almost any disease, and it can be a critical element in many cases (see Chapter 2).	Heart and blood-vessel diseases Hypertension Mental disorders Psychosomatic disorders Asthma
Degenerative Processes	The degenerative processes associated with aging and old age can cause disease. These processes may actually begin as early as infancy or childhood.	Degenerative hearing loss Atherosclerosis Osteoporosis (bone brittleness due to loss of calcium)

Infection is the attack that these exogenous agents wage against the body. Disease occurs only when the infectious agent originally *presents itself* in such great numbers or *multiplies* to such an extent within the infected body that it can cause harm to it. The microbes may produce damage because of their numbers, as is the case with pneumonia, or because they release poisons, or *toxins,* like those given off by the bacteria responsible for tetanus or diphtheria. In other cases, both mechanisms are involved. Disease usually becomes apparent when the body fights the invader. The site of infection may become sore, hot, and swollen. Other parts of the body may become involved as the infection spreads.

Infectious agents are of six main types: bacteria, viruses, rickettsiae, fungi, protozoa, and worms (or metazoa). Many common diseases caused by the six main types of pathogens are described in the Appendix.

Bacteria, a type of single-celled plant life, are the most plentiful of such microorganisms and comprise the major portion of organisms endogenous to humans. Most bacteria are either nonharmful or are vital to human existence. The bacterium *Escherichia coli,* for example, plays an important role in digestion; other bacteria perform such functions as vitamin production and destruction of potential pathogens.

Some diseases are caused by endogenous bacteria that for various reasons get out of hand. For instance, bacteria normally found on the skin may have a role in acne; bacteria endogenous to the mouth are involved in the serious gum disease pyorrhea; and intestinal bacteria, particularly in women, may be transferred from feces to the urethra and cause urinary tract infections. An upset in normal balances between tissues and the flora that inhabit them is thought to play a role in such problems. Harmful bacteria, on the other hand, are responsible for such diseases as gonorrhea, meningitis, tuberculosis, tetanus, and syphilis. Fortunately, bacteria are susceptible to antibiotics, so that bacterial diseases can largely be brought under control.

Viruses are the most minute and primitive form of life. Essentially they consist of a bit of nucleic acid (RNA or DNA, but never both) within a protein coat. Once a single virus enters a cell, it takes over the cell's machinery and directs it to produce many hundreds of new viral particles. A single cell thus engorged with viruses breaks apart, spewing its contents in all directions, each viral particle having the ability to again enter a cell, capture its machinery, and start the cycle again. Among the many virus-caused diseases are smallpox, rubella, measles, mumps, influenza, the common cold, hepatitis, and genital herpes.

Viruses differ greatly in size and shape. The spherical influenza virus is about ten times larger than the tiny cuboid polio virus. In one major respect, all viruses are the same: they cannot multiply outside the cell.

Rickettsiae are considered intermediate between bacteria and viruses. Most of these organisms grow in the intestinal tracts of insects (vectors) that carry them to their human host. Such blood-sucking insects as lice, rat fleas, mites, and ticks spread these infectious agents to humans. Typhus fever is transmitted by fleas, ticks, and lice; Rocky Mountain spotted fever is transmitted by ticks.

Fungi are plants that lack chlorophyll and must obtain their food from organic material—in some cases, from humans. Ringworm and athlete's foot are infections caused by fungi.

Animal parasites, including certain types of *protozoa* and worms, are organisms that have developed the capacity to live in or on the body of another animal, known as the *host.* Most parasites have acquired the remarkable ability of spending part of their life in one host (a human being) and the rest of their life in another host (which can range from a mosquito to a cow, fish being a particularly common host). Protozoa are responsible for such diseases as amoebic dysentery and malaria. Worms that make their homes in humans include pinworms, tapeworms, and flukes.

HOW INFECTION SPREADS

Acne, pyorrhea, and urinary tract infections are examples of endogenous, normally harmless microbes causing their host to become diseased. Or, possibly, the host has become diseased from another source, causing the host's endogenous microbes to proliferate and create further ailments. In any case, the resulting disease remains restricted to that one person. But infectious ailments that derive from exogenous microbes, such as colds, tuberculosis, sexually transmitted diseases, and malaria, can be passed from individual to individual, either directly or through such intermediaries as insects, air, or drinking water: they are *communicable.*

Pathogenic agents may enter the body either through breaks in the skin or through any of the natural openings of the body, such as those of the respiratory tract, the alimentary tract, or the urogenital tract. Pathogens also are often *released* through these same parts of the body, to be transmitted to other persons.

Certain infections are spread by direct physical contact—sexually transmitted diseases, for example. Others may be spread by objects such as clothing or eating utensils that have been touched or used by an infected individual. Some organisms travel through the air attached to dust particles or water droplets. One sneeze can account for approximately 20,000 droplets, which may cover a range of 15 feet and which contain large numbers of microorganisms, many of them capable of causing disease. Food and water can also transmit infectious agents, as occurs in cholera, typhoid, and dysentery. In addition, insects act as *vectors* (intermediaries) for such diseases as plague, yellow fever, and malaria.

THE COURSE OF AN INFECTION

Because all these infections depend upon basically the same mechanism—invasion by foreign organisms and the reaction of the invaded body to them—a common pattern can be recognized when disease develops. The course of an infectious disease has five broad phases:

1. The *incubation period* begins with the invasion. During this phase, the organisms multiply in the host. The length of the incubation period varies from disease to disease and from one person to another for the same disease.
2. The *prodrome period* is a short interval characterized by general symptoms such as headache, fever, nasal discharge, malaise, irritability, and discomfort. Diagnosis is difficult because the symptoms are so similar for most diseases. The disease is highly communicable during prodrome.
3. *Clinical disease* occurs when illness is at its height. The characteristic symptoms appear during this phase, and specific diagnosis becomes possible. A disease that is *subclinical* presents few symptoms and may therefore be undiagnosed.
4. The *decline stage* is marked by subsiding symptoms. The patient may feel well enough to become active before recovery, which may increase the danger of relapse.
5. *Convalescence* is the recovery period. The disease may still be communicable. A patient who recovers but still gives off disease-causing organisms becomes one form of *carrier* of that disease.

BODY DEFENSES

The body is exposed to an almost infinite number and variety of organisms, many of which are capable of causing disease. To combat these agents, the body mobilizes a system of natural defenses. The strength with which these defenses operate is greatly influenced by the health of the whole body—or of the body

Figure 14.2 The chain of infection. A pathogen leaves a human reservoir through a portal of exit, such as the nose, mouth, or urogenital system. It is then transmitted to a portal of entry in another person, where the disease is established. To conquer the disease, one has only to break a link in the chain.

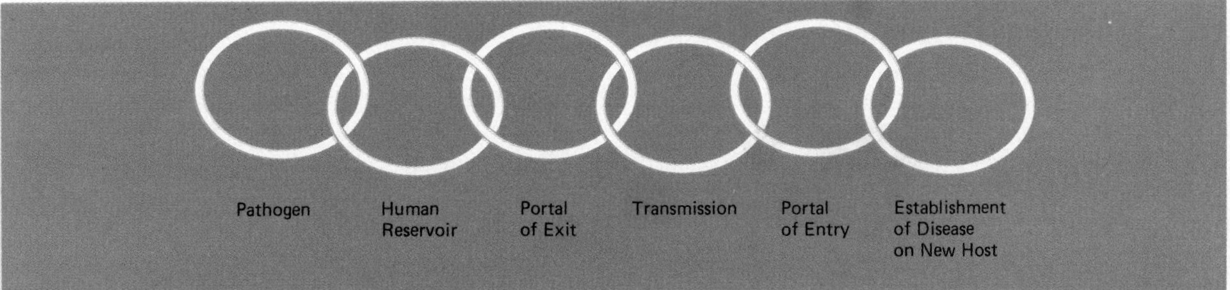

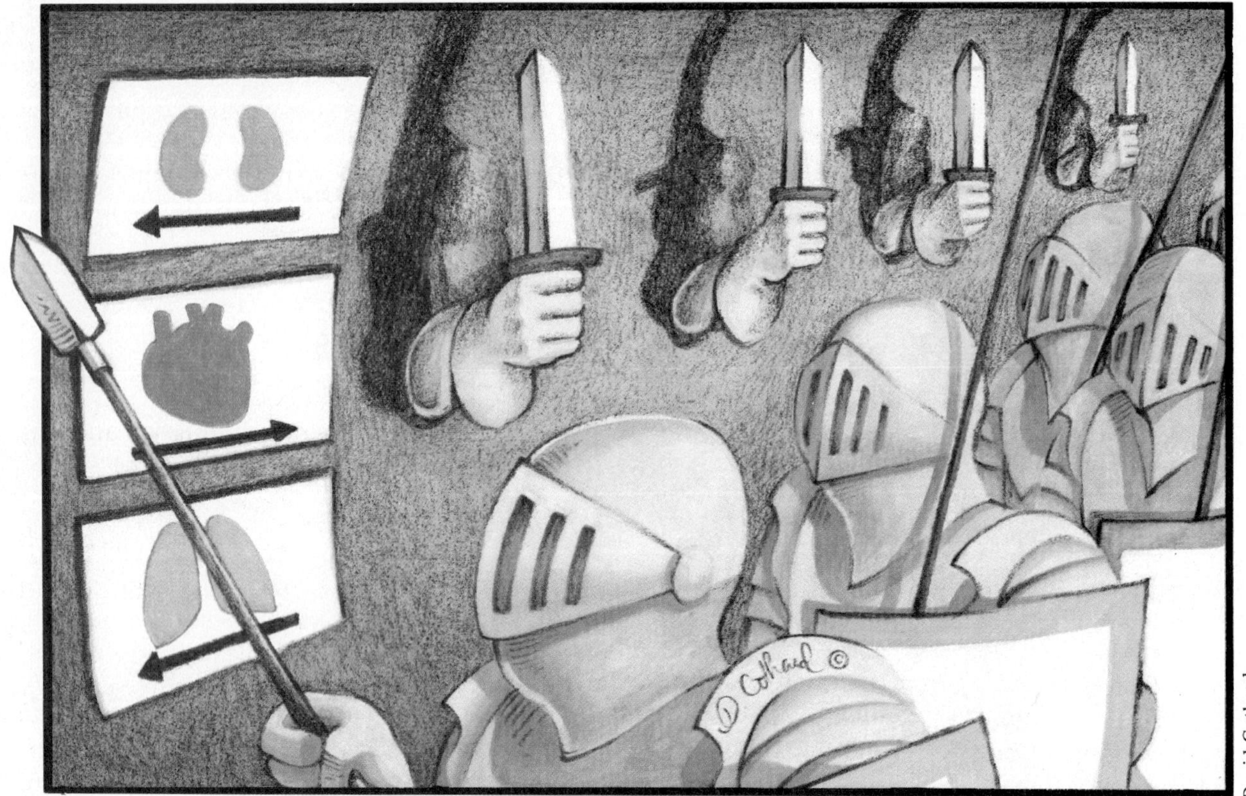

David Gothard

Figure 14.3 The body mobilizes a system of natural defenses to counter the infiltration of disease-carrying organisms. These defenses include the skin and mucous membranes, the white blood cells, and the inflammation process.

systems that are involved in individual defense mechanisms.

The skin is the first line of defense. An invading microbe must find its way through the skin or the mucus-coated membranes that line the respiratory, digestive, and urogenital tracts. Secretions such as tears, perspiration, skin oils, saliva, and mucus have bactericidal chemicals. In addition, respiratory passages have fine, short, moving hairs—*cilia.* Through synchronized beating, the cilia move a carpet of sticky mucus that traps and moves inhaled microbes and foreign matter to the back of the throat, where they are swallowed and disposed of by digestive fluids.

Microorganisms sometimes get beyond these first defenses—through a cut in the skin, for example. They then face a second line of defense in the blood and the tissues. The blood, like some external secretions, contains bacteria- and virus-killing chemicals. It also contains a variety of white blood cells called *phagocytes* that engulf and digest bacteria and foreign particles. These cells can also squeeze through the walls of a blood vessel, migrate to the site in the tissue where microorganisms have entered, and there wage their fight against the invaders. Tissues, too, contain larger phagocytic cells—*macrophages*—that contribute to the local fight. Thus, many bacteria never gain a foothold in the body.

Suppose, however, that microbes do become established and begin to multiply. The body must then resort to a third line of defense, which is part of a complex phenomenon called *inflammation.* The inflammatory response is a response to any irritant or "foreign body." A splinter, for instance, elicits the inflammatory reaction. The blood supply to the endangered area increases while blood flow through it slows down, creating a leakage of tissue fluids into intercellular spaces. These fluids accumulate at the site of infection, together with antibacterial and antitoxic proteins. The rush of blood phagocytes into the tissue is also greatly increased, but other mechanisms continually replace them in the circulating blood. The outward signs of inflammation are usually redness and local warmth, swelling, and pain. The discomfort indicates that the invaders are being counterattacked.

Generalized *fever* is a sign that battle is being waged throughout the body. Fever is caused, at least in part, by toxic materials produced by the invaders or released from them during their destruction. These toxins interfere with the regulatory mechanisms that normally control the temperature of the body. But while elevated temperatures may be harmful to normal body functions, fever also stimulates production of white blood cells to build up the defense forces more quickly. Additionally, most pathogens cannot survive at above-normal body temperatures.

In the most severe cases, this third line of defense folds, and the invaders begin to spread through the tissues and even into the bloodstream. The infection then becomes generalized and highly dangerous. In other cases, the local battle may go on. More and more of the local tissue is destroyed, and a cavity, or *abscess,* is formed that fills with fluid, battling cells, and white blood cells that have died in the attack *(pus).* Resolution to normal occurs when a sufficient number of invaders are killed or inactivated.

The body also has a defense mechanism directed against viruses. This mechanism, still only partly understood, results in the formation of a unique protein known as *interferon,* which is manufactured in the virus-infected cells. Interferon does not protect the debilitated cell that is producing it. It protects uninfected cells by interacting with the cell membrane to block viral invasion. The interferon manufactured under the influence of one virus can be used by the body to protect itself against other viruses. Some bacteria and synthetic chemicals are capable of stimulating the production of interferon. Research is in progress to find a suitable means of producing the substance synthetically, at an affordable price. Hopefully, interferon may eventually serve as the answer to the prevention and treatment of viral diseases.

IMMUNITY

While the inflammation battle rages at the site of invasion, the body is marshaling yet another defensive system, the *immune mechanism.* The immune response has two parts—the previously discussed cell-mediated or phagocytic response and the antibody response. Both depend on the *lymphocyte,* a type of white blood cell.

Manufactured in the bone marrow along with other blood cells, lymphocytes enter the bloodstream and eventually differentiate into T-lymphocytes or B-lymphocytes. T-lymphocytes move throughout the body gobbling up microbes and other foreign substances—the so-called cell-mediated immune reactions.

The B-lymphocytes play the major role in the manufacture of *antibodies,* proteins that are capable of inactivating specific invaders. In the lymph nodes throughout the body, invading microbes stimulate the B-lymphocytes to divide and become *plasma cells,* which in turn produce antibodies. The microbes or other foreign substances that stimulate the production of antibodies are called *antigens.*

The most remarkable thing about these antibody proteins is their *specificity,* a property lacking in the interferon proteins. The body has the capacity to make innumerable antibodies—but each different infectious agent evokes a different kind of antibody. Likewise, each kind of antibody destroys only that antigen (or one closely related to it) for which it was produced. Suppose one is exposed to measles, and the body produces antibodies against the measles virus. If a mumps virus becomes established in the body, the antibodies synthesized against the measles virus cannot attack it. The body must synthesize a new set of antibodies that will inactivate only the mumps virus.

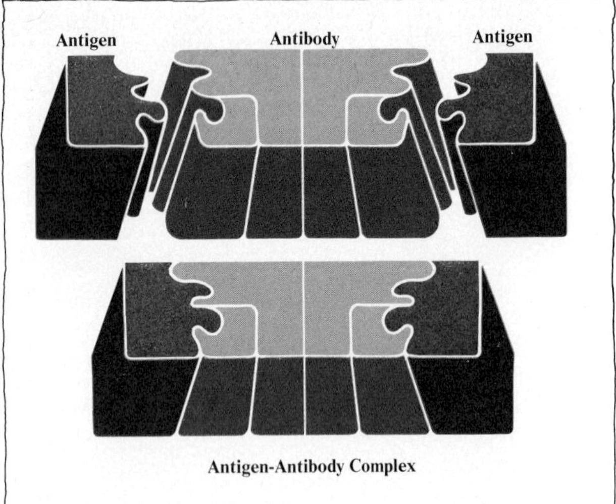

Figure 14.4 Antigen-antibody reaction. Research indicates that an antibody molecule has two identical halves, each with one large and one small component. Each antibody has only one antigen that fits with it. The two surfaces of the antibody molecule fit against the surface of two antigen molecules, thus deactivating them.

Research into immune processes has brought a wealth of information on how natural immune mechanisms work. Enough is now known about them to cause many experts to suspect that malfunctioning of the immune system may be involved in many puzzling medical problems, including those concerned with allergy, rheumatoid arthritis, and cancer (see Chapter 15). Further research should show more about these relationships.

Immunity is acquired naturally when one develops a disease. In the course of an illness, antibodies appear, and one begins to recover. Not many years ago, having the disease was the only way people could develop immunity. Today, immunity may be induced artificially by vaccines. In several days or weeks, specific antibodies circulate in the bloodstream, in large amounts, ready to attack the initiating microbe (antigen).

Some vaccines contain living infectious agents; included in this group are those used against yellow fever and measles, as well as the Sabin oral polio vaccine. These living agents have been weakened *(attenuated)* in the laboratory but still provoke the formation of specific antibodies. Other vaccines contain killed infectious agents; included in this group are the whooping cough and Salk polio vaccines. The killed microbes will not produce the disease but will stimulate production of specific antibodies against the same organism.

Immunity can also be induced against certain microbial toxins. Diphtheria and tetanus produce disease through their toxins. Modified toxins, called *toxoids,* which are no longer poisonous, are used to induce antibodies that will inactivate the poisons if the invading organism strikes.

Having the disease or receiving a vaccine produces *active immunity.* Occasionally, someone is exposed to a disease and cannot wait for antibodies to form. In such cases, antibodies formed by another person or an animal can be given, using the process called *passive immunization.* These antibodies come from a protein fraction of blood serum called *gamma globulin.* Passive immunization is used against diseases, such as infectious hepatitis, for which an effective vaccine for humans has not yet been devised.

Effective and safe vaccines for most common viral diseases are available today. In general, active immunity is long-term and in some cases lifelong, whereas passive immunity lasts only a few weeks or months. Table 4.2 gives a schedule for recommended immunizations and boosters. A physician should be consulted for any variations.

COMMON INFECTIOUS DISEASES

A description of the major human infectious diseases is provided in the Appendix. Nevertheless, some diseases are so prevalent that they warrant special attention in this chapter. These common infections include colds, flu, hepatitis, and mononucleosis. Special attention will be given to syphilis, gonorrhea, and genital herpes, the most commonly reported of the sexually transmitted diseases. In addition, these discussions should help illuminate some of the general points about disease discussed in this chapter.

Table 14.2 Recommended Immunization Schedule

Disease	Age at First Dose	Boosters
Diphtheria Whooping cough Tetanus	6 weeks to 2 months; series: 3 injections one month apart	At 1 year and before entering school; tetanus every 4 years
Polio Sabin (oral)	6 weeks to 3 months; 3 doses 6 to 8 weeks apart	At 12 to 15 months and on entering school
Measles	1 vaccination at 12 months	As yet, no recommendation
Mumps	1 vaccination in preadolescence	As yet, no recommendation
Influenza	Any age past 3 months; series: 2 shots 1 month apart for persons exposed to flu in their work	Annually for person exposed or endangered
Rubella	1 vaccination at 12 months	As yet, no recommendation
Typhoid and paratyphoid A and B	After 3 months; series: 3 shots 1 to 4 weeks apart for persons taking trips where water supply is questionable	One shot every 3 years if visiting frequently or living in typhoid area
Tuberculosis	After 3 months; series: 1 shot BCG vaccine for selected persons unavoidably exposed to continuous contact with TB	BCG only on recommendation of the USPHS
Rabies	Any age; series: up to 14 injections after being bitten by a rabid animal or one suspected of being rabid	None
Yellow fever	After age 6 months; series: 1 shot if going to yellow fever area	One, if remaining in a yellow fever area for prolonged period
Cholera	After age 6 months; series: 2 shots 7 to 10 days apart if traveling to cholera area	Boosters 4 to 6 months apart if living in cholera area; after 4 years repeat immunization

Source: Adapted from U.S. Public Health Service, Communicable Disease Center, Atlanta, Ga.

The Common Cold

The common cold is practically a universal nuisance and contributes heavily to the amount of time lost each year because of viral diseases. One theory suggests that healthy people carry cold viruses in their noses and throats all the time but exhibit cold symptoms only when something like fatigue or lowered resistance produces favorable circumstances for the viruses to proliferate. Cold viruses seem to survive in the air, beginning their journey to another person either in the spray of droplets from a sneeze or in the air exhaled when a cold victim talks or breathes. They are also transmitted by skin-skin contact, as when an infected person shakes another person's hand. The period of time between first exposure to the virus and the appearance of symptoms—the incubation period—is short, usually about eighteen to forty-eight hours.

The average American contracts between four and eight colds per year. One would think that with so many people having colds and so many hours of productivity being lost, scientists would know more about the common cold than they do. But only in the last few years have researchers gained any certain knowledge about the agents responsible for it. For one thing, there are many viruses that cause colds. So far, more than thirty have been implicated, and more may still be discovered.

Cold viruses appear to differ from other viruses in that they do not confer long-lasting immunity. It is also possible that cold viruses mutate rapidly. If that is the case, each successive cold could be caused by a different virus, resulting in an endless series of apparently similar diseases.

The fact that colds are caused by viruses suggests some means of prevention and treatment. Because so many different viruses are involved and because the environmental and physiological circumstances for the development of colds are still so poorly understood, there is little one can do to prevent them beyond avoiding persons with "new colds" (the first twenty-four hours is the most communicable stage) or staying away from others when one has a new cold. It is also useful to maintain one's resistance to infection through adequate nutrition, rest, control of stress, and exercise, although expert opinion on the values of such measures varies widely.

Once a cold has developed, the main concern is to keep it from leading to more serious illness. No chemicals or antibiotics are effective against the common cold, although aspirin may be useful in easing discomfort or reducing fever. There is new evidence, however, that aspirin may also reduce the body's germ-fighting efficiency and cause more viruses to be "shed," thus contributing to greater spread of the infection. In a recent study of cold victims, daily nasal samplings disclosed that aspirin users produced up to a third more viruses than nonusers.

Nasal sprays, nose drops, decongestants, cough medicines, or other proprietary remedies should preferably not be used without medical supervision; most of them are useless, and some may create conditions favoring more serious infection. Some decongestants, for example, may dry and crack the mucous membrane of the bronchi and make it more vulnerable to bacterial infection. Over-the-counter cough medicines are rarely strong enough to offer much relief and on occasion may interact harmfully with other drugs one is taking. Cough drops are relatively expensive and offer no advantages over ordinary hard candy in stimulating saliva flow to relieve a mild tickling cough. Generally speaking, the advantage of any of these remedies is of a psychological nature: sufferers who feel better after using them would in all likelihood have felt better anyway. The same phenomenon is also true for those employing vitamin C megadoses as a "cure" for colds. As noted in Chapter 18, there is *no proof* that this vitamin can either prevent or cure the common cold. While some studies at first indicated that vitamin C might possibly lighten the symptoms or shorten the duration of a cold, attempts by the same researchers to duplicate their own results have been unsuccessful.

Far more helpful is use of a vaporizer to moisten the dry air so common in indoor living, particularly in the winter. Steam breathing is useful in loosening nasal congestion. Blowing the nose should be done gently, with the mouth open, to avoid forcing congestion and infection up the eustachian tubes to the middle ear.

Influenza

Influenza, or flu, is not usually a serious disease when uncomplicated by secondary infection. (Often, in fact, persons thinking they have flu may in reality have only a respiratory tract infection with symptoms more severe than usual.) But when bacteria become involved, or when the flu virus spreads to the lungs, the condition may be lethal, particularly for the very young, the elderly, and those with a low level of health. Several viruses are responsible for influenza. There are three major types, A, B, and C, as well as numerous strains within each type. Type A is far more virulent than the other two. When epidemics occur, the viruses seem to cause more serious forms of the disease than they do during the lulls between major outbreaks.

The early symptoms of influenza resemble those of the common cold, but in addition

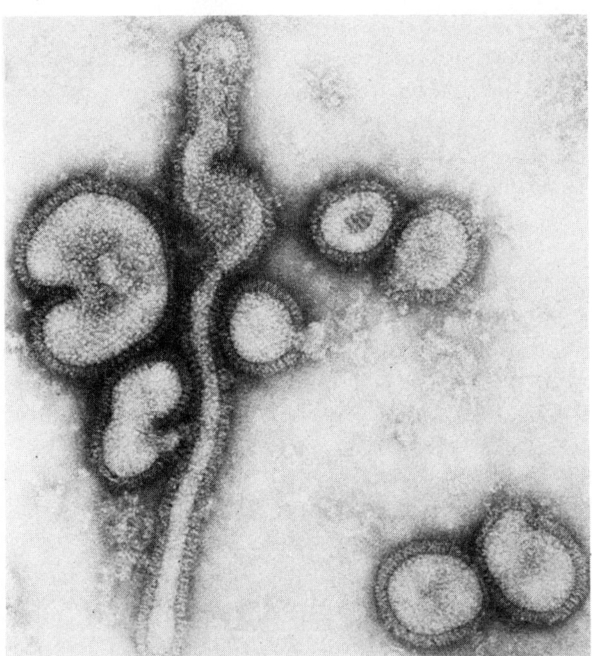

Figure 14.5 An influenza virus.

there is often sudden fever, weakness, coughing, and aching pain in the back and extremities. Incubation is brief, requiring only one to three days. The infected individual is able to communicate the infection to others from the time just before symptoms appear until approximately a week later. Frequently, a great physical and mental depression accompanies influenza, often persisting long after the infection itself is over.

There are vaccines against specific strains of influenza virus, but they are not effective against other strains. Accordingly, vaccination will not protect susceptible individuals if an outbreak involves a different viral strain. Nevertheless, the Surgeon General's Advisory Committee on Influenza suggests that persons over sixty-five, those with chronic cardiovascular disease and certain other diseases, and pregnant women be vaccinated. The components of the vaccine are changed periodically, so individuals must be revaccinated each year.

The influenza virus presents a special problem for medical researchers. The virus appears to mutate readily—to undergo small changes in genetic make-up. An RNA virus that caused an outbreak of flu in the early 1930s was called influenza type A0 virus. In 1947, a slightly altered A1 virus was the culprit, and in 1957 it was the A2 virus. In the late 1960s, an altered form of the A2 began to appear in Southeast Asia and was dubbed the Hong Kong flu. This world traveler, again slightly changed, appeared in England in late 1972 as the London flu. By 1975, the strain in the spotlight was A-Victoria from Australia. In 1976, the notorious swine flu appeared—a variant of a strain that in 1918 had resulted in 500,000 American deaths above the number normally expected.

Hepatitis

Hepatitis (viral inflammation of the liver) has increased significantly in recent years, particularly among young people. Hepatitis A is commonly called infectious hepatitis, and is generally transmitted by fecal contamination of food or water. Hepatitis B is called serum hepatitis and is transmitted through the blood. It is passed on from an infected person through blood transfusion, sharing of needles among drug users, or contaminated tattoo needles.

Both forms of hepatitis have similar symptoms—fever, headache, nausea, and pain in the upper right abdomen. The urine becomes deep yellow, and the individual may become jaundiced. Type A is more common; type B is far more dangerous. Researchers are working on vaccines for both types. Currently, passive immunity can be provided for hepatitis A.

Mononucleosis

Probably every college student has heard of "mono"—infectious mononucleosis. Sometimes it is called the "college disease" or the "kissing disease" because it occurs so frequently during the college years and for a long time was thought to be transmitted principally by kissing.

The greatest incidence of mononucleosis in the United States is among those fifteen to nineteen, followed by the twenty to twenty-four age group. It can produce severe, if relatively short-lived, symptoms, including fever, sore throat, nausea, chills, and general weakness. Some victims exhibit additional symptoms such as a rash, enlarged and tender lymph glands, jaundice, and enlargement of the spleen. Fortunately, except for the rare cases in which the spleen ruptures, permanent disability following mononucleosis is unusual. But a lingering weakness is common and may last a few weeks or months. Jaundice is sometimes stubbornly persistent as well. The symptoms closely resemble those of several more serious diseases, among them polio, meningitis, tuberculosis, diphtheria, and even leukemia. Diagnosis can be made with a simple blood test.

Until recently, the cause of the disease could not be identified. An infectious agent was suspected because of characteristic changes produced in the blood—raised levels and altered appearance of disease-fighting white cells and antibodies. Research in the late 1960s, however, began to implicate a specific organism, the *Epstein-Barr virus,* as the cause of the most common form of infectious mononucleosis.

The poor, both in the United States and abroad, are apparently exposed to Epstein-Barr virus early in life and often contract a mild form of the disease, which usually goes unnoticed. But people who, medically speaking, have more protected lives—middle-class families, for instance—are not generally exposed to the virus until later in their lives and seem to get much sicker when they do contract it. They tend to be exposed as adolescents and young adults, in high school, college, and military service.

The exact methods by which the virus spreads are not known, but kissing is probably only one of several ways. The disease does not spread easily by ordinary contact; in fact, it is rare to have more than one case in a household. Experts generally agree that the disease confers fairly long, if not permanent, immunity. A vaccine to prevent mononucleosis is now being tested, with some optimism as to the results.

SEXUALLY TRANSMITTED DISEASES

Most of the common infectious diseases that now plague the average American are viral in origin—colds, flu, and so on. Bacterial diseases have been largely conquered through the use of antibiotics. It is therefore surprising to find that one of the most common types of infectious disease continuing to ravage the American population is predominantly bacterial in origin—sexually transmitted disease.

Sexually transmitted diseases (STDs) are infectious diseases that are almost always transmitted during sexual intercourse, homosexual relations, or other sexual activity. *Syphilis, gonorrhea,* and *herpes simplex virus Type 2* are by far the most prevalent diseases in this category. Other types of genital infection include trichomoniasis, moniliasis, chancroid, pediculosis pubis, scabies, and genital warts. Collectively, these disorders have been known by the common name of venereal disease or VD. More recently, the term STD has come into use.

In the late 1950s, after a decade of reasonable control of these diseases through antibiotics, syphilis and primarily gonorrhea began showing dramatic increases that have continued, resulting today in a problem of epidemic proportions. In most communities, gonorrhea cases alone outnumber all other reportable infectious diseases combined. The Center for Disease Control in Atlanta estimates that there were 2.5 million new cases of gonorrhea in 1979 (exact statistics are difficult since so many cases go unreported). One in every fifty teenagers will have contracted gonorrhea. At least half of all cases in the United States are among those under age twenty-four, particularly those in their late teens. In 1978, it was reported that some 80,000 women became sterile as a result of gonorrhea.

Figure 14.6 illustrates the spread of syphilis by diagramming a local epidemic. Notice that the disease is not limited to those with many sexual partners. Many of those found to be infected in this epidemic apparently had sexual contact only once, but it was unfortunately with an infected partner.

There seem to be several reasons why STDs have been on the upswing, even though syphilis and gonorrhea can easily be cured with antibiotics if diagnosed early enough: (1) changing life styles that have permitted greater sexual activity; (2) growing mobility, especially among young people traveling about the country, contributing to the spread of infection; (3)

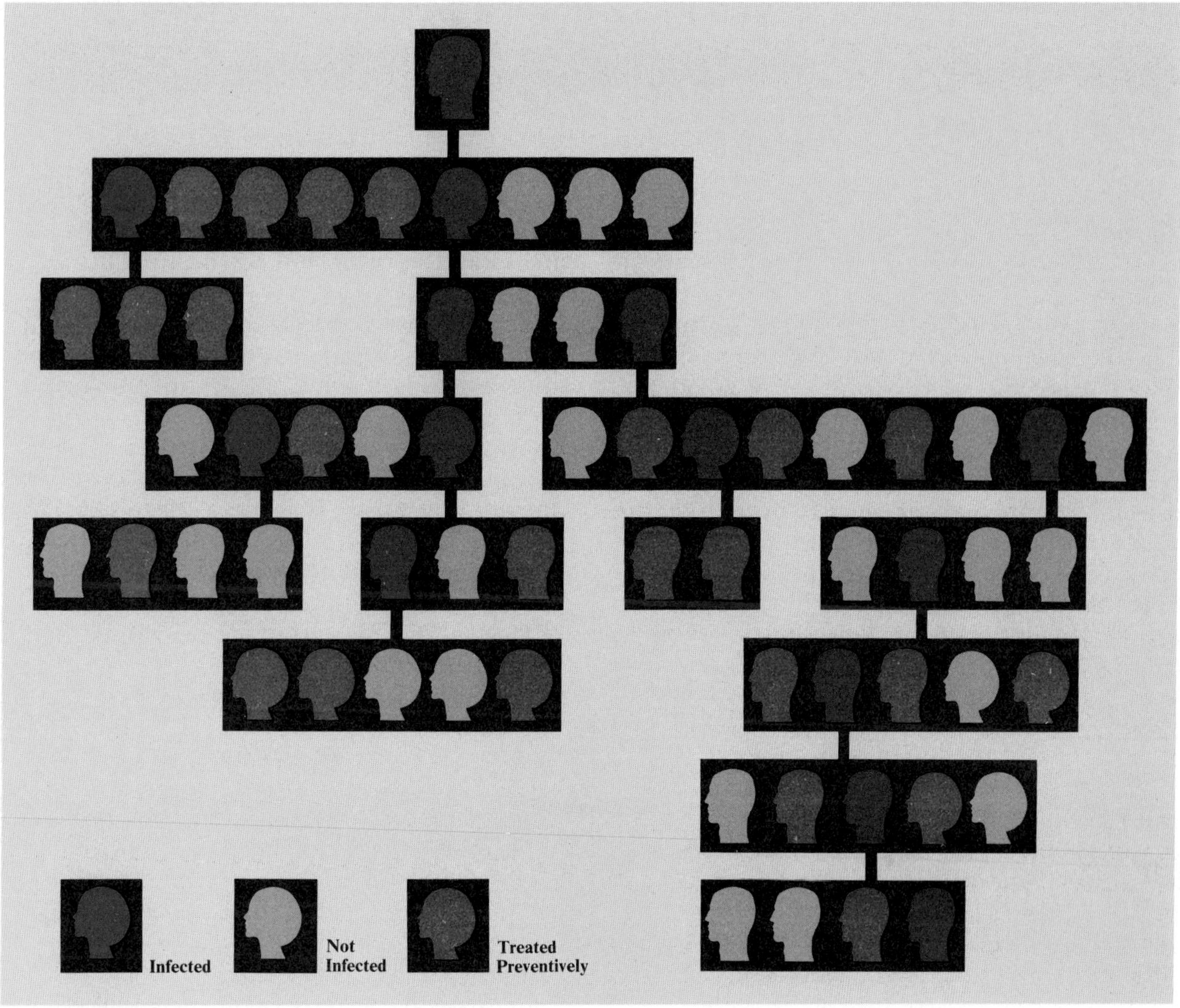

Figure 14.6 How an outbreak of syphilis was spread at a high school. The contacts of each infected person were traced in order to treat them and prevent further spread of the disease.

drug use, often creating a sense of false security and disregard for personal hygiene, precautionary measures, or the need for treatment; (4) increased use of the Pill and IUDs, which do not offer the protection of such older methods of contraception as the condom; (5) complacency about the dangers involved, since many assume STDs are easily and quickly treated with modern antibiotics (which is not true of all types—herpes, for example, is incurable); (6) better diagnostic methods that now reveal more cases than previously; (7) reluctance to seek treatment, even though the victims know that STDs can cause severe, permanent damage if not treated.

Syphilis

The spiral-shaped bacterium (spirochete) that causes syphilis—*Treponema pallidum*—does not long survive the drying effects of air, but it will grow profusely in the warm, moist mucous membranes of the genital tract, the rectum, and the mouth. Sexual intercourse provides the best mode of transmission.

Primary Syphilis The disease begins when a spirochete enters a tiny break in the skin. The infected person may show no sign of the disease for ten to twenty-eight days. The first sign is a lesion known as a *chancre* (pronounced "shank-er"). The chancre is often an open lump or swelling about the size of a dime or smaller, teeming with microscopic spirochetes. The sore is moist, although there is no discharge, and it is generally painless. It usually appears at the site of infection in the genital region—on the shaft of the penis or on the vulva. Unfortunately, it can also develop in the recesses of the vagina, the rectum, or the male urethra. Thus many infected persons, women in particular, never know they have the disease during the initial phase. But visible or hidden, the chancre is dangerously infectious.

At this stage, a diagnosis can easily be made by a doctor and the disease can be treated. Even without treatment, the chancre disappears within several weeks. Many persons therefore gain a false sense of security, but, in fact, the infection has entered the blood and the spirochetes are being carried to all parts of the body.

Secondary Syphilis Secondary-stage symptoms appear anywhere from a few weeks to six months—occasionally even a year—after the appearance of the chancre.

Symptoms of secondary syphilis may include a skin rash; small, flat lesions in regions where the skin is moist; whitish patches on the mucous membranes in the mouth and throat; spotty, temporary baldness; general discomfort and uneasiness; low-grade fevers; headaches; and swollen glands. These symptoms are easily mistaken for those of other diseases. It is therefore important to consult a physician if any of these signs appear, particularly if one has been exposed to syphilis during the preceding six months or so. Secondary syphilis, which lasts from three to six months, can always be diagnosed by blood tests.

The disease is most contagious during the secondary stage. All the lesions are filled with spirochetes; hence any contact with them—even without sexual intercourse—can transmit the disease.

Latent Syphilis The third stage of syphilis is called the latent period. All signs and symptoms of the disease disappear, but it is not gone; spirochetes are invading various organs, including the heart and the brain. This phase sometimes lasts only a few months, but it can also last for twenty years or until the end of life. In this stage, the infected individual appears disease-free and is usually not infectious, with an important exception—a pregnant woman can pass the infection to her unborn child. Although there are no symptoms, a blood test during this stage will reveal syphilis. And within the first two years the highly contagious secondary stage may recur.

Late Syphilis The late stage of syphilis generally begins ten to twenty years after the beginning of the latent phase, but can occasionally occur earlier. In late syphilis, twenty-three percent of untreated patients become incapacitated. They may develop serious cardiovascular disease—many die of severe heart damage or rupture of the aorta—or they may suffer progressive brain or spinal cord damage, eventually leading to blindness, insanity, or crippling.

Congenital Syphilis Congenital syphilis results from the transmission of the disease from pregnant mother to unborn child. If the fetus is exposed to the disease in its fourth month of development, the infection may kill it, produce various disfigurations, or cause an obviously diseased baby. If the fetus is infected late in pregnancy, the infection may not be apparent for several months or years after birth, when the child may become disabled as in late syphilis. Treatment of the infected pregnant woman within the first four months of pregnancy halts the spread of the disease in the unborn child.

Treatment Syphilis is easily cured with antibiotics when the treatment is begun in the first two stages or even in the latent phase. Penicillin is used most often, but other antibiotics may be used when the patient is sensitive to penicillin. In the early 1970s the spirochete began showing some resistance to penicillin, although it still responds readily to other antibiotic treatment. Syphilis confers no immunity to succeeding infections, and there are no preventive vaccines. Thus, continual caution must be taken to ensure prompt and effective diagnosis and treatment after each possible exposure. To reduce the spread of the disease, prenatal and premarital tests are required by law in forty-five states.

Gonorrhea

Gonococci, the bacteria that cause gonorrhea, initially multiply in the lower urogenital tract of both sexes—the urethra of the male and the urethra, vaginal glands, and cervix of the female. There are also anal and oral forms of the disease. It is potentially a serious illness and one that affects many parts of the body. It has a short incubation period (three to fourteen days) and becomes contagious after incubation.

Gonorrhea in Women Gonorrhea affects men and women in different ways due to their anatomical differences. Because early symptoms are frequently not pronounced, women may not be aware of infection. A few days after exposure, a mild burning sensation in the genital region, with or without discharge, may be noticed. If the infected woman is examined, the physician might find a mild inflammation of the vagina and cervix. The disease subsequently spreads from the vagina, through the uterus, and into the Fallopian tubes and ovaries. Inflammation of the Fallopian tubes is often severely painful, but it can be mild enough to be passed off as a stomach upset. If the infection remains untreated, the symptoms may diminish, though the disease continues unabated. The whole pelvis and the lining of the abdominal cavity can become inflamed.

Acute infection can subside after a few weeks. It is followed by a chronic infection that can last for many years, causing extensive damage to the reproductive tract. Sterility frequently follows inflammation of the Fallopian tubes.

Gonorrhea is not as easily diagnosed as syphilis, particularly in women. When a woman suspects exposure to gonorrhea or if she has a vaginal discharge, she should be examined promptly. Her physician will be able to examine the discharge microscopically. If no organisms are found, the doctor may wish to repeat the tests or run other tests. There are many causes of vaginal discharge, and many organisms other than gonococci can be responsible. Nevertheless, the consequences of gonorrhea are so serious that until laboratory confirmation is available a physician may treat the discharge as if it were caused by gonorrhea.

Gonorrhea in Men The early symptoms of gonorrhea are more evident in men. About three to eight days after exposure, men experience a sharp, burning pain during urination. At about the same time, pus begins oozing from the penis, which causes many men to seek treatment. If prompt treatment is not received, the infection spreads to the prostate gland and testicles, where it can cause sufficient damage to produce sterility. In time, the urethra can become narrowed, making it difficult for a man to urinate. If the infection is severe, men can also suffer arthritis as well as heart damage.

Transmission Gonorrhea is almost always transmitted through sexual intercourse. However, the pus is often so laden with gonococci that the infection can be transmitted by hand to susceptible tissues. Personal hygiene is thus important in combating the disease.

Gonorrhea from infected mothers used to be a frequent cause of blindness in children. The bacteria were transferred to the baby's eyes as it passed through the birth canal. Today, newborn babies are routinely treated with penicillin and silver compounds to prevent blindness.

Treatment Gonorrhea is easily treated, particularly in its early stages. Penicillin is the first choice for treatment, despite the recent appearance of strains of gonococci that are partially resistant. Other antibiotics can also be used, particularly for persons who are sensitive or allergic to penicillin. The response to treatment in the early stages is rapid. It is more difficult to treat more severe cases in which complications have appeared.

A patient may be infected with syphilis and gonorrhea at the same time. Although penicillin can kill both gonococci and spirochetes, the amounts required for effective treatment are usually different, and treatment of one disease may leave the other uncured. Therefore, anyone who may have one of these diseases should have routine examinations for both diseases before as well as some time after treatment.

Herpes Simplex Type 2

Until a few years ago, the herpes simplex Type 2 virus (HSV-2) was a rare condition and considered only a minor VD threat compared with syphilis and gonorrhea. Today this painful and highly contagious disease is epidemic throughout the country. Worst of all, it is incurable.

Herpes virus Type 1 is the organism causing the well-known fever blisters or "cold sores," a condition only loosely related to the Type 2 virus, which is also known as *genital herpes.* The blisterlike sores of the latter, however, might be described as fever blisters of the genital area. They appear about six days after sexual contact with an infected person. Other symptoms include difficult urination, swelling of the legs, watery eyes, fatigue, and a feeling of general debility. The symptoms usually respond well to treatment, but the disease does not.

Symptoms recur periodically, often activated by intercourse, though exposure to the sun, lack of sleep, infections, or fever can also bring them on. The disease can be spread anytime during the recurrence. Occasionally symptoms are too mild to be noticeable, and a sexual partner may be infected without any awareness. As a further complication, there is no blood test for herpes, as there is for syphilis.

Pregnant women with genital herpes are likely to suffer even further misfortune: the miscarriage rate is more than three times that of the general population. When miscarriage does not occur, the birth process may expose the infant to the virus, causing death or irreversible brain damage. As a preventive measure, the baby is delivered by Caesarean section (see Chapter 4). Nevertheless, one out of four infants will still develop the infection and have it for life.

As if this weren't enough, several years of reserach indicate a strong relationship between herpes Type 2 and cancer of the cervix and prostate. Women with HSV-2 are eight times more likely to develop cancer of the cervix than are other women. Presumably, the virus penetrates the cervical cells, disrupting normal metabolism and setting off the typical uncontrolled growth of cancer.

A number of different researchers have been hard at work to develop a herpes vaccine. If they are successful, it may be much more than a defense against herpes; it may possibly also shed new light on the continuing battle against cancer.

Other Sexually Transmitted Diseases

Trichomoniasis is caused by a protozoan parasite, *Trichomonas vaginalis,* more commonly known as "trich." The organism produces a profuse white bubbly discharge with a characteristic odor and a general reddening of the vulva. In more severe infections, the discharge becomes greenish-yellow. Trich normally affects only women, although men frequently act as carriers and a few may suffer mild irritation of the urethra.

Diagnosis is easily made by microscopic examination of vaginal secretions (usually the parasite will also appear in a urine specimen). Treatment is with a drug called Metronidazole. Male sexual partners should also be treated to prevent any reinfection.

Moniliasis, also known as *candidiasis* or *thrush,* is a yeast infection of the vagina. Most commonly it occurs from altered conditions of the vaginal lining, such as pregnancy or antibiotic therapy. There has been a recent upsurge of the disorder among Pill users.

Moniliasis is easily recognized by an almost intolerable itching around the entire vulva. The accompanying discharge is white, granular, and lumpy, with a yeasty odor. Treatment is somewhat difficult since individual susceptibility plays a role in the infection. Moniliasis can also occur in the male genitals, and a couple can pass the disease back and forth. Additionally, it may occur in the mouth or anus and on the skin. A sore mouth with white patches on the tongue and cheeks indicates a need for prompt medical attention.

There are a large number of other sexually transmitted diseases. Among the more important are *genital warts, chancroid, pediculosis pubis* (crab lice), and *scabies.* The latter three are described in the Appendix.

Prevention and Control of STDs

STDs produce no immunity, so reinfection is always possible. Their control, therefore, can ultimately be achieved only by preventive measures that will progressively reduce the number of infected persons, hence of carriers and sources of the infectious agents.

It is probably unrealistic to expect total prevention of these diseases. But their incidence could be curbed dramatically if people were to become sufficiently aware of and concerned about their spread. Clearly, the only way to minimize the chances of contracting an STD is to confine one's sexual activity to uninfected partners, or to have none at all. Those with many sexual partners are likely to become infected sooner or later. If one is going to have sexual relations, however, certain precautions may help. Male use of condoms during any and all contact with persons who might be infected reduces the risk of infection, especially if combined with washing. Nevertheless, disease can still be transmitted through kissing or through contact with broken skin or pores. Despite these limitations, the use of prophylactics and washing is recommended when the health status of one's partner is uncertain.

Public health workers also try to reduce the spread of STDs by asking those seeking treatment to name all their sexual contacts. Even when patients are cooperative, tracing contacts is time-consuming and expensive work, further hampered by a shortage of trained personnel. Obviously, all who are infected cannot be discovered. Even though every state requires physicians to report all cases of syphilis and gonorrhea to the health department, case finding is further handicapped by massive failure to report.

STDs represent a major economic and social problem as well as a medical one. For example,

HOW TO

Decrease the Likelihood of Contracting a Sexually Transmitted Disease

Sexually transmitted diseases (STDs), or venereal diseases, as they have been known for many years, may be transmitted during any type of sexual activity. The recent upsurge of all types of STD—particularly gonorrhea, with syphilis not far behind—has generated an urgent need to focus on prevention of these diseases. Following are a few tips for helping to keep STDs under control.

1. Become familiar with the symptoms of all types of sexually transmitted disease, including the ways in which they may differently affect the male and the female.
2. Even though other forms of birth control may already be in use, insist that a condom also be used to avoid the possible spread of an STD. This is particularly important when your partner is not well known to you, or when the possibility exists that he or she may have been unknowingly infected or exposed.
3. Keep alert to the fact that drug use and alcohol tend to promote carelessness in personal hygiene and precautionary measures related to sexual activity.
4. Avoid *any* form of sexual activity with an infected partner. Keep in mind that STDs may also be transmitted by kissing, oral-genital sex, or homosexual activity.
5. Likewise, never, *never* engage in any form of sexual activity if you know—or even remotely suspect—that you have contracted a sexually transmitted disease. Even if you are receiving medical treatment, wait for a go-ahead from your physician before resuming your former activities.
6. If you know or suspect that you have contracted an STD, seek medical attention immediately! Don't delay because you feel embarrassed or think it might "just go away" by itself. Chances are very slim that it will. Most of these diseases are easily cured, however, if treatment is begun early. Delay may cause serious, permanent damage.

HOW TO Build Resistance Against Disease

No one can avoid becoming ill occasionally. But there are ways to reduce the odds and build resistance against disease in general. As you read through the following tips, take a look at your own life style. There may be some changes in order.

1. Eat a well-balanced diet carefully selected from the Basic Four Food Groups. Good nutrition is paramount to good health and disease resistance.
2. Exercise regularly. If you are unused to strenuous exercise, approach it slowly, preferably under a doctor's supervision.
3. Get ample sleep and relaxation. The amount of both needed varies a great deal among different individuals, but both are necessary to one's well-being and ability to ward off infections.
4. If you are a cigarette smoker, think seriously about giving it up *now.* If you cannot give it up, at least cut down—cigarettes are probably society's greatest self-inflicted killer.
5. Keep your consumption of alcoholic beverages down to a moderate level.
6. Avoid habit-forming drugs of all sorts. Never take any type of prescriptive medication unless you are under the care of a physician.
7. Give careful attention to personal hygiene—your self, your clothing, your dwelling place. Always approach food with clean hands.
8. Have regular medical and dental checkups and seek prompt treatment for any illness or suspected disorder.
9. Take advantage of all immunization and disease-screening programs.
10. Strive to get others interested in following these simple principles—your friends, your family, the young, the elderly. Eventually, good health may become habit forming.

hospitalization of the syphilitic insane costs taxpayers about $44 million per year. Unlike most other infectious diseases, STDs still carry a social stigma. And this, along with widespread ignorance, reduces the likelihood that all infected persons will seek treatment promptly, refer their contacts to physicians for treatment, and avoid sexual contact themselves until they are cured. It is important to realize that hot lines and clinics exist throughout the United States that will provide information and support confidentially, without notifying parental authorities. *Anyone* can contract an STD—an awareness of the symptoms, combined with prompt action when they appear, can save much needless anxiety and future agony.

CHANGING PATTERNS OF DISEASE

Examining epidemiological data and the study of disease causation can lead to useful generalizations in the study of disease patterns throughout the world. In regions where people have high standards of living, nutritional and infectious diseases seem to have both low morbidity and low mortality, while heart disease, cancer, stroke, and accidents show high morbidity and mortality (Figure 14.7). Developing nations, on the other hand, must cope primarily with nutritional deficiencies and infectious diseases. Undernutrition (including protein deficiencies), malaria, tuberculosis, and parasites are the greatest killers there. Other nations in various stages of development experience a variety of disease patterns, with the major killers differing from culture to culture.

Influenza, pneumonia, tuberculosis, and diphtheria, leading causes of death in the United States a century ago, no longer take many lives, as Figure 14.8 shows. Both influenza and pneumonia, however, persist as serious acute infections—perhaps the only serious ones, except for the recent upsurge in syphilis, gonorrhea, and genital herpes.

However, as one group of problems comes under some degree of control, something new becomes a significant threat. Today, a new group of diseases predominates among the leading causes of death in the United States: heart disease, cancer, and stroke—the chronic diseases. These diseases are "new" in the sense that centuries, even decades, ago people rarely lived long enough to develop them—nor

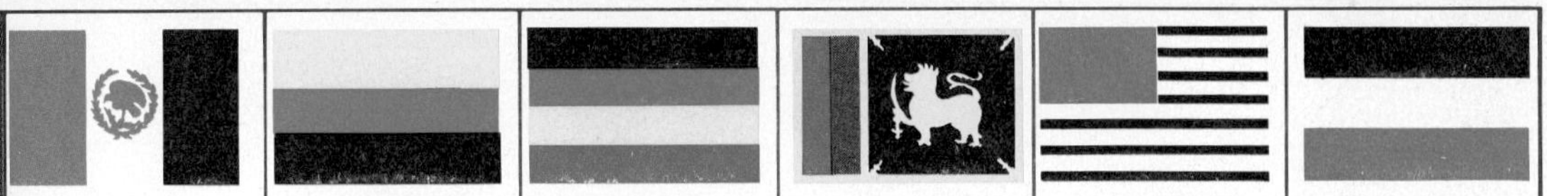

	Mexico Life Expectancy 63	Colombia Life Expectancy 61	Mauritius (Africa) Life Expectancy 66	Sri Lanka Life Expectancy 68	United States Life Expectancy 73	Netherlands Life Expectancy 74
Tuberculosis	14.8	15.8	6.3	4.5	1.6	1.3
Pneumonia	90.1	54.5	37.9	5.9	24.1	18.5
Enteritis	87.5	79.9	60.9	0.9	0.9	1.1
Heart Diseases	73.1	89.1	151.6	60.7	339.2	242.3
Cancers	36.0	46.8	43.7	10.4	171.7	203.3
Cirrhosis of the Liver	19.4	3.7	10.7	4.9	14.8	4.5

Figure 14.7 Death rates by cause for selected countries (per 100,000 population).

did they live in ways that predisposed them to these newly significant diseases.

Perhaps surprisingly, the leading killer of young adults in the United States today is accidents, particularly those related to motor vehicles.

As medicines improve, fewer persons die of infections. But ironically, some of the treatments that must be used for certain other diseases, such as cancer or kidney disease, actually inhibit or knock out one's natural defenses against microorganisms. Patients who have received radiation treatments for cancer, for example, may become susceptible to infections that would normally not make them sick, because the radiation weakens their natural defense mechanisms. Individuals who have received kidney transplants must take drugs that leave them open to infections that doctors have never seen before. Experts say that doctors will see more and more patients with unusual, if not bizarre, infections as medicine continues to develop new ways of manipulating the body's protective mechanisms.

Climate, social custom, technology, and living standards, as well as longevity, affect the patterns of disease, as Figure 14.7 illustrates. Considerable discrepancy also exists between male and female life expectancy, with women generally expected to live longer than men. (While men are more likely than women to smoke and drink heavily, to commit suicide, and to be exposed to stress factors, it is generally believed that there may be inherent sex differences as well.) Although people in the United States had a relatively long life expectancy in 1978 (73 years), it was not as long as that of persons living in many European countries. In contrast to the populations of these advanced nations, the citizens of most South American, African, and Asian countries have short life expectancies.

National figures do have important limitations, however. They do not indicate, for example, the variations that may exist in different parts of the same country. Some of these differences are illustrated in Figure 14.10. When one looks at life expectancy, death rates, and

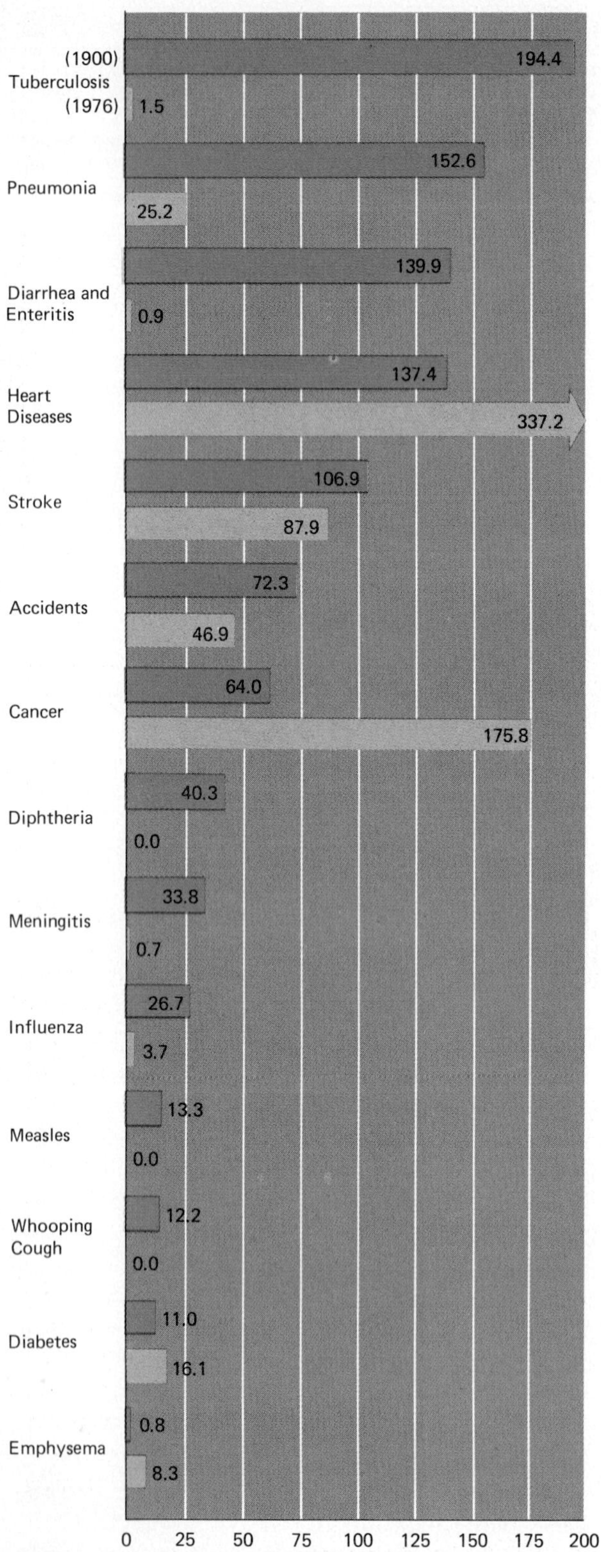

Figure 14.8 Leading causes of death in the United States, 1900 and 1976 (per 100,000 population).

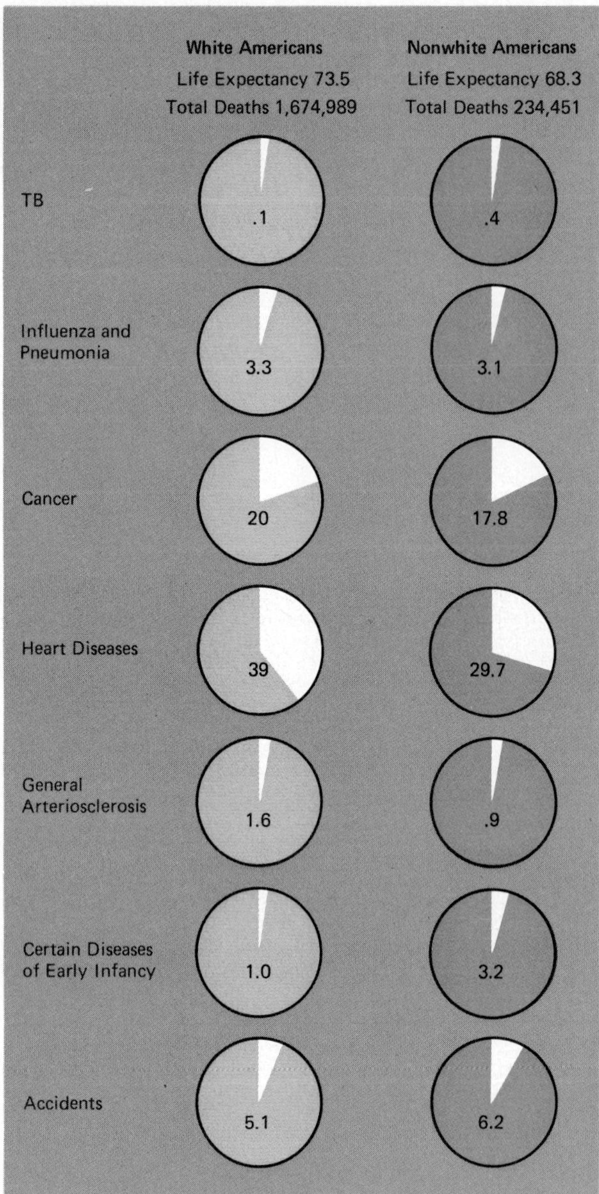

Figure 14.9 A comparison of life expectancy and death rates for different diseases among white and nonwhite Americans, 1976 (per 100,000 population).

the frequency of given diseases, it becomes clear that nonwhite Americans, correlated to a great degree with the lowest socioeconomic levels in the United States, suffer illnesses commonly found in underdeveloped nations. On the average, a nonwhite American can expect to live between five and six years less than

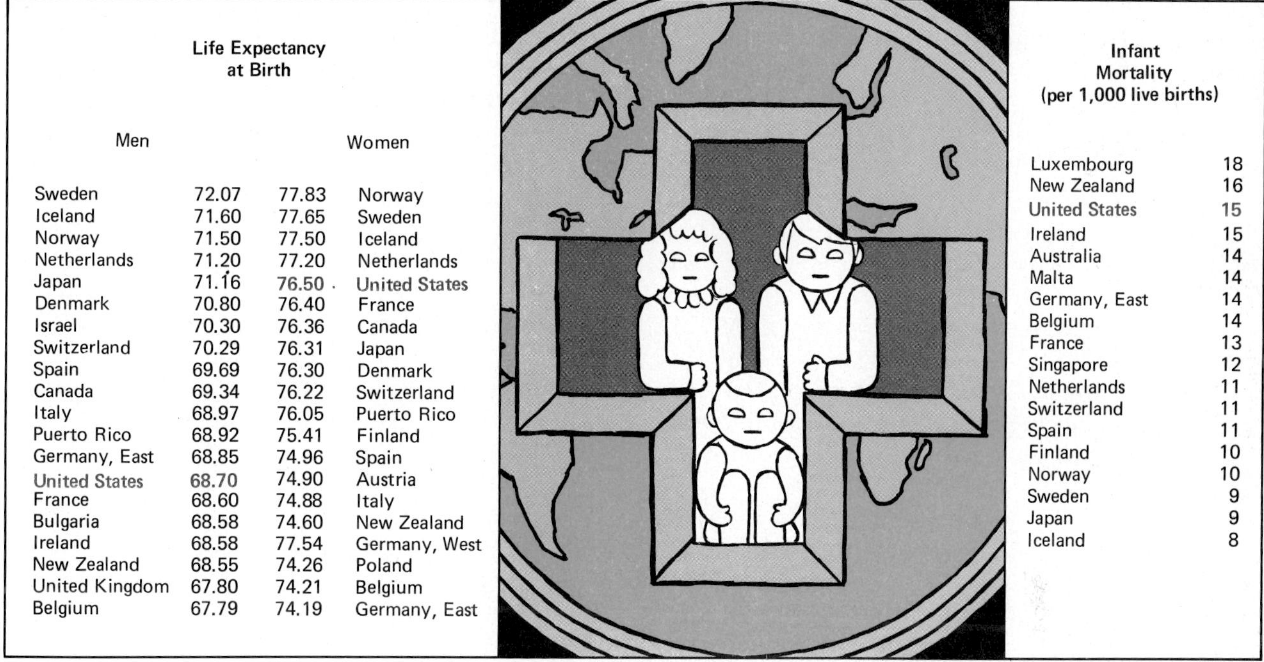

Life Expectancy at Birth

Men		Women	
Sweden	72.07	77.83	Norway
Iceland	71.60	77.65	Sweden
Norway	71.50	77.50	Iceland
Netherlands	71.20	77.20	Netherlands
Japan	71.16	76.50	United States
Denmark	70.80	76.40	France
Israel	70.30	76.36	Canada
Switzerland	70.29	76.31	Japan
Spain	69.69	76.30	Denmark
Canada	69.34	76.22	Switzerland
Italy	68.97	76.05	Puerto Rico
Puerto Rico	68.92	75.41	Finland
Germany, East	68.85	74.96	Spain
United States	68.70	74.90	Austria
France	68.60	74.88	Italy
Bulgaria	68.58	74.60	New Zealand
Ireland	68.58	77.54	Germany, West
New Zealand	68.55	74.26	Poland
United Kingdom	67.80	74.21	Belgium
Belgium	67.79	74.19	Germany, East

Infant Mortality (per 1,000 live births)

Luxembourg	18
New Zealand	16
United States	15
Ireland	15
Australia	14
Malta	14
Germany, East	14
Belgium	14
France	13
Singapore	12
Netherlands	11
Switzerland	11
Spain	11
Finland	10
Norway	10
Sweden	9
Japan	9
Iceland	8

Figure 14.10 Highest life expectancy and lowest infant mortality rates worldwide. The position of the United States, while still relatively low, has improved in the past few years.

a white American—which in part explains the relatively shorter overall life expectancy in the United States compared with other countries (see Figure 14.9). The comparatively high infant mortality rate among the poor also affects these figures.

CONTROL AND PREVENTION OF DISEASE

The dramatic decrease in infectious diseases, and the consequent shift in the United States disease pattern, would not have been possible without the discovery and use of selectively active chemicals, or drugs.

Chemotherapy, the treatment of a disease by chemical means, has become a predominant approach of medical care, extending beyond attack against infectious agents to include treatment of degenerative diseases and mental disorders. (While the term "chemotherapy" is most often used in reference to cancer treatment, it actually includes treatment of any condition in which chemicals or drugs are utilized.)

Certainly the greatest success of chemotherapy has been the development of the *antibiotic* drugs, substances produced by microorganisms that, in dilute solution, can kill or inhibit other microorganisms. After the first of these, penicillin, was introduced in the 1940s, there followed development of many other of these "wonder drugs." Their successful application has served to reduce numerous threats to world health.

Success has not been total, however. In some ways, antibiotics have introduced new problems to medical care. The incidence of directly toxic or allergic reactions to certain antibiotics has shown the need for extreme caution in their use. Another problem, discussed previously, is the appearance of strains of bacteria that are resistant to a given antibiotic. To combat this, doctors must have a series of antibiotics at their disposal so that if one fails, others can be tried.

Although the search for new antibiotics continues, the frontiers of chemotherapeutic research have shifted toward the development of antiviral and anticancer drugs. The most promising of these is a preparation known as *interferon,* a protein produced normally by infected cells, which "interferes" with the spread of infection to healthy cells. At present, preparation for use in humans can be made only from human cells, at very high cost. Efforts are now being made to develop a synthetic version that will successfully combat the common cold—another medical breakthrough. But in spite of the enormous strides of modern medicine, it cannot work miracles. Prevention is still the best means of control.

Disease prevention must take place on many levels. As has been shown, government involvement has proved necessary in many areas: water supply, sanitary facilities, aid to the underprivileged, environmental controls, disease screening, and vaccine programs. Not all such operations function as efficiently as they might.

But one cannot expect governments to shoulder the responsibility alone. Of even greater importance is personal awareness and cooperation. Any kind of medical program is useless if people do not make use of it, or if they do not know *how* to make use of it. Further, the increasing incidence of chronic diseases indicates that some very necessary changes and improvements in life style are in order. Every individual is accountable for following, as far as possible, the principles of balanced, moderate nutrition, exercise, rest, and personal hygiene—and for eliminating, or at least modifying, undesirable habits relating to tobacco, alcohol, drugs, and stress.

Improved health education—on all levels—is imperative. Without knowledge of exactly what constitutes the problem areas, and how to combat them, no solutions are possible.

THE STATUS OF THE COMMUNICABLE DISEASES

Although infectious diseases are not the killers they once were in the United States, they still have a significant impact on the everyday life of the average American. Everyone suffers at least one cold a year, and most people are hit by the flu at periodic intervals. Nevertheless, today's children, through the use of vaccines, are avoiding many of the diseases their parents experienced as a "normal" part of childhood: measles, rubella, and whooping cough, for example. The cases of such formerly feared diseases as polio, diphtheria, and tetanus have dropped to almost nothing. The story of smallpox dramatically illustrates the enormous success that is possible with well-organized vaccination programs. In 1975, the World Health Organization (WHO) announced that fewer than 500 cases of the disease remained worldwide—confined solely to areas of Ethiopia and Bangladesh—compared to the 10 million annual cases of only a decade earlier. For the first time in recorded history, such countries as India were completely free of this killer. No new cases have been diagnosed since 1978, and WHO declared the official end of smallpox on October 26, 1979.

Unfortunately, however, Americans have been lulled into a state of complacency and are failing to keep up their children's immunization schedules. If continued, such negligence could result in new outbreaks of many infectious diseases. At least 80 percent of all children must be immunized in order for any single program to function effectively.

Within the next few decades, scientists will decrease the incidence of many more infectious diseases through the use of vaccines, drugs, and epidemiological methods. But it is up to the public to use these resources. As these diseases, one by one, come under control, medicine can focus more and more on the noninfectious diseases that have become the new killers of humankind. Such diseases are discussed in the next two chapters.

SUMMARY

1. The epidemiologist studies both patterns of disease and patterns of good health in order to reach the ultimate goal of disease prevention. Complicating factors in epidemiological studies include the scientist's bias, the possible

existence of multifactors, and the interpretation and application of the results. The emphasis of epidemiological studies has shifted from infectious diseases to chronic diseases.

2. One's risk of developing a disease is based on the three factors necessary for a specific disorder to occur: environment, contact, and susceptibility. Specific types of disease-causing agents include heredity, environment, infection, diet, drugs, stress, and degenerative processes. Illness often results from a combination of factors.

3. Only a limited number of the billions of microbes in the human body are pathogens—organisms that regularly cause disease. Endogenous microbes reside within the human host and are harmless under normal circumstances; exogenous microbes are outside the body. Infection is the attack of exogenous microbes. Disease occurs when there is a great enough number of exogenous microbes or when they release toxins.

4. There are six main types of infectious agents: bacteria, viruses, rickettsiae, fungi, protozoa, and worms.

5. Infections may be spread either by direct physical contact or through such intermediaries (vectors) as insects, air, or drinking water.

6. The course of an infection has five broad phases: the incubation period, the prodrome period, clinical disease, the decline stage, and convalescence.

7. There are three stages to the body's defenses against disease. The first defense is the skin, the mucous membranes, various secretions, and the cilia in respiratory passages. Second, there are bacteria- and virus-killing chemicals in the blood, phagocytes and macrophages. Third, inflammation and fever indicate that the body is resisting attack. A defense against viruses is interferon, a protein that protects uninfected cells.

8. There are two parts to the body's immune response—cell-mediated response and antibody response. Both depend on the lymphocyte, a type of white blood cell that plays a major role in the production of antibodies—proteins capable of inactivating specific invaders. The microbes that stimulate the production of antibodies are called antigens. Immunity is acquired naturally through illness or may be induced by vaccines.

9. The most common infectious diseases include the common cold, flu, hepatitis, mononucleosis, and sexually transmitted diseases.

10. Sexually transmitted diseases have reached epidemic proportions since the 1950s, as a result of changing life styles, greater mobility, drug use, increased use of the Pill and IUDs, complacency about the dangers involved, better diagnostic methods, and reluctance to seek treatment.

11. Syphilis and gonorrhea are almost always contracted during sexual intercourse. Both can be treated with penicillin or antibiotics if diagnosed at an early stage. Herpes simplex Type 2 is an STD that has reached epidemic proportions and is still incurable.

12. Since there is no immunity from STDs, control can only be achieved by preventive measures to reduce the number of infected persons.

13. Epidemiological data and the study of disease causation reveal certain generalizations about global disease patterns. In regions with a high standard of living, the major killers are heart disease, cancer, stroke, and accidents. In developing nations, undernutrition, malaria, tuberculosis, and parasites are the greatest killers. Climate, social custom, technology, living standards, and longevity affect worldwide patterns of disease.

14. Chemotherapy—the use of selectively active drugs—has been instrumental in the decrease in infectious diseases and the shift in disease patterns. Chemotherapy is now used to treat degenerative diseases and mental disorders. The use of antibiotics, starting with penicillin in the 1940s, has reduced many threats to world health.

15. Disease prevention depends not only on government involvement but also on personal awareness and cooperation.

16. The incidence of infectious diseases has dropped dramatically due to the use of vaccines. However, immunization schedules are often ignored out of complacency. It is the public's responsibility to use the increasing resources that scientists provide.

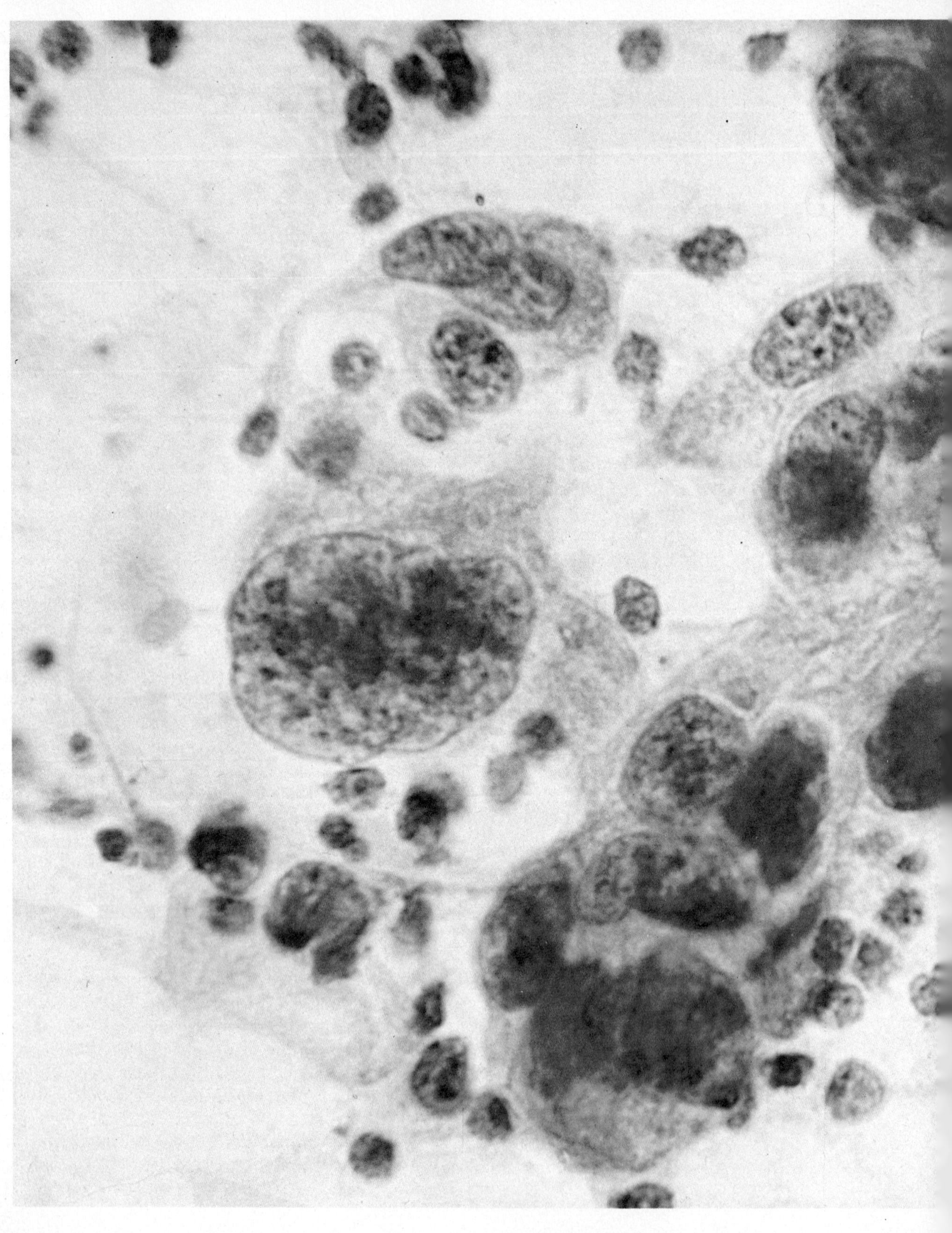

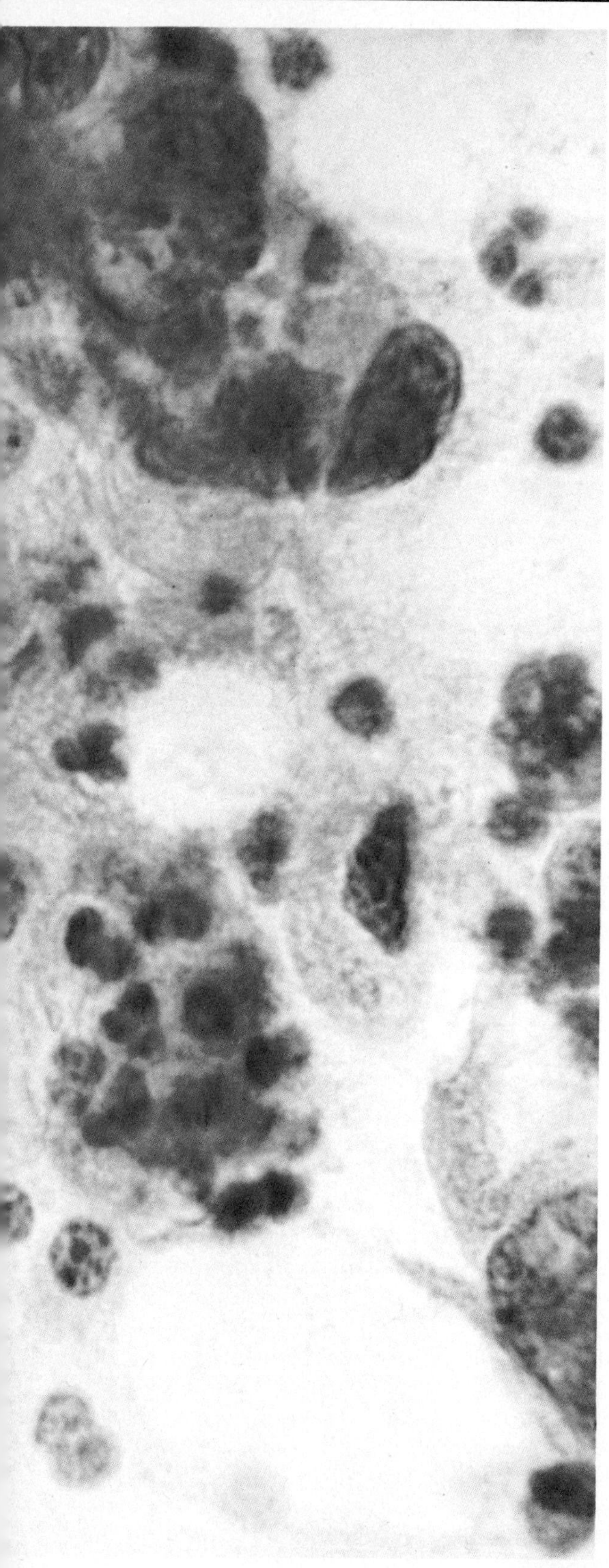

15 Cancer

Although cancer is considered a modern disease, it was not unknown in ancient times. The condition was named by the Greeks from their word for crab, for its clawing, "crablike" growth. But there is no question that incidence of cancer has risen dramatically in recent decades and it is probably our most dreaded disease today. As a cause of death in the United States it is second only to heart disease, accounting for close to 400,000 deaths per year. This figure has risen annually since 1949, and if present trends continue, cancer may well overtake heart disease as the number one cause of death. It is already the leading killer of women in the thirty-to-fifty-four age group.

This increased incidence may be attributed to three factors. First, new techniques permit earlier, more accurate diagnosis than in the past. Second, since the risk of cancer grows with age, our increasing longevity automatically increases the prevalence of cancer. And third, changing life styles have increased exposure to certain causative factors—such as the tobacco in cigarettes.

Although there is still much to be learned, our knowledge about cancer has grown steadily in recent years, both in understanding the disease and in finding ways to cope with it. The struggle to understand and control cancer is complicated by the fact that the term "cancer" actually refers to a number of diseases—each, perhaps, with its own causes and potential cures.

Lung cancer now kills twenty-five times as many men as it did in 1935 (and the incidence has increased steadily for women), while breast cancer—the leading cause of cancer death among women—has had about the same mortality rate for fifty years. Cancers of the uterus and cervix have shown a substantial decrease in women, and cancers of the stomach, rectum, and esophagus have decreased considerably in both sexes. The reasons for these declines are not fully clear, but there are a few possible explanations. For example, improved refrigeration may account for the decline in stomach cancer. Effective screening for cervical cancer —namely, the Pap test—has certainly contributed to decline in deaths from this form of malignancy.

The American Cancer Society estimates that approximately 50 percent of patients with cancer could be saved with existing methods of treatment—instead of the present 33 percent. Why do so many with curable cancer have to die? The problem seems in part to be one of ignorance and fear. Cure depends on early diagnosis and treatment. This is one situation where it is profoundly dangerous to believe that "what you don't know can't hurt you."

Early recognition of the signs of cancer, prompt diagnosis, and aggressive treatment by the appropriate means have made the word "cancer" less terrifying than it used to be. For many cancer victims, hope exists where there was once only despair. Even more important is the fact that some kinds of cancer are preventable. For example, most lung cancer is caused by cigarette smoking and most skin cancer is caused by excessive exposure to the sun. While not all forms of cancer have such obvious associations, where causes have been established it is only common sense to use this knowledge and attempt to reduce the odds of developing those particular forms of the disease.

UNCONTROLLED GROWTH

Cancer is a condition of abnormal cellular growth. One or a few cells initially undergo certain changes and are no longer able to perform their intended functions. Reproduction of these mutant cells becomes highly accelerated; if it continues unchecked, the patient will die. To understand the peculiar nature of cancer, it is necessary to know how the physician (usually a pathologist) distinguishes cancerous tissues from other kinds of tissue.

A *tumor* is a swelling or mass that is formed when cells that normally cooperate with each other in performing a useful function no longer do so. They assume an abnormal size and shape and begin to multiply independently, often rapidly, taking nourishment from normal cells. Such a group of cells, growing in this uncontrolled fashion, is called a *neoplasm.*

Benign tumors are not neoplasms. They generally grow slowly in a capsule that keeps them localized, and they usually do not recur once they are removed. The fact that they are benign, however, does not mean they do no damage. They can cause pressure and subsequent harm to surrounding structures and can rob normal tissues of their blood supply. A benign tumor can have serious consequences if it occurs in a vital organ such as the brain. Benign tumors are usually curable by surgical removal.

Malignant tumors (malignant neoplasms), on the other hand, *are* cancers. Free from the restraints of any capsule, they multiply rapidly and insidiously spread their damaging effects. Surrounding tissues are compressed, invaded, and ultimately killed. Cells break away and enter the lymphatic channels and the blood vessels, both systems then carrying the cancerous cells to distant parts of the body. There they settle, again multiplying rapidly and forming other tumors (see Figure 15.1).

These secondary tumors are called *metastases,* and the process by which they spread is called *metastatic growth.* Such neoplasms may metastasize a considerable distance from the original site, and each metastasis is capable of seeding more new sites. In this way, the entire body can become riddled with cancer.

The cure for cancer involves the complete removal or destruction of *every* malignant cell. When the growth is still *localized* at its original site on the surface of a tissue (cancer *in situ*), treatment is relatively easy. During this time, however, there are few symptoms of the disease and pain is almost never present. Once the metastatic state is reached, removal of all cancer from the body becomes exceedingly difficult. But in many forms of cancer the usual time lag between onset and metastasis permits early diagnosis and treatment before the ma-

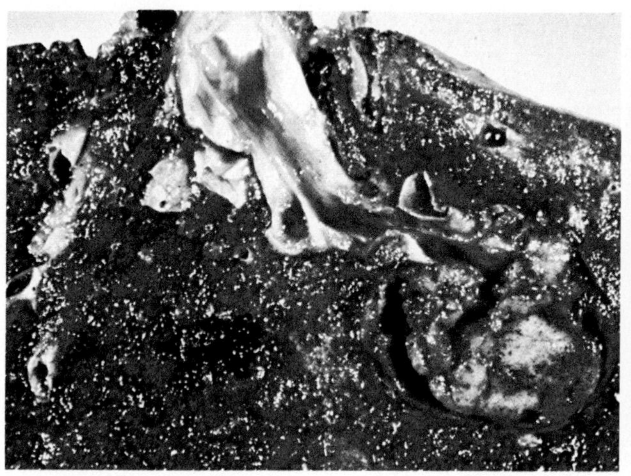

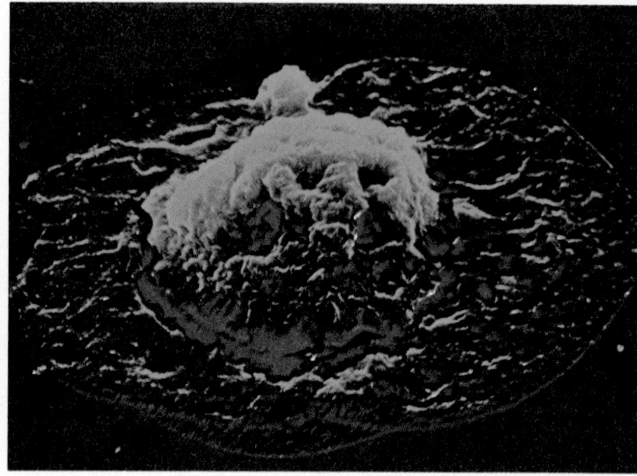

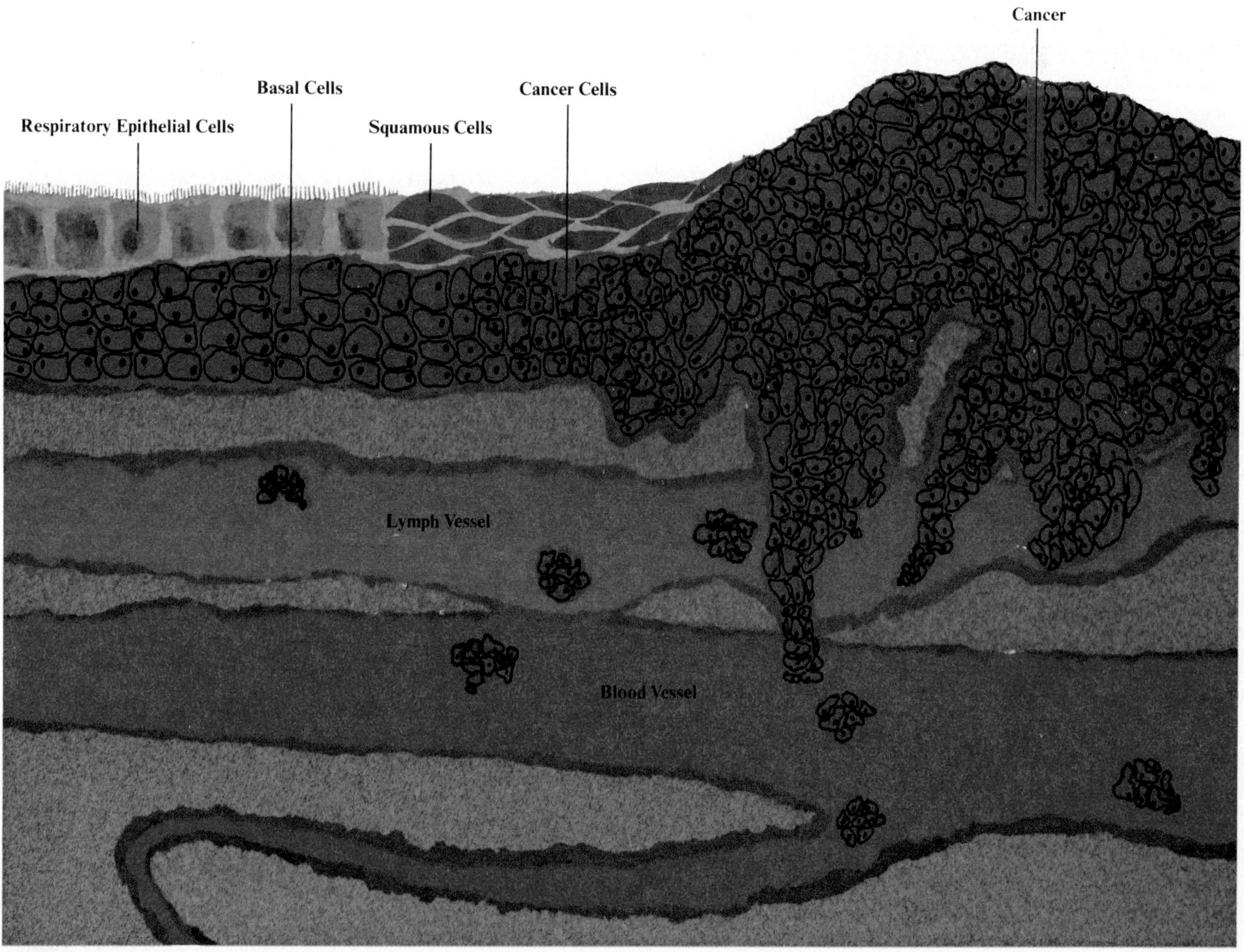

Figure 15.1 *(Top left)* A benign tumor. *(Top right)* A malignant tumor being attacked by the body's immune mechanism. *(Bottom)* How cancer cells multiply and metastasize.

lignancy can spread—*if* discovered early enough by the patient or a physician.

The value of early detection is shown by the different cure rates for certain forms of cancer. Skin cancers are easily seen and frequently receive early attention; in addition, they are readily accessible to treatment. With the exception of melanoma, a cancer of the pigment-carrying cells in the skin that is particularly resistant to treatment, the cure rate is more than 90 percent. For lung cancer, on the other hand, the cure rate is less than 10 percent. This disease is *not* immediately apparent. In fact, it frequently does not produce symptoms that a patient can perceive until the damage has become irreversible. Lung cancers are treated surgically; often one lobe of a lung or an entire lung must be removed. In some cases the tumor at surgery appears to be confined to the lung. Some 15 to 20 percent of these patients will survive five years and be considered "cured," a discouraging figure given that lung cancer occurs so frequently in this country today.

TYPES OF CANCER

There are more than 100 different forms of cancer, about 30 of which are fairly common.

Malignant tumors are classified according to the cells from which they arise and their appearance under the microscope. *Carcinomas* arise from epithelium—the cells forming the skin, glands, and membranes lining the respiratory, urinary, and gastrointestinal tract. *Sarcomas* arise from supporting or connective tissues—such as bones, cartilage, and the membranes covering muscles and fat. These terms are often modified to indicate more specifically the type or location of the disease. In cancer of the breast, for example, cancers derived from cells lining the milk ducts are called *adenocarcinomas,* meaning that they are composed of glandular *(adeno-)* epithelial cells. Other breast cancers might arise from the connective tissue of the breast, in which case they are called sarcomas.

Further subdivisions identify cancers from lymphatic cells as *lymphoma* (Hodgkin's disease is an example) or as *lymphosarcoma;* cancers from blood-forming cells as *leukemia;* cancers from pigment-carrying cells of the skin as *melanoma;* and so on. By these criteria, the more than 100 cancers can be identified. But there are also cancers whose cellular structure is so altered that they no longer resemble the cells from which they originated, and no identification is possible. Such cancers are termed *anaplastic.*

DISTRIBUTION OF CANCER

The most common forms of cancer in the United States are indicated in Figure 15.2. Incidence of all cancers in women exceeds that of men until the age of fifty-five—primarily because the most common forms of cancer in women are those of the breast and genital organs (especially the uterine cervix). Except for these sex-specific sites, and the thyroid and gall bladder, men have more cancer than women in all other sites. After age fifty-five, overall cancer incidence is higher in men.

Most cancers occur more often among older people, the frequency increasing with age. However, some types of cancer also occur rather frequently among children, including acute leukemia and certain cancers of bone, nerve, and kidney tissue. Although some of these cancers are relatively rare, the fact is that in the United States cancer now kills more children between the ages of three and fourteen than any other disease.

CAUSES OF CANCER

Since cancer is actually a group of more than 100 different diseases, it probably has no single cause. However, one causative factor may result in different forms of cancer. Cigarette smoking, for instance, does not precipitate lung cancer alone; it can also lead to cancer of the bladder, larynx, mouth, and other sites. Further, at least some forms of cancer appear to result from a specific combination of factors such as smoking *and* exposure to asbestos.

As in any disease, cancer depends on both the environment and the individual's genetic constitution. A clear example of genetic and environmental interplay is found in carcinoma of the skin. A large proportion of skin cancers is caused by exposure to sunlight, especially

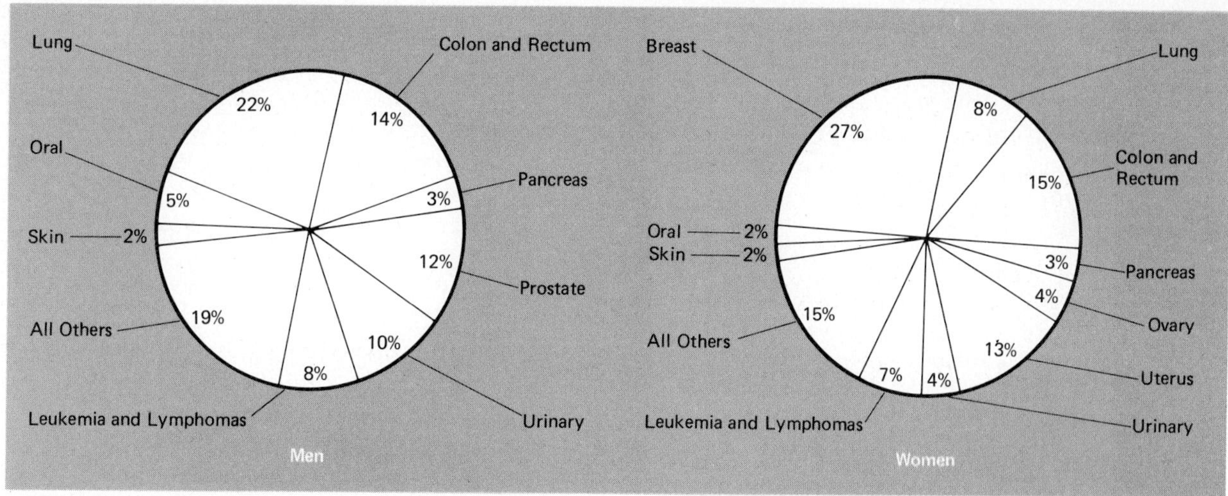

Figure 15.2 Incidence of cancer by sex and site (excluding nonmelanoma skin cancer and carcinoma *in situ* of the uterine cervix).

ultraviolet light. Persons with certain genetic characteristics—light skin, particularly the freckled type—are about ten times more likely to develop skin cancer after excessive exposure to sunlight than are persons with heavy pigment.

Human beings of all races, colors, and environmental habits have been known to develop

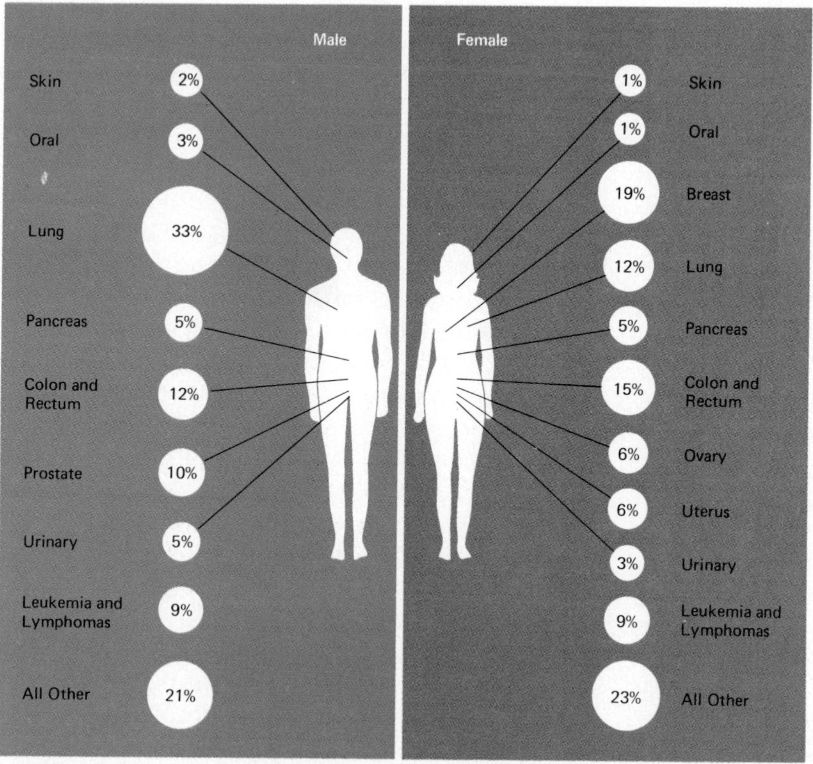

Figure 15.3 Cancer deaths by sex and site: 1978 estimates. The American Cancer Society will provide periodically updated research findings to those who request them.

cancer of one type or another. There are, however, some intriguing differences in the occurrence of some cancers among different human populations. Compared with its incidence in the United States, stomach cancer is more frequent in Scandinavia and Japan; cancer of the cervix and of the penis are much more frequent in India; and cancer of the breast and prostate are one-fourth as frequent in Japan as in the United States. While certain factors are known to play a causative role in these cases, many questions remain. The relative involvement of genetic and environmental factors is an important area for continuing research—and a difficult one, since it is often almost impossible to separate identical genetic patterns from identical environmental patterns.

Heredity

It is known that a few rare types of cancer are definitely hereditary—for instance, cancer of the retina. And evidence continues to build that families tend to inherit a predisposition toward particular types of cancer.

Mothers, fathers, and siblings of persons with cancer of the stomach, breast, large intestine, uterus, or lung have two to four times the risk of also developing the disease, when compared to the general population. Studies also indicate that other blood relatives (aunts, uncles, etc.) show increased risk. One study found that relatives of patients who had contracted breast cancer before the age of forty were *nine times* as likely to develop the disease as the control group.

This familial tendency toward specific forms of cancer is only that—a tendency. One cannot change one's heritage, but an awareness of this risk factor should prompt such persons to eliminate as nearly as possible all other associated risk factors and to be especially attentive to the need for regular checkups.

Diet

Preliminary evidence from a number of studies suggests that a high-calorie, fat-rich diet that is low in fiber may increase the risk of developing cancer of the breast, prostate, colon, and uterus. An interesting example refers to the Japanese cancer patterns mentioned at the beginning of this section. Japanese who migrate to the United States and adopt American dietary habits and cooking methods gradually tend to assume cancer patterns similar to those of the United States; specifically, incidence of stomach cancer declines, while that of breast and colon cancers climbs. Nevertheless, this heredity/environment relationship is not well understood, and further research is needed.

Another possible dietary relationship under study is that between breast cancer and cholesterol—a substance necessary for the body's synthesis of female hormones. Some scientists suspect that elevated cholesterol levels may overstimulate metabolism in the breast tissue.

Tobacco

Currently more Americans (nearly 100,000) die annually of lung cancer than die in automobile accidents. And cigarette smoking has been overwhelmingly indicated as the cause of most lung malignancies. Both the tar and the smoke from tobacco contain specific *carcinogenic* (cancer-causing) chemicals.

The evidence indicates that carcinogenic irritants inhaled over a period of time trigger the cancerous potential in susceptible lung-tissue cells. In the case of cigarettes, inhaled smoke paralyzes the bronchial cilia, interfering with the natural cleansing mechanism. The carcinogenic dusts, gases, and tars linger to irritate and cause precancerous alterations in lung-cell structure, thus eventually triggering the cancer mechanism. Lung cancer has reached near-epidemic proportions, particularly in the male population over forty years of age and most particularly among men who have smoked cigarettes for twenty or more years.

In addition to the danger of lung cancer, cigarette smoking is unquestionably one cause of bladder cancer; this disease appears two to three times as often among smokers as nonsmokers. Apparently the body attempts to excrete the tobacco carcinogens by way of the urinary tract, with consequent irritation of the bladder. Still other forms of cancer associated with cigarette smoking include oral cancers and cancers of the larynx, esophagus, pancreas, and possibly the kidney.

Drugs

Estrogen, one of the female sex hormones, readily triggers cancers of the breast, uterus, and testes in mice and other rodents. Studies of women who use high doses of estrogen to relieve some common symptoms of menopause now indicate an increased risk of cancer of the uterus associated with the medication. Short-term use of low doses of estrogen does not seem to increase uterine cancer risk. Estrogen compounds should be avoided during pregnancy, however, since they may cause cancers in offspring. Past use of one form of estrogen, diethylstilbesterol (DES), to prevent miscarriage resulted in vaginal and cervical cancer and abnormalities in some daughters of exposed women.

Certain drugs used during organ transplants to suppress the immune response and thus lessen chances of the body's rejecting the new organ have now been implicated as increasing the risk of cancer. Results of one study of 6,000 kidney transplants showed development of lymphatic cancer thirty-five times the normal rate.

Chemicals

High-dose, long-term exposure to various occupational chemicals has been shown to increase the risk of certain forms of cancer. Such chemicals include asbestos (insulating and fireproofing), vinyl chloride (plastics), chromates (paint), benzene (rubber), and benzidene (dyes). Generally a long latency period occurs between exposure and onset of disease. Today occupational cancers account for a sizable percentage of cancer deaths in the United States, but extensive safety measures are being implemented to protect the health of workers.

Not only do asbestos workers show an increased incidence of mesothelioma (a rare cancer that attacks the lining of the chest or abdominal cavity) but among *workers who smoke,* there is also increased incidence of lung cancer, beyond expected levels for other smokers. This suggests the possibility that asbestos (and perhaps other chemicals) may exhibit a synergistic effect similar to that of alcohol.

Pollution

Small amounts of carcinogens have been found in the air of America's cities, as well as in samples from some suburban and rural areas. Nevertheless, no firm evidence exists that such carcinogens are a cause of human cancer. The fact that lung cancer death rates are somewhat higher in cities than in rural areas is deceiving: in reality, only *male* rates are elevated, suggesting that the greater use of cigarettes among males may be the actual causative factor here. Similarly, while fossil fuel pollution has been with us for generations, lung cancer rates did not increase until the 1930s—concurrent with increased use of cigarettes.

Oil pollution in both air and water is yet another growing concern. Among a host of other chemicals, oil contains substances known collectively as PAH—a known carcinogen also present in cigarettes, burning garbage, and the fumes from automobile exhausts and power plants.

Radiation

Excessive exposure to the sun's ultraviolet rays can easily precipitate skin cancers, particularly among fair-skinned individuals. Protection with effective sunscreen—*not* suntan—lotions is a must for these persons.

Ionizing radiation—that is, radiation from X-rays, radium, and atomic-bomb explosions, among other forms—indisputably increases the occurrence of leukemia (cancer of the blood), as well as cancers of the thyroid, skin, and bone. Scientists vary in their opinions of avoiding such exposure, some insisting that one rad (a standard X-ray dose) ages the involved cells by one year. See Chapter 17 for a further discussion of the risks of radiation and nuclear energy.

Viruses

An exciting and promising area of cancer research is the study of viruses. Viruses have been found to cause several dozen types of cancers in animals as diverse as frogs, mice, cats, and chickens. Up to the present, viral involvement in human cancer is still somewhat speculative. Yet evidence continues to mount in support of a viral etiology in certain cancers. Specifically, acute leukemia, sarcoma, and melanoma are the cancers most likely to be initially linked with viruses.

As mentioned in Chapter 14, an association exists between cervical cancer and herpes simplex Type 2 virus (HSV-2). New techniques have recently enabled investigators to find HSV-2 nucleic acids (i.e., genetic material) in cervical cancer cells, finally making concrete what before had been only theoretical.

Scientists know that cancer viruses—which are made up of nucleic acids—can establish an intimate relationship with nucleic acids of body cells (that is, with their hereditary machinery). As the virus—or a part of the virus—enters the cell nucleus, it changes the original genetic coding so that all future cells lose any resemblance to the parent cell.

It is also known that certain noncancer viruses or viral gene products can infect cells but remain hidden for a period of time. They multiply only at the fixed rate of normal cell division (mitosis), but each new cell carries the original virus or viral material. Such viruses may remain totally harmless, or at some point they may become activated by radiation, chemicals, or other viruses. Herpes Type 2 appears to react this way.

Knowledge of the mechanisms by which viruses or other agents transform normal cells into cancer cells would offer new approaches in interfering with—or even reversing—the cancer-formation process. The fact that leukemia in cats has been definitely shown to be virally caused, and the fact that an effective vaccine against the disease has been developed, lend great hope to future treatment of human cancer.

Defective Immune Mechanisms

Another theory proposes a relationship between cancer and the *immune mechanisms* of the body. According to this theory, most persons may be harboring individual tumor cells or cancer-causing genes known as *oncogenes* that are destroyed or repressed by normal immunological defenses. Occasionally such defenses may become defective, possibly because of certain cancer-inducing conditions, and active cancer begins to grow. There is a basic difference between the viral and the immune hypotheses. In one, the instructions for becoming an active cancer element come to the cell from a foreign agent, the virus; in the other, they result from an occasional mistake, or mutation, during cell reproduction. However, the viral and immune involvements in cancer need not be mutually exclusive. Either one may play a supportive role for the other, rather than being itself the primary cause.

PREVENTION

Prevention as well as treatment or cure in any disease depends upon three factors: (1) the practical knowledge available at the time, (2) the extent of public education and motivation to use the knowledge, and (3) the availability of an adequate medical system to apply the knowledge. In the case of cancer, the mechanism responsible for the disease is not wholly understood. True prevention, in the sense of totally eliminating occurrence of the disease, is not possible. Nevertheless, the risk of developing many forms of cancer can be significantly reduced by avoiding known carcinogens.

The single most important carcinogen in the U.S. environment is the smoke of tobacco, especially from deeply inhaled cigarettes. It is estimated that at least 80 percent of lung cancer, now the number one malignant killer, could be prevented if this habit were eliminated. This would also result in a corresponding reduction of cancers of the mouth, throat, larynx, esophagus, and bladder.

Chronic, excessive alcohol consumption, a major social and health problem in itself (see Chapter 12), is also related to the higher risk of cancer in the mouth, throat, larynx, and esophagus, when combined with the effects of tobacco smoking and poor nutrition.

While the relationship between diet and cancer is still unclear, moderate eating is beneficial to one's health in general. Excessive amounts of fats and cholesterol should be avoided, sufficient vegetable fiber should be included, and total calories should be kept consistent with the body's needs.

Good hygiene of the genitals, mouth, throat,

HOW TO
Decrease Your Risks of Developing Cancer

There are no guarantees that any one person can forever avoid developing cancer. Nevertheless, there are many ways to minimize the risk.

1. Give up cigarettes—and preferably all other forms of tobacco.
2. Limit fat intake to 80 grams per day and cholesterol intake to a maximum of 300 mgs. per day. Use skim milk products instead of whole. Try low-fat margarines and cheeses.
3. Use more veal, chicken, turkey, and fish. Trim fat from other meats, use lean cuts, and drain well after cooking.
4. Eat more fruits, vegetables, and cereals.
5. Keep alcohol consumption moderate. Avoid alcohol entirely if you smoke—it further enhances the carcinogenic effects of tobacco.
6. If you drink each day, make sure your intake doesn't interfere with eating a well-balanced meal. Make sure particularly that your diet includes sufficient B vitamins and iron.
7. Avoid unnecessary X-rays. If you do need an X-ray, see that modern equipment is available and that proper precautions are taken to minimize exposure. If there is any possibility that you are pregnant, do not submit to an X-ray except in an emergency.
8. Don't broil yourself in the sun. Use a good sunscreen containing PABA. Expose yourself gradually to the sun, avoiding the hours between 11 and 2. Wear protective clothing even on cloudy days.
9. Avoid unnecessary medications, prescriptive and over-the-counter. This is particularly important during pregnancy.
10. If you are a woman and believe that you were prenatally exposed to stilbestrol (DES), tell your gynecologist.
11. If you are a female, postpone sexual intercourse until age eighteen or later. If practical, have your first child prior to age thirty.
12. Maintain high standards of personal hygiene —and make sure your sexual partner(s) does also. If you have many partners, use a condom.
13. If you are exposed to industrial chemicals at work, follow safety instructions.
14. Be very cautious in tearing down structures that could be lined or insulated with asbestos.

Source: Elizabeth Whelan, *Preventing Cancer: What You Can Do to Cut Your Risks by Up to 50 Percent* (New York: W. W. Norton, 1978).

and skin will help reduce the likelihood of cancer in those sites. Early circumcision helps prevent cancer of the penis, but cleanliness may also be effective. Repair of jagged teeth helps prevent cancer of the tongue. In general, being observant about one's body and seeking prompt care when anything unusual develops is sound preventive medicine.

X-rays and other sources of ionizing radiation are to be avoided as much as possible because of the added risk of developing leukemia and cancer of the thyroid, and perhaps of the breast and lung. Such exposure is especially dangerous to children and the developing fetus. This warning does not mean that X-rays should never be used diagnostically, but it does mean that they should be used with discretion and that exposure rates should be kept as low as is practicable.

Individuals with particularly susceptible skin, such as albinos and those with light complexions, should protect themselves from overexposure to the sun by appropriate coverings and sunscreen preparations. Those containing the ingredient PABA (para-aminobenzoic acid) offer especially effective protection from the sun's dangerous ultraviolet rays. Radiation from the sun is not only a primary cause of skin cancer, but also the major cause of premature aging of the skin.

Since most occupation-related cancers today reflect working conditions that existed twenty to thirty or more years ago, industry's growing awareness of such hazards is leading to the use of extensive safety measures. But such measures are effective only if workers adhere to them precisely.

Surgery can be used to prevent cancer. *Prophylactic* (preventive) surgery consists of removing tissue known from past medical experience to have a high potential for developing into cancer. Such tissues include warts or moles in areas that are subjected to constant irritation and abnormalities, such as the mouth, vagina, and rectum.

DETECTION AND DIAGNOSIS

The greatest hope for the cancer victim is in early diagnosis and prompt treatment. Persons who are alert to the signals that may indicate

Would you rather not know these 7 warning signals?

1. Unusual bleeding or discharge.
2. A lump or thickening in the breast or elsewhere.
3. A sore that does not heal.
4. Change in bowel or bladder habits.
5. Hoarseness or cough.
6. Indigestion or difficulty in swallowing.
7. Change in size or color of a wart or mole.

If a signal persists for 2 weeks, see your doctor without delay. Because many cancers are curable if detected and treated early.

American Cancer Society

It's up to you, too.

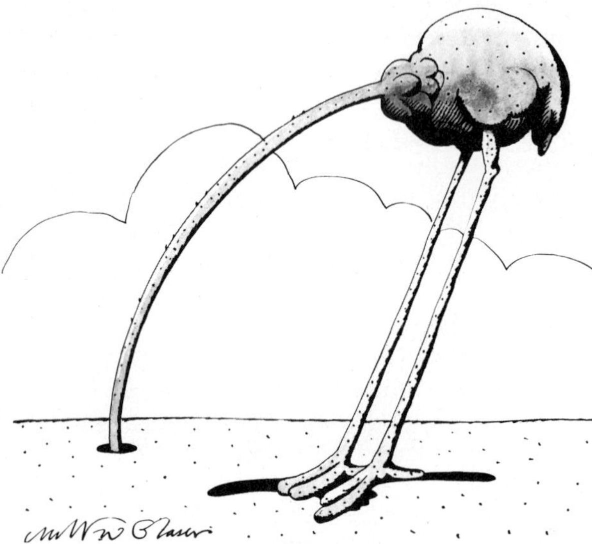

Figure 15.4 The seven warning signals of cancer.

cancer, and to the need for regular medical checkups, are those most likely to have cancers detected early enough to be successfully treated.

The American Cancer Society emphasizes seven warning signals of cancer, shown in Figure 15.4. They should be known and remembered by everyone. *None of these symptoms automatically means the existence of cancer; most often they do not.* But they *are* warning signals, and if they progress or last for longer than *two weeks,* they demand medical attention. Tragically, some people who observe a possible warning sign follow a "maybe it will go away" attitude. Such a reaction is foolish; the importance of early detection cannot be overemphasized.

The most curable cancers are usually those that are detected even before actual symptoms appear. There is a good chance that individuals can detect some of the early warning signs by examining themselves periodically. With the aid of a mirror, they should observe their skin, mouth, and scalp. Men should examine the penis and testes, women the breasts and vulva. Women should make a habit of examining their breasts every month, preferably between menstrual periods. The suggested method is shown in Figure 15.5.

Personal examinations should be supplemented with physical checkups by a physician at recommended intervals. If one of the warning signs develops between visits to the doctor—even shortly after a checkup—it should be reported immediately.

During the physical checkup, the doctor should examine a woman's breasts and cervix. Specimens should be obtained from the vagina and cervix for a Papanicolaou test, or *Pap smear,* to detect early signs of cancer of the cervix. Deaths from cervical cancer could be reduced 90 percent if all women had this test annually and were promptly and adequately treated when abnormalities were noted. Both men and women should periodically have a rectal examination by a procedure known as *proctoscopy.* Cancer of the colon-rectum is the second leading cancer killer of both sexes.

The poor cure rates for lung cancer are due in part to the fact that the usual diagnostic procedures—X-ray and microscopic examination of a specimen of lung tissue—detect the disease too late. Sputum cytology is designed to pick up early signs of cancer and earlier precancerous cell changes. It calls for regular microscopic examinations of sputum coughed up from the lungs by high-risk patients (such as cigarette smokers).

While microscopic examinations of cells taken from a patient by means of a Pap smear or sputum sample can be used to determine the existence of cancer, these methods must be confirmed by *biopsy* of the tumor—examination under a microscope of a bit of tissue suspected to be diseased. Needle biopsy is a newly developed technique whereby tissue material is withdrawn from the tumor by means of a needle, rather than by usual surgical means.

TREATMENT

The key to successful treatment of cancer is to diagnose it at a stage when it can be completely destroyed or removed from the body, leaving

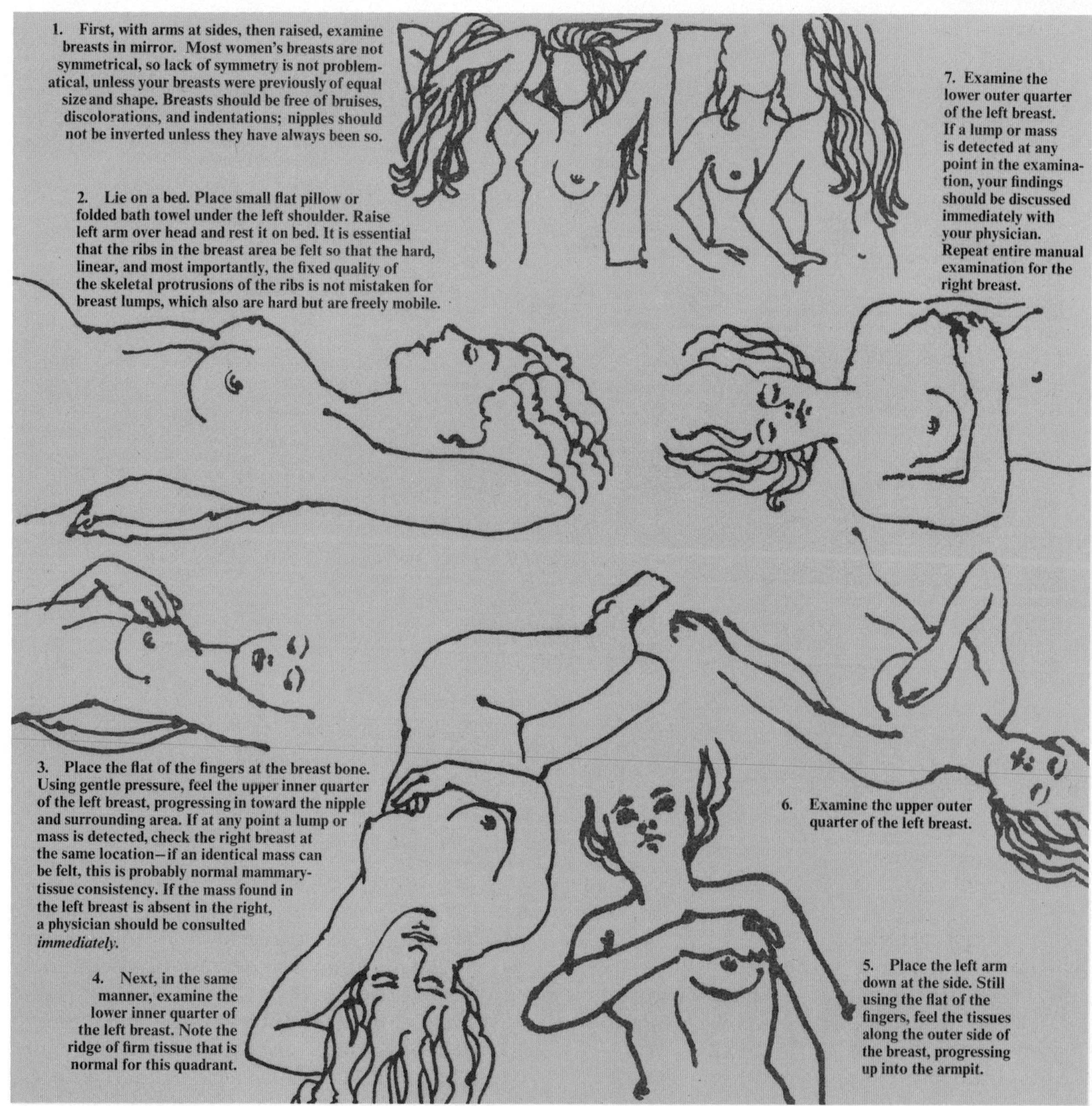

Figure 15.5 Breast self-examination. The breasts should be examined at the same time each month—one week after the end of the menstrual period.

no malignant cell behind. The major problem is, and has always been, to use a therapeutic agent that will kill the malignant cells without interfering with normal cells. To date no such comprehensive agent has been developed, and physicians must rely on the three existing forms of treatment: radiation, surgery, and chemotherapy. Usually various combinations of the three methods are employed.

Modern radiation treatment depends upon powerful sources, such as cobalt machines (utilizing radioactive cobalt), or electronic

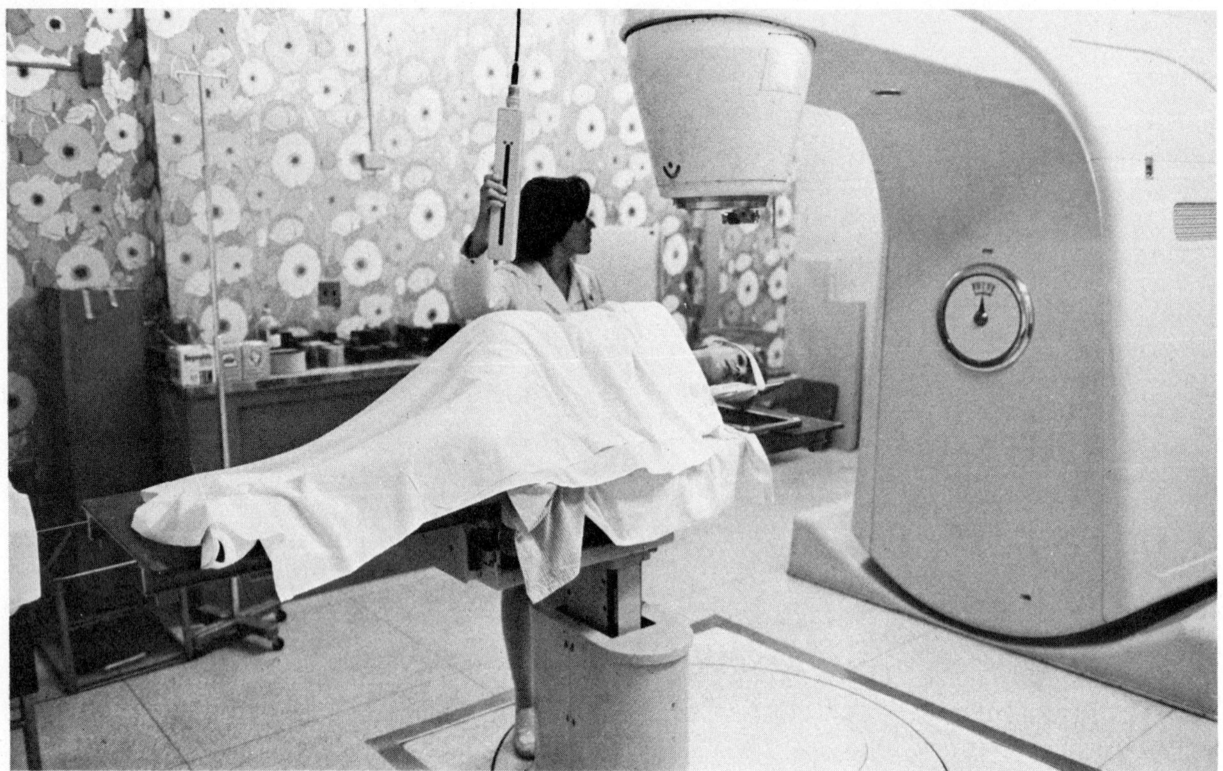

Figure 15.6 Radiation treatment for cancer using a linear accelerator. This machine can more precisely direct the radiation rays to the tumor site, with less of a damaging effect on healthy tissues and skin.

equipment, such as linear accelerators. To avoid exposing normal tissue to radiation, new, highly refined *ultrasound* techniques can locate tumors deep in the body with pinpoint precision. Research is now underway on a new radiation device known as *pion beam* therapy, a series of "miniature nuclear explosions" that cause little or no damage to other organs. With this more specifically focused technique, the malignant growth process can be slowed or stopped with more precision.

Chemotherapy has gained increasing importance in the past few years. Three types of drugs now being used are: (1) hormones, which either by injection or removal of glands may restrict (at least temporarily) growth in such areas as the breast or prostate; (2) metabolic antagonists, which slow down or stop the growth of malignant cells (especially effective in leukemia, where it may lead to remission of five or more years); and (3) cell poisons, highly dangerous compounds that may also affect normal cells. Current research promises to improve greatly the effectiveness of chemotherapy in treating cancer.

Cancer patients require careful management by their physicians. Often the knowledge and skills of several specialists are needed, and the patient may benefit from a team approach that marshals the talents of a surgeon, radiologist (a specialist dealing with all forms of radiation therapy: X-rays, radium, or radioactive isotopes), medical oncologist (chemotherapist), and pathologist. Most cancer patients are best handled in cancer centers or by medical groups whose main focus is neoplastic disease. The American College of Surgeons lists more than 900 cancer clinics in the United States and Canada where proper treatment can be obtained.

The results of cancer therapy are judged by the proportion of patients who survive for at least five years without recurrence of cancer. Unfortunately, some cancers recur even after five years, so that most physicians prefer to avoid the word "cure." All cancer patients should receive periodic examinations to assure that the cancer has been eradicated and to permit further treatments should there be any evidence of recurrence.

QUACKERY

Although methods are available to either cure or arrest many forms of cancer, some victims do not go to physicians and hospitals where they can be treated. They go instead to quacks, on whose advice they spend an estimated $100 million annually for drugs, diets, and all forms of bizarre treatment.

Laetrile is one of the best-known quack cancer treatments. It was illegal in the United States until 1978, when it was federally approved for cancer patients who had been medically certified as "terminally ill." By the fall of that year, seventeen states had legalized laetrile even though it was still prohibited from interstate commerce. Repeated studies at reputable cancer and medical research institutes have failed to disclose any evidence whatever that laetrile will either cure or prevent any form of cancer. Nevertheless, an estimated 70,000 Americans are now using this totally ineffective drug.

Laetrile is not only useless as a protection from or cure for cancer; it may be very dangerous. There are a number of recorded cases of poisoning and death related to ingestion of large numbers of laetrile tablets. This fact is hardly surprising since laetrile contains large amounts of hydrogen cyanide, a classic suicide potion.

Advocates of laetrile and other quack treatments often claim success and offer testimonials of "cured" patients. They do *not* say that the "cure" they attribute to their treatment is most likely the result of a naturally occurring remission of the disease or a standard medical treatment such as chemotherapy.

Cancer quacks prosper not only because people are ignorant but because they are afraid or desperate. Victims who fear they have incurable cancer or who have had those fears confirmed by medical means will often grasp at any straw. The greatest tragedy of cancer quackery is that the victim who might be cured often delays a trip to the doctor and instead relies on useless drugs and treatments. When the victim does finally seek appropriate treatment, it may be too late to curb the disease.

NEW RESEARCH

Some of the most intriguing cancer research today lies in work with viruses and their relationship to human cancer. (As previously mentioned, a definite relationship has already been established in many kinds of animals.) If and when specific viruses are isolated as cancer-causing agents, preventive vaccines may be developed. Needless to say, this degree of progress is probably a long way off, since to date there has been only limited success in developing vaccines against the viruses of infectious diseases.

Experiments with the virus-inhibiting substance known as *interferon* (see the Focus box and Chapter 14) continue to offer hope as a new form of cancer treatment. Interferon also has a strong effect on the immune system, possibly enabling the body to "reject" malignant tumors. Interferon has very recently been synthesized in the laboratory, and it could be generally available in a few years.

Interferon studies are but one part of the research being conducted in the entire field of *immunotherapy.* Scientists hope eventually to marshal the body's own disease-fighting system against cancer invaders. No toxicity is involved, since no "foreign" agents are administered. One compound known as BCG has been proved successful in stimulating the immune defense mechanisms of animals and is now being tried in limited experiments with humans.

Chemoprevention includes the study of new drugs which will stop or inhibit cancer growth. Certain synthetic vitamins known as *retinoids* have successfully reversed the cancer process in animals and are now being attempted in human therapy.

FOCUS

Interferon Versus Cancer–A Ray of Hope?

The battle against cancer has been one of modern medicine's most frustrating challenges. Many treatments have been tried, and though some have worked some of the time, the disease has eluded conquest. As a result, people are disinclined to believe reports of new drugs or therapies that supposedly can cure cancer. One area of very recent research, however, does seem to offer a faint ray of hope.

In 1957, a team of medical researchers in England discovered a protein called interferon, which is produced naturally by body cells to fight viruses. Subsequent research showed that *interferon* slows down the rapid division of tumor cells and performs a role in the body's immunological defense system. It is rare and difficult to isolate, however, and only lately have studies to determine its effects on human cancer become feasible on a significant scale.

Research on interferon with other animals has been promising. In one study, for example, mouse interferon inhibited the growth of highly malignant tumors in living mice. (Interferon seems to protect only members of the same animal species that produced it.) Other experiments with animals have also had positive results.

Early work on the effects of interferon on human cancer has also been encouraging, although the number of patients involved in these studies has been too small to provide definitely convincing results. Interferon therapy was first tested on human beings in Stockholm, Sweden, in 1974. Twenty-one patients with osteogenic sarcoma, a rare but deadly bone cancer that usually affects young people between the ages of ten and twenty-five, were given injections of interferon for eighteen months after an operation to remove the primary tumor. These patients showed approximately twice as many cases with metastasis-free, long-term survival than did control patients.

Interferon has also been found to shrink tumors in studies in Houston, Texas, and at Stanford University in California. In the Stanford study, conducted by Dr. Thomas C. Merigan, prolonged use of interferon caused shrinkage of tumors in three patients with lymphoma, a cancer of the lymphatic system. However, the substance had no beneficial effect on three patients who had the disease in its rapidly progressing later stages. These patients had previously undergone other treatments, such as radiation therapy, and had used anticancer drugs. Merigan suspects that the tendency of these treatments to suppress the body's natural immunological defenses may have contributed to interferon's failure in these cases.

Since interferon is naturally manufactured by the human body, it may be effective against cancer longer than other anticancer drugs before serious toxic side effects appear. This does not mean, however, that the substance is harmless. And again, it must be stressed that, in spite of the promise interferon now holds out, we must await the results of more extensive clinical studies before we learn whether it really is a cure for cancer or just another red herring.

Lastly, there has been some success in the development of a blood test to detect the presence of cancer in its earliest stages. Work is continuing to perfect such a test and to refine it to a point where it will disclose precisely where the cancer is located and/or what type of malignancy it is.

SUMMARY

1. The overall incidence of cancer has increased steadily over the years, but so has the possibility of cure or prolonged life for those who suffer from certain types of cancer. Early diagnosis, preventive measures (such as not smoking cigarettes), and medical treatment have greatly reduced the fatality rate for cancer.

2. Cancer is a condition of abnormal cellular growth. A tumor is a swelling or mass that is formed when cells that normally function usefully together multiply independently, taking nourishment from surrounding normal cells. Only malignant tumors, those that

spread their damaging effects to other parts of the body, are considered cancers. The process by which the malignant tumors spread is called metastatic growth.

3. As in most diseases, the cause of cancer appears to result from an interaction between many hereditary, environmental, and psychological factors.

4. Cultural differences in the incidence of certain cancer types and family patterns of the disease point to both environmental and hereditary contributions. However, the relative importance of environmental and genetic factors is often hard to differentiate.

5. Other factors, which are more under one's control, such as diet, drug and tobacco use, exposure to chemicals, pollution, and radiation, also have a profound effect on cancer incidence.

6. Some scientists believe that some forms of cancer are linked to viruses. Others believe that innate cancer-causing genes (known as oncogenes), normally repressed by immunological defenses, become active when these defenses malfunction, causing malignant tumors. These theories may not be mutually exclusive and together may explain the cancer process.

7. While the risk of cancer can never be eliminated, certain precautions can be taken. Refraining from smoking cigarettes, avoiding excessive consumption of alcohol, fats, and high-cholesterol foods will greatly reduce one's risk of certain types of cancer. Avoiding unnecessary exposure to X-rays, sunrays, environmental carcinogens, and drugs will also be helpful. Good hygiene and regular medical checkups are also important preventive measures.

8. The three forms of cancer treatment on which most physicians rely, either separately or concurrently, are: radiation, surgery, and chemotherapy.

9. Because cancer victims are fearful and distraught, many try ineffective and expensive quack cancer treatments, such as laetrile. Unfortunately, this may prevent them from getting beneficial medical care which could prolong their life.

10. Cancer research continues and many hopeful discoveries have been made. Natural virus-inhibiting substances and drugs and vitamins which stop cancer growth are now being tested. Progress is also being made in the area of early cancer detection.

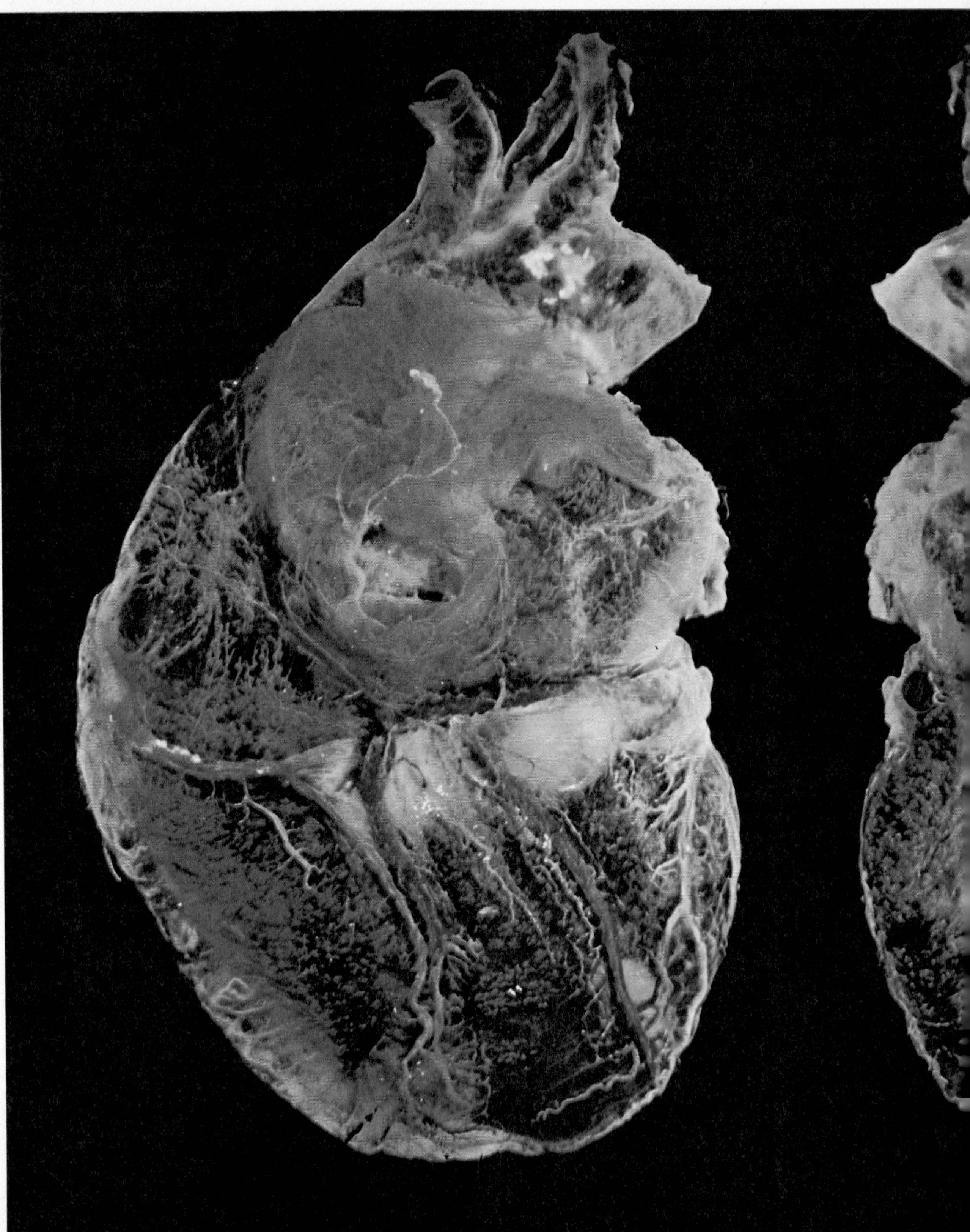

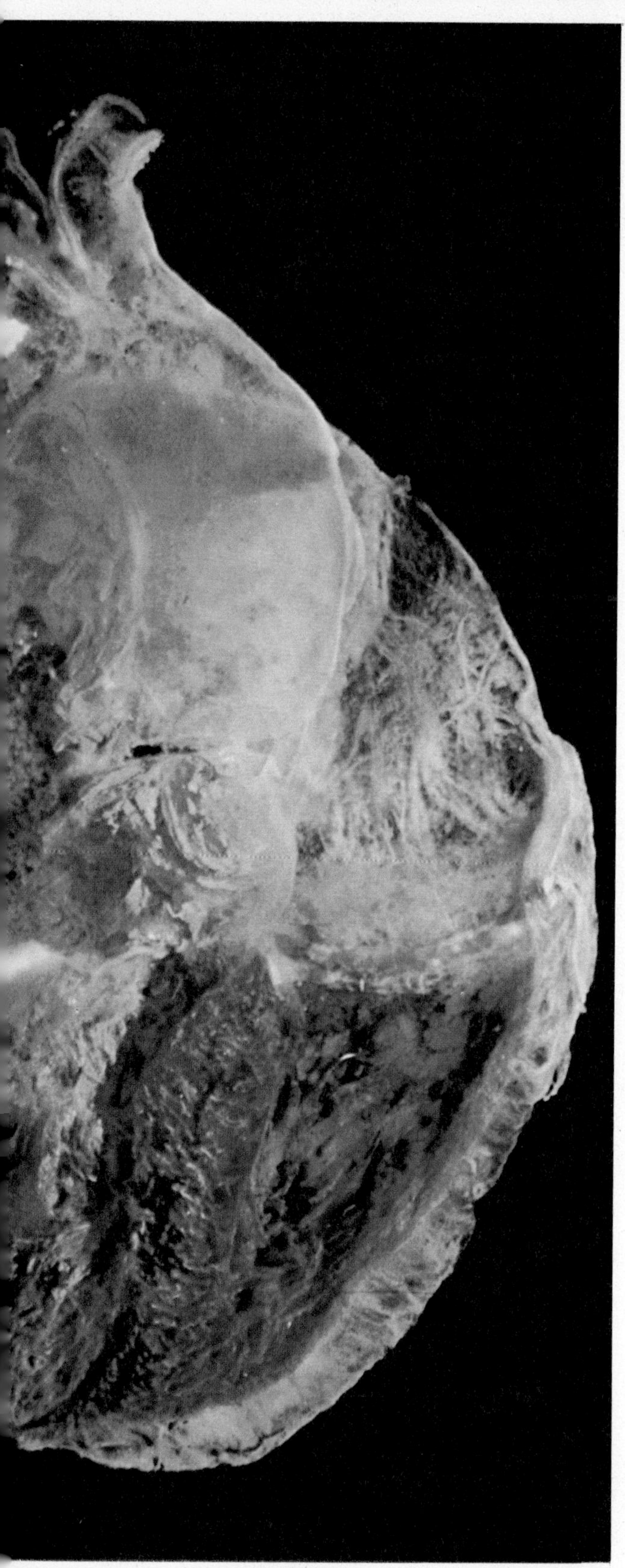

16 Cardiovascular Disease

Modern industrial advances have brought vast changes to both Western and non-Western societies. Peoples of the West have prospered in terms of physical wealth and longer life spans. But economic and technological development has also introduced problems that were of little importance in earlier centuries. Among these are the so-called chronic and degenerative diseases—conditions that can affect entire systems of the body but to date have been most frequently associated with the cardiovascular system.

Cardiovascular disease encompasses a number of disorders involving the heart ("cardio") and the blood vessels ("vascular"). Included are such conditions as atherosclerosis, high blood pressure, rheumatic heart disease, and congenital heart disease—any of which, either alone or in combination with other factors, may lead to heart attack or stroke. Considering the central role of the circulatory system in the body, it is little wonder that impairment of its function will profoundly affect other body systems. And conversely, malfunction of other systems will markedly influence cardiovascular performance and health.

In Western countries, cardiovascular disease is the most drastic killer of modern times. In 1976, this group of diseases was responsible for just over half of all deaths in the United States. Cardiovascular disease and cancer together take the lives of almost three out of four Americans who die each year.

Coronary artery disease is a leading cause of death among American men beyond the age of thirty-five and American women past forty.

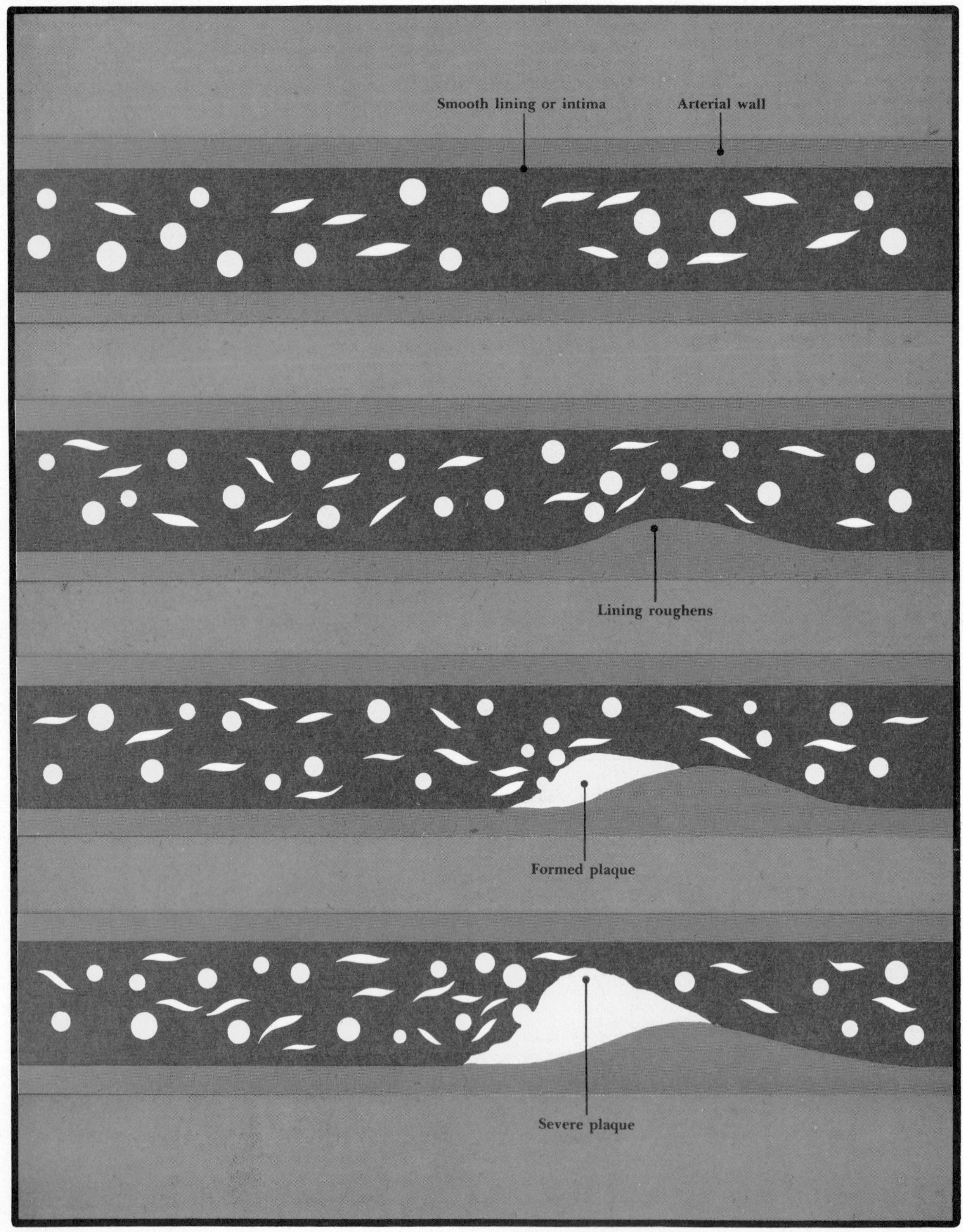
Smooth lining or intima
Arterial wall
Lining roughens
Formed plaque
Severe plaque

These figures dispel two common misconceptions: first, that women rarely have heart attacks, and second, that heart attacks occur only in the elderly. It is true that in each age group women are less likely to have heart attacks than men; nevertheless, heart attacks are still a major cause of death among women in most age groups.

Although these figures are depressing, it is important to note that in the United States, there is a glimmer of hope. The 1970s revealed a slight but gradual decline in heart disease mortality, especially from strokes, after half a century of steady rise. This trend reflects a multitude of advances in diagnosis and treatment, new medications, and improved surgical techniques. Perhaps even more importantly, life-style modification has begun to demonstrate its very real influence in preventing heart attack and stroke among susceptible persons.

The various risk factors associated with cardiovascular disorders—and what each individual can do to reduce them—will be presented. First, however, the many forms of cardiovascular disease will be discussed.

ATHEROSCLEROSIS

Atherosclerosis is the narrowing or thickening of arterial blood vessels through buildup of fatty deposits known as plaque. In the United States and other industrialized nations, atherosclerosis probably begins in most victims before the age of twenty.

Heart attacks, which alone claim more than 600,000 lives in the United States each year, are a complication of *coronary* atherosclerosis—fatty thickening of the inner lining of the coronary arteries that carry the blood supply for heart tissue. During a heart attack, without sufficient blood, part of the heart muscle dies and the remainder may falter in its regular rhythm, beat so irregularly that it is useless, or stop working entirely.

The flow of blood to the heart muscle can easily be halted by a small clot caught in an already narrowed atherosclerotic coronary artery. The result is often a heart attack. A similar clot in the brain can cause a stroke.

Figure 16.1 The mechanism of atherosclerosis. Atherosclerosis may develop when (a) normally smooth intima (the innermost lining of the artery) (b) becomes irregular and attracts fibrin. (c) This fibrin matrix then collects fat particles and other debris, thus producing plaque. (d) Later in this degenerative condition, calcium is deposited and the plaque hardens.

HEART ATTACKS

A heart attack can happen to anyone. Those who have seriously attempted to reduce the risk are less likely to suffer an attack, but they are not immune. Everyone, therefore, should be aware of what happens during a heart attack and how it should be treated.

The symptoms of a heart attack are sometimes mistaken by the patient for something else (frequently indigestion). By and large, they consist of a constricting, squeezing, or crushing pain in the middle of the chest. The pain may radiate down the left arm or to the neck, shoulders, or jaw. The victim becomes pale, sweats profusely, grows short of breath, and may vomit. The symptoms, however, may vary greatly from patient to patient. A heart attack may also be so mild as to go unrecognized. These "silent" heart attacks may be revealed only later when the electrical activity of the heart is studied with an electrocardiograph—or at autopsy.

Angina Pectoris

The symptoms a patient feels during a heart attack are the expression of damage to the heart muscle when the coronary blood flow becomes reduced by a narrowing of its vessels. Pain, pressure, or tightness in the front of the chest may be a sign that the heart is not getting enough oxygen. A person who regularly has such pain following exertion, excitement, or eating may have *angina pectoris.* Angina is not really a disease but is a symptom of oxygen deprivation to the heart muscle.

Angina pains are usually caused by coronary atherosclerosis. The reduced blood flow through the narrowed arteries carries sufficient oxygen for normal, but not for over-

Table 16.1 Warning Signs of Heart Attack and Stroke

Heart Attack	Stroke
Prolonged, oppressive pain or unusual discomfort in *center* of chest	Sudden, temporary weakness or numbness of face, arm, or leg
Pain may radiate to shoulder, arm, neck, or jaw	Temporary loss of speech, or trouble in speaking or understanding speech
Sweating may accompany pain or discomfort	Temporary dimness or loss of vision, particularly in one eye
Nausea, vomiting, and shortness of breath may also occur	An episode of double vision
	Unexplained dizziness or unsteadiness
	Change in personality, mental ability, or pattern of headaches

Source: From Daniel M. Wilner, et al., *Introduction to Public Health* (New York: Macmillan, 1978), p. 397.

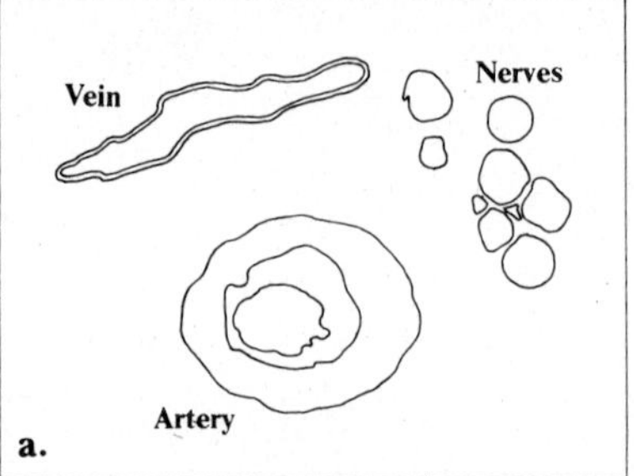

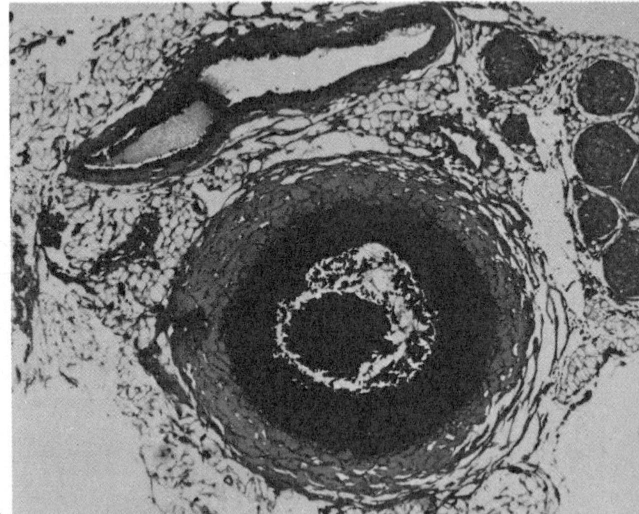

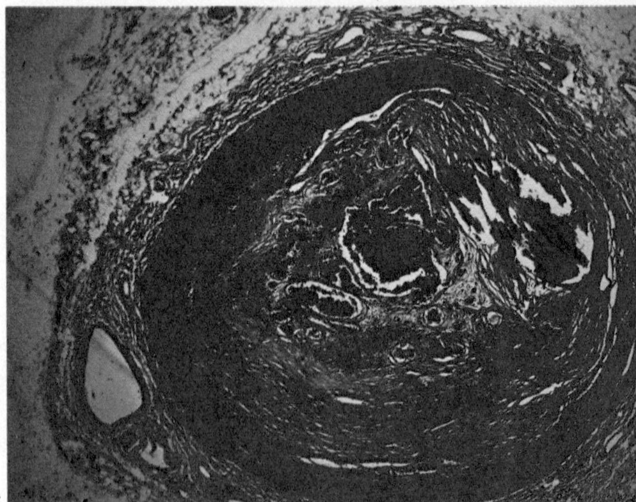

Figure 16.2 (a) Illustrative cross section of a normal artery. (b) Photographic cross section of normal artery. (c) Atherosclerotic artery.

loaded, heart activity. An increased demand on the heart will reveal this deficiency and trigger the angina attack. Pains may occur in persons who have recovered from a heart attack or in those who have never had—and never will have—an attack.

The outlook for persons with angina pectoris varies greatly. They may have to restrict their activity to avoid pain, or they may hardly be aware of the problem. In any case, many people are able to live normally for many years. The use of a nitroglycerin tablet under the tongue gives prompt relief. The drug propranolol is also used with considerable success. Certain surgical techniques are helpful in some cases.

Myocardial Infarction (Heart Attack)

The narrowing of coronary arteries is sometimes associated with the formation of a blood clot, or *thrombus,* which may precede or follow a heart attack. A heart attack is therefore sometimes called a *coronary thrombosis.* Coronary spasm, or temporary contraction of the blood vessel, may also occur. If the damage is serious enough, the part of the heart muscle that has been denied its blood supply may die. The dead area is called an *infarct;* a heart attack is thus termed a *myocardial* (muscle of the heart) *infarction.* When part of the muscle dies, scar tissue forms. Scar tissue does not contract, but if the scar is not too large, the heart may continue to function and the patient may recover. One of the reasons patients are required to rest for some time after a heart attack is to reduce the work load on the heart so that the wound can heal.

Faltering Heartbeat

A heart attack not only damages the muscle physically; it may also drastically alter the rhythm of the heartbeat. The heart is a mechanical pump with its own electrical system. The rate at which the heart beats (normally between sixty and ninety-five times a minute, depending on heart size and cardiovascular fitness) is regulated by a tiny area of specialized tissue known as the *pacemaker.* It sends a current of electricity over the heart. First, the upper two chambers (the right and left atria) contract. After a very slight pause, the lower chambers (the right and left ventricles) follow suit.

Sometimes a heart attack may produce little damage to the heart muscle but still cause the ventricles to go out of control. They beat hundreds of times a minute, so rapidly that the heart is incapable of pumping blood. Unless such *fibrillation* (See Figure 16.3) can be stopped and normal circulation restored, the patient will die. One of the major reasons for getting a heart-attack victim to a hospital as soon as possible is so that ventricular fibrillation can be immediately recognized and treated with special equipment. Carefully controlled electric shock is usually required to stop the fibrillation, and the heart may have to be stimulated electrically before it beats normally. Many heart-attack victims succumb to ventricular fibrillation even though their heart muscle is not permanently damaged.

Figure 16.3 *(Top)* An electrocardiogram (ECG or EKG) exhibiting the regular waves of a normal heartbeat compared with one showing the wild, irregular rhythm of a heart muscle during fibrillation *(Bottom).*

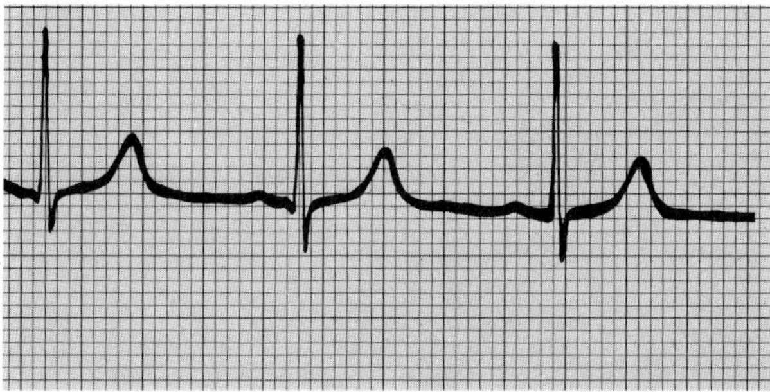

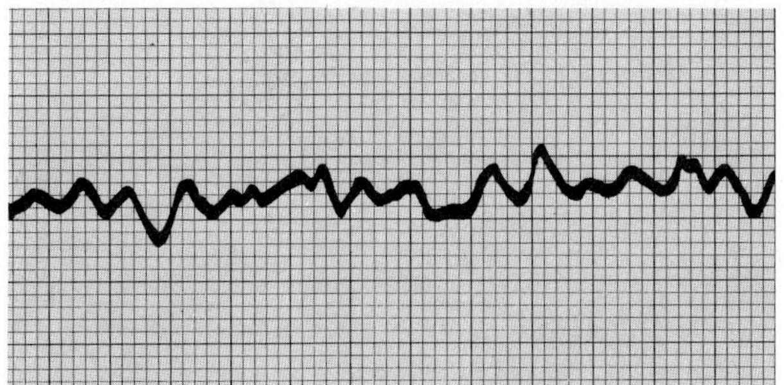

Heart Block

Sometimes a heart-attack victim who seems to be recovering will experience a sudden slowing of the heartbeat. It may also occur for reasons other than a heart attack and usually affects patients in their sixties or older.

Heart block results from failure of the electrical connection between the atria and the ventricles. Impulses do not reach the main pumping chambers often enough. The normal rate can be restored with an electronic pacemaker. Usually the heart can repair itself within a few days, and the natural rhythm returns. When it fails to do so, an artificial pacemaker can be implanted and can take over the job for many years.

Cardiac Arrest and Emergency Treatment

Anytime the heart stops beating, the condition is called *cardiac arrest.* The heart may stop because of a heart attack or for many other reasons—drowning, electrocution, or strangulation, for example. Immediate action is

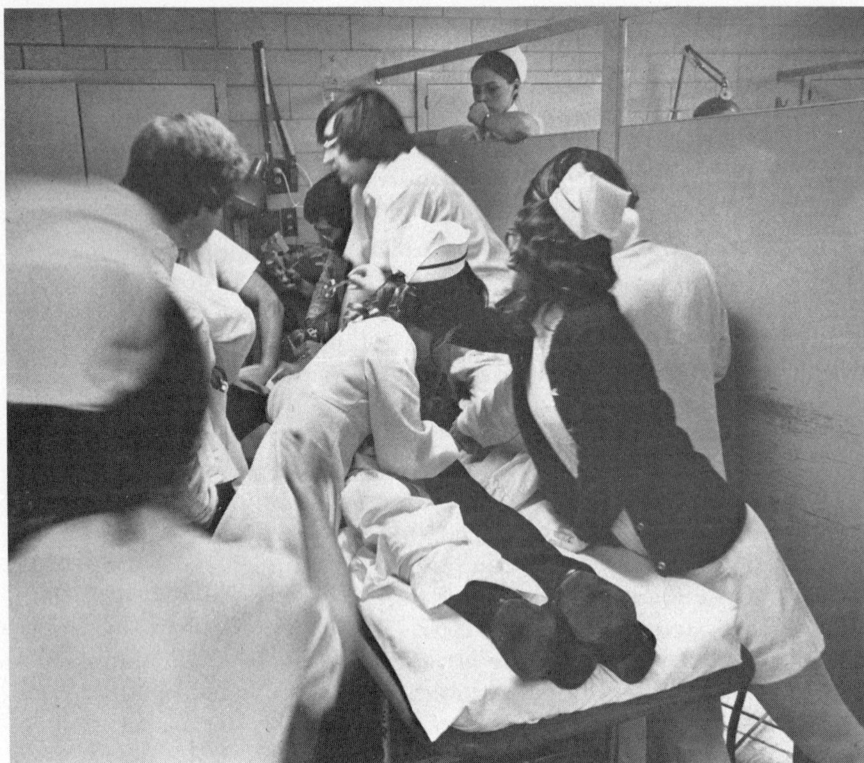

Figure 16.4 A medical team giving cardiac massage and oxygen ventilation to a man in cardiac arrest. Immediate medical attention increases chances of survival and lessens the risk of brain damage due to lack of oxygen to the brain.

necessary or the patient may die, for the brain can survive without damage for only about four minutes after circulation is stopped.

In the absence of immediate medical attention, *cardiopulmonary resuscitation (CPR)*—external cardiac massage and resuscitation that includes ventilating the lungs—can save the patient. Cardiac massage squeezes blood out of the heart and forces it into the arteries and thus to the tissues. Mouth-to-mouth breathing forces the victim's lungs to continue supplying the needed oxygen to the body. These techniques should be known by all adults, but should *not* be performed without proper training. (See Chapter 18 for an elaboration of mouth-to-mouth resuscitation.)

Postcardiac Rehabilitation

Many people survive heart attacks and live for many years afterward. To maximize chances for recovery and prevent future attacks, it is imperative that the victim heed the risk factors indicated later in this chapter. Particularly, careful attention must be given to diet; cigarette smoking must be eliminated. Situations of stress should be kept to a minimum. Most heart patients can benefit from a moderate exercise program under the direction of a physician. Any medication should be taken exactly as prescribed, and regular medical examinations—again, according to doctor's instructions—are a must.

Following these common-sense rules for good heart health will greatly increase one's chances of enjoying a longer, fuller life.

OTHER HEART PROBLEMS

Heart Failure

Heart attack is but one example of a condition that might lead to congestive heart failure. The term *congestive heart failure* does not refer to a heart that has stopped but to a heart that cannot pump enough blood to meet all the demands put on it. Almost every known type of heart disease may produce congestive heart failure. Sometimes it can be triggered by high blood pressure, which forces the heart to work extra hard to deliver sufficient blood to the body's organs and tissues. At other times it can be caused by defective heart valves, a damaged heart muscle, or weakening of the entire heart by disease or poison. The patient with congestive heart failure may be short of breath, have swelling of the ankles, or exhibit certain abnormal physical signs or shadows in chest X-rays.

Some of these defects can be alleviated by surgical procedures or medical treatment. When the underlying disease cannot be remedied, the physician can improve the action of the heart by administering digitalis or a similar drug that strengthens the heart's contractions. Excess water can be removed by administration of certain drugs and restriction of dietary salt intake. A promising new therapy for severe heart failure—termed "unloading" —uses drugs that decrease vascular tone, thus lowering the resistance to pumping blood out of the heart and increasing cardiac output.

Congenital Heart Disease

Congenital defects can affect all structures of the heart or its emerging vessels. They may occur in combination as well as singly. *Septal* defects are small holes in the walls separating the left and right chambers of the heart. One of the most common congenital defects is a hole in the atrial septum or the ventricular septum. For a period of time, at least, these defects appear to have little effect on the circulation; but overall efficiency of the heart is reduced. Some of the blood flows back from the left to the right chamber; some may also flow directly from the right to the left chamber, diluting the oxygen-rich blood coming from the lungs with deoxygenated blood from the veins.

Much more serious are defects involving an obstruction or narrowing of the valve between the right ventricle and the pulmonary artery, known as *pulmonary stenosis.* Often it is coupled with septal defects, the most common combination being the *tetralogy of Fallot,* which includes four distinct defects: a ventricular septal defect, pulmonary stenosis, a consequent thickening of the right ventricle, and a shifted position of the aorta (the main artery leading away from the heart). The seriousness of these defects derives from the fact that a considerable portion of the blood is prevented from entering the pulmonary artery. Instead it is diverted directly into the left ventricle and pumped out to the body without having had a chance to become oxygenated. This poorly oxygenated blood mixture reaching the tissues gives a baby (particularly at the lips and fingertips) a dusky, bluish color instead of its normal pinkishness. Such a child is commonly called a "blue baby." The degree of *cyanosis,* or bluish color, depends on the severity of the heart defects.

New techniques of diagnosis and surgical therapy are saving many individuals with congenital heart defects from early death or a lifetime spent as an invalid. Sophisticated X-ray methods and techniques for sampling pressures within the heart now enable physicians to identify defects precisely and to determine whether they can be corrected. Open-heart surgery—made possible by the development of the heart-lung machine, which takes over the functions of these two organs—can be used to correct many defects so that affected persons can lead normal lives.

Rheumatic Heart Disease

Rheumatic fever is an inflammatory disease of connective tissues that may occasionally follow a streptococcal infection, usually of the throat. Rheumatic heart disease accounts for much of the heart disease found in young children and adults. Approximately one-third of all rheumatic fever victims are left with heart damage, particularly of the valves.

Rheumatic fever is usually regarded as a disease of childhood, mostly affecting children between the ages of five and fifteen, although it does occur in older people as well. It has a great tendency to recur, however, and thus becomes a chronic ailment affecting all ages. Rheumatic fever affects many parts of the body —joints and muscles in particular—but damage to the heart from scarring of heart muscle and valves is its greatest danger. Depending on the extent of the scarring, rheumatic heart disease will interfere with the normal functioning of the heart, which will then be forced to do more work in supplying the body's needs. An attack of rheumatic fever does not necessarily mean that one is left with a damaged heart. Nevertheless, with each recurrence of the disease there is an increased chance of damage to the heart.

Rheumatic heart disease is virtually 100 percent preventable. Penicillin can cure streptococcal infections, and early treatment of the infection with antibiotics totally prevents heart damage. It is therefore extremely important to consult a physician if one develops a sudden severe sore throat (which may be "strep throat" or tonsillitis), ear infection, or is known to have been exposed to a strep infection of any type. Patients who have had rheumatic fever once are given penicillin (or another appropriate antibiotic) for several years to prevent recurrence of the disease. Surgical operations are used to correct or remove already damaged valves.

HIGH BLOOD PRESSURE

When the powerful left ventricle pumps blood into the body, it produces a pulse and blood pressure. When the heart relaxes in preparation for the next contraction, the pressure drops somewhat. These two pressures are determined by a blood-pressure cuff placed around an arm. They are the *systolic pressure,* produced when the heart contracts, and the *diastolic pressure,* which remains after the heart dilates and its muscle relaxes. Young adults have a normal systolic pressure of between 100 and 120, older adults from 120 to 140. Diastolic pressure is usually below 90 in a healthy individual. Thus, a good average blood pressure for a college student might be 120/80.

The systolic pressure represents a marked increase in the arteries with each heartbeat, but healthy arteries are elastic and expand to accommodate the load. Blood-pressure readings normally vary from time to time. They may increase during excitement, decrease during rest. High blood pressure, known medically as

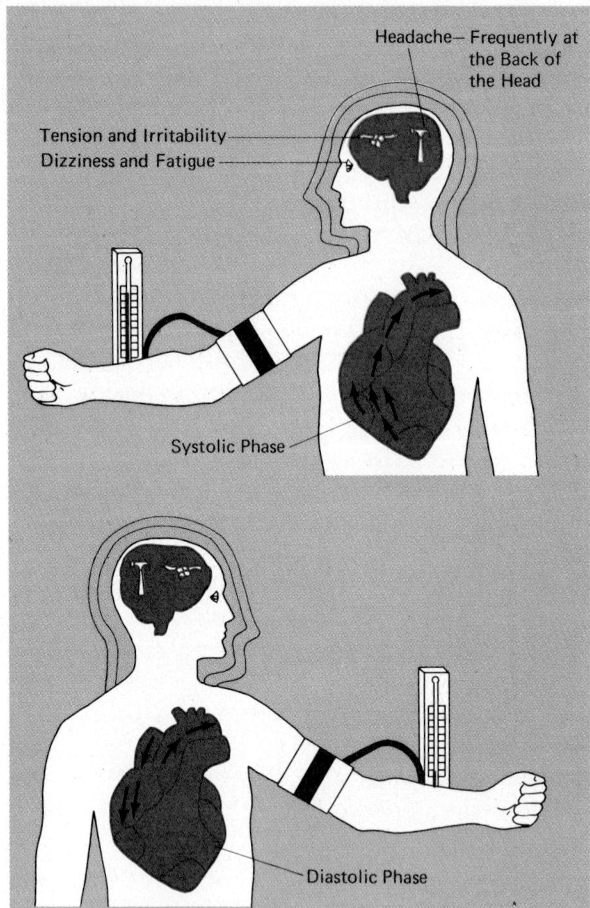

Figure 16.5 High blood pressure. The heart exerts its greatest pressure when pumping in a fresh supply of blood (systolic phase, *top*) and the least pressure when pausing between beats to fill with blood (diastolic phase, *bottom*). The blood pressure is the measurement of pressure on the arterial wall at the extreme points of the systolic and diastolic phases. High blood pressure usually causes no symptoms until complications occur.

hypertension, refers to a condition in which the blood pressure is always higher than it should be. Generally speaking, a continued blood pressure above 145/90 is considered abnormal for people of all ages.

Over 23 million people in the United States have hypertension in some form. One-half of them are not aware that they have it; one-quarter are receiving no treatment for it; and an additional one-eighth are receiving inadequate treatment. Thus, only one person in eight is receiving adequate hypertension therapy.

While hypertension is rarely found in persons under twenty years of age, systolic blood pressure tends to increase with advancing years. By age fifty, approximately one-half of the population has the disorder to some degree, although many are free of symptoms and learn of their problem only during a routine physical checkup. Until the age of about fifty to fifty-five, women are far less likely than men to have high blood pressure. Nonwhites are two to five times more likely to be affected than are whites.

Perhaps one of the greatest difficulties in treatment of hypertension is the lack of awareness that even moderately elevated levels must be controlled. Too often, the lack of discomfort lulls its victims into thinking that the condition can be safely ignored. But the danger is very real. Persons with high blood pressure have ten times the risk of stroke of normal individuals. High blood pressure is the leading cause of congestive heart failure, a condition in which the heart enlarges, loses its strength, and can no longer pump blood effectively. In addition, hypertension speeds up the accumulation of cholesterol and other fatty materials in the inner walls of the arteries. This condition, known as atherosclerosis, can produce a lessening of or complete interruption in the blood supply to a certain portion of the heart muscle. Additionally, risk is greatly increased for possible congestive heart failure and kidney complications. With proper treatment to control blood-pressure levels, studies have shown that the risk of all three disorders can be cut by two-thirds.

By far the most common form of hypertension is *essential hypertension.* About 90 percent of persons with hypertension fall into this category, and it is present in about 10 percent of the population (about 20 million Americans). Today it is known that essential hypertension is caused by the sustained constriction of the smallest arteries all over the body, decreasing the amount of blood carried by the vessels.

Since hypertension rarely causes symptoms, it is necessary for individuals to have their blood pressure recorded by a physician, nurse, or some other trained person. Modern drugs are very useful in controlling the condition.

STROKES

Strokes occur because of hemorrhage, clots, or some other blood-vessel obstruction *(occlusion)* in the brain, causing the destruction of a significant amount of brain tissue. Also known as *cerebrovascular accidents,* they are the third leading cause of death in the United States. In addition, about two-fifths of persons over age fifty have severe atherosclerosis of vessels in or serving the brain. This means that one or more arteries are narrowed by at least 50 percent.

Medical terms used for various kinds of strokes are *cerebral hemorrhage, cerebral thrombosis,* and *cerebral embolism.* An *embolus* is a mass of abnormal material carried by the bloodstream to clog a blood vessel. Often the material is a fragment of a clot (thrombus) or an atherosclerotic thickening (plaque) broken away from its original location. A diseased heart may be a cause of cerebral embolism in a brain having quite normal arteries.

Cerebral hemorrhage, or uncontrolled bleeding, is generally caused by the bursting of a diseased artery in the brain. Nearby cells, no longer fed by the artery, are deprived of oxygen and begin to die. Frequently such hemorrhage is due to bursting of an *aneurysm,* a blood-filled pocket that bulges out from a weak spot in an arterial wall.

But in many strokes, as in many heart attacks, the underlying disease begins developing long before the critical, crippling event occurs. A stroke may have been "incubating" for thirty or forty years before symptoms appear. Preventing atherosclerosis, or treating diseases such as hypertension that may lead to strokes, can greatly reduce the mortality rate from these attacks. The presence of two or more such factors enormously increases the risk of stroke.

When some of the nerve cells in the brain are deprived of their blood supply by a stroke, the parts of the body controlled by these nerve centers can no longer function normally. As a result, a stroke patient may be partly paralyzed, may suffer some loss of memory—especially short-term memory—or may exhibit general confusion. Often there are difficulties in comprehension and the ability to speak coherently,

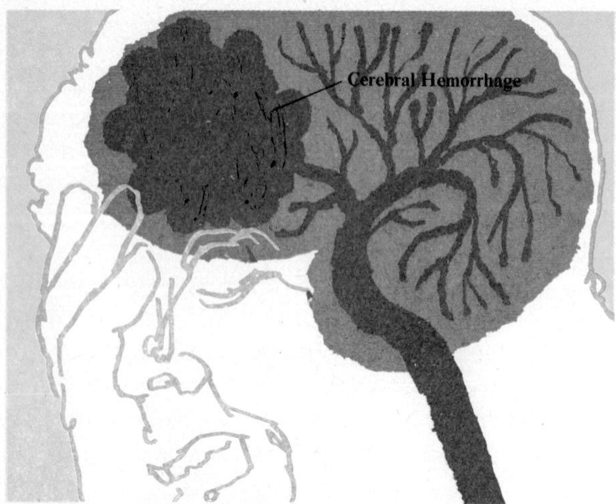

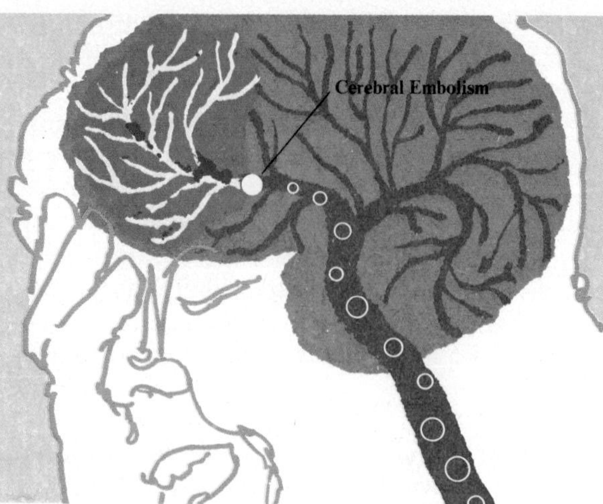

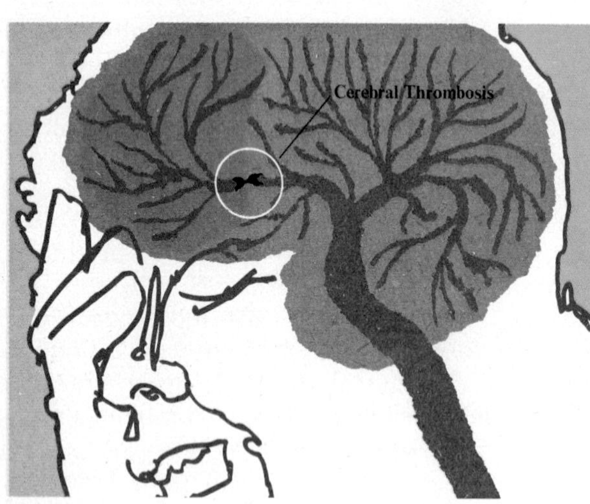

Figure 16.6 Three types of strokes. *(Top left)* Cerebral hemorrhage, in which blood flow to the brain is impaired due to rupture of a diseased cerebral blood vessel. *(Top right)* Cerebral embolism, in which a mass of abnormal material clogs a blood vessel. *(Bottom left)* Cerebral thrombosis, in which a blood clot forms in a cerebral blood vessel. In all cases, oxygen transport to parts of the brain is impaired, resulting in the death of some brain tissue.

known as *aphasia. Emotional lability*—sudden and extreme mood fluctuations or inappropriate emotional reactions—is fairly common. The amount and location of damage to the brain will determine the extent and types of involvement.

Transient Ischemic Attacks

A temporary attack with symptoms similar to stroke is known as a *transient ischemic attack* (TIA). Such an attack may last anywhere from a few minutes to twenty-four hours. It serves as a warning signal for possible impending stroke, since at least 40 percent of the victims later suffer a major attack. (The figure may actually be much higher since many TIAs go unrecognized by their victims.)

Symptoms that indicate TIA include any unexplained numbness, tingling, unusual weakness, or paralysis of any part of the body; difficulty in swallowing, speaking, phrasing sentences, or thinking clearly; sudden dizziness, fainting, altered vision, or severe headaches. Any such symptoms indicate a need for immediate medical testing. Prompt treatment of causative conditions (such as hypertension or disease in the carotid arteries of the head, which carry blood to the brain) may prevent a future stroke.

Treatment

Some patients recover quickly and can resume normal activity; others may never recover completely. Partial recovery takes a long time if serious damage has occurred. If the stroke is induced by a blood clot or a narrowed blood vessel, anticoagulants are sometimes prescribed. Occasionally surgery is useful. Often an extensive period of retraining is required.

When one stroke, even a transient one, has occurred, the chances of a second stroke are increased tenfold. Newest in prevention of second attacks among stroke victims is the use of simple aspirin. An extensive Canadian study has shown a 50 percent reduction in death and disability among men with normal blood pressure. Apparently aspirin has just enough anticoagulant ability to slightly, but effectively, alter the clotting of blood platelets, thus making it safer to use than stronger preparations (such as heparin), which are often difficult to adjust to optimal dosage. As few as two aspirin per day may be useful in preventing TIAs among susceptible persons. Testing is also underway to discover whether aspirin can also ward off second heart attacks as well.

As of this writing, it is still too soon for scientists to ascertain the precise cause-effect relationship here. Aspirin therapy of this type should never be undertaken without the advice of a physician. In any case, unless other risk factors (hypertension, obesity, cigarette smoking, for example) are controlled, the use of aspirin is likely to have little preventive effect.

On the whole, rest, good nursing care, and encouragement of earliest possible activity are the major forms of initial treatment. Proper exercise and other forms of therapy can do much to help the patient recover speech and the use of muscles.

RISK FACTORS

The incidence of heart attacks and strokes may be increased by a number of risk factors to which the potential victims have been exposed. Specialists do not always agree which of the many factors involved in the disease are most important, but they have identified several. Fat content, particularly saturated fat, in the diet is one, along with obesity, excessive eating, and lack of exercise. Cigarette smoking and high blood pressure contribute seriously to the likelihood of a heart attack. Hereditary factors and diabetes have been implicated. Psychological stress may also play a role. The reduction of risk factors, in the opinion of most physicians, could considerably decrease the number of heart attacks. The emphasis here, of course, should be on preventable risks—cigarette smoking, a fully voluntary risk, and high blood pressure, which is at least in part voluntary because it can be effectively controlled if diagnosed early.

Cigarette Smoking

Persons who smoke one pack of cigarettes a day are twice as likely to have heart attacks as nonsmokers. Those who smoke more heavily are more prone to atherosclerosis. The preventive value of not smoking has been clearly demonstrated. Three years after a smoker has given up cigarettes entirely, the risk of having a heart attack can drop back to that of a nonsmoker. The role of smoking in heart disease is also discussed in Chapter 13.

Diet

Many specialists regard diet as the single most important factor in atherosclerosis. Many aspects of the diet are involved. Scientists know that one of the major constituents of atherosclerotic fatty deposits is cholesterol. Whether cholesterol actually *causes* narrowing and hardening of the arteries is questionable, but it may be an accomplice in the crime.

During the past few years, much has been written about the ill effects on the heart of dietary cholesterol and saturated fats (fats from which the body synthesizes its own cholesterol). But careful analyses of these studies reveal little, if any, correlation. While disease of the coronary arteries occurs more frequently among individuals with high cholesterol levels, there is no indication that the elevated levels are due to *dietary* intake. Additionally, some individuals with extraordinarily high cholesterol levels never show any signs of coronary heart disease.

More recent studies indicate a relationship between heart disease and *lipoproteins*—substances containing both fat and protein which transport fat molecules, including cholesterol. The heaviest of these is known as *high-density lipoprotein* or *HDL. Low-density lipoprotein (LDL)* is lighter because it contains less protein and is the medium by which most cholesterol is transported through the body. Greater concentrations of HDL than LDL appear to offer protection from heart disease, although the reasons are not yet clearly understood.

As persons reach adulthood, their concentrations of HDL are lowered and those of LDL proportionately raised, thus theoretically accounting for the greater risk of heart disease as age increases.

The significance of this for the healthy individual is still unclear. Therapy by means of HDL injection is not yet a reality. Concerning diet regulation, until further investigation suggests otherwise, there is probably no need for the average person to avoid moderate amounts of either fats or cholesterol.

Another diet-related risk factor is *obesity.* However, there is little indication that obesity itself is a cause of heart disease. More likely it is the interrelationship between obesity, hypertension, blood fat levels, and possibly diabetes that significantly contributes to increased risk of heart disease and atherosclerosis. The middle-aged, overweight person is two to three times more susceptible to coronary heart disease than a similar person of normal weight.

Similarly, *diabetes* is not considered a cause of cardiovascular disorders. However, heart disease is significantly more common among diabetics and tends to appear at an earlier age than in nondiabetics.

Exercise

People who are physically active seem to be less prone to heart attacks and tolerate them better than those who lead sedentary lives, as has been suggested many times in studies comparing active and less active workers, often in the same occupational field. The sort of physical activity involved is also important; cardiorespiratory endurance training of the sort described in Chapter 10 may provide some protection.

Research is now underway to determine what value exercise may have in preventing heart attacks. It is known that certain forms of strenuous exercise, such as running, cycling, and swimming, lead to the development of extensive *collateral circulation*—that is, growth of additional coronary blood vessels. The value here is that a possible blocked coronary artery can be immediately bypassed and circulation continued by way of the additional collateral arteries. Death and disability from heart attack are virtually unheard of under such circumstances.

Running or other strenuous sports do not suit or appeal to everyone. Nevertheless, there are enough data to justify recommending controlled, regular exercise as a general health measure for all.

Stress

As with other studies involving the relationship of stress and disease, no actual proof exists that stress in itself helps to cause heart disease. However, extensive research to determine a possible association has divided all persons into high-risk "Type A" individuals or low-risk "Type B." Type A is characterized by a competitive, aggressive, impatient, fast-paced life style that is constantly under pressure. Type B is totally the opposite, showing personality traits of far greater complacence. Most persons, of course, are a combination of both types, but generally one set of traits is dominant. One extensive study showed that 90 percent of all patients below the age of sixty who were treated for heart attack were Type A.

Whatever the influence of stress on the possibility of heart attack, it is the *degree* of significance that must also be considered. It is highly unlikely that stress will prove to be as important a factor as smoking, diet, or hypertension.

The Pill

Oral contraceptives themselves do not cause heart disease. But knowledge of their safety and side effects was greatly clarified recently with the release of an international series of medical reports confirming a deadly, synergistic relationship of Pill use and cigarette smoking. Cigarette smoking has already been established as a causative factor in heart disease. What *synergistic* means in this case is that the

Situation	Joe (Type A)	Roscoe (Type B)
Oversleeps—awakes at 7:30 instead of 6:30	**Action:** Gulps coffee, skips breakfast, cuts himself shaving, tears button off shirt getting dressed. **Thoughts:** I can't be late again! The boss will be furious! I just know this is going to ruin my whole day. **Results:** Leaves home anxious, worried, and hungry.	**Action:** Phones office to let them know he will be late. Eats a good breakfast. **Thoughts:** No problem. I must have needed the extra sleep. **Results:** Leaves home calm and relaxed.
Stuck behind slow driver	**Action:** Flashes lights, honks, grits teeth, curses, bangs on dashboard with fist. Finally passes on blind curve and nearly collides with oncoming car. **Thoughts:** What an idiot! Slow drivers should be put in jail! No consideration of others!	**Action:** Uses time to do relaxation exercises and to listen to his favorite radio station. **Thoughts:** Here's a gift of time—how can I use it?
Staff meeting	**Action:** Sits in back, ignores speakers, and surreptitiously tries to work on monthly report. **Thoughts:** What a waste of time. Who *cares* what's going on in all those other departments? I have more than I can handle keeping up with my own work. **Results:** Misses important input relating to his department. Is later reprimanded by superior.	**Action:** Listens carefully, and participates actively. **Thoughts:** It's really good to hear my co-workers' points of view. I can do my work a lot more effectively if I understand the big picture of what we're all trying to do. **Results:** His supervisor compliments him on his suggestions.
Noon—behind on deskwork	**Action:** Skips lunch. Has coffee at desk. Spills coffee over important papers. **Thoughts:** That's the last straw! Now I'll have to have this whole report typed over. I'll have to stay and work late.	**Action:** Eats light lunch and goes for short walk in park. **Thoughts:** I'll be in better shape for a good afternoon with a little exercise and some time out of the office.
Evening	**Action:** Arrives home 9 P.M. Family resentful. Ends up sleeping on couch. Does not fall asleep until long into the morning. **Thoughts:** What a life! If only I could run away and start over! It's just not worth it. I'll never amount to anything. **Results:** Wakes up late again, feeling awful. Decides to call in sick.	**Action:** Arrives home at usual time. Quiet evening with family. To bed by 11 P.M., falls asleep easily. **Thoughts:** A good day! I felt really effective at work, and it was nice reading to the kids tonight. **Results:** Wakes up early, feeling good.

Figure 16.7 A day in the life of Type A (Joe) and Type B (Roscoe). People like Joe do not adapt well to stress and have been shown to be particularly prone to heart attacks.

Pill acts in some not yet understood way to increase the effects of cigarette smoking. Women who smoke moderately or heavily *and* use the Pill run significantly higher risks of heart disease (myocardial infarction) than do nonsmoking Pill users.

Factors Beyond Our Control

As with many chronic diseases, heredity tends to play a part in the risk of heart disease, particularly that which occurs in the younger years.

We have already established that heart disease is more common among men than women up to a certain age level, and that risk of heart attack increases with advancing years. None of these factors can be changed. Logically, therefore, the risk factors that *can* be controlled become more important than heredity, sex, and age.

Multiplying the Risks

Any one of the risk factors so far discussed adds significantly to the chances of a heart attack. But when several of them are combined, the danger is greatly multiplied—up to seven times with high cholesterol, multiplied by up to seven times more for high blood pressure, and multiplied by two for smoking a pack of cigarettes a day. When the risks are multiplied this way, one can see even more clearly the dire consequences of the life style of affluent societies.

There is no scientific proof that these are the only or even the most important factors involved in atherosclerotic heart disease. Only with controlled experiments with large numbers of human subjects over a period of many years can science hope to understand the causes of this disease. Until more is known, however, the principles of living outlined above represent the best current medical knowledge. Following these recommendations will not guarantee protection against heart disease, but it will substantially reduce the risks and will certainly be beneficial in general.

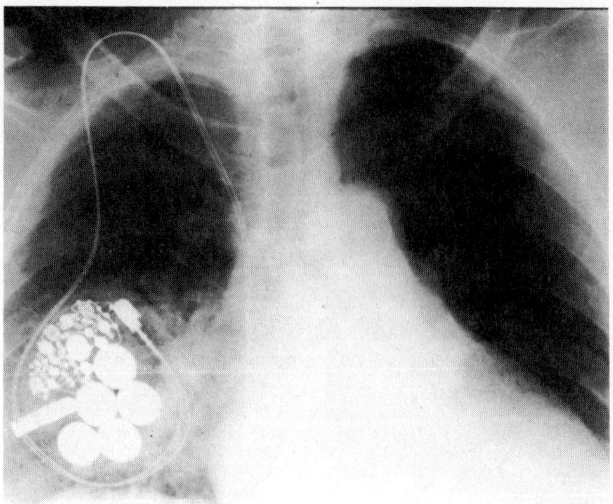

Figure 16.8 This X-ray shows an artificial pacemaker positioned in the chest. The pacemaker has proven to be highly successful in patients whose cardiac electrical system no longer delivers electrical impulses strong enough or regular enough to maintain the rhythmic contractions of the heart.

CARDIOVASCULAR SURGERY

The development of the artificial pacemaker was a breakthrough in the control of heart disease. It functions much the same as a natural pacemaker, transmitting electrical impulses over a specific pathway of the heart and causing it to pump at a steady pace. The device is operated by a battery, which must be replaced periodically—a procedure that can be performed only by additional surgery.

Vascular surgery has become increasingly important in the treatment of damaged arteries. In 1977, 70,000 coronary bypass operations were performed in the United States. The most common procedure is to use a tiny segment of the patient's own vein, one end of which is stitched to the healthy portion of the damaged artery and the other end to the aorta. Advanced detection techniques permit the surgeon to plan in advance exactly where to construct the bypass. The results of bypass surgery have thus far been encouraging—in the hands of an experienced surgeon the overall risks are small. However, in cases where the coronary arteries are extensively damaged and the heart muscle is weakened as a result, the risks of this type of surgery may be considerably greater.

Other types of vascular surgery include artery transplants, or replacement of damaged arteries with flexible synthetic tubing. Microvascular bypass surgery for stroke victims enables an artery from the scalp to be attached to another on the surface of the brain by means of an operating minimicroscope and microinstruments.

Apart from repair or replacement of blood vessels, still another technique for relieving clogged arteries is insertion into the vessel of a "roto-rooter" type device which simply cleans out the obstruction.

Congenital heart disease is gradually being

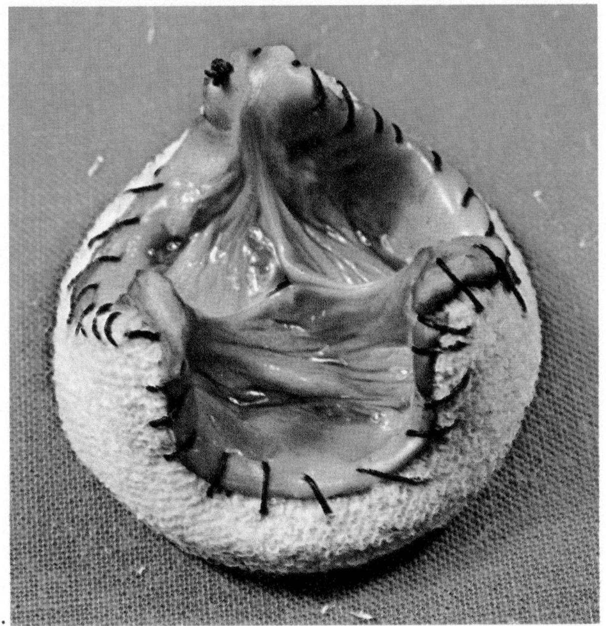

a.

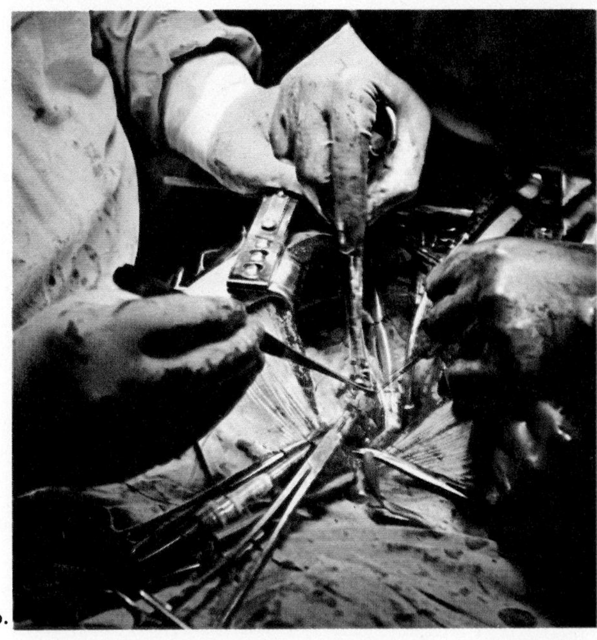

b.

Figure 16.9 Recent advances made in medical science have afforded normal lives to many heart patients. (a) A human heart valve taken from the heart of an accident victim has been sutured to a Teflon collar. This type of valve has been found to be the least damaging to the blood. When a human heart valve is not available, totally fabricated "ball-type" valves (which work like a ping-pong ball in a snorkel) are used. The metal that is used in this valve, unlike the human-Teflon valve, causes the blood to clot, and patients with ball-type valve replacements must be medicated with anticoagulant drugs. (b) The valve is sutured into place. The whitish tissue to the left of the instruments is the heart. The large plastic tube leads to a heart-lung (coronary bypass) machine.

reduced by new surgical techniques. One such procedure, known as a *transcatheter closure,* requires only thirty minutes to repair atrial-septal defects having holes up to the size of a quarter. A stainless steel umbrella-shaped device with mesh covering is anchored to the heart wall, which then becomes the framework for growth of new heart tissue. The procedure can save the lives of the estimated 10,000 babies who are born every year with this defect. Other forms of congenital heart defects that were previously impossible to correct surgically can now be repaired by means of a technique known as *cold-packing.* The baby's body is attached to a heart-lung machine, then cooled to 77°F and anesthetized. At that point, heartbeat and circulation stop, enabling successful surgery to be completed on the tiny heart and blood vessels.

Heart valve surgery is still another area of new surgical techniques. This includes the repair of existing valves or transplant operations utilizing either human or artificial valves.

The most dramatic form of heart surgery is the heart transplant. Heart transplant has encountered the same problems as many other forms of organ grafting, most of them resulting from the body's natural tendency to reject foreign tissue, even when it represents a beneficial replacement. Medicine is gradually improving its techniques for dealing with graft rejection, but it is still a major stumbling block for organ transplant. Most physicians believe that many more years of research are needed before heart transplant can become a practical form of treatment.

Small mechanical pumps have been used as auxiliary circulatory devices to relieve diseased hearts temporarily while the heart muscle heals itself. The long-term potential of such equipment is uncertain, however. A true artificial heart, capable of functioning inside the body indefinitely, has not yet been developed. Although many investigators are studying the possibility, it seems unlikely that such a device will become a reality for many years.

PREVENTION

Prevention is still the best weapon modern medicine has against heart disease, since CVD cannot be cured. It is far easier to eliminate many of the risk factors than to have to resort to surgery or medication after the fact.

Some congenital heart defects may be avoided during pregnancy by carefully following good health practices, preventing disease, and avoiding alcohol abuse. Rheumatic fever can be caught and treated before it attacks the heart. *Cor pulmonale* (or pulmonary heart), a condition induced by the high capillary resistance of diseased lungs, is aggravated if not actually caused by tobacco smoking; eliminating smoking can reduce the risk. With hypertension, early recognition and treatment are now possible.

Prevention is never perfect, however. Even individuals who eat properly, have normal blood pressure, do not smoke, and exercise regularly may still have heart attacks (though the chances are much smaller). Every adult should be familiar with the early warning signs of heart attack and stroke, and should be taught how to perform mouth-to-mouth resuscitation and cardiac massage. Greater emphasis should be placed on the need for prompt emergency treatment. Mobile units and special coronary care units in hospitals, utilizing both medical and paramedical personnel, have already contributed greatly to the present declining rate of cardiovascular diseases.

Many people still consider the afflictions of cardiovascular disease to be an inevitable part of middle or old age but irrelevant to children and young adults. As has been shown, however, even small children may be on their way to heart attacks if various factors—such as heredity and diet—are working against them. Modified life-style habits may help such children to eliminate heart difficulties throughout their lives. At the very least—for both children and adults—the practice of minimizing all known risk factors will help raise the odds for a longer, healthier life.

SUMMARY

1. Cardiovascular diseases involve the heart and blood vessels and include conditions such as atherosclerosis, high blood pressure, rheumatic heart disease, and congenital heart disease.
2. Coronary artery disease is a leading cause of death among American men over age thirty-five and American women past age forty. Some middle-aged and young people also show early signs of atherosclerosis.
3. The symptoms of a heart attack include a constricting or crushing pain in the middle of the chest, paleness, profuse sweating, shortness of breath, and sometimes vomiting. Heart attacks are caused by insufficient coronary blood flow to the heart due to the narrowing of the blood vessels. Sometimes a blood clot, or thrombus, may precede or follow a heart attack. The part of the heart muscle that has been denied its blood supply may also die. This dead area is called an infarct; a heart attack is thus called a myocardial (heart muscle) infarction.
4. A person who regularly has pain, pressure, or tightness in the chest may have angina pectoris. This is a condition resulting from oxygen deprivation to the heart muscle.
5. Heart attacks drastically alter the heartbeat. The normal tissue, known as a pacemaker, which emits electrical impulses to control the heartbeat, may be disturbed. If so, fibrillation, a dangerously rapid heartbeat, may result.
6. Sometimes heart-attack victims or elderly people have heartbeats that are too slow. This means that a heart block has developed due to the failure of the electric connection between the atria and ventricles. To remedy this, it is often necessary to surgically implant an artificial pacemaker to regulate the heartbeat.
7. Whenever the heart stops beating, due to a heart attack or accident, the condition is called cardiac arrest. The brain can only sur-

vive for four minutes without oxygen or blood, so immediate cardiopulmonary resuscitation (CPR) is essential. This involves external cardiac massage and ventilation of the lungs using mouth-to-mouth resuscitation.

8. When the heart cannot pump enough blood to the rest of the body, a condition known as congestive heart failure results. This causes shortness of breath, swelling of the ankles, and abnormalities in chest X-rays. Certain drugs are useful in ameliorating, but not curing, these difficulties.

9. Congenital heart defects, such as small holes in the cardiac wall or defects in the heart valves, can sometimes be remedied by open-heart surgery.

10. If left untreated, rheumatic fever, an inflammatory disease of connective tissues, can result in heart damage, particularly of the valves.

11. High blood pressure, or hypertension, is detected by a simple blood-pressure test. When the systolic pressure and/or diastolic pressure is above normal limits, hypertension is diagnosed. People over the age of fifty and nonwhites are more likely to suffer from hypertension. Left untreated, high blood pressure can cause strokes, congestive heart failure, atherosclerosis, increased cholesterol levels in the blood, and kidney disease.

12. Strokes occur because of hemorrhages, clots, or some other blood-vessel obstruction. A stroke victim may be partly paralyzed, suffer memory loss, or exhibit general confusion. Emotional lability or an inability to comprehend or speak coherently (called aphasia) is also common.

13. A temporary attack with symptoms similar to stroke is known as a transient ischemic attack (TIA). These episodes may involve temporary numbness, paralysis, and difficulty in speaking or thinking clearly. A TIA is a warning of a possible impending stroke.

14. The risk factors implicated in both heart attacks and strokes are: high-cholesterol foods, obesity, excessive eating, lack of exercise, cigarette smoking, hypertension, psychological stress, hereditary predisposition, and diabetes. All of these risks increase geometrically when more than one is present in the same person.

15. Pacemaker implantation, coronary bypass surgery, artery transplant or replacement, transcatheter closure, the surgical unclogging of arteries, and heart transplants are some surgical techniques that have been developed to remedy cardiovascular difficulties.

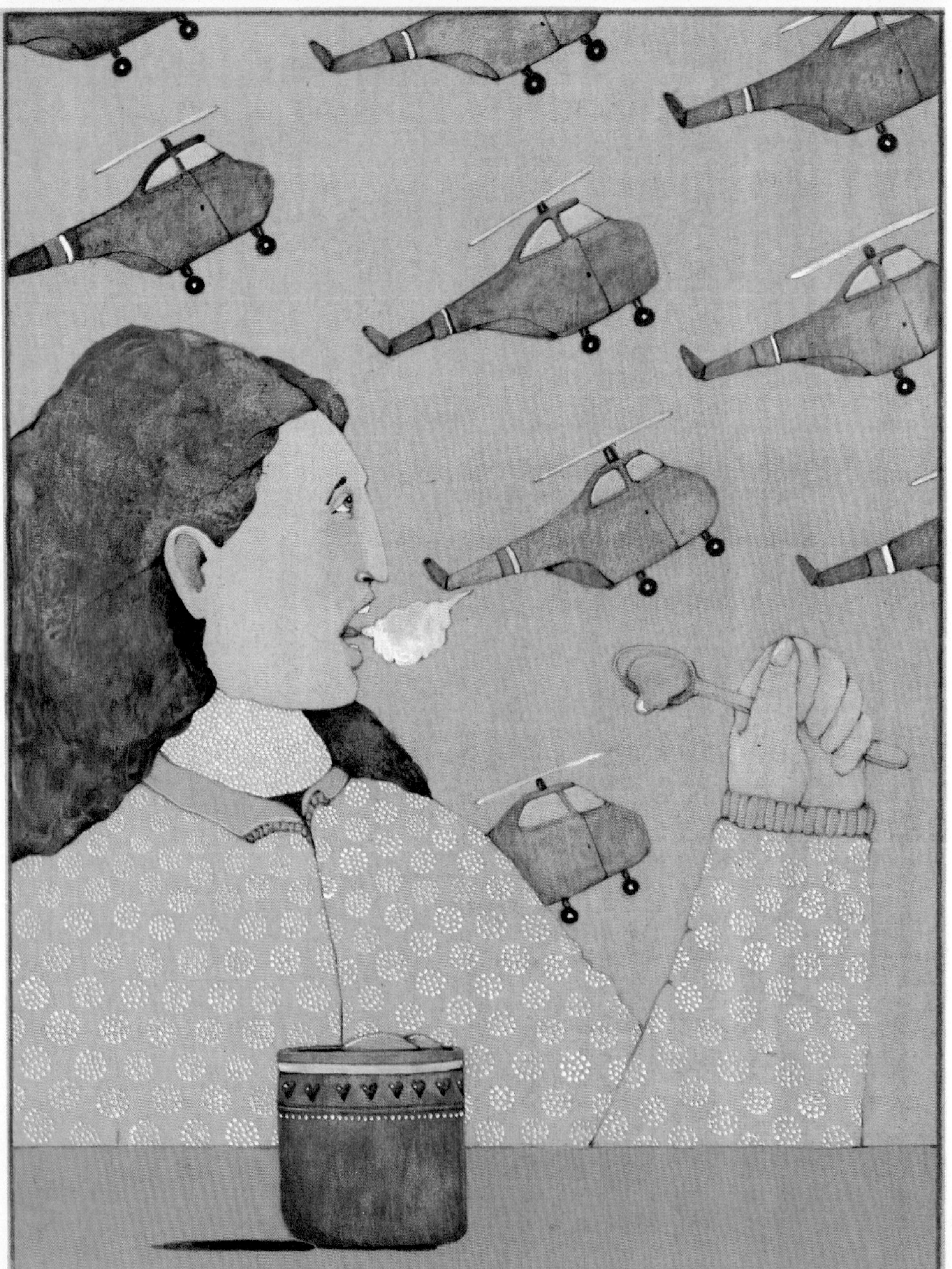

Dagmar Frinta

VI HEALTH AND SOCIETY

In order to remain creative and productive, any society depends upon the optimal health—physical, mental, and emotional—of as many of its members as possible. In Part VI we turn to aspects of health for which society is largely responsible.

In the United States today, we benefit from a technologically advanced society. Most of us take the basic necessities of life—food, clothing, and shelter—for granted, we enjoy a high standard of living, and we can go anywhere in the world in a matter of hours. Chapter 17 takes a look at the *other* side of progress—the manufactured chemicals, pollutants, and radiation that threaten not only our health but of our entire planet's ecosystem.

Until recently, quality medical attention was regarded as a privilege of a few people rather than as everyone's right. Our system of medical care, which offers the best facilities and equipment in the world, is still inaccessible to many Americans. And, partly because our health-care system has grown so expensive and impersonal, many others are turning to *self-care:* looking after themselves when they are sick and knowing when to see a doctor. The plusses and minuses of both our health-care system and the self-care movement are covered in Chapter 18.

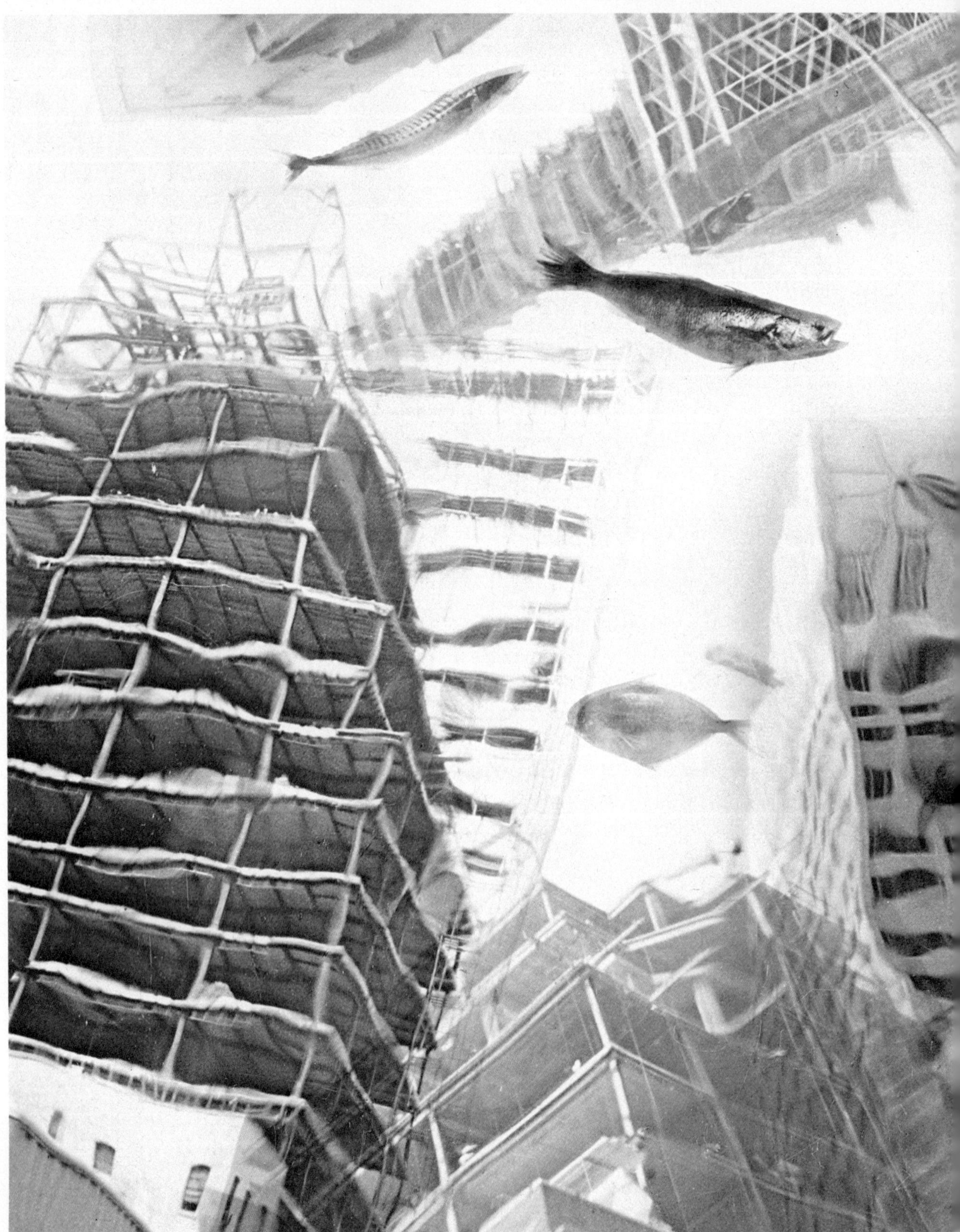

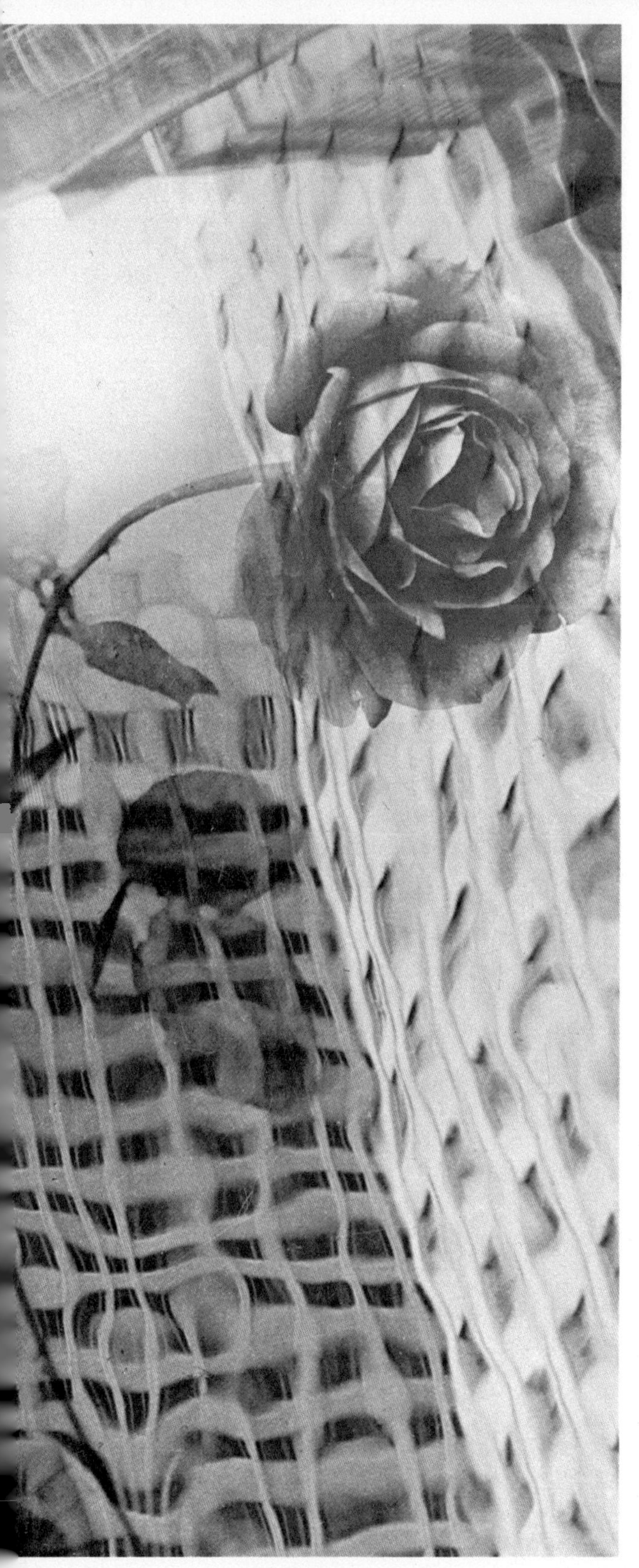

17 Health in the Environment

Human life as we know it has always depended on the deliberate manipulation of the natural environment. And in the industrialized nations, where this manipulation has been more extensive and more successful than anywhere else, people enjoy the highest living standards in the world.

But it is becoming clear that all of this progress has a cost. In the last quarter of the twentieth century, the industrialized nations of the world have begun to struggle with a new health problem: the negative effects of technological progress on the natural environment. It almost seems as if each technological solution for human problems creates more difficulties. Nuclear power plants produce radioactive waste materials, some of which will be dangerous foı half a million years—and no one has yet come up with a satisfactory disposal plan. Advances in medicine, public health techniques, and food production continue to lower world mortality rates, while fertility rates increase and overpopulation threatens the quality of life worldwide. The highways are choked with automobiles that travel fast enough to kill any occupant on impact. The roadsides are littered with aluminum cans that will virtually last forever.

Americans have become more and more aware that their efforts to improve living conditions through technology and industrialization have simultaneously spawned or magnified a variety of health problems, such as pollution, obesity, stress, heart disease, cancer, and mental disorders. In this chapter, we consider the major environmental influences on health in

America today, examine the extent of their threat, and suggest actions that the individual might take to lower the risks of these problems. We will also touch on the complexities involved in efforts to solve these problems, including the technological, economic, and political realities.

THE CHEMICAL ENVIRONMENT

One technological development that has brought great benefits to humanity has been the discovery and synthesis of thousands of chemical compounds. These chemicals range from prescription drugs, pesticides, and fertilizers to dyes, plastics, and industrial substances. Without them, many comforts that we take for granted would be missing. Food would be harder to come by, and infectious disease would remain a deadly killer. But these benefits must be weighed against the hazards involved in the production, use, and disposal of chemicals within the context of the environment.

The hazards of a particular chemical depend on a number of factors: the volume at which it is produced; the rate at which it is released into the environment; the intrinsic properties—such as water solubility—that determine its movement through the environment; the extent to which it accumulates; its chemical stability; and its toxicity.

What Makes a Chemical Harmful?

People often refer to specific chemicals as being "safe" or "poisonous," but such labels may be misleading: even common table foods have an intrinsic toxicity. For example, the refined sugar sucrose in a half pound box of candy could theoretically kill a twenty-pound child. And some chemicals that are beneficial at a low dose are toxic at higher doses. For example, very small amounts of the element selenium are essential to the human diet; yet too much selenium can cause severe liver damage and possibly cancer. The difference between the dose needed for a beneficial effect and the dose that produces an adverse effect is known as the *margin of safety*.

There are two reasons why a person can be exposed to potentially toxic chemicals without any harmful effect. First, the body has many enzyme systems—particularly in the liver—that break down or metabolize unwanted or toxic chemicals. Second, the body has repair mechanisms that are constantly replacing damaged enzymes, cell parts, and even whole cells. If the damage from a toxic chemical occurs within the normal rate of breakdown and replacement, it is not considered harmful.

If the dose is increased so that the rate of breakdown exceeds the rate of replacement, there may be a loss of function that can lead to a permanent disability. As Figure 17.1 shows, a chemical can produce a series of thresholds for chronic effects, such as weight loss or changed level of enzyme activity, until the ultimate threshold—death—is reached. This entire pattern is called the *dose-response effect* of a drug.

The federal and state governments regulate the dose or amount of many of the chemicals to which people are exposed. Workers in certain occupations are permitted higher exposure for shorter periods of time than is the general public. Government regulations also control the chemicals discharged into the air people breathe, the water they drink, and the food they eat.

Setting a "safe" level is difficult. Allowances must be made for the responses of the very young, the very old, the sick, the disabled, and others who are especially susceptible because of some genetic, developmental, nutritional, physiological, or psychological characteristic. Scientists sometimes disagree about the safety of a given dose level of a particular chemical, especially when they are trying to determine the effects of small doses over very long periods of time. The complexity of these issues can best be appreciated by looking at specific examples.

Asbestos

Asbestos is a naturally occurring mineral that can be processed to form fibers that are fireproof and practically indestructible. These fibers are used in a wide variety of products, including cement pipes, shingles, floor tiles, paper goods, insulating and packing materials,

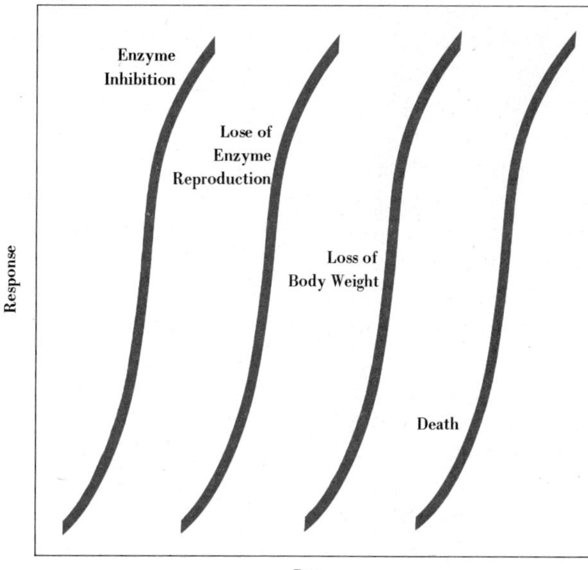

Figure 17.1 Dose-response effects occur in a series. With increasing doses, each condition becomes worse and new conditions are produced.

and so on. More than 300 million tons of asbestos are produced every year.

Working with asbestos is a significant occupational hazard. People who inhale asbestos dust are susceptible to asbestosis, a crippling and sometimes fatal lung disease. Studies have shown that workers who are continually exposed to asbestos fibers also have a much greater incidence of both lung cancer and cancer of the intestinal tract. An obvious dose-response relationship is involved, since the incidence of tumors is related to the length of exposure. The situation seems to be worst for cigarette smokers. In a study of 370 asbestos insulation workers, no lung cancer deaths were observed among nonsmokers, whereas lung tumors claimed the lives of 24 smokers.

Recently some authorities have become concerned about the danger of relatively small amounts of asbestos fiber to the health of the general public. One London study found that one-third of patients who died of an asbestos-related cancer had no known history of direct exposure to asbestos dust. Asbestos fibers are commonly present in the lungs of urban dwellers, who breathe the fibers in with the air. Asbestos has also been found in wines that are filtered with asbestos mesh, in baby powder, and in water supplies. Most of our homes and cars contain some asbestos in insulation, water pipes, brake linings, and the like. Are all of these materials hazardous?

It is extremely difficult to measure low concentrations of asbestos in the environment because the fibers are so small that they can be detected only with high-magnification electron microscopes. Furthermore, the time that elapses between exposure to asbestos and the appearance of an asbestos-related disease is typically anywhere from fifteen to fifty or more years. These conditions make it very difficult to study the effects of low-level asbestos exposure on the general public.

Nevertheless, authorities and consumers are moving to reduce the use of asbestos products, especially those that generate airborne particles. For example, the use of asbestos soundproofing materials in schools and other public buildings has been prohibited. Such measures, combined with strict regulation of asbestos dust in the workplace, will help to reduce the most obvious hazards while further studies are conducted.

Mercury

Mercury is a naturally occurring element that is widely distributed in the earth's crust. From a general chemical point of view, release of mercury into the environment would not produce any undesirable health effects. However, certain microorganisms can convert mercury into an organic form, methyl mercury. Unfortunately, this fact was not discovered until several years after a tragic incident for which it was responsible.

From the early 1930s until 1971, certain Japanese factories released industrial wastes containing substantial quantities of mercury into the Pacific Ocean. Marine microorganisms metabolized the mercury to its organic form, which became progressively more concentrated as it passed along the food chain to higher organisms. The highest organisms in the chain were human beings—residents of a fishing village on Minamata Bay, whose diet consisted almost solely of fish. The level of

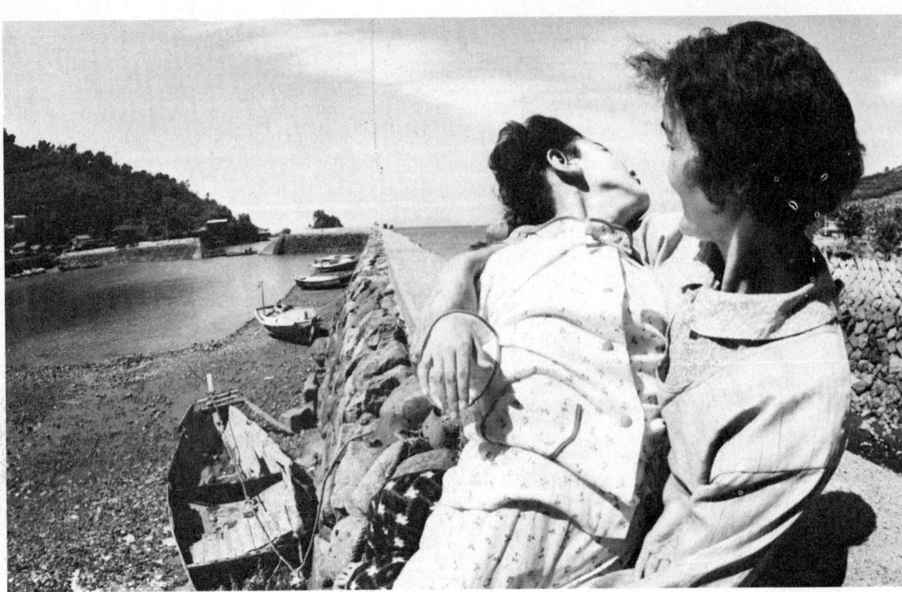

Figure 17.2 Many victims of Minimata disease, like the Japanese girl shown here, suffer numbness of the arms and legs.

mercury in the fish they ate resulted in fifty-two deaths, and more than a hundred other people became ill with the characteristic symptoms of methyl mercury poisoning.

Because of this incident, such mercury poisoning is now usually referred to as *Minamata disease.* It is characterized by such symptoms as inability to speak, mental retardation, numbness of the arms and legs followed by deterioration of muscle tissue, gradual loss of vision and hearing, disruption of equilibrium, loss of coordination, and emotional disturbance. Many victims are permanently disabled, and children born to mothers who have consumed contaminated seafood are severely deformed (see Figure 17.2).

Other cases of mercury poisoning have come to light since the Minamata episode. Between 1971 and 1972, thousands of people in Iraq were poisoned by bread made with flour contaminated by a methyl mercury fungicide; of these victims, some 500 died. Among Canadians whose diet is mostly fish, authorities found many people with Minamata symptoms in the early 1970s. In 1975, the French Institute of Medical Oceanography reported that the mercury content of common fish species caught in the Mediterranean Sea off the French and Italian Rivieras had reached three times the maximum acceptable limit for fish fit for human consumption. People who ate an average of five pounds of such fish a week were warned that they would be chronically ill within seven years and dead in twenty years.

As a result of such incidents, most industrialized nations have instituted strict regulations prohibiting mercury pollution, and acute mercury poisoning from contaminated food is now far less likely than it was a decade ago. However, mercury continues to be mined, used, and released into the environment. Some authorities are now concerned with the chronic effects of long-term exposure to relatively low levels of mercury, especially mercury vapor and mercury particles in the air. As is true of asbestos, the hazards of human exposure to relatively low levels of mercury have not been clearly established.

Lead

Lead, like mercury, is a naturally occurring element, usually distributed in low concentrations. Since the introduction of the automobile, however, the lead content of the atmosphere has greatly increased, for lead is an additive in most gasolines. Furthermore, lead is commonly used in paints, ceramics, glassware, pipes, and many other manufactured goods.

The effects of lead poisoning are known: weakness, loss of appetite, anemia, and damage to the nervous system. Lead poisoning through the use of lead cooking utensils is thought to have contributed to the decline of the Greek and Roman civilizations, especially by causing brain damage, miscarriages, and stillbirths in the upper classes. The effects of long-term exposure to low concentrations of lead are not known, however. Responding to outside pressure, oil companies are now making unleaded gasoline, thus reducing the risks of atmospheric lead poisoning.

Of even greater danger is the poisoning that occurs when children eat lead-based paint and putty, usually off walls and woodwork. Hundreds of children have died from this type of poisoning, and thousands of others have suffered chronic symptoms related to it. A 1977 study found that children whose blood contained even slightly elevated levels of lead scored lower on intelligence tests than a carefully matched group of children with normal blood.

Pesticides and Herbicides

Pesticides have become a pervasive part of the American environment. Low levels of some pesticides may be found in the air, in water, in food, and in the bodies of animals—including human beings. As was noted earlier, these chemicals have played a major role in increasing food production and in controlling disease throughout the world. It is estimated that millions of lives have been saved by using DDT to destroy mosquitoes carrying malaria and yellow fever. Yet pesticides such as DDT become a problem because they are easily spread; they persist in the environment since they are not easily broken down; and they tend, like PCBs, to accumulate in living tissues, especially in the fatty tissues of the human body.

Like mercury, DDT becomes more concentrated as it moves up the food chain. And it has been so thoroughly dispersed that even penguins in the Antarctic have measurable quantities of DDT in their fatty tissues. Although no human fatalities have been recorded from the proper use of DDT, the long-term effects of DDT exposure are still largely unknown.

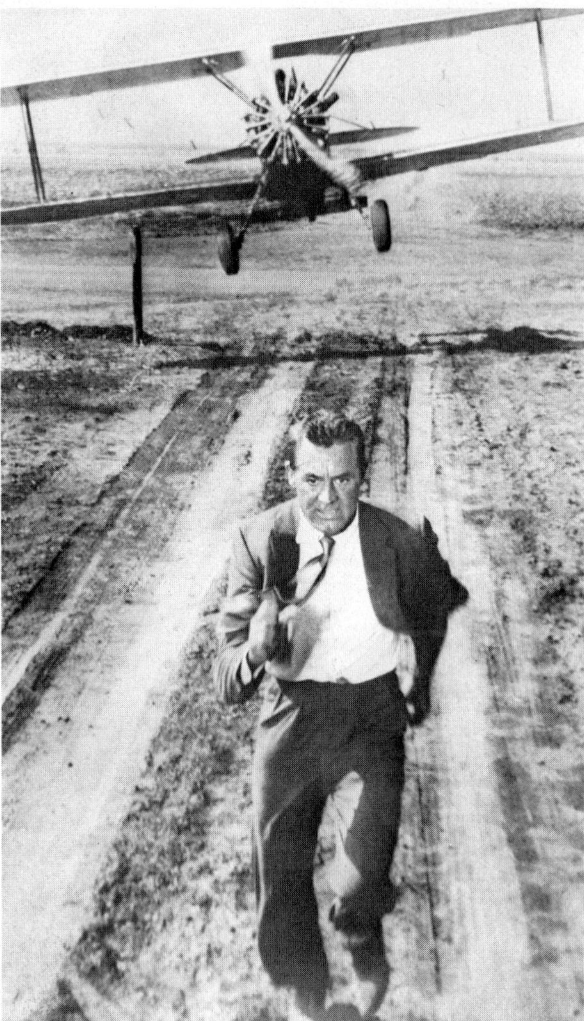

Figure 17.3 In Alfred Hitchcock's film *North by Northwest,* the character played by Cary Grant sees a crop-dusting plane that appears to be spraying distant cornfields with a powdered insectide. Unexpectedly, the plane flies toward him and begins spraying bullets instead. When the film was released in 1958, the irony of this directorial twist lay in the suddenly realized lethal potential of a seemingly innocent activity in a seemingly innocent setting. Two decades later, the recently discovered health-threatening potential of many insecticides (including chlordane and heptaclor, used in cornfields) adds another layer of irony to the scene.

In 1973, the Environmental Protection Agency imposed a ban on the use of DDT in the United States. Two other widely used pes-

FOCUS

Carcinogens in the Workplace

The discovery that even minute amounts of certain industrial chemicals can cause cancer has led to regulations limiting the presence of these substances in the workplace. The federal agency most involved in setting these standards is the Occupational Safety and Health Administration (OSHA). To date, OSHA has sharply reduced the allowable on-the-job exposure to carcinogenic substances such as asbestos dust, vinyl chloride, and coke oven emissions.

However, the cost to industry of complying with these regulations is enormous. For example, one standard proposed for the presence of acrylonitrile, a chemical used in textile plants, in the air during an eight-hour workday is 2 parts per million (ppm). The engineering changes required to meet this standard would cost the textile industry $3.52 million. But to eliminate all risk of cancer, the exposure limit would need to be about .2 ppm. This would cost the industry an additional $126.2 million a year. Understandably, the textile industry has balked at such a standard.

Another risk chemical is benzene, which is used mostly in the chemical, tire manufacturing, and petroleum industries. About 629,000 workers in the United States are exposed to benzene vapors on the job. It has been known since World War II that these vapors are dangerous. In 1946, an exposure limit of 100 ppm was recommended, and this limit was further reduced several times until, in 1971, OSHA adopted a 10-ppm standard.

However, more recent studies have indicated that long-term exposure to benzene may cause leukemia. The most important of these studies was a follow-up on workers at two Goodyear Company plants in Ohio in the 1940s. Of the 748 workers who had been exposed to benzene, 9 died of leukemia—a mortality rate seven times greater than that of both the population at large and the workers who had not been exposed to benzene. It is likely that exposure levels at these plants were generally around 100 ppm, but they may occasionally have gone much higher.

In light of these studies, OSHA is now pressing for a reduction of the benzene limit to 1 ppm. The industry, led by the American Petroleum Institute, has protested. The cost of putting this new standard into effect—estimated at $500 million by OSHA and twice as much by the industry—is one factor. But the industry also feels that since the studies were conducted when exposure to benzene was far higher than under the present 10-ppm standard, reducing the limit even more is unnecessary. The Fifth Circuit Court of Appeals in New Orleans agreed, ruling that OSHA was trying to impose an immense financial burden on the industry without any strong evidence of resulting benefits.

At the heart of the matter is the controversy surrounding risk quantification—a method of estimating how much risk a given substance poses and balancing this risk against various benefits. OSHA contends that risk quantification is too imprecise and may allow unnecessary incidence of cancer. Labor unions such as the AFL-CIO support this view, claiming that risk quantification puts a dollar value on employees' lives. Industry—and other government agencies—disagrees, advocating standards that are "reasonably necessary."

OSHA has appealed the New Orleans court's decision, and the Supreme Court will soon review the case. Its ruling may be crucial to the formulation of a national policy on occupational safety.

ticides, aldrin and dieldrin, were banned in 1974. Like DDT, these compounds were found to accumulate in fatty tissues when taken into the body in the food chain. Government action was taken in 1975 against chlordane and heptaclor, pesticides used primarily in cornfields, but also around houses and gardens, after measurable amounts were found in dairy products, fish, and poultry. Chlordane and heptaclor are suspected of causing cancer.

The United Nations is advocating an integrated attack on pests that includes many nonchemical components. This campaign would include genetic control techniques, control of breeding habitats, breeding crops and animals resistant to pests, biological control, and behavioral control using aroma-controlling pheromones that can attract or ward off other animals. If these methods can be developed to the point where they can be used to control a variety of insects, the use of chemical pesticides can be reduced.

POLLUTION

The term *pollution* refers to biological, physical, and chemical wastes that contaminate the environment. Much of what might be termed pollution is *natural,* resulting from processes such as volcanic activity, dust storms, erosion, sea spray, animal waste products, and the like. Only one-fifth of atmospheric emissions comes from human sources. The significant difference, however, is that human pollutants are concentrated in confined areas—primarily cities—where people are subjected to their own effluents (waste materials poured into the environment) in great volume.

Normally, the environment can cleanse itself of pollutants. Chemical reactions, air movements, water flow, dilution, and microbial activity tend to break down, disperse, and recycle poisonous substances. However, these processes cannot keep up with the volume of pollutants produced in urban areas. Furthermore, some human-made substances—PCB, for example—tend to resist environmental breakdown. Substances that more readily lend themselves to breakdown and assimilation by the environment are considered *biodegradable;* substances that are more persistent are designated *nonbiodegradable.* Some of the major pollutants that pose a threat to human health enter the body through the air we breathe and the water we drink. Other hazards take the forms of solid wastes and noise.

Air Pollution

The greatest threat of air pollution seems to come from the cumulative effects of long-term exposure to specific pollutants. The major sources of air pollution in the United States are fuel combustion, chemical processing, and the burning of wastes. Motor vehicles account for more than half the air emissions. Air pollutants with the greatest health-threatening potential are sulfur oxides, nitrogen oxides, carbon monoxide, hydrocarbons, particulate matter, and fluorocarbons.

Sulfur oxides, produced primarily by combustion of *fossil fuels,* such as coal, petroleum, and natural gas, are thought to be a principal cause of excessive deaths during major smog incidents. Sulfur dioxide in particular has been implicated in bronchitis, emphysema, and asthma. The sulfur oxides irritate the eyes, throat, and lungs, causing coughing and choking. Fortunately, the past forty years have seen an increase in control of emissions and a reduction in the burning of high-sulfur fuels, resulting in a significant decrease in the sulfur oxide content of the air in urban areas.

Nitrogen oxides come from motor vehicle emissions and the burning of fossil fuels. They are thought to contribute to respiratory difficulties and to reduce the oxygen-carrying capacity of the blood. *Carbon monoxide* is released from automobile exhausts at the rate of 60,000 tons a year in the United States and constitutes more than half of all human-made air emissions. This deadly gas, which is colorless and odorless, hampers the oxygen-carrying capacity of red blood cells. Exposure to significant doses of carbon monoxide causes oxygen deficiency in the blood, resulting in impaired respiration and malfunctioning of the brain and the heart. Other effects include impaired hearing, vision, and thought. Excessive exposure can lead to unconsciousness and death. Carbon monoxide levels are also high in dense traffic, at intersections, and in enclosed areas such as garages and tunnels.

Hydrocarbons, also produced primarily by automobile emissions, result from incomplete burning of fuel. Hydrocarbons are a significant factor in photochemical smog. *Particulate matter* includes dust, ash, and other fine particles that are by-products of fuel combustion, other types of burning, and abrasion milling. These particles irritate the eyes, throat, and lungs, may be carcinogenic, and are observable components of smog.

Although *fluorocarbons*—chemical compounds that were used for a number of years in many aerosol spray cans—are not known to have a direct effect on human beings, they are nevertheless considered a threat to world health by a growing number of scientists. Evidence has accumulated to suggest that these compounds, because they are inert and do not react with what is shot out of the cans in which they are used, float up unchanged to the stratosphere, where they may be contributing to a gradual depletion of the ozone layer, ten to

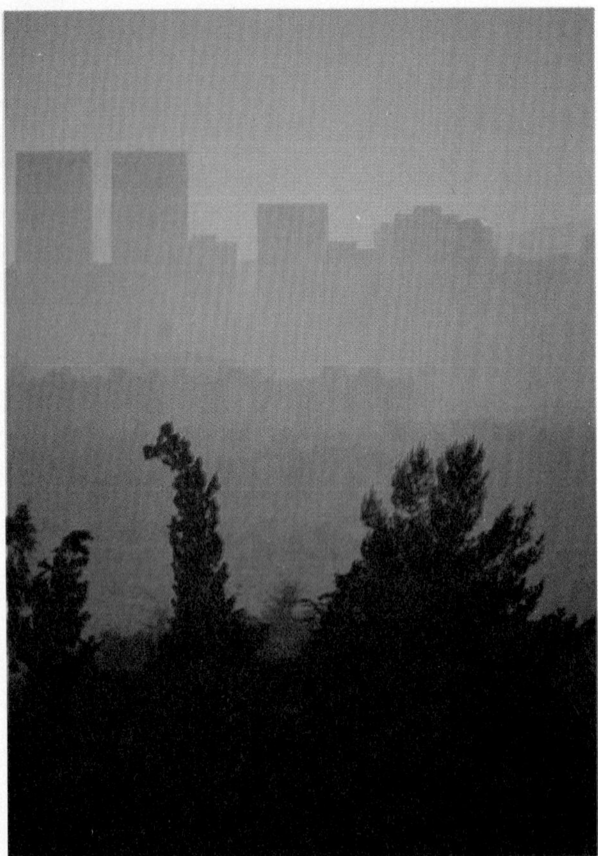

Figure 17.4 Photochemical smog surrounding Los Angeles. Automobile exhaust emissions are trapped by weather conditions, thus causing air pollution.

forty miles above the earth. Among the possible consequences of ozone depletion, scientists fear an increase in the incidence of skin cancer and an alteration of world climates.

Since 1974, when fluorocarbons first gained public attention, consumer awareness of their potential threat appears to have been a major factor in declining sales of aerosol spray cans. Indeed, shipments of such cans in the United States dropped 26 percent over the first six months of 1975 as a result of decreasing demand. In 1978, federal agencies banned the manufacture of fluorocarbon propellants, and in 1979, the shipment of aerosols containing fluorocarbons was prohibited in interstate commerce. This action is a good example of the growing awareness of pollution dangers on the part of scientists, consumers, and regulatory agencies.

Smog There are actually two types of smog—the London type and the Los Angeles type. The London variety, blamed for thousands of deaths in Europe and the eastern United States, is more correctly termed *sulfur-dioxide smog.* The burning of fossil fuels (primarily coal with high sulfur content) has been a major pollution problem in European cities for centuries. Sulfur-dioxide smog inhibits the action of the cilia in respiratory passages, allowing smog particles to remain and irritate sensitive tissues. These particles and chemicals so impair breathing that people with chronic respiratory problems may die. Impaired breathing can also aggravate heart problems. Reduction of the use of high-sulfur fuels has significantly decreased the occurrence of London-type smog.

Los Angeles-type smog, more properly called *photochemical smog,* results from the interaction of two prime factors: exhaust emissions from automobiles and temperature inversion. This type of smog occurs in areas characterized by poor air circulation (a valley, for example), sunny weather, and low humidity. In Los Angeles, a layer of cool ocean air may slip in under the normally warm, stable air above the city, thereby causing a *temperature inversion.* Motor vehicle emissions rise through the cool air but cannot penetrate the warm layer, which acts like a lid on the Los Angeles basin. The pollutants are therefore trapped and subjected to the action of sunlight, which produces additional pollutants (such as ozone). The emissions gradually dissipate, but while they remain, they can cause extreme eye and nose irritation in city inhabitants.

For otherwise healthy people, air pollution may be more of a temporary irritant than a major health threat. It is wise for city dwellers to avoid going outdoors and engaging in strenuous activity on smoggy days and to heed smog alerts.

Water Pollution

Throughout history, waterways have been popular dumping grounds for garbage and human wastes. Such indiscriminate use made water a major means of disease transmission—particularly of typhoid and cholera. Sewage continues to be a major water pollutant in a number of American communities, but modern sewage treatment plants are greatly reducing threats to public drinking supplies.

Water pollution comes not only from human wastes but also from industrial processing, radioactive substances, agricultural runoff, and oil seepage. Of additional concern is thermal pollution, which occurs when power plants use water for cooling and consequently raise the temperature of a nearby body of water. Thermal pollution can change the ecological balance of a lake—for example, by killing certain species of fish and promoting the proliferation of other species.

Several kinds of water pollution, including thermal pollution, contribute to the process of *eutrophication*—the depleting of oxygen in a body of water. The worst culprits in this process appear to be nitrates and phosphates from fertilizers and municipal sewage. Nitrates encourage the growth of algae; excess nitrates can cause massive *algal blooms,* which grow quickly and then die. Bacterial decay of these algal blooms depletes the oxygen supply in the water, causing fish and other organisms to die. This process has occurred in Lake Erie to such an extent that a layer of nitrogen- and phosphorus-rich mud covers the lake bottom in thicknesses ranging from 20 to 125 feet. The lake water has been rendered unfit for drinking, recreation, or industrial purposes.

Lake Michigan has also suffered major contamination from the dumping of industrial wastes and municipal sewage, as well as from DDT and other pollutants. Efforts have been made to clean up the lake over a period of more than twenty years. Industrial and municipal discharges have declined in response to stricter regulations; the state of Indiana has banned phosphate detergents; and, as we saw earlier, the federal government has banned DDT. As a result, the near-shore areas of Lake Michigan are improving. Some public beaches have opened again. The lake's fish contain 90 percent less DDT than they did before the ban was imposed. Phosphorus concentrations along the Indiana shoreline have been greatly reduced.

However, eutrophication continues in the lake's open waters. The concentrations of PCBs in lake fish have not declined, despite a PCB ban. Chlorine levels are rising in the lake due to runoffs from salt used to treat icy highways. The effects of these higher levels are not known, but it is feared that they could change the lake's biological systems irreversibly. The history of Lake Michigan demonstrates how persistent and complex a problem water pollution can be.

Solid Wastes

Solid waste pollution consists of garbage, litter, abandoned cars, and other discarded materials, along with the solid waste products of agriculture, mining, and manufacturing—together a formidable and growing problem in highly technological societies. In recent years, the solid products of pollution-control devices (the toxic sludge that remains after water used in chemical processing has been detoxified to meet government regulations, for example) have been added to the list of industrial pollutants.

Nontoxic trash and litter are problems primarily because they are ugly and because there are not enough places to dispose of them without contaminating the environment. Open dumps provide a breeding ground for rats and flies. Incineration can lead to air pollution, while dumping in natural waters contributes to water pollution. The discarding of these materials also represents a loss of resources, since many of the substances that make up trash and litter could be salvaged and recycled. For example, 50 percent of municipal trash in the United States is waste paper, which could be reclaimed, pulped, and made into useful fiber.

Many of the solid wastes from mining and industry are potentially dangerous unless they are properly managed. When toxic substances are simply dumped on the land, they can leak into the groundwater near the dump and contaminate drinking water sources. This happened in 1972, when almost all the employees of a newly constructed office and warehouse in Minnesota suddenly developed arsenic poisoning. They had been drinking water from a new well drilled near the site of an abandoned village dump. Forty years earlier, neighborhood farmers had discarded the pesticide arsenic trioxide at the dump. Some of the soil samples taken near the well contained arsenic concentrations of up to 40 percent.

Nobody knows how many tons of toxic solid wastes have been dumped on the land and buried in landfills around the country. Government regulations for the safe handling of such wastes have only recently been implemented. This is another pollution problem which has been identified and will be regulated, but people still have to deal with the results of previous mismanagement.

Noise Pollution

Noise is now recognized as another form of pollution that can be hazardous to human health. The loudness, or strength, of a sound is measured in *decibels.* The sounds encountered by human beings range from zero decibels to about 150 decibels. (Some common noise levels are shown in Figure 17.5. Note that the decibel scale is a logarithmic scale, so that the sound level of a vacuum cleaner is *10 million* times more intense than a barely audible sound.) Noises at 130 decibels and higher cause pain; prolonged exposure to sounds at 80 decibels and above can cause hearing loss. Each year more noises encroach upon our everyday lives. The main sources of excessive noise in the environment are modes of transportation (cars, motorcycles, planes, trains), construction, industry, and household appliances. In addition, rock musicians and their fans, who subject themselves to amplified music (usually in the 110–120 decibel range), may suffer permanent hearing impairment.

Besides developing hearing problems, persons exposed to noise pollution may suffer from fatigue, loss of sleep, and emotional stress. Excess noise produces bodily changes such as increased heart rate, digestive spasms, blood vessel constriction, and pupil dilation. In animal studies, continual noise has led to heart, brain, and liver damage. Noise may be a factor in such human stress-related disorders as peptic ulcers, high blood pressure, weight loss, and emotional disturbances.

Control of noise pollution is difficult. European countries have instituted a number of an-

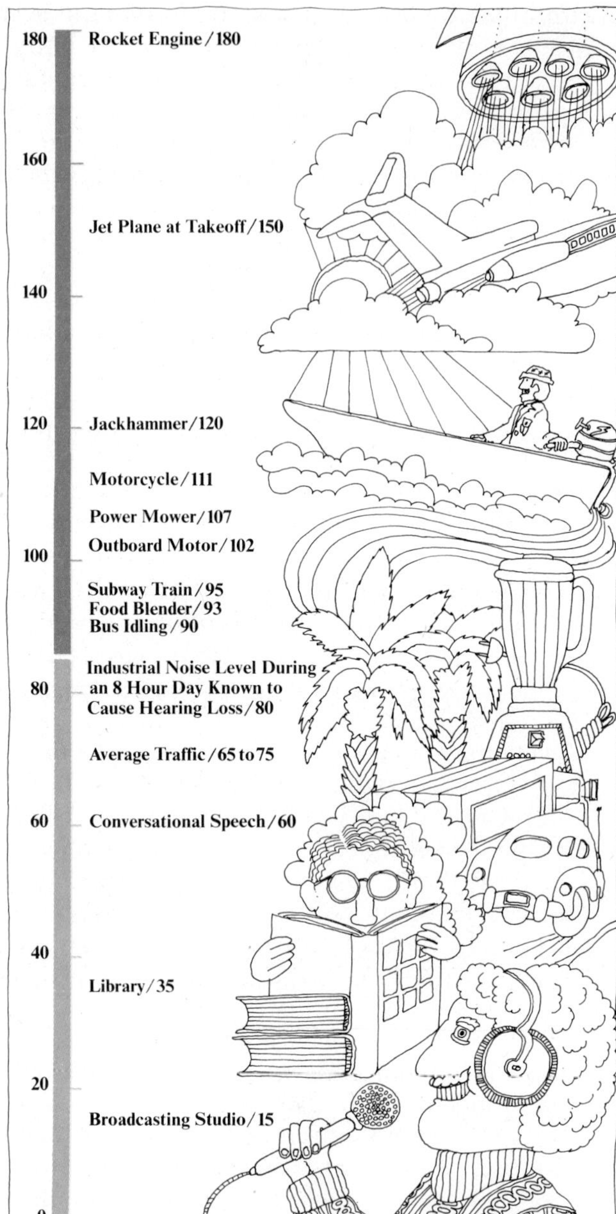

Figure 17.5 Noise pollution. The types of sounds that contribute to the noise level in urban communities, as measured in decibels. Sounds in the top half—the danger area—can lead to hearing losses.

tinoise laws that appear to be successfully curbing harmful noise. The Japanese carefully monitor the noise levels at busy intersections in urban areas. However, in the United States, where average noise levels have increased greatly in the last twenty years, few communities have dealt with the problem successfully. Industries have fared better in protecting employees. Workers in high-noise occupations are outfitted with special headgear. Soundproofing and wise architectural planning help to separate office workers from noisy machinery. Nevertheless, the problem is a long way from being totally solved, and insurance companies continue to pay out millions of dollars to workers who have gone deaf from exposure to excessive noise on the job.

RADIATION AND PUBLIC HEALTH

Since the oil embargo of 1973, energy issues have been debated around the world with increasing intensity. No issue arouses more strongly opposing views than the use of radioactive materials to fuel nuclear power plants. On the one hand are experts who claim that nuclear power is *the* answer to the world's energy crisis, an advance that will rescue us from economic and social disaster. On the otherhand, equally qualified persons say that nuclear power has the potential to become the greatest technological disaster of all time.

Everyone agrees on one thing: sooner or later, the world is going to run out of fossil fuels—the coal, oil, and natural gas that provide almost all the energy we use today. In 1976, 93 percent of the total energy used in the United States came from fossil fuels. It is difficult to calculate how much longer these nonrenewable resources will be available. One must estimate population growth, energy consumption, the number and capacity of new fossil fuel sources that will be discovered, and patterns of distribution. Several recent studies indicate that world production of petroleum will peak and begin to decline by the end of this century.

One solution to the eventual decline of fossil fuels is to increase the energy provided by nuclear sources. The nuclear power plants now in use and those envisioned for the future are designed to generate electricity. The energy they produce can be used to replace fossil fuels wherever electrical power can be substituted. A home that is now heated with oil, for example, could be heated with electricity instead. However, electricity cannot be used to power large, high-speed automobiles or planes, for example, so changes in our patterns of energy consumption would be required.

Are Nuclear Power Plants Safe?

In March 1979, the Three Mile Island nuclear power plant near Harrisburg, Pennsylvania, was dangerously out of control for at least forty-eight hours. This incident riveted the public's attention to the question of how safe nuclear power plants really are. Anything designed and operated by human beings is subject to human error. Nuclear power plants have been designed with this principle firmly in mind. They have backup cooling systems, monitoring devices to keep track of radiation levels, and many other safety features. Whether these measures are adequate is, of course, at the heart of the public debate about nuclear reactors. We cannot settle that question here, but we will examine some of the hazards that are presented by the generation of nuclear power.

The isotopes that are released in the nuclear fission reaction are highly radioactive substances. These waste products are extremely dangerous. Plutonium, the most toxic of them, can produce lung cancer when quantities as minute as a millionth of a gram are inhaled. The *half-life* of plutonium (the length of time required for half of any amount to decay and turn into another substance) is 24,400 years; the plutonium being produced in nuclear power plants today will be around for approximately half a million years.

If there were a serious accident in a nuclear power plant, the radioactive waste products of the fission reaction might be released into the environment surrounding the plant. Even if such an accident never occurs, there are no permanent, safe methods of disposal, transportation, or storage available now for these substances.

Other hazards are also associated with nuclear power. The uranium ore from which nuclear fuel comes emits radon, a radioactive gas that causes lung cancer when it is inhaled—for example, by workers in uranium mines and refining plants. The milling and refining pro-

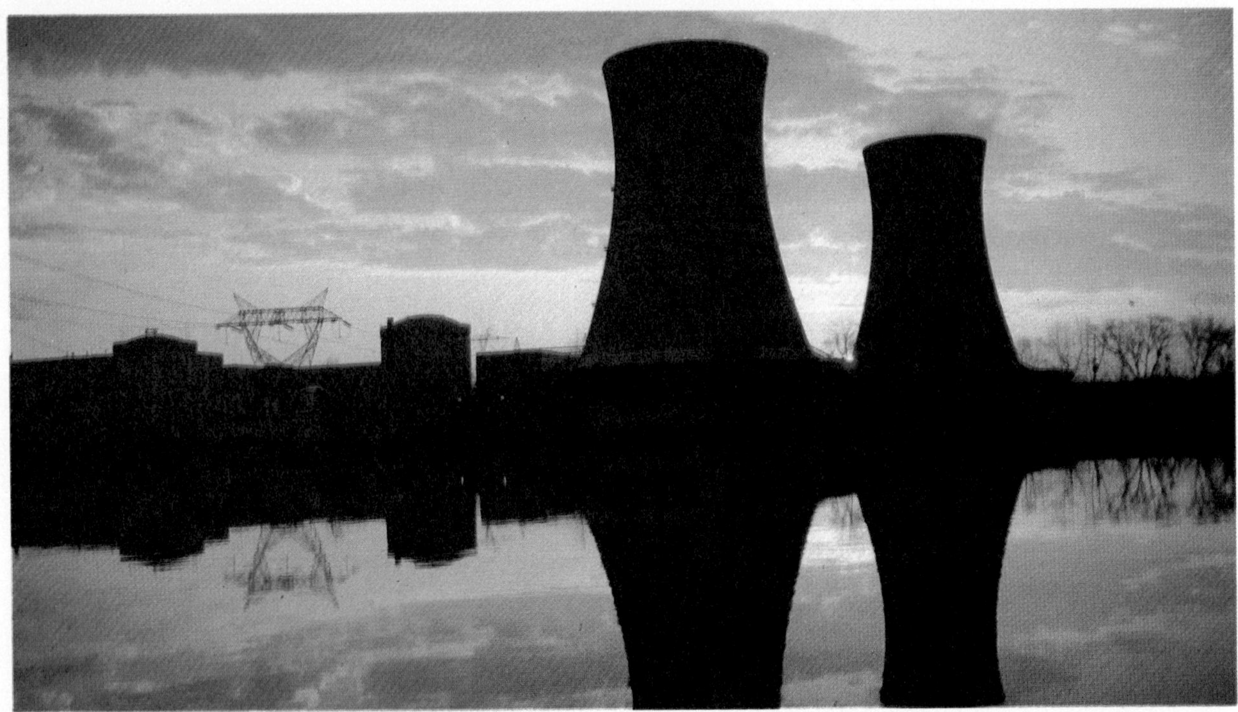

Figure 17.6 Despite claims of fail-safe backup systems for nuclear power plants, the accident at Three Mile Island (shown above) uncovered the risks inherent in nuclear power. The health effects of radiation emitted into the air during and after the Three Mile Island incident will not be fully known for many years. Increased incidence of cancer, genetic mutations, and leukemia are possible long-term consequences.

cess produces thousands of tons of waste ore, called tailings, which are left in heaps in areas surrounding the refining plants; these waste heaps also emit radon. Furthermore, nuclear plants emit low levels of radiation during normal operation, and some experts believe that these emissions can be dangerous over a long period of time.

Biological Effects of Radiation Exposure

Radiation has always been a part of the natural environment in the form of radioactive mineral deposits, cosmic radiation, and similar natural sources. Human-made radiation comes from such sources as medical X-rays and radiation therapy, microwave ovens, color television sets, industrial isotopes and X-rays, the radioactive wastes from nuclear power, and nuclear fallout from weapons testing.

Natural radiation represents about 58 percent of an average person's exposure to the environment. Human-made radiation accounts for 41 percent, and the remaining 1 percent comes from fallout.

Radiation may enter the body directly through the skin, but it is usually inhaled or ingested. The effect of radiation exposure depends on the dose, the length of exposure, the type of radiation, and the individual's degree of sensitivity. Prolonged exposure produces *radiation sickness* in most people. Symptoms of this disease come in stages: first, nausea, diarrhea, vomiting; second, loss of hair, hemorrhaging below the skin surface, ulcers in the mouth and digestive system; third, eye cataracts, high susceptibility to infections, and possible leukemia. Radiation has the most serious effect on those tissues in which cells normally reproduce rapidly—the lining of the digestive tract, the blood-forming tissues, and so on. Of particular susceptibility are sperm and egg cells and developing fetuses. Radiation is thus a major factor in genetic mutations, and significant doses are known to cause infertility, miscarriage, and birth defects.

In doses below those that cause radiation sickness but above normal (such as those experienced by workers who deal with radiation), radiation is thought to be carcinogenic. Because radioactive particles act primarily to alter or destroy individual cells, long-term exposure at normally "nondangerous" levels may promote cancerous growth. Recent studies indicate that there may be no safe level of radiation exposure, no dose of radiation so low that the risk of cancer is zero.

POPULATION AND HEALTH

Obviously, pollution would not be the problem it is today without the incredible population explosion of the past 150 years. In the early 1800s, the world's population reached 1 billion. It took about 100 years for the population to double—it reached 2 billion in 1925. In the last fifty years the population doubled once again, reaching 4 billion. Taking various growth factors and trends into account, another 2.5 billion persons will be added to the population in the next 25 years.

Populations have not been exploding at equal rates around the world, however. By 1975 a great disparity in growth trends had become apparent. The rich industrialized nations of the world were growing at a much slower rate than the poorer, less developed nations. The U.S. birth rate in 1977, for example, was 15 per 1,000; the death rate was 9 per 1,000; the rate of natural increase was 0.6 percent; and the time it would take to double the existing population was 116 years. In the same year in Latin America, the birth rate was 36 per 1,000; the death rate was 9 per 1,000; the rate of natural increase was 2.7 percent; and the doubling time was only 26 years.

These very different rates of population growth can be broadly attributed to two trends. (1) Birth rates tend to drop as the standard of living rises, so that the most affluent populations have the lowest birth rates. (2) In the less developed nations, greater control of disease, better sanitation, safer water supplies, better housing, and improved nutrition have contributed to lower infant mortality. Decreased death rates, combined with high fertility, have brought spectacular population increases in Asia, Africa, and South America.

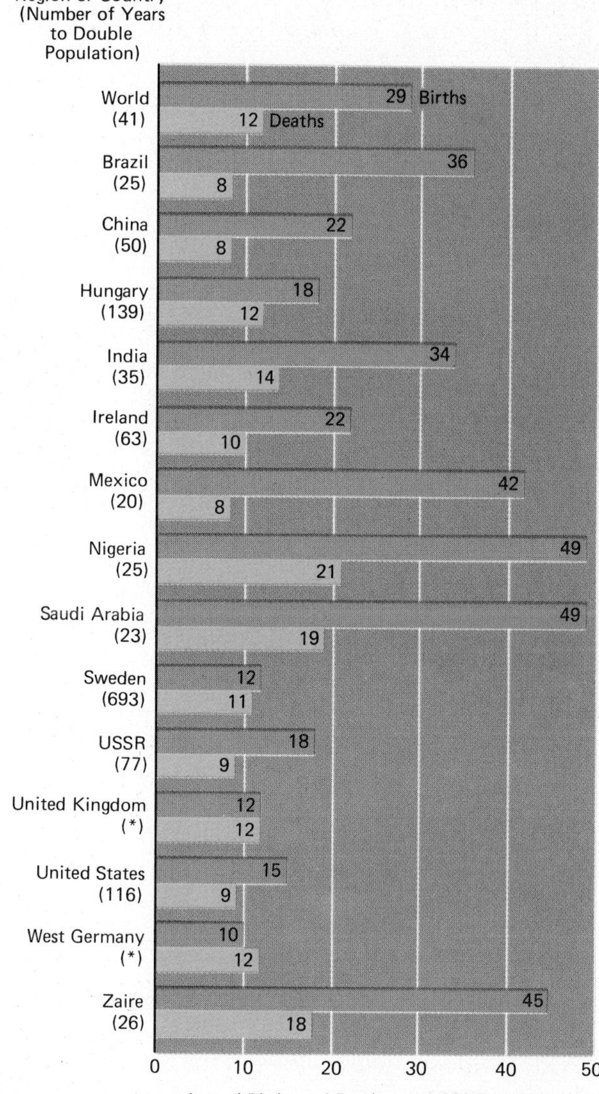

Figure 17.7 World population figures for selected countries, 1978. Note that in the United Kingdom and West Germany, the birth rate and the death rate are so close that these countries are experiencing zero or negative population growth.

*Indicates zero or negative growth.

Humanity at the Crossroads

The addition of millions of new human beings to the earth each year brings numerous prob-

VIEWPOINT

Solar Energy—A Viable Alternative?

In the past decade or so, as concern about the environment has become widespread and our traditional energy sources—notably oil—have become scarcer and more costly, growing numbers of Americans have become interested in developing new types of energy that are clean, inexpensive, and "home grown" (to free us from dependence on imported fuels). Probably the best known of the proposed alternatives is *solar energy*—energy from the sun.

The sun is a virtually limitless source of energy. The sunlight that reaches the earth in *one day* can meet the whole planet's energy needs for *fifteen years!* And sunlight is clean. Unlike fossil fuels such as coal and oil, which must be burned to generate heat, the sun's rays need only be trapped by plates called *collectors* to achieve the same effect.

Several foreign countries are already harnessing solar power very extensively. Japan, for example, has over 2 million homes with solar water heaters, and Israel has 250,000. Niger, a developing nation in arid West Africa, requires solar water heaters in all new hospitals, hotels, schools, and housing for government personnel.

In the United States, solar energy has been put to use, but we are lagging far behind these other countries. In spite of the increasing arguments for solar energy, it has not yet become a substantial part of our energy program. A major factor is economics; solar energy is still inefficient and expensive compared to conventional sources of power. But many Americans are also heavily committed—both economically and psychologically—to our prevailing forms of energy and are reluctant to consider solar as a realistic option.

The federal government now offers tax incentives to individuals and businesses who install solar energy systems, ranging from simple collectors for heating water and home or work spaces to far more complex projects, such as power plants, that convert sunlight into electricity. Thirty-seven states are also awarding tax credits to encourage use of solar power. California's incentive is by far the largest, so, not surprisingly, about one-third of all solar systems in the United States are located there, supplying power to homes, apartment complexes, and a wide variety of industries—including a winery.

Of course, California receives more direct sunlight than most other states, but solar energy is feasible even in areas that receive relatively little sunshine, such as New England. Although solar power is less efficient in less sunny areas, home heating requirements in these regions are generally greater, so it can be used as a cost-effective supplement to conventional types of energy.

Solar energy is still a revolutionary idea to many people, but it is likely to begin to fulfill an increasing proportion of our energy requirements—possibly as much as 10 or 15 percent by the year 2000. Not only is solar power clean and inexhaustible, but it has another point in its favor. As former Secretary of Energy James R. Schlesinger has commented, "Solar has captured the public's imagination."

lems. How are these people to be fed, clothed, and sheltered? How can energy be made available to everyone, and how can increased waste products be disposed of? What, if any, responsibility do the rich nations have to the poor nations? How will political stability, environmental conditions, and worldwide public health be affected by these population trends?

The food problem is one of the most significant of these questions. The gap between the rich and poor nations is certainly clear in terms of the food that people have available to eat. One-third of the world's population lives in the industrialized nations, uses about 85 percent of the world's annual resources, and enjoys an overabundance of many different kinds of food. By and large, these populations are well nourished, even overnourished. The other two-thirds of the people in the world live in the less industrialized nations, use about 15 percent of the world's resources, and suffer from chronic poverty, lifelong malnutrition, and starvation.

Part of the solution to the food problem

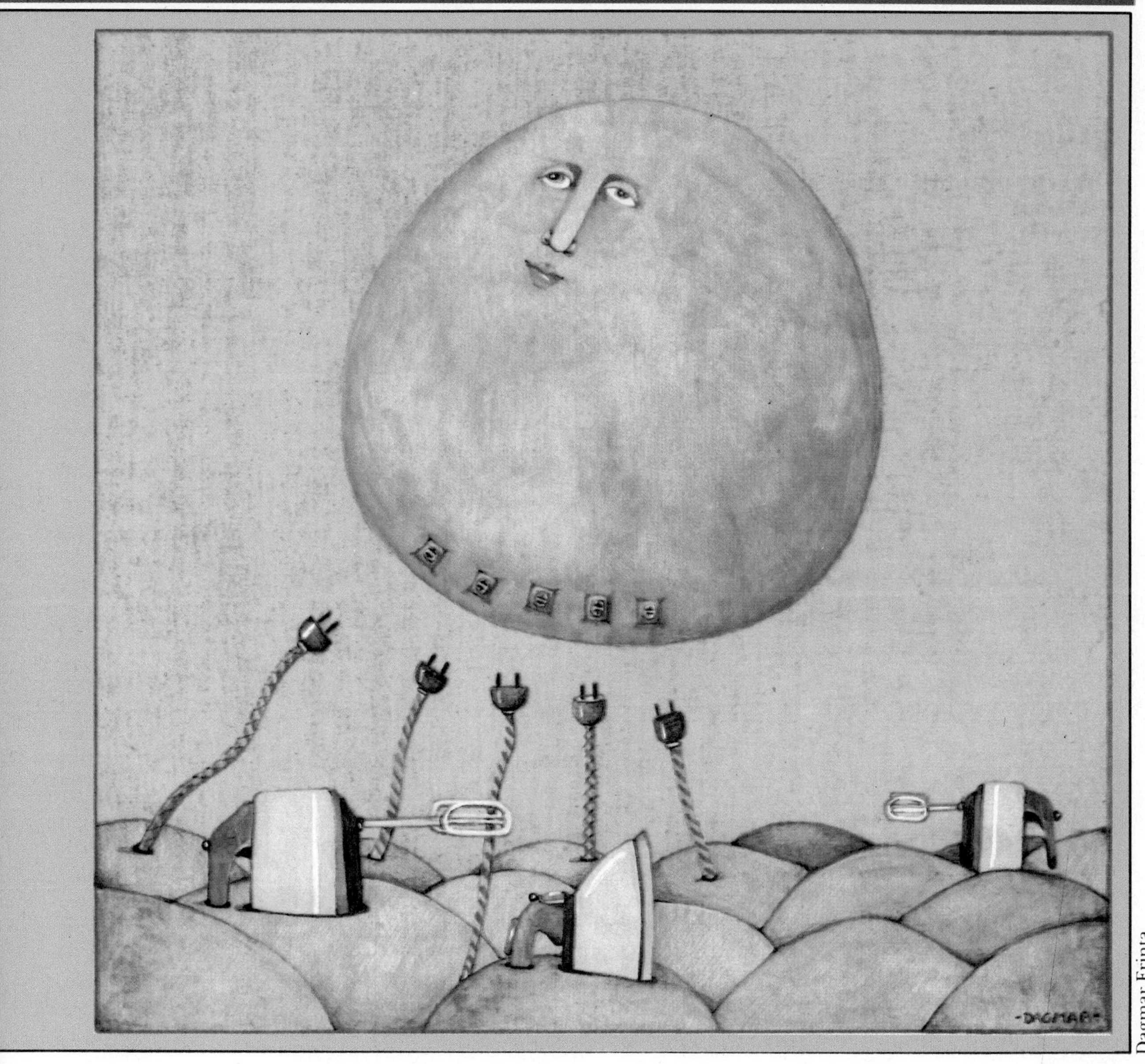

Dagmar Frinta

could be to create the economic and political climate that would allow excess food to be sold or given to the poor nations and to develop the transportation and distribution facilities needed to get the food to hungry people. Another part of the solution could be to increase food production so that it outstripped population growth. In recent years, population growth has offset whatever gains have been made in food production.

What is being done to increase food production so that it can outstrip population gains? Advances in agricultural technology—the "Green Revolution"—have been significant in the past few decades. New crop varieties that are high in yield and adaptable to different climates have been bred. Pesticides and herbicides have helped reduce insect and plant pests. New fertilizers, improved methods of irrigation and cultivation, and more sophisticated weather forecasting have all contributed to the production of more food. This technology has contributed to dramatic rises in food production in some areas. Unfortunately,

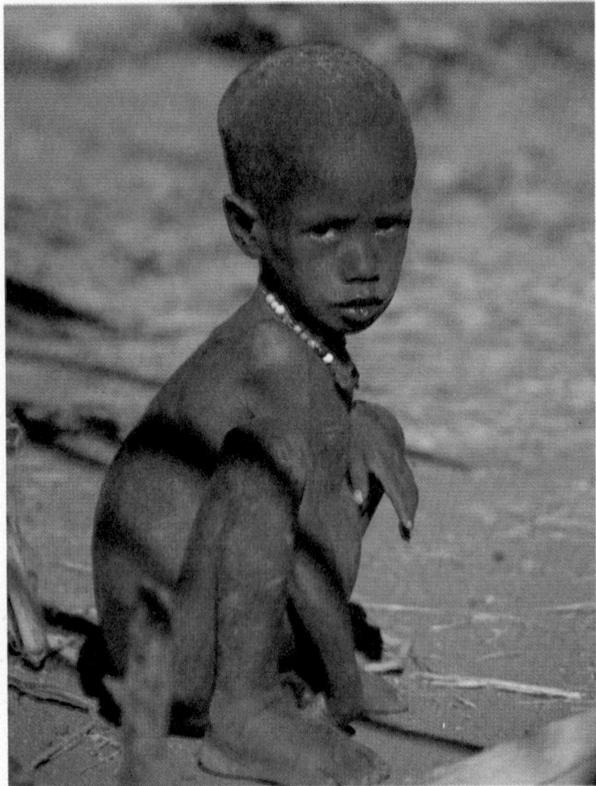

Figure 17.8 A majority of the people in the world live in chronic poverty and suffer lifelong malnutrition despite surplus food production in the more industrialized countries. The "Green Revolution," which through agricultural advances has produced healthier and more abundant crop yields, will only be meaningful when food can be produced and distributed in those areas where it is most needed.

many of these advances are least available where they are most needed, and none of them is useful in every agricultural situation.

SOLVING THE PROBLEMS OF THE ENVIRONMENT

The problems surveyed in this chapter are among the most persistent and pressing ever faced by humankind. It is tempting to think in terms of sweeping answers, and rather simplistic solutions are often offered. But these problems are incredibly complex, not only in themselves but in their economic and political ramifications. This section touches briefly on some of the complexities involved in solving the problems of health in the environment. Some people believe that all environmental problems can be solved with new technology, but technological solutions may create new difficulties. Sometimes the technology has an unexpected side effect; earlier we mentioned the development of insect strains that are resistant to pesticides. Sometimes the solution involves a tradeoff; the new high-yield crops, for example, need careful management because they are not as disease and pest resistant as the lower-yielding varieties they have replaced. And in some cases, a technological solution may be worse than the problem; some experts who opposed the banning of DDT fear that the chemicals developed to replace it will be even more dangerous to the environment.

Another practical dilemma raised by the search for solutions to environmental problems has to do with the credibility of the scientific community. Sometimes experts simply disagree about what the facts are. We have seen that some scientists believe that low-level radiation is harmless, while others insist that it could be extremely hazardous. Experts also disagree about whether there is a threshold level beneath which exposure to carcinogenic substances will not cause cancer. When disagreements such as these are publicly aired, people may become confused and cynical because they do not know who to believe. Once science loses credibility, it also loses some of its ability to participate in the education needed to solve environmental problems.

INDIVIDUAL ACTION

The consequences of most environmental problems are long-term. As long as the average person has air, water, and food and feels relatively healthy, the highly publicized dangers do not seem very real. And the effects that are most immediate and noticeable (odors, noise, dirt) are often easily tolerated. Thus many people may make an effort to contribute to some collective action (recycling programs, antilitter campaigns), but most people are not strongly motivated to make changes in their lives as precautions against environmentally induced disease.

Theoretically, each individual has an "optimal environment"—one that meets all needs for space and for physical and mental health. To a certain extent, then, each person must see to it that the environment caters to these specific needs. A person with respiratory difficulties will be concerned about breathable air; a person with high sensitivity to certain chemicals will need to be careful in handling chemical products; a critic of the automobile can find alternate means of transportation.

One need not be an environmental expert to make intelligent use of information such as that provided in this chapter. Once sensitized to the types of health hazards prevalent in the environment, the individual can take greater precautions in using pesticides, can eat a varied diet to avoid overexposure to certain chemicals, and can avoid noxious gases and noises in the working environment. Positive activities of all sorts are possible. You can use a smaller car and therefore less gas; car-pooling is another way to conserve our petroleum resources. Becoming aware of overpackaging and planned obsolescence might lead a person to boycott products that are overwrapped—such as the fast-food hamburger, which is wrapped in paper, placed in Styrofoam, and put in a bag, only to be unwrapped and eaten minutes later. One can use cloth napkins instead of paper. The possibilities are endless.

The knowledge that we are able to deal effectively with some environmental hazards not only helps to take away some of the fears that have been generated in past years but also contributes to feelings of self-worth and efficacy. And it reinforces the will to apply our own ounce of pressure toward changing collective ways.

SUMMARY

1. The hazards of a particular chemical depend on the volume at which it is produced, the rate at which it is released into the environment, the intrinsic properties that determine its movement through the environment, the extent to which it accumulates, its chemical stability, and its toxicity.
2. Setting a "safe" level of exposure to chemicals is difficult; people differ in their sensitivity to chemicals and scientists sometimes disagree about the safety of a given dose level of a particular chemical.
3. Hazardous chemicals in the modern environment include asbestos, mercury, lead, pesticides, and herbicides. Workers in contact with these chemicals are under particular danger. Technology is being developed to identify carcinogenic substances before workers are exposed to them.
4. Pollution refers to biological, physical, and chemical wastes that contaminate the environment. Biodegradable substances lend themselves to breakdown and assimilation by the environment; nonbiodegradable substances are more persistent.
5. Major air pollutants include fuel combustion, chemical processing, and the burning of wastes. Those with the greatest health-threatening potential are sulfur oxides, nitrogen oxides, carbon monoxide, hydrocarbons, and fluorocarbons.
6. The long-term effects of specific pollutants are unknown. The damage of air pollutants is exerted on the eyes, throat, and circulatory system. Those suffering from chronic bronchitis or emphysema are subject to the greatest danger.
7. Several kinds of water pollution contribute to the process of eutrophication—the depleting of oxygen in a body of water.
8. Solid waste pollution includes discarded materials; solid waste products of agriculture, mining, and manufacturing; and the solid products of pollution control devices.
9. Noise pollution may result in hearing problems, fatigue, loss of sleep, and stress.
10. Nuclear power has presented a series of hazards including the possibility of mishap, the disposal of radioactive waste products, the emission of radon, and the emission of low levels of radiation during normal operation.
11. The effect of radiation exposure depends on the dose, the length of exposure, the type of radiation, and the individual's degree of sensitivity. Studies indicate that there may be no safe level of radiation exposure.
12. To meet food needs of the future food production must increase more than population growth. Possible solutions may lie in agricultural technology or in more equitable worldwide distribution of food.

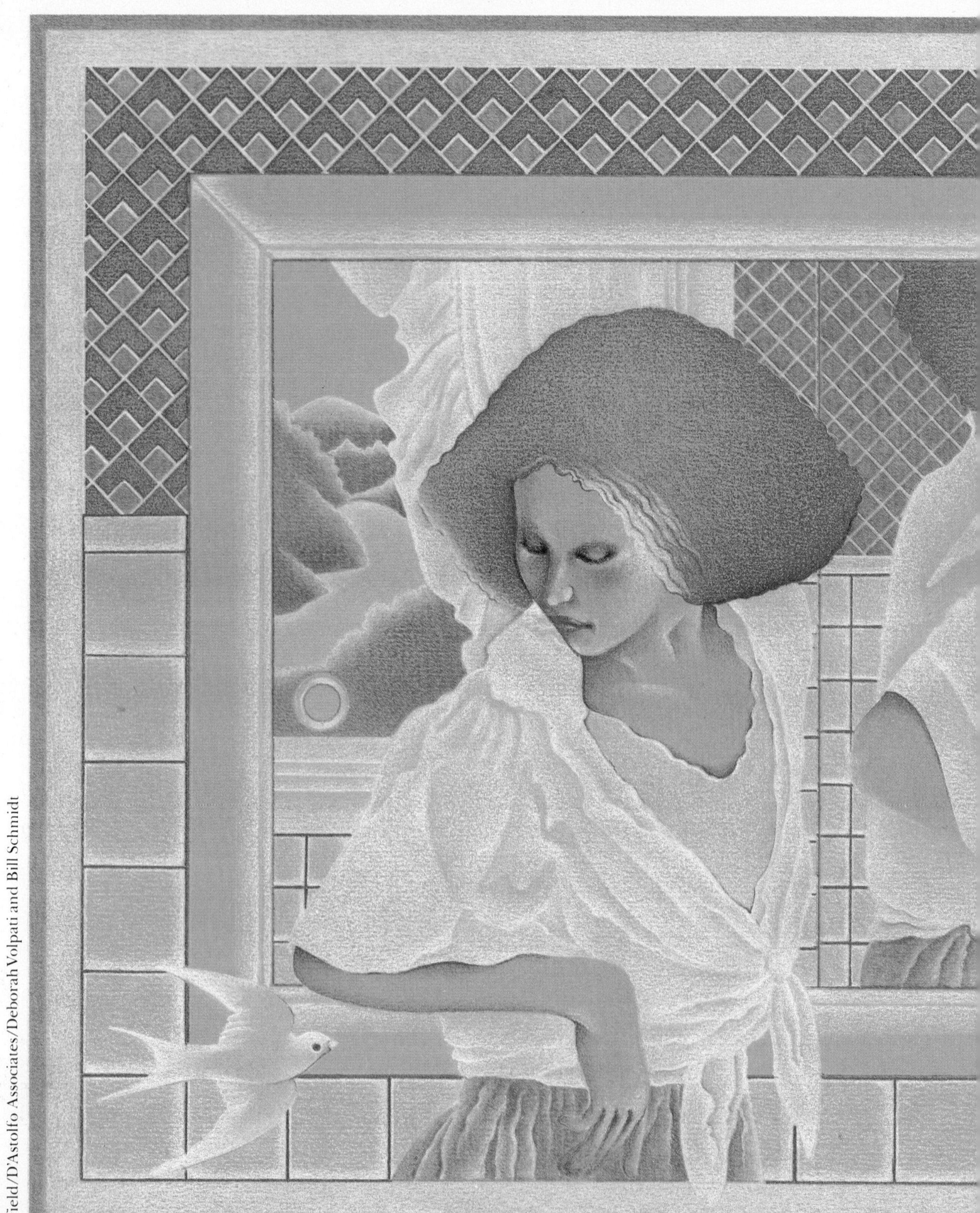

Infield/D'Astolfo Associates/Deborah Volpati and Bill Schmidt

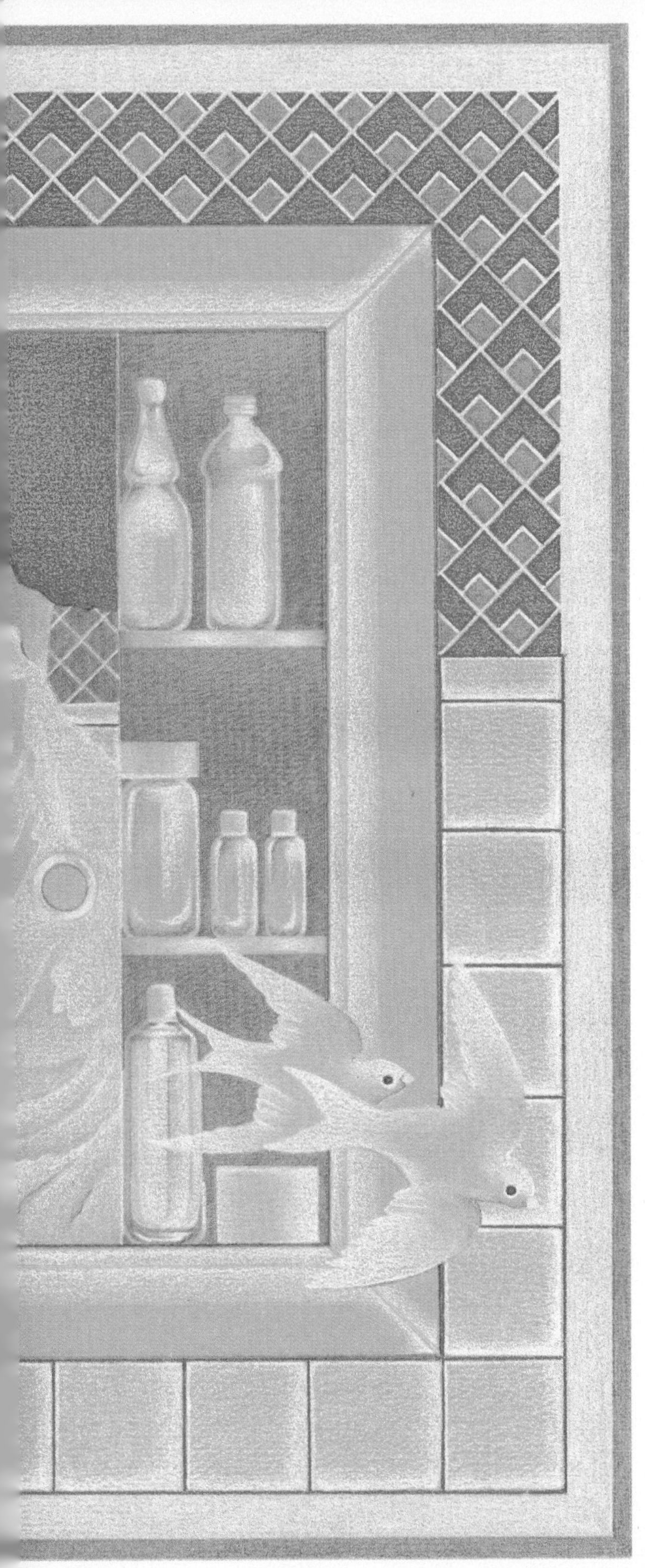

18 Health Care and the Consumer

Health care is big business in the United States —and it's getting even bigger. Americans spend more on health care than any other people, and costs continue to skyrocket. In 1965, the nation spent $38.9 billion ($198 per person) on hospital bills, physicians' fees, laboratory tests, and other health care. This year the figure is over $200 billion—nearly 10 percent of the Gross National Product—and this upward trend shows no sign of slowing down.

The rising costs of health care have contributed not only to a growing scrutiny of our health-care system, but also to the return of self-care. The medical advances of the twentieth century led many people to think that pills could magically cure every ailment and to accept whatever their doctors told them. In the past few years, however, more and more people have begun to take an active role in their own care and to ask their doctors more and better questions. People are realizing that we all have primary responsibility for our own well-being.

In this chapter we will examine the benefits and drawbacks of our health-care system. We will look at the community's role in health care, the quality of medical care in the United States, the complex problems of health-care delivery, and suggestions that have been proposed for improving the system. We will also look at the goals and pitfalls of self-care, the skills you need to develop, how to choose and talk to a doctor, and how to protect yourself against quacks.

HEALTH CARE AS A HUMAN RIGHT

Is health care a right or a privilege? Translated into dollars and cents, the question is: Who should pay for health care—the individual, the employer, the community, or the government? In the United States the view that health care is a basic human right and that society, rather than the individual or the family, is responsible for providing it has evolved only within the last few decades. This new concept of health care has developed out of many changes in our society: advances in medical technology, increased national affluence, increases in medical costs, the greater availability of effective health remedies, evolving social organizations, and an intensified awareness of our dependence on one another.

Our attitudes and, indeed, our health problems were quite different at the turn of the century. Then, average life expectancy was forty-seven years, and our most serious medical problems were acute infectious diseases such as diphtheria, tuberculosis, rheumatic fever, typhoid, influenza, and pneumonia. Most Americans lived in small towns and were served by a general practitioner who made house calls and dispensed affordable—but not very effective—medical care from a little black bag. At that time, it was not unusual to know most of the people in your town. If you needed assistance, you turned first to your neighbors. Welfare, social security, unemployment insurance, and health insurance were all unheard of.

Today, on the other hand, we can prevent many infectious diseases by immunization and cure infections when they do develop. The major killers are the chronic degenerative conditions such as heart disease, cancer, and stroke—diseases of life style, which no vaccination can prevent. Most Americans now live in large cities, often far from their extended families. Many of us do not even know our neighbors. In time of illness, few of us can look to relatives or neighbors for help and care. And there are few general practitioners. Most physicians are specialists and provide expensive medical care in offices, clinics, or hospitals, where elaborate equipment and supporting staff are available (see Table 18.1). The relationship between the health-care system and the public is marked by paternalism rather than partnership.

Table 18.1 Estimated Number of Persons Employed Within Each Health Field, 1974

Health Field	Number
Administration of health services	48,200
Anthropology and sociology	1,700
Automatic data processing in the health field	4,000–5,000
Basic sciences in the health field	60,000
Biomedical engineering	12,000
Chiropractic	16,600
Clinical laboratory services	172,500
Dentistry and allied services	279,800
Dietetic and nutritional services	72,700
Economic research in the health field	400
Environmental sanitation	20,000
Food and drug protective services	47,900
Funeral directors and embalmers	50,000
Health and vital statistics	1,350
Health education	22,500–23,000
Health information and communication	7,400–10,500
Library services in the health field	10,300
Medical records	60,000
Medicine and osteopathy (M.D. and D.O.)	362,700
Midwifery	4,300
Nursing and related services	2,319,000
Occupational therapy	13,500–14,500
Opticianry	12,000
Optometry	25,100–25,300
Orthotic and prosthetic technology	2,800–3,800
Pharmacy	132,900
Physical therapy	26,100
Podiatric medicine	7,100
Psychology	35,000
Radiologic technology	100,000
Respiratory therapy	18,000–19,000
Secretarial and office services in the health field	275,000–300,000
Social work	38,600
Specialized rehabilitation services	11,250–13,250
Speech pathology and audiology	27,000
Veterinary medicine	33,500
Vocational rehabilitation counseling	17,700
Miscellaneous health services	323,950
Total	4,672,850–4,707,-650

Source: Department of Health, Education, and Welfare, *Health United States, 1976–1977* (Washington, D.C.: U.S. Government Printing Office, 1977), p. 304.

It is not only the form but the very nature of

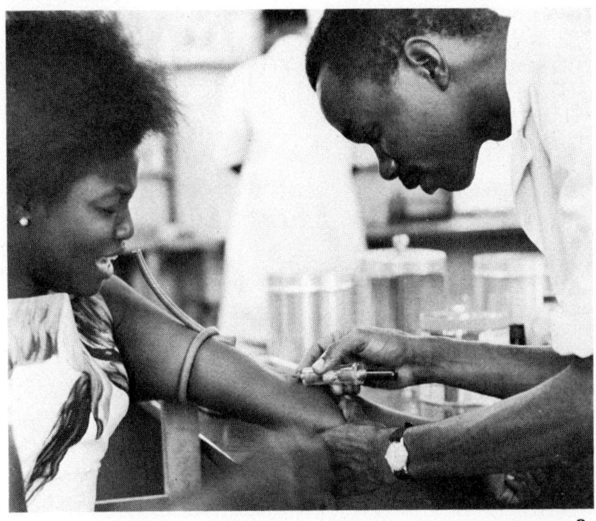

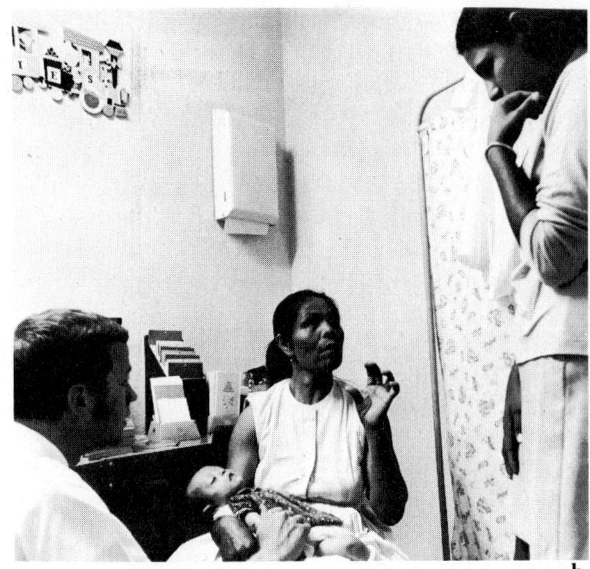

Figure 18.1 Free clinics have enabled the poor to receive good health care, as well as information about preventive care (a). These and other community-based clinics are responsive to the special health needs of the population that they serve. Here a mother at the free clinic for migrant workers in San Joaquin Valley, California, describes her health problems with the aid of an interpreter (b).

our health problems that has changed. Population growth, industrial expansion, and great leaps in technological development have all contributed to serious pollution problems and other ecological changes. Increasingly we face a host of new medical problems that transcend individual, familial, or communal powers—notably cancers and other diseases caused by pollutants and radiation (see Chapter 17). Thus, we have begun to think about how to rework our system of health care so that care will be provided and guaranteed for all. Given the escalating cost of medical care, finding viable solutions is especially urgent.

THE ROLE OF COMMUNITIES

The community can no longer be primarily responsible for the health care of its members, as it was at the turn of the century, but community action can sometimes bring swift and significant health-care reforms. Indeed, a new kind of health activism is growing in communities across the country. For example, in New York City, thousands of children in poorly kept buildings have suffered lead poisoning from eating the lead-based paint that peeled off cracked walls and windowsills (see Chapter 17). Residents brought pressure on the city government to provide free testing for slum children so that the poisoning could be detected early, before brain damage occurred. This testing was promised but was slow in being established, until a group of young Puerto Rican activists managed to put mobile units on the streets to test children for poisoning. This action aroused enough publicity to ensure that the city's program would be made more effective and instituted more promptly.

One of the most promising expressions of this new community involvement is the "community clinic" program. Community clinics have sprung up in most major cities, especially in poor areas. These clinics are largely community run, often with the aid of volunteer doctors and nurses, and much of the record-keeping work is done by local, nonprofessional people who are known and trusted. These clinics are often better able than large urban hospital clinics to bring people in for treatment before their problems become acute. But community clinics do not always succeed; many are very short-lived. And many other neighborhood health centers remain in operation only as long as grant subsidies from government or private agencies are able to support them. Although the full effectiveness of community clinics is far from proven, they undoubtedly demonstrate the changing attitude of communities toward the health care of their members.

Future Role of the Community

It appears clear that community health efforts are developing in two important directions. First, *consumer representation* in decision-making bodies is growing, particularly with regard to the identification of community health problems and the allocation of resources to deal with them. The effectiveness of health institutions requires renewed cooperation between communities and health-care providers, as well as the reduction of bureaucratic procedures that tend to alienate organizations and people.

Second, *community organization* of individuals and agencies sharing similar health concerns is developing. Such organizations plan and exercise sharply focused programs and also rally political support. In this way, they break through traditional and bureaucratic resistance to change. For example, Ralph Nader's Public Interest Research Group has branches throughout the nation, which use both consumer representation and community organization to effect needed change in a variety of health areas. This group has been responsible for remarkable and speedy upgrading of the care of chronically ill patients in nursing homes.

HEALTH-CARE DELIVERY: A HOST OF PROBLEMS

The deficiency in the American medical-care system is not one of quality; the United States has the finest facilities anywhere in the world, and American medical research is second to none. The deficiency lies in the *delivery system*—the inability to bring this excellent medical care equally to *all* people. A close look at the present system reveals that this inability stems from a whole set of problems, ranging from inefficient distribution of personnel to skyrocketing costs.

Inefficient Distribution of Physicians

American physicians have long been allowed, if not encouraged, to practice where and for whom they want. As a result, the availability of physicians varies greatly from state to state and from one area to another within a given state, and there are often gross inadequacies and inefficient distribution of personnel. South Dakota, for example, has about one-third as many physicians relative to its population as has New York State—78 per 100,000 people compared with 198 per 100,000. A study of four upper Midwest states disclosed that more than 1,000 remote towns, because of their small size and declining economic condition, do not have a single physician. One area in Los Angeles County has a physician-population ratio of 9 per 100,000 compared with about 1,800 per 100,000 in Beverly Hills and 175 per 100,000 for the whole country. The shocking truth is that today millions of Americans are receiving inadequate health care—or none at all.

This haphazard availability of medical service cannot be blamed solely on the physicians. Being in business for themselves, physicians tend to establish their practices where they most want to live and where they are assured of patients who can pay their bills. Unless incentives are provided for physicians to practice in underserviced areas, the inequitable distribution of health services must be expected to continue, if not intensify.

When we consider the availability of physicians to the average patient, we must also remember that specialists outnumber general practitioners by approximately four to one. The ratio of specialists to general practitioners will, if anything, worsen, because only 12 percent of medical school graduates in recent years have been entering general practice.

Inadequate Health Insurance Coverage

More people than ever before—80 percent of the population—are covered by some form of health insurance, but there are still 18 million Americans without any coverage and most policies have severe limitations—many cover only hospital care and not visits to a doctor's

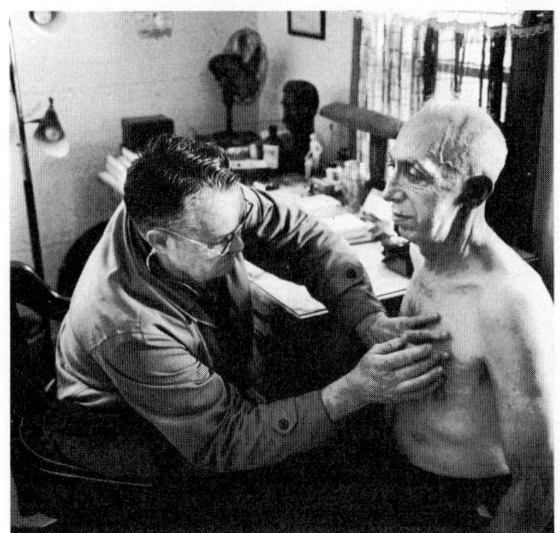

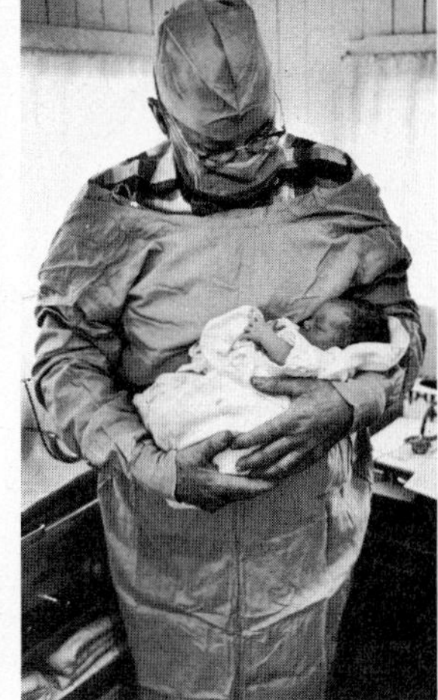

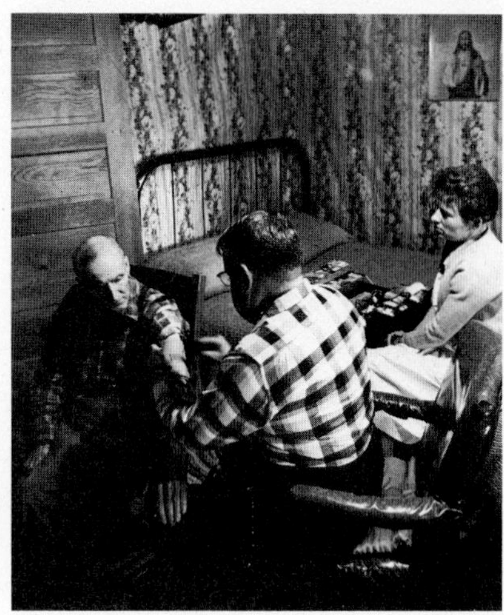

Figure 18.2 In the three photographs above are pictured the diverse tasks of the rural doctor. The rural doctor must, by necessity, practice general medicine, whereas the urban doctor can have a specialized practice in one area of medicine.

office, for example. Income and employer are major factors in determining how much and what kind of health insurance protection a family has. Of all persons in families with incomes of $15,000 or more, 92 percent carry some insurance, but only 41 percent in families with incomes between $3,000 and $5,000 and 37 percent in families with incomes under $3,000 have any health coverage.

There are more than 1,700 different insurance carriers, offering a bewildering array of health insurance policies that are beyond the comprehension of most Americans. The result is that millions of people who believe they are covered have serious gaps in their health protection. Many others have double, or overlapping, coverage. More than 22 million have double coverage for hospital expenses, more than 20 million have double coverage for surgical expenses, and nearly 11 million have double coverage for regular medical expenses. Yet most insurance companies will not pay a claim if it is paid by another company, so double coverage is usually a complete waste of money.

What portion of the health-care bill does health insurance pay? The government pays 55 percent of hospital bills, 24 percent of doctors' bills; consumers pay approximately 6 percent of hospital bills, 39 percent of doctors' bills; and private health insurance pays only about 37 percent of hospital and doctors' bills. It is not surprising, therefore, that medical bills are the leading cause of bankruptcy in the United States today.

The High Cost of Health Care

We have already touched upon the high cost of health care in the United States. In 1979, the nation was spending 9.1 percent of its Gross National Product on health care—more than $920 per person. Many factors are involved in the escalation of health-care expenditures. Some parallel national inflationary trends. But others are specifically related to health-care activities, so health costs are inflating faster than other prices. Between 1950 and 1977, physicians' fees rose 43 percent faster that the prices of nonmedical goods and services. Let's take a look at some of the major components of health care and examine why costs are so high and whether resources are wasted or misused.

Hospitalization *Hospitalization* accounts for the largest portion of health expenditures, and its costs are among the fastest rising—increas-

Table 18.2 Personal Health-Care Expenditures, By Source of Payment, 1976

Type of Expenditure	All Personal Health-Care Expenditures	Direct Payment	Third-Party Payment			
			Total	Private Health Insurance	Government	Philanthropy and Industry
			Amount in Millions			
Total	$120,431	$39,099	$81,332	$31,359	$48,417	$1,556
Hospital care	55,400	4,909	50,491	19,443	30,396	652
Physician services	26,350	10,198	16,152	9,502	6,632	18
Dentist services	8,600	6,970	1,630	1,160	469	0
Drugs	11,168	9,423	1,745	721	1,023	0
Other health services	18,913	7,598	11,316	533	9,896	886
			Per Capita Amount			
Total	$551.50	$179.05	$372.46	$143.61	$221.72	$7.13
Hospital care	253.70	22.48	231.22	89.04	139.20	2.98
Physician services	120.67	46.70	73.97	43.51	30.37	0.08
Dentist services	39.38	31.92	7.46	5.31	2.15	0.00
Drugs	51.14	43.15	7.99	3.30	4.69	0.00
Other health services	86.61	34.79	51.82	2.44	45.32	4.06

Source: Department of Health, Education, and Welfare, *Health United States, 1976–1977* (Washington, D.C.: U.S. Government Printing Office, 1977), p. 364.

ing three times as fast as the general cost of living. Why?

There are several good reasons why hospitals are so expensive. First, regardless of how many beds are filled, there are many fixed costs that a hospital must pay: emergency rooms with expensive equipment that sits idle most of the time but that must be ready twenty-four hours a day; operating rooms; salaries for administration, nurses, and supporting staff; heating, cooling, lighting, and custodial costs; and so on. Second, a hospital is a workshop for doctors, who need and expect up-to-date, sophisticated equipment to be available. Third, hospital patients count on first-rate care; the average patient is attended by three to five highly qualified staff members.

However, hospital costs are probably a good deal higher than they need be. For one thing, hospitals have traditionally been built without careful regard to need. We now have some 100,000 unused hospital beds in the United States, and the cost of maintaining these empty beds is between 60 and 70 percent of the cost of maintaining the occupied beds! The problem is not only that we have overbuilt, but also that, again, distribution is haphazard; we don't make the most efficient use of the beds we have.

There is another complicating factor: many patients in hospitals today do not need to be there. It is believed that approximately 30 percent of the patients in hospitals could be adequately cared for in less expensive facilities, or even at home. Furthermore, because most health insurance policies do not cover out-of-hospital expenses, physicians often admit their patients to the hospital for routine tests that could be performed on an outpatient basis. And acute, or short-term, hospital care is the most expensive type of health care available—currently more than $200 a day (and charges of $500 a day are not unusual).

Third, many hospitals seem to be in an equipment arms race. Each hospital wants to have its own equipment no matter how expensive it is or how infrequently it will be needed. Yet some equipment could be shared with minimal inconvenience by several adjacent metropolitan hospitals. Such cooperation would increase usage and reduce costs and waste significantly.

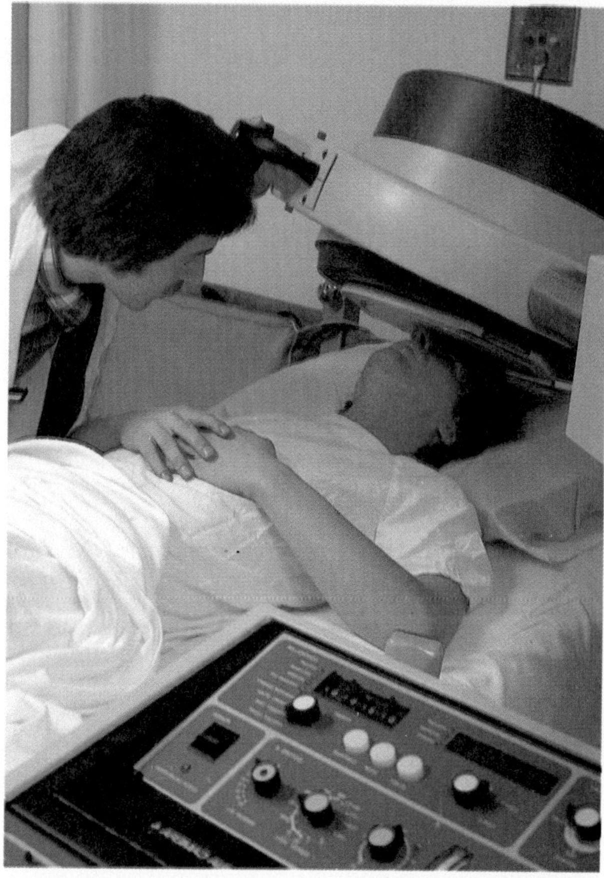

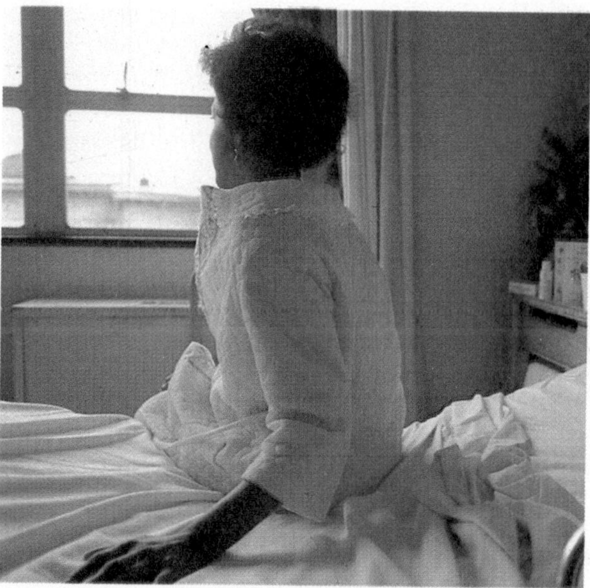

Figure 18.3 Hospital care is extremely expensive partly because of the cost of the complex machinery needed for diagnosis and treatment. Expenses could be reduced if hospitals shared equipment and treated as outpatients those people who require simple tests or procedures.

Surgery Surgery is a second major area of medical care, and some critics believe that it is needlessly encouraged by our present system of health care. They point to the fact that while most insurance policies do not pay for medical services provided outside the hospital, they do provide dollar allowances for surgery. In addition, surgeons' incomes are generally dependent on how many operations they perform. And many patients feel more satisfied—and healthier—if they undergo some surgical procedure. Thus, there are more pressures—from all sides—to operate than there are not to operate.

There is evidence that a good deal of unnecessary surgery is performed in the United States. When surgeons are on salary and the decision to operate is based solely on medical considerations, the incidence of surgery has been seen to drop to 50 percent of the amount of surgery performed by physicians paid on a fee-for-operation basis. And in the United States, tonsillectomies—usually elective operations—amount to 6 percent of all operations; in Sweden, where surgeons are on salary, the same operation accounts for only 1 percent of total surgery. Unnecessary surgery means unnecessary surgeons' fees, unnecessary hospitalization, and unnecessary risk to the patient's health or life.

Unnecessary operations in the United States have a high price tag—an estimated $4 billion and 10,000 deaths each year. In light of these figures, a 1978 government report recommended that HEW require Medicare and Medicaid patients to consult a second doctor before undergoing elective surgery (e.g., nonessential hysterectomy or removal of the gall bladder, adenoids, or tonsils). And many health insurance carriers have begun to pay for second opinions when elective surgery is involved.

THE QUALITY OF MEDICAL CARE

Because of the complex and demanding nature of medical care, it is difficult for the average person to judge its quality. In the past, therefore, it was always the professionals themselves who policed their own members by exercising exclusive control over the education, licensing and certification, and practice of their skills. In recent years, however, several other factors have become important in promoting the quality of medical care.

1. The federal government is playing a more active role in determining whether the public is getting its money's worth.
2. The public is more concerned with nonscientific aspects of the quality of care—for example, having a Spanish-speaking person available during the examination of a Spanish-speaking patient, having medical offices open in the evening to serve working people, or having doctors explain their findings to patients in everyday language.
3. The rising costs of medical care are making it difficult for many families to afford expensive treatments.
4. Medical care has evolved into a business, and financial considerations may influence a health worker's judgment about a particular problem.
5. The expanding use of malpractice suits by the public has raised questions about negligence in the practice of medicine.

IMPROVING THE SYSTEM

Improving Distribution of Health Care

Most physicians have avoided practicing in poor or rural areas for a variety of reasons, primarily economic. However, it is now possible for physicians to earn almost as much money in such areas as they can in urban or well-to-do communities. The main barrier to a more efficient distribution of physicians is now essentially one of preference: urban areas tend to provide a doctor with better facilities, more opportunities to socialize with colleagues, a better school system for his or her children, and so on. It is also easier for an urban physician to arrange for free time because other doctors can take over patients for short periods.

One way to improve distribution of physicians is to grant scholarships and fellowships to students who agree to practice in underserviced areas upon qualification or to cancel the educational debts of physicians and dentists serving in such areas. A second possibility is to make it more financially rewarding for physicians and allied professionals to set up practice in needy areas. The Canadian province of Ontario, for example, provides financial assistance to doctors and dentists who establish and maintain a practice in areas designated as underserviced. The province guarantees them an annual net income when assigned to one of these areas, making up any deficit in this assured income. Of course, the practitioner keeps any income that exceeds the guaranteed amount.

Group Practice

One suggestion for reforming our health-care system is the concept of group practice. A *group practice* is an organization of full-time physicians and other health professionals who work as a team, sharing their skills and knowledge and using the same buildings, equipment, laboratory, and technicians. They divide their total group income according to a prearranged plan, which may be a fee-for-service system for each doctor, a salary system for all the doctors, or some intermediate arrangement. Group practice is cooperative rather than competitive medicine. It is a method of organization already used by a number of leading clinics and medical centers associated with educational or charitable institutions.

Some advantages of group practice for the patient are these:

1. Most services are provided under one roof.
2. The consumer can be assured of having a physician who has been selected by other doctors and who performs under the watchful eyes of colleagues, an effective promoter of quality care.
3. Physicians may be on salary, so medical decisions are less dependent on monetary considerations.

4. Services are available on a twenty-four-hour basis every day of the year.
5. If a patient's personal physician is not available or moves away, a competent doctor from the same team will be at hand, with direct access to the patient's medical records.
6. Referral for consultation is easily arranged, usually with minimal stress to the patient.

Health Maintenance Organizations

An approach that combines improved medical practice and improved financial coverage is the *health maintenance organization,* or *HMO.* HMOs are usually group practices in which patients receive their health care in return for a monthly fee that is paid in advance. Three well-known examples of HMOs are the Health Insurance Plan of Greater New York, the Group Health Cooperative of Puget Sound, in the Seattle area, and the Kaiser Foundation Medical Care Program based in San Diego, California. Together the three plans care for about 5 million patients. In the United States, there are now approximately 175 HMOs functioning in thirty-six states. They service over 6 million patients.

For the consumer, HMOs offer special advantages. Administrative red tape (claim forms and bills, for example) is virtually eliminated. Consumers know what their medical care and hospitalization costs are going to be because they are on a fixed monthly rate. This opportunity to budget is an advantage regardless of who pays for the health coverage—the individual, the employer, the community, or the government.

HMOs encourage preventive medicine. With prepayment, each potential patient contributes to a fund in advance. Caring for illness takes money out of that fund, so that each case prevented or hospitalization avoided allows more money to remain in the fund. The physician may earn more money by promoting health, whereas under the fee-for-service system he or she earns income only when the patient is sick; conversely, the patient benefits from more extensive and costly treatment when needed, without exorbitant payments. HMOs offer about one-third more services per dollar than traditional programs offer.

Studies have shown that patients under HMOs have less frequent hospitalization, shorter periods of hospitalization, and less surgery than those under sole practitioners. In one study, the rate of appendectomies dropped 59 percent when teams of salaried physicians replaced practitioners paid on a fee-for-service basis. Another study compared utilization rates under Blue Cross/Blue Shield coverage with those of HMOs. The HMOs had 40 percent less hospitalization.

HMOs also stimulate competition. The hospitalization rate goes down when an HMO enters a community. Also, traditional health insurance companies expand their range of services to remain competitive. Unlike Blue Cross and other health insurance carriers, HMOs have been quite successful in limiting their cost increases, largely because people are treated on an outpatient basis whenever feasible.

Of course, HMOs are not a magical solution to health-care reform. Especially in its early years, the typical HMO is far from self-sufficient; it is likely to depend heavily on large federal grants or other subsidies.

Health Care vs. Sickness Care

The traditional medical-care delivery system has evolved slowly and randomly. In spite of remarkable medical advances in recent years, it remains virtually unchanged. Even though the population has increased and the problems have changed over the years, the point of entry into the medical-care system is still the physician. Under the traditional fee-for-service system, the patient has to pay for each visit to the doctor. This fee puts most people off seeing their doctor until they are really sick. It has effectively discouraged early entry into the system, which is essential for early treatment and preventive care. On the other hand, if the fee is replaced by a monthly payment, as in the HMOs, the physician is likely to spend far more time examining healthy people, which often frustrates doctors who have been trained to cure the sick.

One proposed solution to this problem is *triage,* a low-cost system for determining the

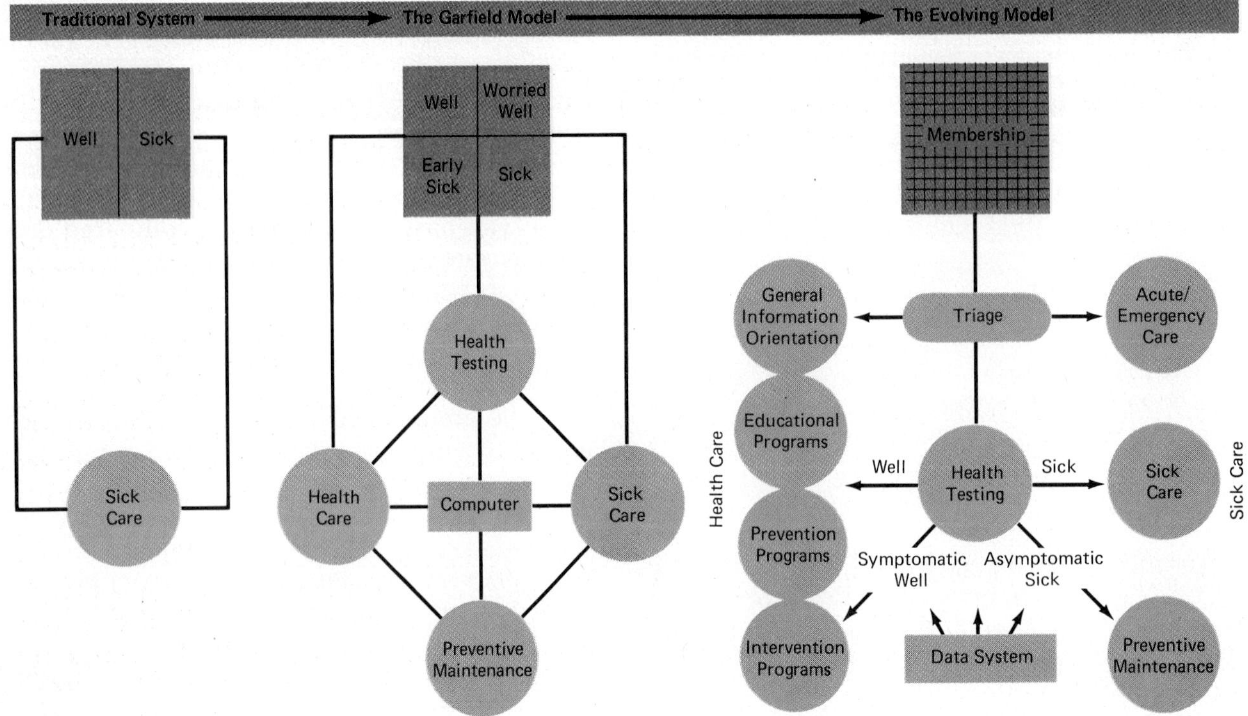

Figure 18.4 Evolution of a health-care delivery system. This diagram represents a model of the changing health-care delivery system as envisioned by researchers at the Kaiser-Permanente HMO program in San Jose, California. Note the presence of the "health care" component, as opposed to the "sick care" component, in the evolving model. Built into the model is the assumption that patient care in the medical system is improved when risk factors are identified and appropriate intervention is recommended at an early stage.

immediate needs of a patient and making an initial patient referral. Personnel on triage determine whether the patient needs acute or emergency care, health testing, or merely general health information that can be given over the telephone in the form of brief taped messages on specific topics.

Health testing takes the form of *multiphasic screening,* which combines a detailed computerized medical history and a series of diagnostic tests administered by paramedical personnel. These tests include a variety of measures, ranging from heart and thyroid function to neuromuscular and hearing checks. X-rays are taken, as well as a series of twenty blood-chemistry measurements. A computer indicates whether additional tests are needed or whether an immediate appointment with a doctor is advisable. Multiphasic screening also detects symptomless and early illness and provides doctors with a preliminary survey and a basic health profile for future reference.

Triage and multiphasic screening separate the well from the sick, and establish entry priorities. They permit maximal use of paramedical personnel, free physicians to treat patients who are seriously ill and require expert medical training, and considerably reduce doctor and hospital costs. Figure 18.4 illustrates the evolution of a delivery system that makes use of triage and health testing as the entry point.

The triage approach is based on two basic principles of health care:

1. The earlier an illness is detected, the greater the probability of effective diagnosis and treatment.
2. The greater the accuracy in predicting which individuals are likely to contract a given illness, the greater the chances of preventing that illness from developing.

National Health Insurance and a National Health Service

The United States is the only industrialized country without a comprehensive program of government health insurance or a national health service. National health insurance was instituted in Germany in 1883, in the United Kingdom in 1911, in France in 1928, and so on. Americans have been debating about it since 1912.

Traditionally, the United States has tried to solve the financial aspect of medical care by private insurance. But the poor cannot afford insurance, and insurance companies do not want to cover the elderly because of their high rates of illness. So in 1965, the government instituted Medicare and Medicaid. Medicare pays 38 percent of the total medical-care bills of those over sixty-five. Medicaid covers the cost of care for the poor, but many physicians will not treat Medicaid patients and underfinancing has forced many states to cut back on services offered. These are the only two forms of government health insurance we now have.

Unfortunately, even if national health insurance (NHI) became a reality, it would not solve the major problems of our medical-care system. As presently conceived, NHI seems to be merely a method of financing medical care—that is, paying those who provide health-care services. It will not change the basic structure that has evolved. Moreover, even the most progressive NHI proposals have serious limitations on drugs, dental care, psychiatric care, and skilled nursing home care. This is one of several reasons that support has been developing in some quarters for national health service.

Proponents of a *national health service* view it as the only sensible long-term solution to our health-care problems. Such a service would eliminate our present health insurance industry, Medicare, Medicaid, and most other types of coverage. It would provide comprehensive care for all, with no payment required at the time of service. It would be paid for by tax dollars and employer contributions, and administration of the program would be under direct public control and accountability. Most doctors would be on salary or some other

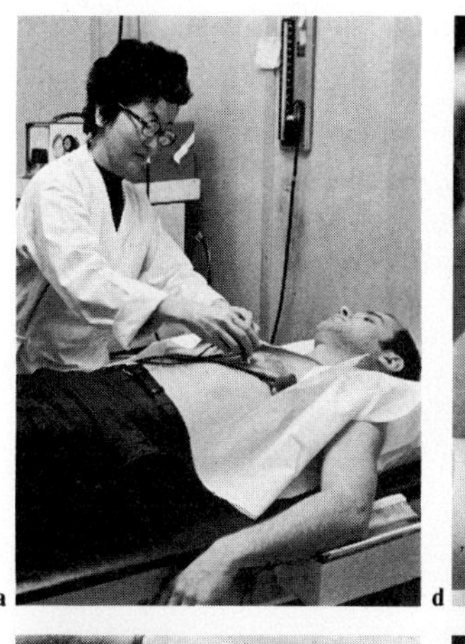

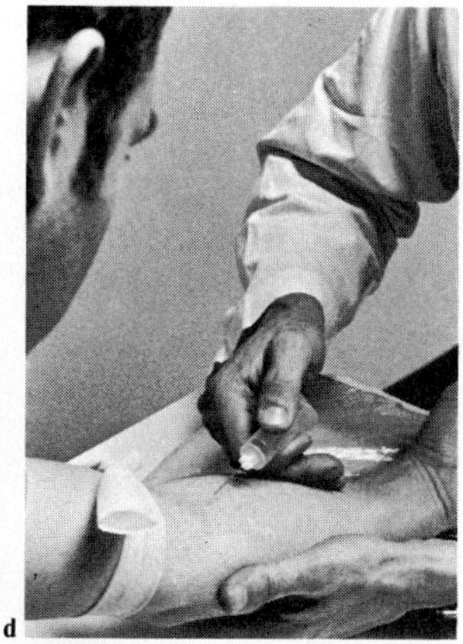

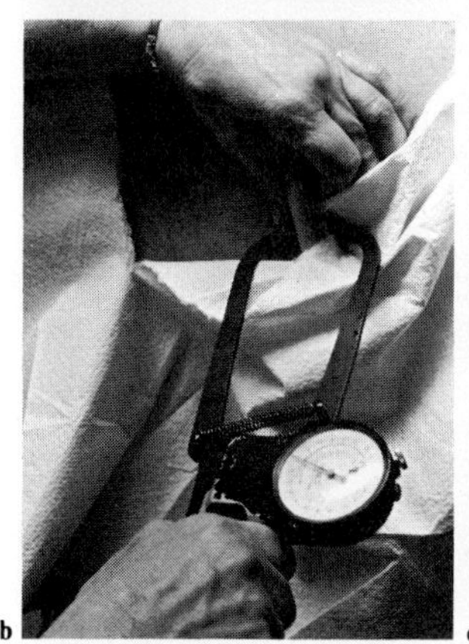

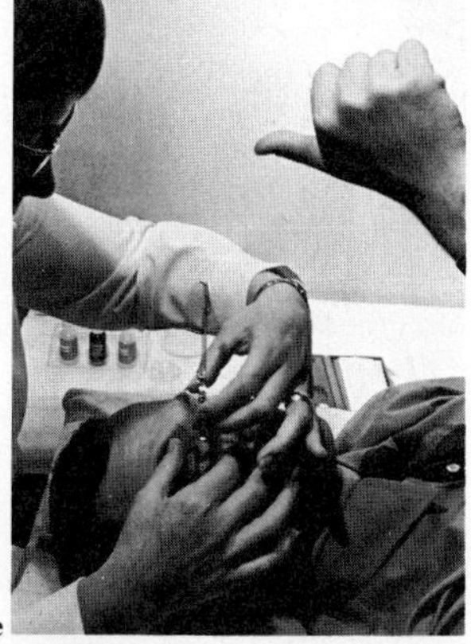

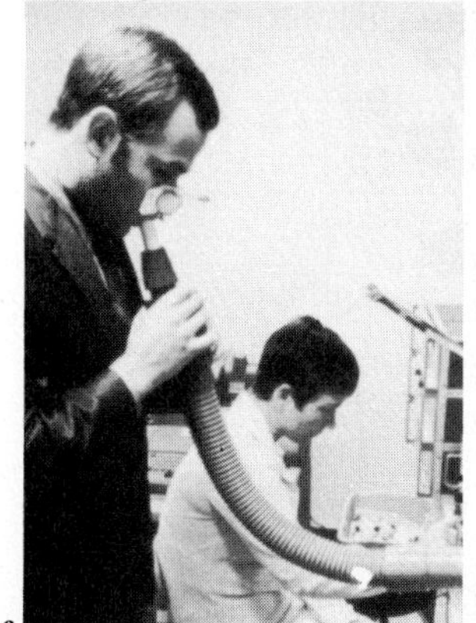

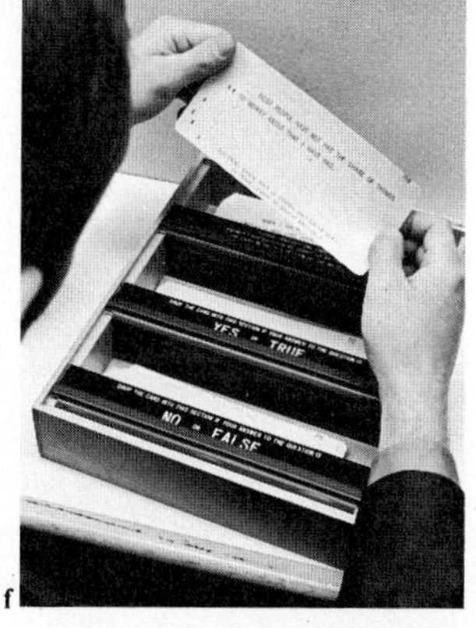

Figure 18.5 Several steps of the multiphasic screening test: (a) an electrocardiogram is taken; (b) skin-fold test measures body fat; (c) lung capacity is measured; (d) blood sample is taken for analysis; (e) the eyes are checked for glaucoma; (f) patient receives set of cards for psychological evaluation.

FOCUS

Health Care in the Year 2003

What will our system of health care be like in the year 2003? There have been many speculations. Stanley Matek of the Health Planning Council (Orange County, California) presented one scenario at an annual meeting of the American Public Health Association:

> It is the year 2003, Citizen Jones has not been feeling well over the weekend, but believing that he will feel better later in the day, decides to go to work on Monday.
>
> His route happens to take him within range of one of the ubiquitous "health monitoring sensors" which have been installed throughout the city to perform biological tests once done in clinical laboratories.
>
> As Jones passes the sensors, a deviation from acceptable health norms is registered; instantaneously, a signal is flashed to a remote central station. Jones is identified at the station by a kind of electronic fingerprint. His health problem is immediately diagnosed and triaged along with hundred of diagnoses received that morning.
>
> Found to have only a minor problem, Jones is contacted several days later by the "Contact Monitoring Council" and directed to visit a "public health intervenist."

To citizens of the twenty-first century, surveillance and follow-up procedures such as these will be routine. By then, according to Matek, health education, early detection, and preventive medicine will be the dominant aspects of our health care. This emphasis on prevention and early detection will be reflected in a variety of self-care kits and equipment as well as a wide range of self-care courses. Drugs, alcohol, and tobacco will be rationed, and our national health policy will encompass laws for institutions and industries as well as individuals. All public health workers will be assigned to schools or factories or research work.

Among the most interesting changes predicted by Matek will be the increasing status of biologists and chemists over that of physicians. Primary care will now be dispensed by a new type of professional—a combination of pharmacist and nurse practitioner—providing "over-the-counter health care."

If this scenario doesn't suit you, perhaps Dr. Robert Kane's vision of the future may seem more persuasive. Dr. Kane, senior researcher of the Rand Corporation, believes that even in 2003 we will still have "a system dominated by emphasis on medical care."

National health insurance will be a reality, but, says Dr. Kane, costs for medical care will be extraordinarily high: 25 percent of the Gross National Product (compare this with 9.3 percent in 1978). Thus, tight controls on health-care spending will require that citizens on welfare work within the medical industry. Those who smoke, consume alcohol, or engage in other risk behavior will have their benefits reduced. Triage . . . will be used extensively and most of us will have "only limited access to certain kinds of treatment."

In this national health insurance system, physicians will have a secondary role. Their services will be too costly in most cases. According to Dr. Kane, by 2003 the services of the physician will, for the most part, be accessible to wealthy citizens who have the option of a private fee-for-service system, which will exist alongside the national health insurance system.

Notice that these two very different projections into the future have something in common: in both, the physician's role and status have changed significantly, and paramedical personnel play a much greater part in our health-care system. But 2003 is a long way off and perhaps you have a scenario of your own.

Source "Two Futuristic Scenarios," *Urban Health* (October 1978), pp. 10-11.

method of payment that discourages overservicing and unnecessary surgery.

A national health service would encourage preventive services and emphasize community health centers rather than hospitals and doctors' offices. It would cover acute and chronic care, intermediate and skilled nursing home services, and hospices for the terminally ill.

Supporters of a national health service emphasize that profit making in the health-care field should not be allowed. Victor and Ruth Sidel, in their book *The Healthy State,* say:

> We reject it [profit making] as a basis for the organization of any part of health care or medical care in the United States; a national health service must not permit investors to gain wealth or income at the expense of the sick or at the expense of the rest of society. This, of course, extends to insurance companies and drug companies as well as to profit-making entrepreneurs in hospitals, nursing homes and ambulatory care.

Obviously such a proposal threatens the interests of the major groups currently providing our medical care. In the United States, a national health service is a very long-term goal.

Of course, if national health insurance or a national health service were instituted, we would still pay dearly for health care. We may envy countries with government-supported health care, but we should not overlook the staggering tax burdens on these countries' citizens. In Sweden, for example, government-sponsored medical care costs nearly 12 percent of the Gross National Product—a higher percentage than we pay under our current system.

THE SELF-CARE MOVEMENT

As we have seen, the focus of our present health-care system is treatment, rather than prevention. However, there is a growing public awareness of and belief in preventive medicine. These forces have spurred the rise of the self-care movement. The impetus toward self-care also comes from sources such as the consumer movement, sparked by consumer advocate Ralph Nader; the women's movement, which has made women more aware of caring for their own bodies; and community clinics, which have spread the philosophy that people can do much for their own health.

The self-care movement manifests itself in myriad books and magazine articles about the phenomenon and in an outpouring of self-care courses. Many community clinics conduct health education programs to teach self-care skills. In the early 1970s, at Georgetown University, Dr. Keith Sehnert developed a thirty-four-hour course in which he taught patients how to use such tools of the medical trade as stethoscopes and blood-pressure cuffs. Sehnert called it the "Course for Activated Patients," whom he defines in his book *How to Be Your Own Doctor—Sometimes,* as "a kind of hearty hybrid who is three-quarters patient and one-quarter physician," and who has "learned to speak the doctor's own language, and ask him questions rather than passively sit, honor and obey." Sehnert's course has since become a model for many similar courses across the country.

The fact is that to a considerable extent you can do more for your own health than a doctor can. Doctors tend to be trained to practice *crisis medicine*—that is, to intervene after disease strikes—rather than *prospective* (or preventive) *medicine*—that is, to maintain health and head off disease before it strikes. Actually, doctors can do very little to prevent illness, other than giving immunization shots for certain diseases. Only you can maintain your health and prevent disease by proper eating, sensible alcohol or drug use, getting enough sleep, exercising sufficiently, not smoking cigarettes, driving carefully, and avoiding accidents of all sorts. As the age-old aphorism puts it: "An ounce of prevention is worth a pound of cure."

And only you—not your doctor—can have a "holistic" view of your health within the context of your own life. Only you can understand your overall social and economic situation and be aware of possibly conflicting motivations on your part.

The goal of self-care is *not* to replace your doctor. Medicine is a highly complex, technical, and specialized field of learning, and physicians have the know-how and the technology to make diagnoses and perform treatments far beyond the capability of any layperson. The goal, instead, is to consult physicians as advisers—to use them as a resource—while recognizing your primary responsibility for your own health. And by learning more about what you can care for yourself, you may be able to save yourself the time and expense of unnecessary trips to the doctor. The idea, says Sehnert, is "knowing how to stay healthy and how to prevent minor illnesses from becoming major ones"

Limitations to Self-Care

However, there are real pitfalls in the self-care movement. One is ignorance or misinformation. Many people do what they think is right, without any scientific basis for their self-diagnosis or self-treatment, and they may actually be doing themselves or their loved ones outright harm. A related hazard is that self-care draws unscrupulous quacks. Some people react so strongly against the medical establishment that they foolishly shun sound, established medical care and may be more likely to waste their money—and risk their health—on worthless remedies. There is also a legal pitfall: a layperson who attempts to treat other people—an unlicensed person, for instance, who delivers a baby at a home—can be prosecuted under the laws of many states for practicing medicine without a license.

THE SCOPE OF SELF-CARE

In order to practice self-care, whether just for yourself or for your family or household, you need to build up a library of current health-care and first-aid reference books, keep systematic medical records, and stock certain basic medications and equipment and learn how to use them.

You should develop competence in performing *emergency care:* you should be prepared to perform first-aid for such emergencies as poisonings, breathing difficulties, heart stoppage, and accidental injuries involving bleeding, shock, and broken bones. You should learn enough about *pharmacology* to use over-the-counter drugs sensibly and also to understand why and how to take prescription drugs. You should be able to self-diagnose and self-treat *common minor ailments* and also participate in the care of more serious *chronic disorders.* And you should know how to maintain your own mental health.

It is beyond the scope of this chapter to detail all the information you will need for this endeavor. It would be a good idea to take a course in self-care. If there is no such course in your community, you might consider helping to initiate one through an adult-education pro-

HOW TO Perform Mouth-to-Mouth Resuscitation

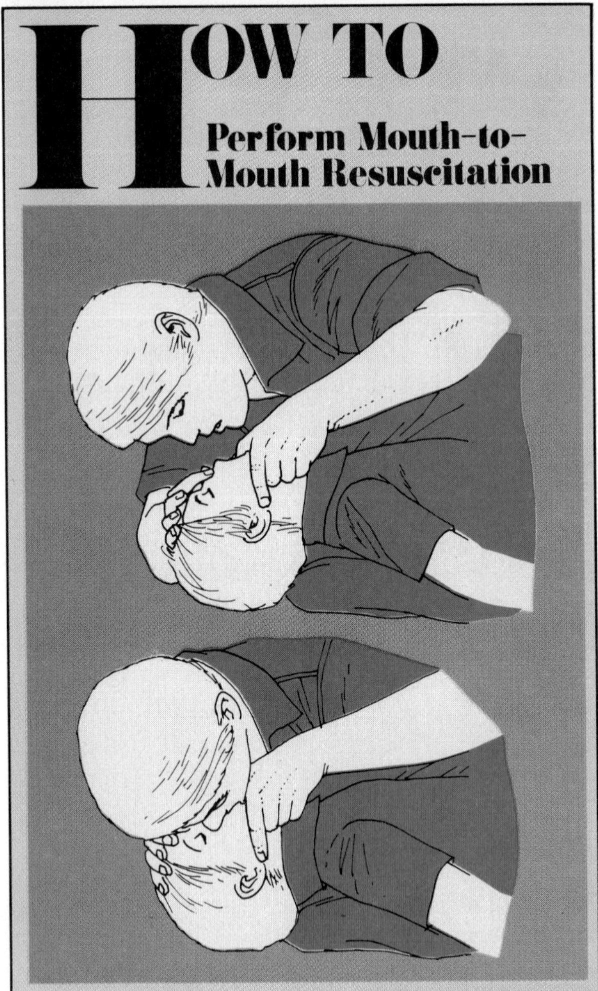

1. Lay the victim on his back, turn his head to one side, and remove any mucus, vomit, or gum from his mouth. Then turn the head forward.
2. Place one hand under the victim's neck and the other on top of his head. Tilt his head back so that the chin is pointing up.
3. Take a deep breath, open your mouth wide, and place it over the victim's mouth. Pinch the victim's nostrils closed as you do this. Exhale into the victim's mouth. Remove your mouth and listen for a return of air from the victim. Repeat this procedure again, listening for a return of air. If there is no return, check for possible blockage of the respiratory tract.
4. Continue this breathing at a regular rate of approximately 12 breaths per minute.
5. If the victim begins to breathe on his own, time your breathing with his to allow for exhaling. Once breathing has returned and is sufficiently strong, resuscitation can be stopped.

Source: William Fassbender, *You and Your Health* (New York: Wiley, 1977).

gram. The course naturally should be taught by a qualified health educator, physician, nurse, or other health professional.

Accident Prevention

Accidents probably touch the lives of more people than almost any other single trauma. In the United States, accidents are the fourth leading cause of death, after heart disease, cancer, and stroke. Within the fifteen to twenty-four age group, accidents claim more lives than *all* other causes combined.

A simple sequence of facts illustrates the dimensions of the accident problem. In the time it takes to deliver a ten-minute speech on safety, 2 people will die in accidents and approximately 200 others will be disabled

Broadly speaking, accidents result from enviromental hazards or unsafe behavior, or a combination of the two. Many different variables are involved. People can be injured not only by various objects and forces in the environment but by their own unsafe thinking or action, or by that of other human beings.

One factor in unsafe behavior is the exercise of bad judgment—insufficient seeking of adequate information, faulty expectations, impulsive decision making. Another is an exaggerated sense of invulnerability, leading to lack of anticipation or actual disregard of other people's actions or reactions and to a deficient sense of responsibility for one's own actions. A third factor is overconfidence in one's ability, causing inadequate attentiveness and neglect of safety precautions.

By far, the greatest number of accidents involve motor vehicles, but the second largest catagory involves the home.

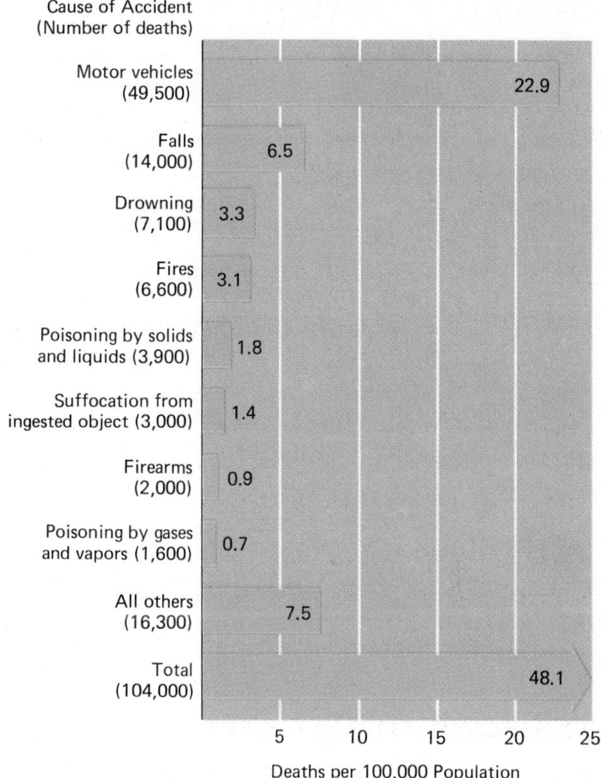

Figure 18.6 Accidental deaths in the United States, 1977.

MOTOR VEHICLE ACCIDENTS

The motor vehicle is the most dangerous machine with which most of us come in daily contact. Accidents involving motor vehicles kill and cripple, and change the lives of more people than any other kind of mishap. In fact, for young people between the ages of fifteen and twenty-four, it is the leading cause of deaths

Motor vehicles include not only automobiles, but mopeds, motorcycles, snowmobiles, and power boats. Although all these motor vehicles have become increasingly popular in recent years, the greatest hazard remains the automobile.

The automobile industry has made a number of changes: improved headlights for greater illumination; windshields of tempered glass to reduce jagged shards; recessed steering wheel hubs and knobs, padded surfaces, head rests, lap and shoulder belts.

However, none of these mechanical and technical improvements can counteract the human element that enters into virtually all motor vehicle accidents.

The National Safety Council estimates that one-half of all fatal motor vehicle accidents involved drivers who had consumed alcohol. The drivers may not have all been drunk, but some alcohol was in their systems. Because of the sharp increase in traffic accidents since the

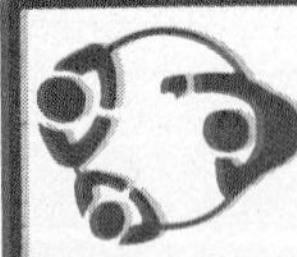

EDITH

Don't wait for smoke and fire to surprise you. Plan your home fire escape now. If you live in an apartment, ask the management to schedule drills. Practice during Fire Prevention Week and once or twice more during the year. If you move, make a new plan right away!

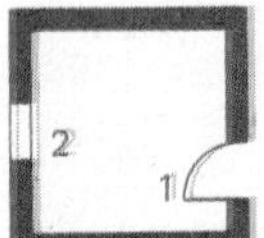

Discuss and Plan Ahead

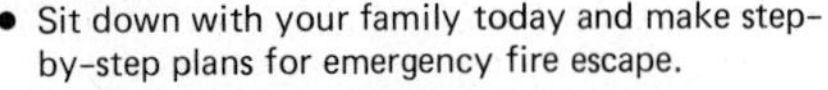

- Sit down with your family today and make step-by-step plans for emergency fire escape.

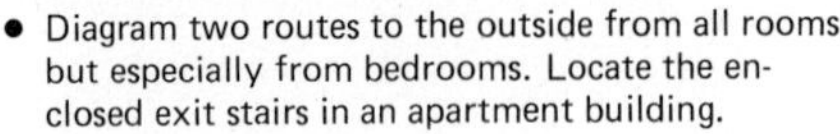

- Diagram two routes to the outside from all rooms, but especially from bedrooms. Locate the enclosed exit stairs in an apartment building.

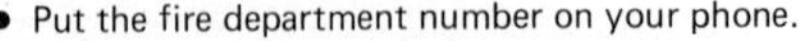

- Put the fire department number on your phone.

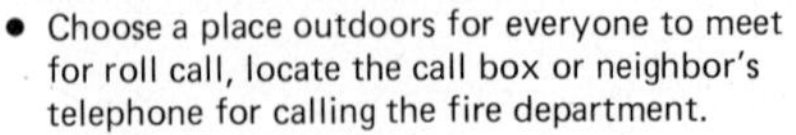

- Choose a place outdoors for everyone to meet for roll call, locate the call box or neighbor's telephone for calling the fire department.
- Discuss why you shouldn't go back inside once you're out. (People have died returning to a burning building.)

You May Need to Make a Purchase

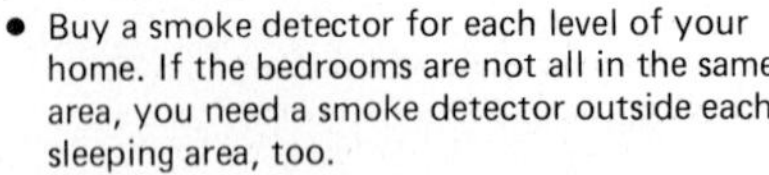

- Buy a smoke detector for each level of your home. If the bedrooms are not all in the same area, you need a smoke detector outside each sleeping area, too.

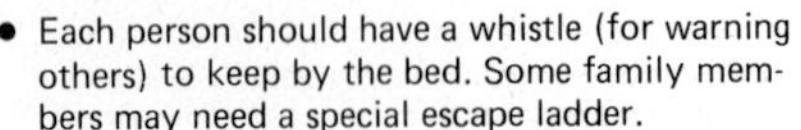

- Each person should have a whistle (for warning others) to keep by the bed. Some family members may need a special escape ladder.

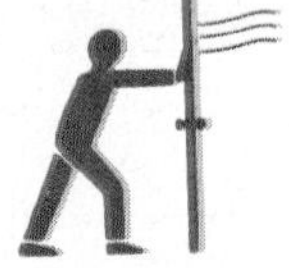

Practice

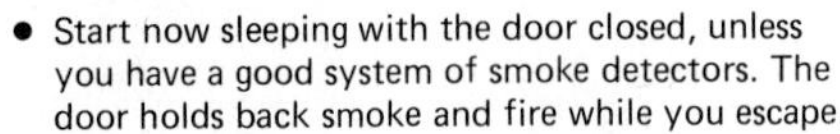

- Start now sleeping with the door closed, unless you have a good system of smoke detectors. The door holds back smoke and fire while you escape.

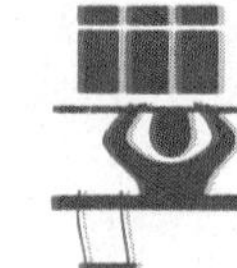

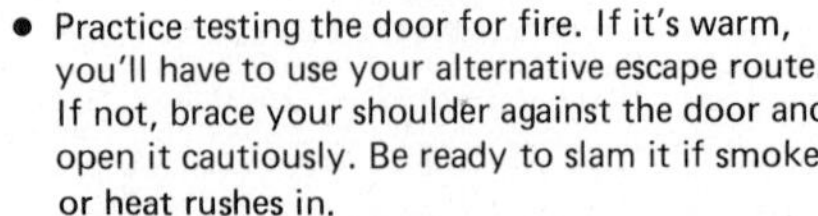

- Practice testing the door for fire. If it's warm, you'll have to use your alternative escape route. If not, brace your shoulder against the door and open it cautiously. Be ready to slam it if smoke or heat rushes in.

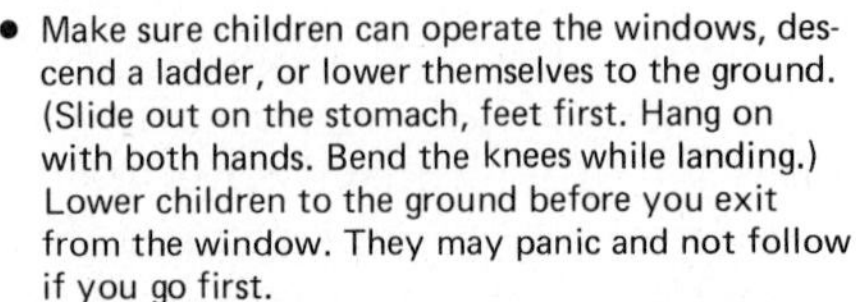

- Make sure children can operate the windows, descend a ladder, or lower themselves to the ground. (Slide out on the stomach, feet first. Hang on with both hands. Bend the knees while landing.) Lower children to the ground before you exit from the window. They may panic and not follow if you go first.

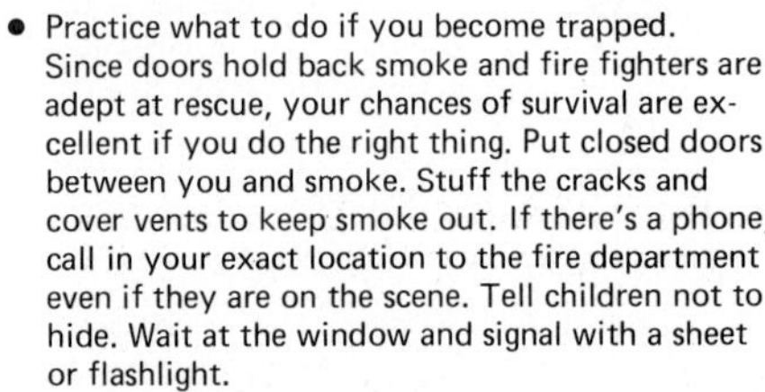

- Practice what to do if you become trapped. Since doors hold back smoke and fire fighters are adept at rescue, your chances of survival are excellent if you do the right thing. Put closed doors between you and smoke. Stuff the cracks and cover vents to keep smoke out. If there's a phone, call in your exact location to the fire department even if they are on the scene. Tell children not to hide. Wait at the window and signal with a sheet or flashlight.

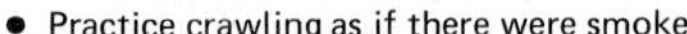

- Practice crawling as if there were smoke.
- Have children practice saying the fire department number, the family name, street address, and town into the phone.

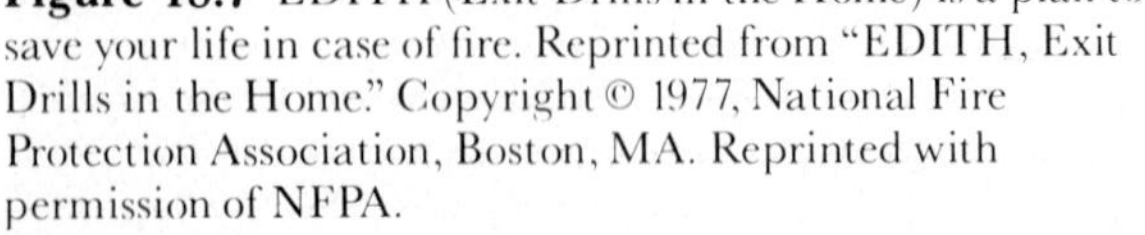

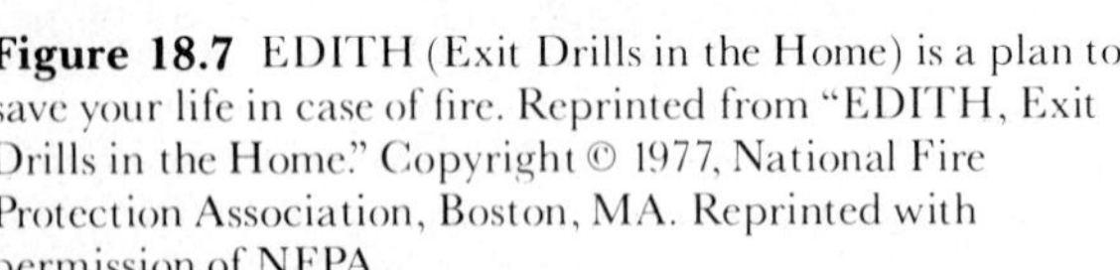

Figure 18.7 EDITH (Exit Drills in the Home) is a plan to save your life in case of fire. Reprinted from "EDITH, Exit Drills in the Home." Copyright © 1977, National Fire Protection Association, Boston, MA. Reprinted with permission of NFPA.

lowering of the drinking age, many states are changing the minimum drinking age back to twenty-one.

HOME ACCIDENTS

Home is not always the refuge from harm it is thought to be. Consider the case of John Glenn, the first American to orbit the earth. Glenn was able to complete his mission without harm. It was in a home accident that he suffered a serious head injury; he slipped and fell in the bathtub. Some 22 percent of all accidental deaths are the result of home accidents —that is, accidents that occur either in the home or on the premises surrounding the home. The majority are caused by falls and fires.

A few simple precautions can minimize falls: adequate lighting, firm handrails for stairways, and grab bars and traction mats or strips for bathtubs and showers. Today nonskid throw rugs and nonskid floor wax are also available.

Many fire hazards have been eliminated through the more widespread use of noncombustible building material. In private homes, fire and smoke detector and alarm systems are being installed in increasing numbers. Efficient lightweight extinguishers for home use are also available. In addition to minimizing fire hazards, every family should have rehearsed a set of fire-safety procedures in the event of fire. (See Figure 18.7, which explains the plan known as EDITH [Exit Drills in the Home].)

Serious burns can also result from the improper use of flammable liquids. Today many nonflammable, nonexplosive cleaning fluids are available for home use.

Call your doctor immediately. If he or she can't be reached, call one of the following: local poison control center if available, hospital, pharmacist, police, or fire department. If possible, begin first-aid treatment while another person calls for help. The nature of the poison or overdose will determine the first-aid measure to use—*until medical help is obtained.*

If the patient is unconscious or in convulsions:

- Do *not* force liquids on him or her, and do *not* induce vomiting.
- Provide artificial respiration if necessary, keep patient warm, and take him or her to the hospital immediately.
- Take along the poison container, label, remaining contents, or any vomited material to help identify the poison.

If the patient swallowed a corrosive or petroleum product:

- Do *not* induce vomiting.
- Dilute the poison with water or milk. *Dosage*: 1 to 2 cups for patients under 5 years of age; up to 1 quart for patients 5 years and older.
- Get patient to the hospital immediately. Take along the poison container, label, or remaining contents to help identify the poison.

If the patient swallowed an overdose or poison that is *not* a corrosive or petroleum product:

- Dilute with water or milk. *Dosage*: 1 to 2 cups for patients under 5 years of age; up to 1 quart for patients 5 years and older.
- Induce vomiting. *To induce vomiting*: 1 tablespoon (½ ounce) of syrup of ipecac, plus at least 1 cup of water. (If no vomiting occurs within 20 minutes, dose may be repeated *only once.*) If syrup of ipecac is unavailable, induce vomiting by placing the blunt end of a spoon or your finger at the back of the victim's throat. *Do not give salt water.* When vomiting begins, keep patient face down with head lower than hips to prevent choking; place a small child across your knees in a "spanking" position.
- If no vomiting occurs within 20 minutes, repeat syrup of ipecac dose *only* once as already described—but don't waste time waiting any longer. Call doctor or hospital again for further instructions. If you can't get those instructions, take patient to hospital immediately. Bring along the container, label, or remaining contents to help identify the poison. If vomiting occurs, bring a sample of the vomited material.

Examples of corrosives: sodium acid sulfate (toilet bowl cleaners), sulfuric acid, nitric acid, oxalic acid, hydrofluoric acid (rust removers), iodine, silver nitrate (caustic pencil), sodium hydroxide or lye (drain cleaners), sodium carbonate (washing soda), ammonia water, sodium hypochlorite (household bleach). *Examples of petroleum products*: gasoline, kerosene, lighter fluid, naphtha, mineral seal oil (furniture polishes), petroleum solvents and cleaners.

Figure 18.8 First aid for accidental poisoning.

Other fatalities are caused by drowning, suffocation, and poisoning. Since more than four-fifths of all fatal poisonings occur in the home, it is essential to know something about the various solids, liquids, gases, and vapors that can result in poisoning. Poison first-aid charts for the home are available, and prescription items and children's vitamins are packaged with safety tops that cannot be opened by youngsters. In many communities there is an emergency number (usually of a poison control center). The dangers of suffocation among young children can be minimized by destroying all polyethylene plastic trash, food, and garment bags. And, of course, all home swimming pools should have adequate enclosures.

Dangers from electric current, hazardous equipment and flammable materials in home workshops, and power lawn mowers also exist.

Evaluating Health Literature

There is an overwhelming amount of health-care literature available on the market. Not only are there many health books for laypersons, but many companies, professional groups, and government and voluntary health agencies also publish useful pamphlets and brochures. There is also no guarantee that the information in a given publication is accurate. Different books often give conflicting advice. How can you tell what to believe? Here are some guidelines for judging the soundness of a publication:

1. Who are the authors? What are their qualifications? Are they physicians? This alone does not guarantee accuracy, but it's a start. Do the authors represent a special interest group or have any apparent biases? Are they trying to sell something? Much of the information might be sound, but you should be alert to these vested interests.
2. When was the book published? In the field of health, a ten-year-old or even a five-year-old book can be out of date.
3. Do the authors document their claims? This is particularly important when they are discussing new or controversial treatments or other practices. If the data are not

all in on a new product or practice, the authors should make this situation clear.
4. Is the material clearly organized and presented in a way that will make it easy for you to find what you need in an emergency?
5. Is the content to the point and not burdened with superfluous material?
6. Is the terminology clear? While some medical terminology is necessary, too much can be confusing. In some cases, baffling jargon may mask inaccurate or quack literature.

One thing to keep in mind about any health literature, as Drs. Donald M. Vickery and James F. Fries point out in their own book *Taking Care of Yourself, A Consumer's Guide to Medical Care,* "If you are under the care of a physician and receive advice contrary to this book, *follow the physician's advice* [italics added]; the individual characteristics of your problem can then be taken into account."

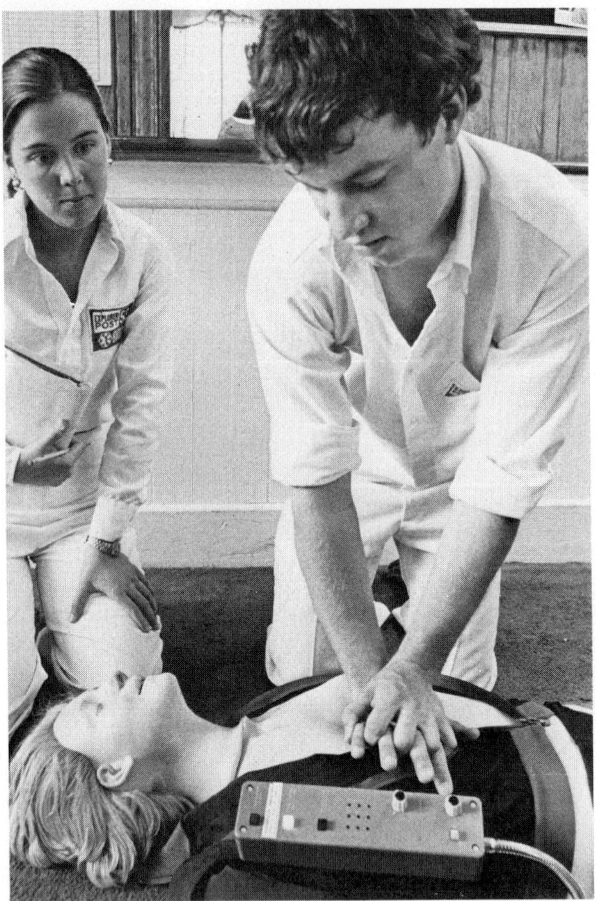

Figure 18.9 Here a young man is instructed in the technique of cardiopulmonary resuscitation, using a specially designed mannequin. This procedure can help save another person's life when medical care is not immediately available.

Self-Care Skills

The purpose of developing simple self-care skills is "not so that you can compete with your doctor or challenge his or her diagnosis," explains Sehnert, "but so that you can anticipate and help prevent medical problems." You should become familiar with the normal appearance and readings of your own body and those of the members of your household, so that you will know when they change. This will help you avoid calling your doctor unnecessarily, and when you do call, you will be able to describe the symptoms better. The tools in a home "black bag" are for preliminary observations only, Sehnert points out, "for screening out the person who needs to see a doctor from the one who may only need to take some simple preventive measures to prevent a spark from becoming a bonfire." Here is how to make these observations.

Temperature While normal mouth temperature is 98.6°F (37°C), it actually can vary several degrees. Temperatures above 100.4°F or below 96.8°F are usually, however, symptoms of disease. You should not ignore high fevers, particularly in children: prolonged high temperature can cause brain damage.

Throat Have the person whose throat you are examining tilt his or her head back slightly, open the mouth wide, and say "Ahhh!" With a tongue depressor or spoon handle, flatten the back of the tongue and shine a penlight down the throat until you get a clear view.

You should look at healthy throats to become familiar with their appearance. If someone in your household complains of a sore throat, look to see how red or swollen it is and whether it has any white or yellow patches, so that you can describe its appearance when you call the doctor.

Eyes Remove glasses or contact lenses. By simply looking at the whites of the eyes, you can see whether they are yellowish or reddish. By gently drawing down the lower lid, you can also see the mucous lining, which should look moist and pink. If it is swollen or reddish or grayish, or if there is any discharge or crustiness around the eyelashes, there may be an infection.

To check pupil size, darken the room enough so that the pupils dilate. Hold a penlight about a foot above the person's head and pass the beam down across one eye, flashing the beam directly into the pupil. Repeat for the other eye. As the light flashes into the eye, the pupil should constrict. If it does not, or if it remains constricted when the light is removed, this may indicate a head injury.

Pulse (Heart Rate) You—or your "patient"—should be completely at rest, since the heart rate increases with physical exertion and with stress. With the "patient's" palm up, press your fingers down on the thumbside of the wrist until you feel the artery throbbing. (Do not use your thumb; it has a pulse of its own that will confuse your count.) Using a watch with a second hand, count the number of beats you feel in fifteen seconds. Multiply this number by four to get the heart rate in beats per minute. (If you try to count for a full minute, there is a tendency to lose track of the count.)

In a healthy, resting adult, the heart normally beats between 60 and 80 times a minute. Athletes may have rates of 40 to 60 a minute; young children, 90 to 120.

Breasts Breast cancer kills more women in the United States—33,000 each year—than any other cancer. Yet if it is detected and treated early, nearly 85 percent of its victims recover. And more than 95 percent of all breast cancers are discovered by women them-

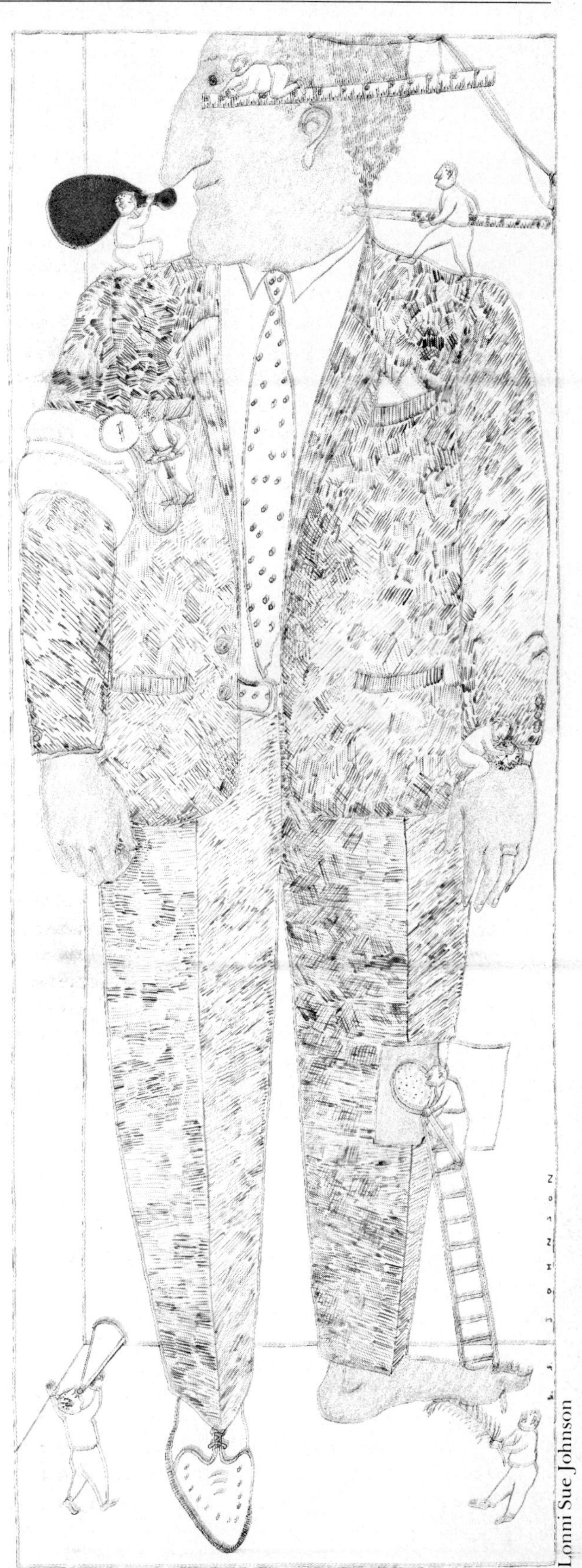

Figure 18.10 The vital signs are those measurable and observable functions that indicate the overall condition, either healthy or unhealthy, of the body. These signs—pulse; respiration rate; temperature; ability to move, feel, and respond to verbal and physical stimuli; the size of the eye pupils; and the color and the condition of the skin—can easily be noted by the layperson and alert him or her to a possible medical problem.

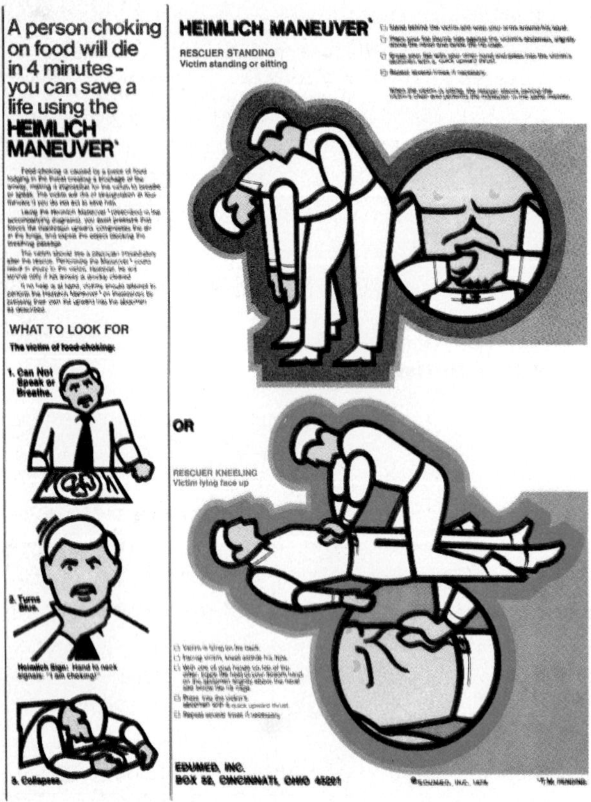

Figure 18.11 The Heimlich technique, or maneuver, has been extremely effective in saving the lives of choking victims.

selves. The American Cancer Society recommends that women examine their own breasts every month. Instructions for doing this are given in Chapter 15, Figure 15.5.

Taking Care of Yourself

Dr. Lowell Levin of Yale University School of Medicine, in his book *Self-Care; Lay Initiatives in Health,* points out that perhaps 75 percent or more of health care in this country is actually undertaken without professional intervention. On the other hand, physicians complain that some 70 percent of the patients jamming their waiting rooms do not actually need to see a doctor—they could just as well take care of themselves, save their own time and money, and free the doctor to concentrate on people who do need professional expertise.

According to the 1973 National Health Survey, at least half of all acute minor illnesses seen in the doctor's office are caused by respiratory diseases such as the common cold, pharyngitis, laryngitis, rhinitis, bronchitis, and sinusitis. Physicians know that many of these and many other common ailments—minor headaches, stomach aches, diarrhea, nausea, vomiting, muscle pains, coughs, and mild fevers—are self-limiting diseases that usually run their course within a short period of time no matter what anyone does about them. Many of them are caused by viruses that cannot be killed by antibiotics or other drugs. (Antibiotics are effective primarily against bacterial diseases.) Doctors generally cannot cure these ailments; they can only tell you what you can do for yourself—rest, ease symptoms with over-the-counter drugs if necessary, or drink fluids as appropriate. The idea of self-care is to become sensitive enough to the subtle signals your body sends that you recognize when you need to take care of yourself and allow your body's immune system to fend off an invading "bug" before it develops into something more serious. However, this does not mean that you should neglect these common ailments, since sometimes they are indeed symptoms of serious conditions.

An aspect of self-care that we usually take for granted is personal cleanliness. Such simple sanitary measures as washing our hands after going to the toilet and before preparing food prevent the transmission of infectious diseases. Another simple sort of self-care is avoiding overexposure to the sun; its rays are a major factor in aging the skin—producing wrinkles, growths, and mottled pigmentation—and causing skin cancer. Likewise, flossing the teeth and meticulously brushing them after meals prevent tooth decay and periodontal (gum) disease.

Another important area of self-care is the chronic disorders, such as hypertension, diabetes, arthritis, kidney disease, and hemophilia. Many of these conditions require that patients and their families learn how to administer, under medical supervision, fairly elaborate self-care over long periods of time: giving injections, taking blood-pressure readings, adhering to complex drug or dietary schedules, or performing kidney dialysis.

An additional facet of self-care is making wise decisions about when to stop taking care of yourself and seek professional care from a physician, a subject that will be discussed in the following section. You should also think through ahead of time what you would do in an emergency, at night or on a weekend, or whenever you could not get your own doctor fast enough. Is there a police emergency number in your community? Where is the nearest hospital emergency room? How would you get there? Many times an ambulance, for instance, might be slower than your own car or a taxi.

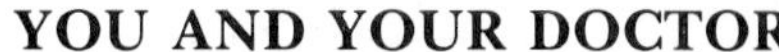

YOU AND YOUR DOCTOR

How to Choose a Doctor

Don't wait until you get sick. While you are well, you should seek out and establish a relationship with a physician. It is often not easy to find a competent and caring practitioner, particularly if you have just moved to a new community. Many areas of the country have shortages of doctors, and doctors in these places may be reluctant to accept new patients. If you plan to move, you could ask your present doctor to recommend a physician in your new area.

Otherwise, ask your friends, neighbors, relatives, or colleagues at school or work who they find satisfactory—but keep in mind that they may not necessarily be qualified to evaluate a doctor's competence. County medical societies will usually give out the names of doctors willing to take new patients—but they carefully avoid evaluating them for you. You could also locate the nearest good hospital and find out the names of the physicians who practice there. If you live near a university medical center and school, find out the names of the physicians on staff.

Libraries have reference books in which you can check out a physician's educational background, training, and other credentials. The American Medical Association publishes a directory of physicians, organized by state, and the *Directory of Medical Specialists* lists doctors

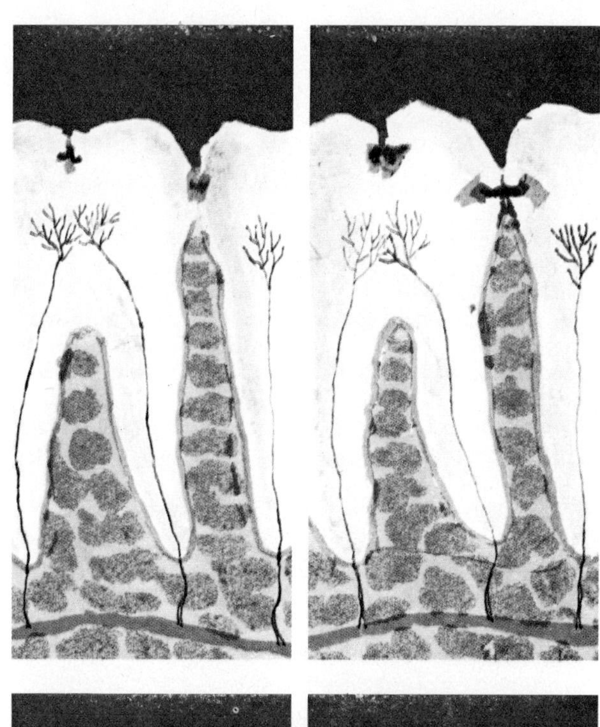

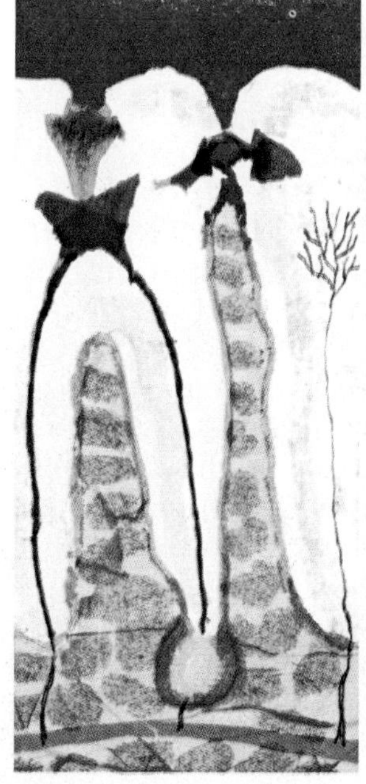

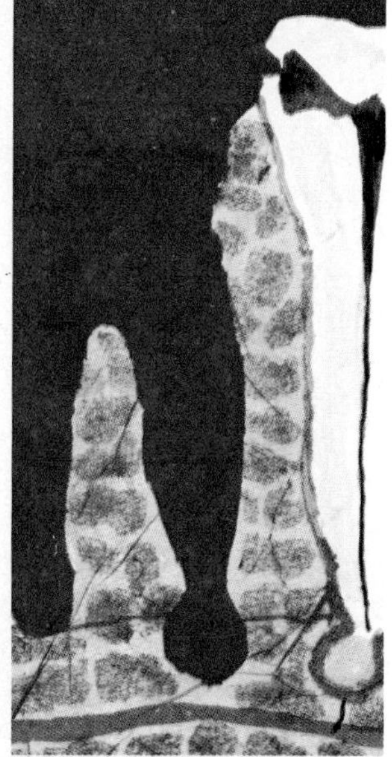

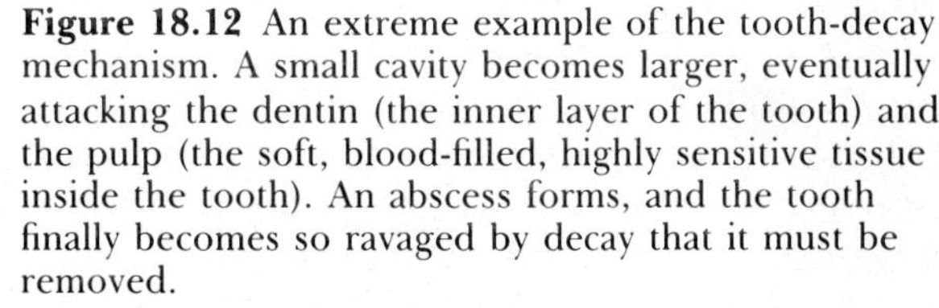

Figure 18.12 An extreme example of the tooth-decay mechanism. A small cavity becomes larger, eventually attacking the dentin (the inner layer of the tooth) and the pulp (the soft, blood-filled, highly sensitive tissue inside the tooth). An abscess forms, and the tooth finally becomes so ravaged by decay that it must be removed.

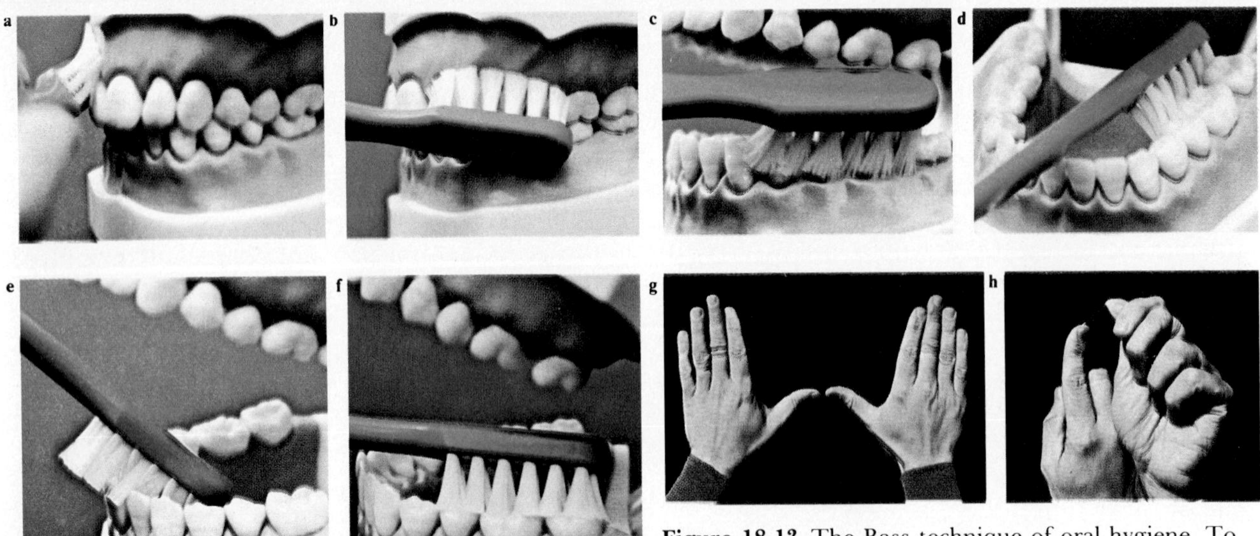

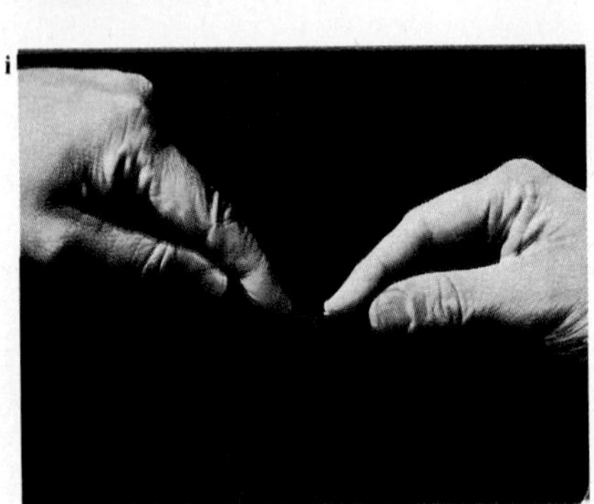

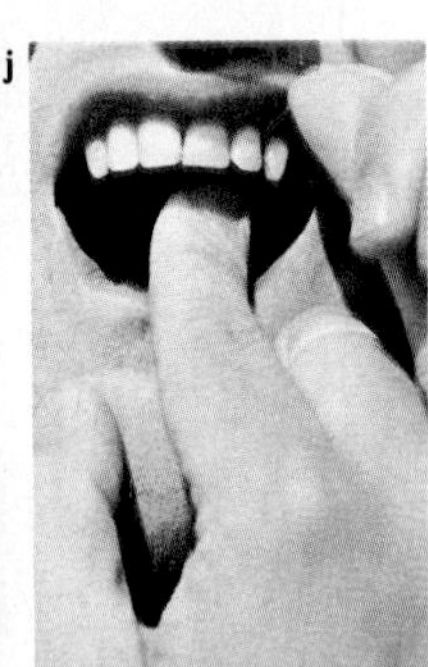

Figure 18.13 The Bass technique of oral hygiene. To clean the outside surfaces of all teeth and the inside surfaces of the back teeth, position the brush at the junction between the teeth and gums (a). Use short back-and-forth strokes. Do the outer surfaces first (b, c), and then do the inner surfaces (d, e) in the same manner. To clean the inner surface of the upper front teeth, hold the brush vertically, using several gentle back-and-forth strokes over gums and teeth. Brush back and forth on biting surfaces (f). After brushing, rinse the mouth vigorously to remove the loosened plaque from the teeth and mouth. The use of dental floss is encouraged for getting into the crevices between teeth. Pass the floss over the left thumb and the forefinger of the right hand for cleaning the upper left teeth (g); reverse the hold for the upper right. Clean the bottom teeth by holding the floss between the forefingers of both hands.

who are certified by the professional board of their specialty.

One good way to establish a relationship with a physician before you get sick is to make an appointment to discuss your needs, desires, and expectations for health care.

Physical Examinations

Physical examinations vary considerably in their complexity. Some involve extensive, "multiphasic" screening, lengthy questionnaires, multiple observations by physicians, many laboratory tests of the blood and urine, and monitoring tests such as an electrocardiogram as we discussed above. Other physicals are simpler and may involve only a few key tests and observations.

There is a difference of opinion among physicians as to whether extensive, routine, annual checkups are worth the time and expense for healthy adults. Some doctors do recommend annual physicals, and many schools and employers require them; other doctors point out that such regular examinations rarely reveal any previously undetected disease in which early treatment makes any difference.

The general rule of thumb is that as we grow older, the regular checkup has greater potential for spotting adverse conditions. While you are young, you should have enough physicals to establish a baseline of what is normal for you; you may have had these at school or camp or at work. Prior to age thirty, routine annual checkups may not be worth the money, since they rarely find an illness that has not already revealed itself by some symptom. It is probably better to rely on prompt response to any unusual symptoms by either phoning or visiting your physician. However, it is wise for a woman of any age to have a general physical examination before becoming pregnant (see Chapter 4). Between the ages of thirty and forty, recommends Sehnert, people who have no specific complaints and are not taking any medication should have a physical examination every five years. Between forty and fifty, people should be examined every three years; between fifty and sixty, every two years.

However, at all ages, people who do have any abnormal symptoms or who are taking any medication (including the Pill) should have physicals more often. And there are specific things that *should* be checked regularly, particularly in high-risk people. According to Vickery and Fries, the most essential are the following.

Blood Pressure Everyone—even healthy adults with no symptoms of heart disease or hypertension—should have his or her blood pressure checked every year or so. Hypertension, which is both dangerous and treatable, often does not reveal itself by any overt symptoms.

TB Test You should have a skin test (called the Mantoux or PPD test) for tuberculosis every three to five years, unless you have been exposed to TB, in which case you should have it more often. This test involves introducing a small amount of tuberculin (a sterile extract from the TB bacterium) under the skin. If the skin turns red or swells, it may mean that you have active tuberculosis. In that case, your doctor would probably suggest a chest X-ray.

Pap Test Sexually active women and women over twenty-five should have a "Pap smear" once or twice a year to screen for cancer of the uterine cervix. In this procedure, the physician uses an instrument called a speculum to spread the walls of the vagina and gently scrapes the cervix to obtain a sample of vaginal cells. These are subsequently examined under a microscope. Cervical cancer is usually completely curable if caught early. At the same time, the physician will generally also check for breast cancer, as mentioned earlier in this chapter.

Glaucoma Test Glaucoma is a condition in which the pressure inside the eyeball increases. If not treated, it can lead to blindness. You should have your eyes checked for this disease every two years after the age of thirty-five.

Miscellaneous Vickery and Fries also recommend that you take your doctor's advice about whether or not you need to have your urine checked and (for people over thirty) be screened for bowel cancer. You should also have your eyes, ears, and teeth checked periodically.

When to See a Doctor

Again, it is beyond the scope of a single chapter to detail all the circumstances in which you should see a doctor. This is why you should try to take a self-care course or, at least, acquire some reference books. The books (mentioned previously) by Sehnert and by Vickery and Fries both deal with the question—symptom by symptom—of when you should call the doctor. It is not always an easy decision to make, and many people—out of ignorance or fear—do not always make it wisely. Studies show that people suffering heart attacks often jeopardize their lives because they delay for hours before seeking medical care, and many people with cancer die because they fail to get proper treatment in time (see Chapter 15).

Nevertheless, some simple guidelines can be given. Only doctors can prescribe antibiotics for bacterial infections, treat cancer, and perform surgery. There are also certain emergency situations in which almost anyone would intuitively know to see a doctor immediately: massive bleeding that cannot be stopped, major burns, suspected broken bones, suspected poisoning. You should also get immediate medical help if a person is in severe pain; has cold sweats, particularly if combined with lightheadedness or chest or abdominal pain; is short of breath at rest, other than due to exertion; or is unconscious, in a stupor, or so disoriented that he or she cannot tell you what happened or does not know his or her name or whereabouts.

It is also recommended that you call a doctor if you have been running a fever for more than a week, find a lump in your breast, have an unexplained weight loss, cough up blood, find blood in your feces or urine, or if any problem that you are taking care of yourself persists beyond a reasonable length of time.

You need to see a doctor or other health professional for immunization shots. You should also see a doctor if you suspect you are pregnant or if you have any of the seven warning signs of cancer described in Chapter 15, Figure 15.4. And if any doctor tells you that you need surgery, you should consider getting a second opinion from another doctor. A congressional subcommittee has charged that physicians perform 2 million unnecessary operations—with a loss of more than 10,000 lives —each year. While this charge is disputed by the American Medical Association, many medical insurance policies are now paying for second surgical opinions.

How to Talk with Your Doctor

When you call or visit a doctor, be prepared to explain why you are seeking medical assistance. Organize ahead of time how you will describe your symptoms. Be explicit. Don't say, "I feel terrible," or "I ache." Do say, for instance, "I have a temperature of 103°F and my throat is swollen," or "Johnny's pulse is such-and-such, and his eardrum looks red."

Depending on the complexity of the problem you might even write out some notes for yourself and take them along so that you won't forget any symptoms. You might also take along your home medical records, so you can refresh your memory and add new notations. You should also have, on paper or in your mind, a list of questions that you want to ask the doctor, as well as paper and pencil for writing down the answers. (See Figure 18.14.)

Tell the doctor—whether or not he or she asks you—if you are also seeing another doctor for another problem. Be particularly sure to say whether you already are taking any drugs, whether recreational, prescription, or over the counter. Even such drugs as aspirin, caffeine, antacids, laxatives, and vitamins could be contributing to your symptoms or might affect your treatment. You should also mention any allergies you may have. People who are allergic to eggs, for example, cannot safely receive certain inoculations.

Before the visit, ask yourself these questions:	
1	Why am I going to the doctor? (the main reason or "chief complaint")
2	Is there anything else that worries me about my health? If so, please list.
3	What do I expect the doctor to do for me today? (in ten words or less)

During the visit, complete with help of your doctor:	
1	What is the diagnosis?
2	What exactly does that mean? (If you already understand the diagnosis, omit this question.)
3	Why did I get it, and how can I prevent it next time?
4	Are there any helpful patient-education materials available for the condition? or special organizations I should look into (for example, the Diabetic Association, Muscular Dystrophy Association, and so on)?
5	Are there any medications for me to take? If so, are there any special instructions, concerns, or possible side effects I need to know about the medicine?
6	When am I to return for another visit, if any?
7	What should I do at home in the way of activity, treatments, or precautions?
8	Am I to phone in for lab reports? Will you notify me even if my lab tests are negative?
9	Should I report back to the doctor for any reason?

Figure 18.14 The ask-the-doctor list.

One of the most difficult aspects of talking with physicians can be the technical terminology they use. Some of this is necessary for precision, and you should make some effort to learn the basic vocabulary relevant to your particular medical problems, particularly if you have a chronic condition that you and the doctor will be dealing with over a long period of time. You might even find a medical dictionary useful. If you don't understand what your doctor is saying, speak up and ask questions. Doctors often don't realize that they are failing to communicate clearly, and patients often don't let the doctor know that he or she is not being clear.

Before you leave the doctor's office, make sure you understand the diagnosis of your problem and what the treatment will be. Find out what to expect as the treatment progresses and what side effects to watch for. You should ask whether you should return for another visit and, if so, how soon. And if the doctor prescribes a drug, you should also ask additional questions (see Chapter 11).

YOUR RIGHTS AS A PATIENT

As part of the movement toward greater responsibility on the part of patients, there is also a new emphasis on your legal rights as a patient, in relationship both to individual doctors and to hospitals. The American Hospital Association has drawn up a Patient's Bill of Rights, which—while not a legal document—is useful in setting forth guidelines for both patients and health professionals (see Figure 18.12). Another, more complete discussion of the subject is contained in the excellent book by law professor George J. Annas, *The Rights of Hospital Patients* (Avon, 1975). While both of these sources deal primarily with hospital patients, they are also useful for ambulatory patients.

MAKING CONSUMER DECISIONS

Although we are surrounded by health information, our decisions as health consumers are not always wise. We not only neglect the signs of cancer and heart disease, but we also spend more than $2 billion a year in the United States on quackery. Lack of knowledge about health and medicine makes many people vulnerable to health misinformation, quackery, and health fads. Consumers commonly have an array of misconceptions, ranging from thinking that vitamins are cure-alls or that venereal disease can be transmitted nonsexually to believing that "an apple a day" literally "keeps the doctor away." Unwise consumer decisions also often result from poor decision-making skills or lack of time to do the necessary study. The protection of the individual must depend upon better consumer and health education that

1	The patient has the right to considerate and respectful care.
2	The patient has the right to obtain from his physician complete current information concerning his diagnosis, treatment, and prognosis in terms the patient can be reasonably expected to understand. When it is not medically advisable to give such information to the patient, the information should be made available to an appropriate person in his behalf. He has the right to know, by name, the physician responsible for coordinating his care.
3	The patient has the right to receive from his physician information necessary to give informed consent prior to the start of any procedure and treatment. Except in emergencies, such information for informed consent should include but not necessarily be limited to the specific procedure and/or treatment, the medically significant risks involved, and the probable duration of incapacitation. Where medically significant alternatives for care or treatment exist, or when the patient requests information concerning medical alternatives, the patient has the right to such information. The patient also has the right to know the name of the person responsible for the procedures and/or treatment.
4	The patient has the right to refuse treatment to the extent permitted by law and to be informed of the medical consequences of his action.
5	The patient has the right to every consideration of his privacy concerning his own medical care program. Case discussion, consultation, examination, and treatment are confidential and should be conducted discreetly. Those not directly involved in his care must have the permission of the patient to be present.
6	The patient has the right to expect that all communications and records pertaining to his care should be treated as confidential.
7	The patient has the right to expect that within its capacity a hospital must make reasonable response to the request of a patient for services. The hospital must provide evaluation, service, and/or referral as indicated by the urgency of the case. When medically permissible, a patient may be transferred to another facility only after he has received complete information and explanation concerning the needs for and alternatives to such a transfer. The institution to which the patient is to be transferred must first have accepted the patient for transfer.
8	The patient has the right to obtain information as to any relationship of his hospital to other health care and educational institutions insofar as his care is concerned. The patient has the right to obtain information as to the existence of any professional relationships among individuals, by name, who are treating him.
9	The patient has the right to be advised if the hospital proposes to engage in or perform human experimentation affecting his care or treatment. The patient has the right to refuse to participate in such research projects.
10	The patient has the right to expect reasonable continuity of care. He has the right to know in advance what appointment times and physicians are available and where. The patient has the right to expect that the hospital will provide a mechanism whereby he is informed by his physician or a delegate of the physician of the patient's continuing health care requirements following discharge.
11	The patient has the right to examine and receive an explanation of his bill regardless of source of payment.
12	The patient has the right to know what hospital rules and regulations apply to his conduct as a patient.

Figure 18.15 The patient's bill of rights.

Table 18.3 Health-Consumer Protection Agencies

Agency	Affiliation	Role
Food and Drug Administration (FDA)	Federal government	Bans false and misleading statements on drug labels; requires that active ingredients be listed on labels; demands that all manufactured foods, drugs, and cosmetics be proven safe before they can be marketed; evaluates new drugs for safety and effectiveness.
Federal Trade Commission (FTC)	Federal government	Protects consumers against injuries that could result from false advertising and unfair selling practices; investigates cases of deceptive practices.
Consumer Product Safety Commission	Federal government	Develops and enforces safety standards for thousands of household products.
United States Postal Service	Federal government	Guards the public against sale of fraudulent products by mail.
Better Business Bureau (BBB)	Private nonprofit organization	Helps resolve consumers' complaints against businesses.
Consumers' Union	Private	Impartially tests and rates consumer products; publishes *Consumer Reports,* which compares price, performance, and safety of brand-name items including drugs and other health products.
Consumer reporters	Local radio and television stations	Use the power of publicity to resolve consumer complaints.

provides a basis for sound, independent decisions about health choices and purchases. For a listing of the leading agencies that protect consumers against unsafe and ineffective health products, see Table 18.3.

Another factor that contributes to poor consumer decisions about health is fear—of pain, of illness, or of death. Frequently this fear leads to a counterproductive reaction in which people delay seeing a doctor for their symptoms because they don't want their fears confirmed. Quacks take advantage of such fears by advertising "cures" that they claim are both painless and fully guaranteed. Often these "cures" seem to work because of the so-called *placebo effect.* (Placebos are inactive substances, such as "sugar pills," that are often used as controls in drug research; they sometimes improve a patient's condition simply through their suggestive, psychological value.) Wishful thinking, hope, the charisma of a quack therapist, and his or her promises all have a placebo effect, and people may seem to get better from these alone.

HOW TO RECOGNIZE QUACKERY

It is appalling that sick people waste their money—or, worse, risk their very lives—by taking useless medicines and following the advice of a health quack. The best line of defense against quackery is to learn both about health generally and about how quacks work, since quackery often follows certain patterns. If the answers to the following questions tend to be "yes"—watch out.

1. Does the sponsor of a product or service claim to be battling the medical profession, which is supposed to be trying to suppress the wonderful discovery? Does he or she maintain that surgery, X-ray, or medication prescribed by reputable physicians will do more harm than good?
2. Is the remedy sold from door to door by a self-styled "health adviser" or advertised in public lectures? Is it promoted in a sensational magazine, by a faith healer's group, or by a crusading organization of lay people?
3. Does the sponsor use scare tactics, predicting all sorts of harmful consequences if you do not use the product?
4. Is the product or service offered as a "secret remedy"?
5. Does the promoter show testimonials to demonstrate the wonders that the product or service has performed for others?
6. Is the product or service claimed to be good for a vast array of illnesses, or guaranteed to provide a quick cure?

"Guarantees in medicine," point out Vickery and Fries, "are almost a guarantee that the product or service is worthless. In medicine, a guarantee is not possible. . . . No worthwhile medical service is accompanied by a guarantee. . . . The offer itself strongly suggests a suspicious product."

People with certain diseases are particularly likely to fall prey to health quacks. Probably the biggest—and certainly the cruelest—area of quackery today is the field of cancer. Cancer quacks take advantage of fearful people, who often delay proper treatment so long that the cancer does become incurable. Or else quacks raise false hopes among people with terminal cancers—and fleece them of their money for worthless "cures." For a discussion of specific forms of cancer quackery, see Chapter 15.

Another disease that attracts quacks is arthritis. For every dollar spent on arthritis research, fifteen are spent on arthritis quackery. The reason for such rampant quackery is that arthritis is both chronic and—as yet—incurable. Although it is highly treatable—simple aspirin often reduces some of the pain and inflammation—quacks have invented a variety of worthless devices and "cures." One of the most common is the copper bracelet, which, quacks claim, cures arthritis magnetically. Millions of these are sold every year. Another quack treatment for arthritis involves vibrators. These may relieve some minor muscle pain and soothe temporarily, but aspirin is more effective.

A LIFELONG RESPONSIBILITY

As we have seen, most Americans are fortunate enough to have an excellent health-care system at their disposal. But this system is geared toward treatment. Maintaining good health and preventing disease are largely *your* responsibilities. Caring for the body that you are going to live in for, hopefully, the next half-century or so is a long-term activity that no one else can perform for you. As the Talmud puts it, "If I am not for myself, who will be for me? . . ."

SUMMARY

1. In the United States, health care is becoming more widely regarded as a basic human right and social responsibility.
2. Community health efforts have been developing in two main directions, consumer representation and community organization. Community clinics are one of the more promising results of community involvement.
3. The deficiency of the American medical-care system lies in its inability to bring excellent medical care to all people. Reasons for this include inefficient distribution of physicians, inadequate health insurance coverage, and the high cost of health care.
4. Hospitalization accounts for the largest and fastest-rising portion of health expenditures. Many reasons for high hospital costs are legitimate, but others result from inefficiency.
5. There is evidence that much unnecessary surgery is performed in the United States, causing a huge waste of lives and money.
6. Organizations outside the medical profession are now taking a greater interest in the quality of medical care.

7. Means of improving the health-care system include health systems agencies, personnel reforms, more equitable distributions of health personnel, health coverage reforms, such as HMOs, and an improved delivery system providing for an easier and more accurate entrance into the system.

8. Even national health insurance would not change the basic structure of our health system. Some believe that the answer lies in a national health service.

9. We all have primary responsibility for our own well-being, and we can generally do more for our own health than a physician can. It would be a good idea to take a self-care course.

10. Most common illnesses—such as colds, stomach upsets, aches, and mild fevers—are self-limiting diseases that usually run their course within a short period of time. Doctors generally cannot cure these ailments.

11. There is a difference of opinion among physicians as to whether routine, annual physical examinations are worth the time and expense.

12. Among the circumstances in which you should seek prompt medical attention are massive bleeding, major burns, broken bones, and suspected poisonings. If another person is in severe pain, has cold sweats, is short of breath, or is unconscious or disoriented, you should get medical help for him or her.

13. To protect yourself against quackery, you should be suspicious if sponsors claim that the medical profession is trying to suppress their wonderful discovery, that the product or service is good for a vast array of illnesses, or that it is guaranteed to provide a quick cure.

Appendix of Common Diseases

A

Addison's disease A disease produced by underactivity of the adrenal glands and an insufficient supply of the adrenal hormones aldosterone and hydrocortisone in the body. It is caused by destruction of the adrenal cortex by unknown factors or by an infective process such as tuberculosis. Aldosterone deficiency is characterized by the inability of the body to retain the salts necessary to maintain blood pressure. When hydrocortisone is deficient, symptoms include weakness, loss of appetite, and low blood sugar. There also is a characteristic pigmentation of the skin. The disease can be fatal if an "adrenal crisis" occurs and the patient enters a state of shock and general collapse. The presence of Addison's disease is confirmed through blood and urine analyses, and treatment consists of the administration of supplementary amounts of the deficient hormone.

amebiasis Better known as amoebic dysentery, amebiasis is a protozoan infection of the lower intestine resulting in abdominal pain and diarrhea. It is transmitted through food contaminated by infected insects or persons or through water contaminated by sewage. It has an incubation period of from five days to three months, and it can last for many years. Symptoms range from mild discomfort and loose bowel movements to acute diarrhea and dehydration, sometimes resulting in death. Amebiasis confers no immunity, and there is no vaccination process. Preventive measures consist mainly of attempts to decrease the modes of transmission.

amoebic dysentery *See* amebiasis.

angina pectoris *See* text, Chapter 16.

appendicitis An infection of the appendix, a tubelike extension from the first segment of the large intestine. The appendix becomes swollen, tense, and markedly congested. There is a sharp localized pain. As pus production increases, an abscess may form on the wall of the appendix, causing the wall to rupture (perforate). Rupture of the wall creates a generalized infection (peritonitis) of the peritoneum, the abdominal lining that envelops most of the abdominal viscera. These serious, and occasionally fatal, complications can be avoided by timely surgical removal of the diseased appendix (appendectomy).

arthritis A chronic, disabling, systemic inflammation of the joints. The first symptoms include early fatigue, fever, morning stiffness, and swelling in the small joints of the hands and feet. Gradually, the affected joints become more deformed and swollen, and in extreme cases the limb can be rendered useless. The causes of arthritis are not understood, although it is thought to be an autoimmune disease. There is no cure and the best treatment includes rest, heat, aspirin, and use of certain antiinflammatory drugs that are reserved for severe attacks. Surgical treatment for rheumatoid arthritis has returned many hands to almost normal functioning by replacement of damaged joints with plastic ones.

asthma A symptom of severe irritation of the lungs and bronchial tubes resulting from an allergic reaction, particle irritation, or microbe infection. It is characterized by coughing, wheezing, and shortness of breath. The causes of asthma are unknown, but allergic asthma can be precipitated by several substances, including pollen, dust, and animal hair. Treatment of asthma involves inhalation or injection of adrenalin. Asthma attacks are best prevented by avoiding substances that will precipitate a reaction.

atherosclerosis *See* text, Chapter 16.

athlete's foot The common name for edinaphitos. It is a fungal infection characterized by blistering, scaling, and cracking of the skin between the toes. It is a common, universally occurring disease, more prevalent in men than in women or children. Athlete's foot is usually transmitted indirectly through contact with contaminated clothing, shower stalls, or gymnasium floors; it has an incubation period of from ten to fourteen days; and it may never disappear completely. Thorough washing and drying of the skin around the toes and prolonged exposure of the feet to the drying effects of air will usually eliminate the fungus. In extreme cases an antifungal drug may be used to fight the infection. *See also* ringworm.

B

bacillary dysentery *See* shigellosis.

bacterial endocarditis An infection of the inner heart lining that can be either acute or subacute and that creates growths on the heart valves. It is usually a complication of minor surgery or of respiratory infections such as pneumonia, and it is most common in persons with congenital heart valve defects or with valves otherwise damaged by such childhood diseases as rheumatic fever. Symptoms of the acute form include high fever and chills eventually leading to death; symptoms of the subacute form, which is more common, include fatigue, weakness, anemia, and mild fever. As the disease advances, emboli composed of portions of the growths on the valves begin to close up arteries throughout the body. Treatment consists of the administration of antibiotic drugs such as penicillin, and prevention of the disease in susceptible persons is accomplished by the administration of antibiotics prior to and after minor surgery.

bacterial pneumonia An acute infection and vasocongestion of the lung characterized by fever, coughing, chest pain, and difficult breathing. In most cases it is caused by the pneumococcal bacteria and is better known as pneumococcal pneumonia, but other common types of bacteria from the mouth and throat can produce pneumonia as a complication of other diseases. Pneumonia is transmitted through the mouth or by nasal discharges associated with coughing or nose blowing; it has an incubation period of from one to three days; and it usually lasts from seven to ten days if untreated. Medical treatment consists of isolation and rest for the patient and treatment with antibiotics.

botulism A deadly food poisoning produced by an anaerobic bacterium that grows in the soil and in the intestines of some animals. It is contracted by the ingestion of a toxin produced by bacterial spores sealed inside improperly canned food and allowed to multiply. Symptoms, which occur within twelve to thirty-six hours and vary in severity depending on the amount of toxin ingested, include headache, weakness, and paralysis; death can be rapid due to the inability to breathe. Treatment consists of the administration of a specific antitoxin. The poison can be avoided by boiling canned foods for three minutes, which destroys the toxin.

Bright's disease *See* nephritis.

bronchitis *See* text, Chapter 13.

brucellosis *See* undulant fever.

bubonic fever *See* plague.

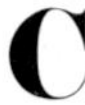

cancer *See* text, Chapter 15.

cerebral palsy The name for a wide variety of physical defects that result from brain damage occurring before or shortly after birth. Exact cause of the damage is often unknown, but such conditions as Rh-blood factor clash between mother and fetus, maternal kidney disease, or high-fever infections of an infant may lead to it. Symptoms of the disease depend on the degree of brain damage and range from partial weakening of one limb to general loss of motor ability and mental retardation. The most common manifestation of the disease is loss of coordination due to imbalance of opposing muscular groups. Cerebral palsy is noncontagious and noncurable. Treatment consists of lessening the severity of the muscular defects through supportive bracing and physical therapy.

chancroid A sexually transmitted disease characterized by the presence of a soft chancre (an open sore) on the genitals and severe, painful swelling of the lymph nodes of the groin. The disease is transmitted through sexual intercourse with infected persons, has an incubation period of from one to three days, and is contagious until healed. Treatment consists of administration of antibiotics, and prevention is best accomplished, but not assured, by thorough washing immediately following intercourse with an infected person. No immunity is conferred, and no artificial immunity is available.

chickenpox A viral disease found throughout the world and endemic to almost all large urban areas. Symptoms include moderate fever, headache, and a characteristic rash, which develops first on the trunk and spreads to the extremities. The rash is composed of blisterlike eruptions that break, form a crusty scab, and finally fall off. Chickenpox is transmitted by droplet infection, is communicable from one day before to six days after the first appearance of the rash, has an incubation period of from two to three weeks, and usually lasts about five days. Because the disease confers a lifetime immunity against reinfection, it is most prevalent in children. Treatment is symptomatic, and secondary infections are prevented through washing and restricting unnecessary movement. Prevention of the spread of chickenpox is accomplished by isolation of infected persons; artificial immunization is unavailable.

cholera A severe bacterial infection of the small intestine found most often in temperate underdeveloped countries such as India. Symptoms of the disease include unceasing diarrhea, vomiting, loss of kidney function, and extreme thirst. Cholera is transmitted through contaminated food or water, has an incubation time of from five to six days, and usually results in death through dehydration and uric acid poisoning. When death does not occur, recovery usually takes place within two weeks. Immunization is achieved through inoculation. Cholera is no longer a problem in the United States.

cirrhosis A systemic disease usually caused either by excessive consumption of alcohol or by the nutritional deficiencies associated with alcoholism. It is characterized by a hardened, enlarged liver filled with scar tissue. As the amount of scar tissue increases, more functioning liver cells are lost, and liver failure develops. Muscles waste and abdominal fluid collects. Jaundice occurs as the diseased liver can no longer supply the body with enough protein to build new tissue and retain fluid within the vascular bed. Treatment is based on good nutrition and avoidance of alcohol. Sometimes this treatment is successful in the motivated individual, but usually the disease is preterminal and little can be done to reverse it.

Clostridium perfringens A bacterium, from the same family as those responsible for botulism and tetanus, that causes a mild food poisoning through spoiled meat dishes. Symptoms of the disease include abdominal pain and diarrhea occurring within six hours after ingestion of the toxin. The disease usually lasts less than one day and is nonfatal. Ingestion of the toxin can be avoided by heating and cooling meat dishes as rapidly as possible and by not eating meat that has been long at room temperature.

colitis *See* ulcerative colitis.

common cold *See* text, Chapter 14.

conjunctivitis An acute, usually bacterial, infection of the conjunctiva. It is characterized by dilation of the blood vessels of the sclera, secretion of pus from the eyes, swelling of the eyelids, and light sensitivity of the eyes. The disease is highly contagious and is transmitted by direct contact or by indirect contact with soiled articles such as towels, handkerchiefs, or bed linen. The incubation time is from one to three days, and conjunctivitis is communicable until symptoms disappear. Applications of tetracycline ointment quickly relieve the symptoms, but the disease may remain infectious for several days.

coronary artery disease *See* text, Chapter 16.

cystic fibrosis A chronic hereditary disease characterized by malformation or absence of the excretory duct of any of several glands. The organs most commonly affected are the pancreas, liver, sweat glands, mucus-producing glands of the lung and throat, and the testicles. Symptoms depend on the gland affected, but the usual course of the disease is chronic and progressive respiratory infection resulting in early death. Antibiotics can prolong the life of the patient and decrease the severity of lung infections. Special diets are often necessary to assure the normal development of affected children.

D

diabetes A systemic disease caused by a deficiency of insulin, a hormone produced by specialized cells in the pancreas. Insulin deficiency interferes with sugar metabolism, obstructs the body's efforts to store carbohydrates as glycogen, and causes excessive accumulation of sugar in the blood, resulting in the excretion of excessive sugar in the urine. The utilization of fat is also impaired. There are two basic types of diabetes—juvenile and adult. The juvenile type occurs during childhood or early adulthood, with the average age of onset being ten to twelve years of age. Juvenile diabetes appears to be a genetic defect resulting in a severe deficit in the synthesis of insulin by the pancreas. The adult type of diabetes most commonly develops in obese individuals after age forty. This diabetes appears to be caused by insufficient insulin production rather than lack of insulin and is not as severe as the juvenile type. Some forms of diabetes may be due to the destruction of insulin-producing cells as a consequence of pancreatic diseases rather than a genetic defect. Common symptoms include increased urinary output, increased thirst and appetite, and fatigue. The complications of diabetes affect all body systems, particularly the cardiovascular, endocrine, and nervous systems. Diseases of these systems are exacerbated by diabetes. The objective of treatment is to correct the disturbed metabolism by the administration of insulin and the restriction of dietary carbohydrates, to maintain normal nutrition and reasonable weight by dietary alterations and exercise, and to prevent or slow down the progress of any complications.

diphtheria An acute bacterial infection characterized by mild fever, sore throat, and a runny nose; it sometimes lasts several weeks. It has an incubation period of from one to six days, is usually contagious for about two weeks beginning three days before the onset of symptoms, is fatal 5 to 10 percent of the time, and is transmitted through contact with nasal or throat discharges of an infected person. Though the symptoms are not severe, the toxin released by the bacterium can permanently damage the heart or nervous system. Diphtheria usually confers a lasting immunity, and children born to immune mothers retain a passive immunity for about six months. Active immunization can also be induced through vaccination.

Down's syndrome *See* text, Chapter 4.

dysentery *See* amebiasis; shigellosis.

E

eczema A term used to lump together all skin irritations characterized by redness, itching, blisters, or scales. If the conditions persist, the skin will eventually become tough and leathery. The application of creams and ointments containing cortisone or the oral administration or injection of cortisone can usually improve the condition.

emphysema *See* text, Chapter 13.

endocarditis *See* bacterial endocarditis.

enterobiasis (pinworms) An infection of the intestinal tract characterized by disturbed sleep, irritability, and itching of the anal area. It is common among children and affects about 20 percent of the United States population. Pinworms are transmitted by the ingestion of eggs laid on the perianal skin and transferred to clothing or hands and eventually to food. The disease is communicable for two to eight weeks after infection and disappears spontaneously. The spread of pinworms is best prevented by strict cleanliness and good toilet habits.

epilepsy An expression of irritation within the brain, frequently caused by a small piece of brain tissue that begins to produce abnormal electrical activity when stimulated. The abnormal activity can spread to neighboring pieces of tissue, gradually involving larger areas of the brain, causing loss of consciousness and often uncontrollable body movements. The symptoms can now be fully controlled by appropriate drug treatment, and when properly handled, the epileptic can lead an essentially normal life. Another procedure that has been quite successful is the removal of the abnormal piece of brain tissue in which the seizure begins.

G

gallstones Accumulation in the gall bladder of stones composed of cholesterol, bile pigment, and calcium. They often are painless and do no harm. They occur in about a quarter of the older people in the United States and cause chronic inflammation of the gall bladder. Occasionally a stone will pass out of the gall bladder into the common bile duct and obstruct the flow of bile into the duodenum. Severe pain in the lower right chest, nausea, and often vomiting follow; jaundice is present in some cases. When these symptoms occur, the presence of gallstones is confirmed by X-ray. Treatment consists of the surgical removal of the gall bladder and stones; preventive measures are unknown.

gastritis Inflammation of the stomach accompanied by gastric indigestion. Gastritis is a catchall term for chronic or acute afflictions caused by many different and sometimes unknown agents. It is most common in older people and is characterized by irritation and reddening of the stomach lining. Symptoms of acute gastritis are nausea, headache, temperature increase, and finally vomiting to remove the irritant, followed by fatigue. Treatment consists of avoidance of irritating substances. Symptoms of the chronic condition, which often indicates a developing ulcer, are similar to those of acute gastritis but are less severe. Chronic gastritis has been attributed to various vitamin deficiencies, secretory malfunctions, and the mild abuse of alcohol. Treatment of the chronic form consists of bed rest, a bland diet, and medication to reduce the acid level of the stomach.

gastroenteritis A catchall term for a variety of severe gastrointestinal inflammations that may be symptoms of another disease or may be an independent infection caused by a number of bacterial and viral agents. Symptoms include nausea, vomiting, diarrhea, and abdominal cramps, and treatment usually consists of a change of diet and in severe cases, surgery. Gastroenteritis may result from food poisoning, chronic alcoholism, hepatitis, or malaria, among others. When it results from infection by a microbial agent, the disease usually lasts from one to two days and is more likely to be fatal among infants than among other age groups. It is endemic in many underdeveloped areas of the world and is transmitted primarily by fecal contamination of food.

German measles *See* rubella.

glaucoma *See* text, Chapter 18.

gonorrhea *See* text, Chapter 14.

ground itch *See* hookworm.

H

Hansen's disease An infectious bacterial disease that affects the skin, the mucous membranes of the mouth, and the testes. The disease is universal but is most prevalent in Asia, Africa, and South America. It is characterized by ulcerous lesions of the skin in which the cutaneous nerves are destroyed, leading to eventual death of the tissue. Only moderately infectious, the disease is transmitted by direct contact with an infected person and has an incubation time of from a few months to twenty years. The disease cannot be cured, but its progress can be slowed through the use of sulfa drugs and antibiotics. Isolation of diseased persons is essential to prevent the spread of Hansen's disease.

hay fever A hypersensitive reaction (allergy) to normal pollens in an environment. During seasons when pollen is prevalent, preformed antibodies bind the inhaled pollens, resulting in upper respiratory distress. Symptoms include swelling of the mucous lining of the nose and throat, wheezing and sneezing, redness in the eyes, and blurred vision. The skin also may become red, itchy, and swollen. A susceptible person can avoid pollens either by changing locations or by taking antihistamines to diminish the allergic response. Also available are a series of desensitization injections that familiarize the body to the specific allergen, thus reducing the allergic response. This treatment is usually reserved for severe allergies, however, because the time required for successful desensitization is quite long.

hemophilia *See* text, Chapter 4.

hemorrhoids (piles) Varicose veins of the rectum. They can be caused by prolonged constipation, excess straining at defecation, diarrhea, or pregnancy. Hemorrhoids are characterized by small folds of swollen skin around the anus; these folds are often painful or itchy. Because hemorrhoids are more annoying than dangerous, treatment usually consists of measures to prevent their irritation through stool-softening medication or soothing ointments and suppositories. In extreme cases, hemorrhoids can be removed surgically.

hepatitis *See* text, Chapter 14.

hernia The protrusion of any organ beyond the space it normally occupies. The term is most often associated with protrusions of an abdominal organ through the abdominal wall. The abdominal wall is weak in the areas of the groin, the navel, and the center of the diaphragm where the esophagus enters the abdomen. If undue strain is put on these weak areas by coughing or by lifting heavy objects, there is a possibility that the wall will rupture and a portion of the intestines or stomach will protrude through the muscle layer. If the hernia is inguinal (groin) or umbilical, a portion of the small intestine will protrude, causing swelling at the site; the swelling will often disappear when the patient lies on his back. In the case of an esophagial hernia, the stomach or a portion of it will protrude into the chest cavity, interfering with the functioning of the heart or lungs. Esophagial hernias are characterized by heartburn and indigestion after meals or when lying down. The danger of a hernia is the possibility that the protruding organ will be strangulated and die because of inadequate blood supply. Treatment of hernias consists of trussing to hold in the protruding organ or surgery to close the hole in the abdominal wall.

herpes simplex *See* text, Chapter 14.

herpes zoster Better known as shingles, a viral infection of a cutaneous nerve root characterized by pain, redness, and blisters along the nerve. It usually affects a nerve of the trunk of the body, and the rash and blisters follow the nerve around the body in a beltlike manner; it can also affect the eyes. Herpes zoster usually affects adults and is caused by the same virus that produces chickenpox in children. Because the disease is self-limiting, pain-relieving measures usually are the only treatment, but cortisone is occasionally used to arrest its progress, and antibiotics are used to treat secondary infections of the blisters. The disease confers a lasting immunity against reinfection and is extremely rare in persons who have had chickenpox during childhood.

histoplasmosis A common fungal infection of the lungs characterized by weakness, mild fever, mild chest pains, and cough; the disease often passes unnoticed. The histoplasmosis mold grows in soil and animal excrement and is transmitted to humans through inhalation or ingestion of the fungal spores; it is not communicable from person to person. The incubation period is from five to eighteen days after exposure, and excessively high doses of the spores can result in a rare and fatal form of the disease. Susceptibility to the disease is general, and the best means of prevention is avoidance of contaminated areas or adequate sanitary precautions when near such areas. Treatment is symptomatic, and the disease confers an immunity against serious reinfection.

hookworm A serious intestinal infection resulting in anemia and malnutrition. The disease is contracted through the skin, usually the feet, and initially produces a severe local irritation called ground itch. The hookworm larvae, which live in the soil, penetrate to the lymphatic system or to a blood vessel and travel to the lungs. From within the lungs they migrate to the throat and are swallowed. Once in the digestive tract the larvae mature into worms and fasten themselves to the intestinal wall. The worms feed on the blood of their host. Eggs appear in the stools of the host about six weeks after infection and continue to be present as long as the infection continues. Administration of specific drugs eliminates the worms. The best means of prevention is adequate sanitation and sewer facilities.

hypertension *See* text, Chapter 16.

I

influenza *See* text, Chapter 14.

K

kidney stones *See* urolithiasis.

kwashiorkor *See* text, Chapter 8.

L

leprosy *See* Hansen's disease.

leukemia A cancer of the white blood cells that can be either chronic or acute. Early symptoms of the chronic condition, which develops slowly and has a long duration, include loss of appetite, weakness, general atrophy, and night sweats. As the chronic condition progresses, symptoms become acute and include high fever, sores and bleeding gums, and severe weakness. The number of white blood cells can be from 15 to 100 times that found in normal blood, and anemia and an enlarged spleen usually accompany the disease. The cause of leukemia is unknown, as is any cure, but it is possible to prolong the life of the patient through the use of cortisone, therapy with radioactive substances, and blood transfusions. *See also* text, Chapter 15.

liver-fluke disease *See* schistosomiasis.

lockjaw *See* tetanus.

lousiness *See* pediculosis.

M

malaria An infectious protozoan disease characterized by remittent fever alternating with chills. Because the disease is transmitted by the bite of a mosquito, it is most prevalent in tropical areas. The incubation time is two weeks. Symptoms begin with general muscular aches and fever, rapidly progressing to chills accompanied by violent shaking and cyanosis. Administration of quinine or a similar drug eliminates the symptoms, but patients can usually recover without medication. Prevention of malaria is best accomplished through eradication of the vector mosquito; daily small doses of quinine will also prevent the disease.

measles (rubeola) An infectious viral disease common in children and characterized by severe rash. It is transmitted through contact with discharges from the nose or throat of an infected person, who can spread germs by sneezing or coughing. It is infectious from a week to eleven days after it is contracted. Early symptoms, which appear about ten days after exposure, include fever, coughing, and swelling and congestion of the mucous membranes of the nose and throat. White spots appear in the mouth, and the following day a rash begins to develop on the scalp and forehead, gradually spreading over the entire body in about four days. As the rash, which is composed of red blisterlike eruptions, progresses, the fever begins to subside. The rash disappears after five days. Treatment consists of isolating the patient and guarding against secondary infection. Measles confers a lifetime immunity, and injections of gamma globulin will provide an artificial immunity for two to six weeks.

meningitis An acute inflammation of the meninges, the membranes enclosing the brain and spinal cord. The disease usually results from a bacterial infection following an injury to the head or as a complication of several infectious diseases. Incubation time for the disease is two to ten days, and symptoms include fever and general aching and pain in the entire body, progressing to severe headaches, vomiting, and intense pain. Treatment of meningitis includes hospitalization and the administration of antibiotic drugs. The disease can usually be prevented or diagnosed early by careful attention to infections of the nose and throat and by the administration of antibiotic drugs to anyone exposed to the disease. Meningitis is rarely fatal if treated properly.

migraine Headaches caused by vasodilation of the arteries of the brain; they are usually severe. Migraine attacks affect a specific area of the head and progress in a characteristic sequence. Headaches begin with a dull building pain and progress to symptoms of confusion, depression, temporary blindness, abdominal pain, or nausea. Treatment of migraine consists of immobilizing the patient in a darkened room and making him or her as comfortable as possible. There is no known way to prevent a migraine headache, but an early awareness and treatment of an impending attack can lessen its severity.

mononucleosis *See* text, Chapter 14.

multiple sclerosis A chronic degenerative disease of the central nervous system, usually affecting people between the ages of twenty and forty. Symptoms of the disease include weakness and loss of coordination in the legs and hands, problems with speech and vision, or loss of certain autonomous functions, such as digestion. Symptoms result from the destruction of the myelin sheaths that cover nerve fibers in the brain and spinal cord. The patient usually retains complete mental facility, but because nervous impulses cannot be properly transmitted, he or she loses muscular control. Multiple sclerosis is marked by long periods of seemingly good health alternating with the manifestations of symptoms that usually become more severe with each occurrence. Because the causes of the myelin sheath destruction are unknown, there is no cure or method of prevention for multiple sclerosis, but proper care and otherwise good health can reduce the frequency of attacks.

mumps An acute viral infection of the parotid and salivary glands located beneath the angle of the jaw bone. It is common and mild during childhood and usually confers a lifelong immunity. Symptoms include swollen glands, puffiness in the side of the face, difficulty opening the mouth, and mild to moderate fever. The disease is transmitted by direct contact with the nasal or throat discharges of an infected person and has an incubation period of from two to three weeks. Complications are rare in children, but mature males often develop a secondary infection in the testicles that can lead to sterility; the disease may also affect the ovaries and breasts of women. For this reason adults who have not had mumps as children should be vaccinated.

muscular dystrophy A chronic condition characterized by gradual weakening, atrophy, or paralysis of a muscle, muscular group, or entire limb. The condition usually results from a disorder of the nerves controlling the affected area. There are several forms of muscular dystrophy affecting different age groups and different areas of the body. There is no known cure for muscular dystrophy.

myasthenia gravis A chronic nervous-system disease of unknown cause. It primarily affects the voluntary muscles of the face, mouth, and eyes and results in slack facial expression, difficulty in eating and talking, and strained vision. Muscles become extremely weak and tire quickly. The disease usually affects adults and develops slowly. The administration of specific drugs can lessen the severity of the disease, and facial exercises can strengthen the muscles involved. Occasionally the thymus gland is removed surgically or treated with X-rays with some beneficial effect.

mycoplasmal pneumonia An acute infection and vasocongestion of the upper respiratory tract characterized by fever and coughing. It is caused by the Eaton agent, a viruslike organism. Mycoplasmal pneumonia is transmitted through the mouth or nasal discharges of an infected person, has an incubation period of from one to three weeks, and can last from three days to several weeks. Treatment consists of isolation and rest for the patient; maintenance of general good health is the best means of prevention.

N

nephritis A general term for any condition marked by inadequate excretory functioning of the kidney due to inflammation of the blood vessels in the nephrons. Common symptoms include the presence of the protein albumin in the urine, swollen ankles, fatigue, and headaches. If the condition becomes severe it can include such symptoms as nausea and vomiting, swelling of the abdomen, and unconsciousness. Acute nephritis is most commonly called Bright's disease and can become chronic if not treated promptly.

Treatment consists of bed rest and limitations on fluid and protein consumption.

nephrosis A chronic childhood disease of unknown cause characterized by degeneration of a noninflamed kidney. Symptoms include remittent edema alternating with periods during which the child seems perfectly normal. During the periods of edema, severe swelling occurs in the face, abdomen, and feet. Swelling subsides quickly with the excretion of large amounts of urine, and the symptom-free periods can last from a few days to months or may even be permanent. Nephrosis usually affects a child for several years and disappears spontaneously. Treatment consists of a special diet and the administration of certain adrenal hormones.

P

paralysis agitans *See* Parkinson's disease.

paratyphoid fever An acute bacterial infection of the intestines similar to typhoid fever. Symptoms include sudden and continuing fever, diarrhea, and the appearance of red spots on the body. The disease is transmitted by direct contact with an infected person or carrier or by contact with food contaminated by an infected person. Paratyphoid has an incubation period of from one to ten days and is communicable from the onset of symptoms to several days after recovery. Susceptibility is general, and the disease usually confers a lasting immunity against reinfection. Treatment consists of isolation and the administration of antibiotic drugs.

Parkinson's disease (paralysis agitans) A chronic condition of old age characterized by progressive paralysis and eventual death. Symptoms begin with a palsy or rigidity of a single limb that spreads to both limbs on one side, then to all the limbs, and finally to the muscles of the trunk and face. The disease seems to originate in the brain, and surgery to reduce the activity of concerned areas of the brain is often performed. Specific chemotherapy can reduce the severity of symptoms and in some instances may improve the patient's condition.

pediculosis Infestation with lice. Two common species of lice attack humans, the body louse and the crab louse; humans are not bothered by animal lice. The body louse infests only the head, beard, and body, and the crab louse infests the pubic region. Lice are transmitted by direct contact with an infested person or by contact with the clothes of an infested person. Symptoms of pediculosis include extreme irritation and itching of the infested area. Eradication of lice is usually accomplished through bathing and applications of poison dusting powder.

peptic ulcer An ulceration of the stomach membrane caused by excess gastric acid. In a healthy stomach, there is a balance between the chemicals that digest the food and the mucus that coats and protects the stomach lining. Excess acid production and/or a defective or insufficient mucus production may combine to upset the protective balance, and localized lesions, known as ulcers, can develop. Emotional stress appears to contribute to the formation of peptic ulcers. The acid first destroys the surface membrane. If the production of acid continues in excessive quantities, the ulcer invades the underlying muscle tissue. An ulcer causes gnawing pains in the stomach that can be relieved by either antacids or milk. Unfortunately, ulcer victims find they are comfortable only when they keep food in their stomachs, since pains often occur during the night. Ulcers sometimes erupt blood vessels, causing hemorrhage and vomiting of blood. Eventually, if allowed to go untreated, a peptic ulcer will perforate the stomach wall, and gastric juices will escape into the abdominal cavity. At this point, surgery is necessary to close the perforation, or the ulcer may be fatal.

pertussis *See* whooping cough.

phenylketonuria (PKU) *See* text, Chapter 4.

piles *See* hemorrhoids.

pink-eye *See* conjunctivitis.

pinworm *See* enterobiasis.

plague An acute, bacterial infection of two types, bubonic fever and pneumonic plague. If untreated, one-quarter to one-half of the cases are fatal. Symptoms of both types include fever, low blood pressure, delirium, and coma. Bubonic plague is further characterized by swelling of the lymph nodes of the groin. The disease exists in wild rodents in several areas of the world and is transmitted to humans through the bite of an infected rat flea; pneumonic plague can also be spread by droplet infection. The incubation period is from two to six days, and susceptibility is general. The disease confers a temporary immunity; and a temporary artificial immunity is available through vaccination. Treatment of plague involves the administration of antibiotics. The best means of prevention is the eradication of urban rat populations.

pneumonia *See* bacterial pneumonia; mycoplasmal pneumonia.

pneumonic plague *See* plague.

poliomyelitis An acute viral infection of a part of the spinal cord. It can vary in severity, but it usually strikes in one of three recognizable forms. Symptoms of the most mild form include fever, headache, diarrhea, and aching muscles; this form often is not recognized as polio. The second form of the disease is known as nonparalytic and is characterized by temporary paralysis of the limbs. A final form, known as paralytic, can be permanently disabling or cause death. The disease is usually transmitted through droplet infection or contact with the feces of a person infected with the mild form of the disease. The incubation period is from one to three weeks, and the disease is communicable from two days to six weeks after infection. Polio cannot be treated, but vaccination provides a lifetime immunity against infection.

psoriasis A chronic skin disease of unknown cause characterized by recurrent eruptions of local inflammation, composed of patches or red spots that increase in size until they resemble a thick scaly welt. As the welt heals the skin is temporarily discolored and the scales begin to fall off the eruption. Psoriasis is usually found on the feet, hands, and knees, but it also can occur on the scalp and chest. Treatment of the disease is aimed at reducing the severity of the skin eruptions and includes special low-fat or low-alcohol diets, hormone injections, radiation therapy, administration of sedatives or tranquilizers, and the application of special ointments. Psoriasis cannot be spread from one person to another, but little else is known about its cause or the means to prevent it.

puerperal fever *See* streptococcal puerperal fever.

R

rabies (hydrophobia) A viral disease transmitted by the bite of an infected animal. From the bitten site, the virus travels up the nerve fiber until it reaches the brain. Along the way it produces pain and spasms in associated muscles; after reaching the brain it develops into a frank encephalitis, with the frightening symptom of hydrophobia (fear of water) that causes the person to convulse at the sight or taste of fluid. Once the disease sets in it is fatal. Proper wound care and vaccination, which consists of up to fourteen injections, must be quickly performed if an infection is suspected.

rheumatic fever *See* text, Chapter 16.

ringworm A fungal infection of the skin characterized by blistering, scaling, and loss of hair. It is highly contagious and exists in several different forms. The disease is most prevalent in children and in persons living in warm, damp climates. Ringworm can be transmitted directly or indirectly through contact with an infected person's clothing, and it has an incubation period of from ten to fourteen days. A common source of transmission is an infected household pet. Thorough washing and drying of the affected areas and the application of antifungal ointments eliminate the infection. When hairy parts of the body are involved, the hair is usually clipped short or removed. *See also* athlete's foot.

Rocky Mountain spotted fever A tick-borne rickettsial infection most prevalent in the Rocky Mountain states but also occurring infrequently throughout the United States and parts of Canada and Mexico. Symptoms include fever, a rash starting on the wrists and ankles and spreading over the entire body, headache, and infection of the conjunctiva. The disease is common in wild rodents and is transmitted to man by the bite of an infected wood tick or dog tick. The incubation time is from two to ten days. If untreated, spotted fever lasts for about two weeks and is fatal 20 percent of the time. The administration of tetracycline until the fever disappears usually assures recovery. The best prevention is avoidance of tick-infested areas and careful and prompt removal of any ticks from one's person or pets.

rubella (German measles) A mild, highly contagious viral infection common between the ages of four and nineteen. Symptoms include fever, rash, and swollen glands in the throat and neck. The disease is transmitted by direct contact or by droplet infection and has an incubation period of from two to three weeks. Rubella is infectious from seven days before until about ten days after the appearance of the rash. Treatment consists of isolating the patient and guarding against secondary infection. Rubella confers a lifetime immunity, and vaccination is available but rarely administered. If contracted during the first trimester of pregnancy, the adult form of the disease can cause serious birth defects. Vaccination of pregnant women is advised. *See also* text, Chapter 4.

rubeola *See* measles.

S

salmonellosis An acute food poisoning produced by several types of salmonella bacteria. Symptoms include fever, sudden pain of the abdomen, diarrhea, loss of appetite, nausea, and vomiting. A common disease, the infection is usually contracted through ingestion of contaminated meat or poultry, but it can be spread from person to person by direct contact. The incubation period is from six hours to two days. Salmonellosis is rarely fatal, and treatment usually consists of keeping the patient as comfortable as possible while the disease runs its course. The best means of prevention is thorough cooking of all meat dishes and eggs.

scabies An infection of the skin by a small mite. Symptoms include intense itching along small lesions at the base of the fingers and toes, in the armpits, on the breasts of women, and on the genitals of men. The female mites burrow under the skin, creating tunnels about a quarter of an inch long in which eggs are laid. As the eggs hatch, the burrow opens to the surface and the mites escape. The disease is transmitted by direct contact and has an incubation time of from one to two weeks. It is communicable until the mites are eradicated. Treatment consists of frequent bathing in hot water followed by applications of a special ointment to the affected areas.

scarlet fever A streptococcal infection characterized by fever, sore throat resembling tonsillitis, rash, and swelling of the glands of the neck and tongue (strawberry tongue). The disease is transmitted by direct contact, droplet spread, or contact with clothing of an infected person. It has an incubation period of from one to three days and is usually communicable for two to three weeks after infection. If untreated the disease can have serious complications, including nephritis, scarring of the valves of the heart, and severe arthritis. The administration of penicillin decreases the severity of the symptoms and usually prevents complications. Scarlet fever confers a lifetime immunity.

schistosomiasis Liver-fluke disease. It is common in most underdeveloped areas of the world. The worms deposit eggs in various organs of the body, and as each egg matures it produces a small scar in the tissue. The long-term effect of this process is gradual deterioration of any organ involved. The disease is contracted by contact with water containing the worm larvae, which enter the body through the skin. The larvae migrate to the liver and mature before entering the veins of the abdomen as adult worms. Eggs discharged in the urine and feces hatch into larvae, which must invade a fresh-water snail. After living within the snail for several weeks, the larvae become free-swimming and can attack humans. Symptoms appear from four to six weeks after infection, and the disease is communicable as long as eggs are discharged from the body, sometimes for twenty-five years. The worms and eggs are killed by the injection of a specific drug. The best means of prevention is avoidance of endemic areas.

shigellosis (bacillary dysentery) An acute bacterial infection of the intestine. Symptoms include fever, vomiting, abdominal cramps, diarrhea, and often the passing of blood. The disease occurs throughout the world but is more severe in warmer climates. It is transmitted by contact with food, water, or objects contaminated by the feces of an infected person, and it has an incubation period of from one to seven days. Shigellosis is infectious as long as bacteria are present in the feces, usually two weeks. Water and salt are given to replace that lost by diarrhea, and the patient is made as comfortable as possible; in severe cases antibacterial drugs can be used to combat the infection. The best prevention consists of adequate disposal of feces and purification of water supplies.

shingles *See* herpes zoster.

sickle cell anemia *See* text, Chapter 4.

smallpox A highly contagious viral disease known for the disfiguring pockmarks that it produces. Symptoms of the disease include fever, headache, and pain of the abdomen lasting from three to four days. As these symptoms pass and temperature returns to normal, a rash of small red blisters forms over the body. The blisters form scabs and fall off in about three weeks, leaving characteristic scars. Smallpox is transmitted by direct contact with an infected person, by contact with the scab of a smallpox blister, or by droplet infection. The incubation period is from seven to sixteen days, and the disease is infectious from the time symptoms appear until all the scabs have fallen off. The disease is fatal about 30 percent of the time but confers a lifetime immunity to survivors. Artificial immunity is recommended in special situations only, since the disease has been all but eradicated.

staphylococcal disease A general term referring to infection of any of several parts of the body by staphylococcus bacteria. The disease is universal but is more prevalent in crowded living areas, infant nurseries, and hospital wards. Symptoms depend upon where the disease occurs: in the community, staphylococcal disease is usually characterized by fever, headache, and widespread skin lesions that can lead to conjunctivitis or pneumonia; in infant nurseries, skin lesions are common and such complications as abscess of the breast or brain, pneumonia, and septicemia (the invasion of the bacteria into the bloodstream) occur; in hospital wards, the elderly are usually victims and suffer from lesions that may develop into pneumonia or septicemia, or cause death. The disease is transmitted by direct contact with an infected person or a carrier or by contact with the clothing or bed linen of an infected person, and it has an incubation period of from two days to several weeks. It is contagious until all lesions disappear. The administration of appropriate antibiotic drugs hastens recovery and decreases the severity of symptoms. Prevention is best accomplished by personal hygiene and avoidance of infected persons.

staphylococcal food poisoning An acute reaction to toxins produced by several strains of staphylococcus; it is not an infection. Symptoms include abdominal pain, diarrhea, nausea, and vomiting. It is contracted by eating foods in which staphylococci have grown and produced toxic wastes; such foods are commonly pastries, salads, and sliced meat products. The incubation period is from two to four hours, and the disease usually lasts less than two days. It is rarely fatal, and treatment consists of making the patient as comfortable as possible.

strep throat *See* tonsillitis.

streptococcal puerperal fever An acute bacterial infection of the genital tract of women who have recently given birth or undergone abortion. Symptoms include fever, headache, and pain in the lower abdomen. The disease is transmitted by direct contact with a streptococcal carrier or infected person or by contact with contaminated clothing or bed linen. Incubation time is from one to three days, and the infection is communicable for about three weeks. Penicillin is used to treat puerperal fever. Fatal cases are now rare.

syphilis *See* text, Chapter 14.

T

tapeworm A parasitic infection of the digestive tract characterized by the presence of worm segments, or proglottides, in the feces. Symptoms may be absent or may include abdominal pain, diarrhea, constipation, anemia, or weight loss. The disease is contracted by eating inadequately cooked beef or pork containing the worm larvae. The proglottides first appear in the feces from eight to ten weeks after infection and may continue to appear for as long as forty years. Tapeworm eggs are passed with the proglottides and hatch into larvae after being eaten by cows or hogs. A major complication of pork tapeworm is invasion of the larvae into the muscles or nervous system of the host. Drugs are available that can kill the intestinal worms, but no therapy is available to eliminate the larvae. The best means of prevention is avoidance of raw meats.

Tay-Sachs disease *See* text, Chapter 4.

tetanus (lockjaw) An acute bacterial infection of the central nervous system with a fatality rate of about 35 percent. The bacteria responsible for the disease live in the intestines of horses, cattle, and humans, in animal feces, and in soil. The bacterial spores enter the body through a cut or puncture wound and incubate from four days to three weeks. Tetanus symptoms include infection at the site of entry, painful muscular spasms, fever, headache, stiffening of the muscles of the neck and jaw, and eventual stiffening of the entire body. The best prevention is through vaccination and the administration of a booster injection when danger of infection is suspected. For unvaccinated individuals, antitoxin serum is available. Tetanus does not always confer an immunity against reinfection.

tonsillitis (strep throat) Usually a streptococcal infection of the tonsils, the spongy lymph glands located in the back of the mouth on either side of the throat. Symptoms include fever, headache, nausea, pain and redness of the throat, and swelling of the lymph glands of the neck. The disease is transmitted by direct contact with a carrier or an infected person, by contact with the clothing or bed linen of an infected person, or by droplet infection. The incubation time is from one to three days, and the disease is communicable for ten days after infection. Tonsillitis is rarely serious unless it becomes chronic, and in the absence of treatment symptoms usually disappear within nine days. The administration of penicillin shortens the course of the disease and reduces the potential for spread. The best means of prevention is avoidance of infected persons.

trachoma A chronic viral eye disease characterized by inflammation of the eyes, excessive tearing, small scarring, blisters on the eyelids that eventually cause them to become deformed, light sensitivity, and the growth of blood vessels into the cornea leading to possible blindness. The disease is highly contagious and is transmitted by direct contact with the tears of an infected person or indirectly through contact with soiled articles. The incubation time is from five to twelve days and trachoma is infectious until symptoms disappear. Applications of tetracycline ointment usually eliminate the infection. No immunity is conferred. The best prevention is avoiding infected persons.

trichinosis A roundworm infection of the muscles

characterized by abdominal pain, nausea, fever, muscular pain, and sometimes swelling of the eyelids. The disease is usually contracted by eating larvae-infested pork. The ingested larvae develop into worms in the small intestine. As the adult worms reproduce, second-generation larvae penetrate the intestinal wall and migrate in the blood and lymphatic systems to various muscles, where they form small painful cysts. As the cysts become embedded in the muscles, they are surrounded by scar tissue and the symptoms disappear. The parasite is most common in the United States and eastern Europe, and susceptibility is general. No treatment exists, and no immunity is conferred against reinfection. Adequate cooking or freezing of all pork products is the best way to avoid the disease.

trichomoniasis *See* text, Chapter 14.

tuberculosis An infectious disease that may affect almost any tissue in the body, especially the lungs.

typhoid fever An acute bacterial infection characterized by fever, headache, slow pulse, body rash, constipation or diarrhea, and enlargement of the spleen. The disease is transmitted by direct contact with an infected person or through water contaminated by infected feces or urine. The incubation period is from one to three weeks, and susceptibility is general. If untreated, typhoid fever lasts for about three weeks, is infectious throughout its course, and is fatal about 10 percent of the time. Specific antibiotic chemotherapy reduces the fatality rate to 2 percent and relieves the severity of the symptoms. Typhoid fever confers a high immunity against reinfection, and artificial immunity is available through vaccination.

typhus fever An acute rickettsial infection characterized by fever, headache, and a rash that spreads from the inside of the thighs and armpits over the entire body. Two major types of typhus fever exist, epidemic louse-borne and endemic flea-borne, differing in the severity of their symptoms and mode of transmission. The disease is transmitted from rats, which are the reservoir of infection, to humans via the feces of feeding lice or fleas. The incubation time is from one to three weeks. The fatality rate for untreated epidemic typhus is from 10 to 40 percent; for untreated endemic typhus it is about 2 percent. Tetracycline reduces the fatality rate of both types and relieves the severity of the symptoms. Typhus fever confers a limited immunity for several years, and artificial immunization is available through vaccination. Additional preventive measures consist of attempts to eliminate rats, lice, and fleas from crowded residential areas.

U

ulcer *See* peptic ulcer.

ulcerative colitis a catchall term describing any condition in which the large intestine is inflamed and extensively ulcerated and the cause is unknown. Symptoms include severe, often bloody, diarrhea, moderate fever, and general atrophy of the body and weight loss. A bland diet accompanied by medication to slow the diarrhea is the usual treatment in mild cases. If inflammation persists and becomes severe, the colon is surgically removed.

undulant fever (brucellosis) An acute bacterial infection characterized by remittent fever, sweating, headache, constipation, and pain and weakness of the entire body. The disease is common among domestic farm animals and is transmitted to humans by contact with an infected animal or by drinking unpasteurized milk from an infected goat, sheep, or cow. Incubation period is from five days to three weeks, and although the fatality rate is only 2 percent, the infection and symptoms can persist for several years. Antibiotics are used to combat the disease, but the relapse rate is high. The degree of immunity conferred by undulant fever is unknown, and no means of artificial immunity exists.

urolithiasis (kidney stones) The formation of stones in any part of the urinary tract. Stone formation is thought to result from the precipitation of urinary sediment from too highly concentrated urine and is promoted by urinary infection and infrequent urination. Symptoms of kidney stones include pain in the lower abdomen and progressive uric acid poisoning. The disease is treated by administering drugs to dissolve the stones or by surgery to remove the stones.

W

whooping cough (pertussis) An acute bacterial infection of the throat and lungs that primarily affects children. Symptoms include mild fever and a characteristic violent cough that can last as long as two months. Whooping cough is transmitted by direct contact, droplet infection, or indirect contact with mouth or nasal discharges of an infected person. It has an incubation period of from one to three weeks and is contagious during the early stages. Antibiotics reduce the period of communicability but do little to relieve the symptoms. Whooping cough confers a lasting immunity, and artificial immunization is available through vaccination.

Y

yellow fever An acute viral disease characterized by early fever, headache, and vomiting, followed by subnormal temperatures, intestinal bleeding, and jaundice. The disease is transmitted by the bite of an infected mosquito, and the incubation period is from three to six days. The fatality rate of yellow fever can be as high as 40 percent during an epidemic, and no method of treatment is known. In nonfatal cases recovery takes place in about ten days, and the patient is immune for life. Artificial immunization is available through vaccination.

Further Readings

Chapter 1 Mental Health

Aguilera, D. C., and **J. M. Messick.** *Crisis Intervention.* St. Louis, Mo.: C. V. Mosby, 1978.
How to take appropriate action in crisis situations.

Alvarez, A. *The Savage God: A Study of Suicide.* New York: Random House, 1970. This is a well-researched yet highly personal and emotional study of suicide. Alvarez explores the way that thoughts of suicide color the world of creative persons, recounts his own attempt at suicide, and traces the history of myths surrounding the phenomenon.

Bach, G. R., and **H. Goldberg.** *Creative Aggression.* New York: Avon Books, 1974.
These two psychologists contend that suppression of natural anger and aggression is dangerous to mental health. They provide methods for using aggression constructively and for dealing with suppressed hostility in other people.

Barnes, M., and **J. Berke.** *Mary Barnes: Two Accounts of a Journey Through Madness.* New York: Harcourt Brace Jovanovich, 1971.
This book consists of interspersed chapters by Mary Barnes, who went on a journey through madness, and by Joseph Berke, the psychiatrist who helped Mary out of it.

Benson, H. *The Mind/Body Effect.* New York: Simon & Schuster, 1979.
A presentation of the psychological factors inherent in all health and disease processes. The book offers practical guidance and discusses the effects of behavioral medicine.

Chessick, R. D. *How Psychotherapy Heals.* New York: Science House, 1969.
Chessick discusses the complex methods of long-term psychotherapy. Although intended primarily for specialists, this book also will aid the general reader in understanding the work of psychoanalysts and psychotherapists.

Erikson, E. H. *Childhood and Society.* 2nd ed. New York: W. W. Norton, 1963.
In this classic work, Erikson discusses his eight stages of psychological development in the light of Freud's theory of infantile sexuality. Also included are fascinating chapters on American Indian societies, Adolf Hitler, and Maxim Gorky.

Glasser, W. *Positive Addiction.* New York: Harper & Row, 1976.
An application of the theories of addiction to positive health habits and life styles. It presents a fascinating rationale for becoming "addicted" to practices that are good for us.

Glasser, W. *Reality Therapy.* New York: Harper & Row, 1965.
A presentation of psychotherapy based on the principle that people do not act irresponsibly because they are "ill"; rather, they are "ill" because they act irresponsibly.

Green, H. *I Never Promised You a Rose Garden.* New York: Holt, Rinehart & Winston, 1964.
This sensitive and powerful novel of a brilliant and schizophrenic young girl and her struggle with reality is an often frightening account of life in a mental institution.

Kaplan, B. (ed). *The Inner World of Mental Illness.* New York: Harper & Row, 1964.
A fascinating collection of first-person accounts of what it is like to experience severe mental disturbance. The last section of the book consists of excerpts from literary classics and from the diaries of well-known authors and thinkers.

Kesey, K. *One Flew over the Cuckoo's Nest.* New York: Viking, 1964.
A sometimes funny and often frightening novel about one man's experience inside a mental institution. An important work because it forces the reader to confront the issue of the value of therapy.

Lindner, R. *The Fifty-Minute Hour.* New York: Bantam Books, 1954.
A psychologist has put together a

fascinating and informative collection of short "stories" that are adapted from case histories of people he has treated in therapy.

Maslow, A. *Toward a Psychology of Being.* 2nd ed. Princeton, N.J.: Van Nostrand, 1968.
The fundamental concepts of Maslow's humanistic psychology are contained in this classic work.

Newman, M., and **B. Berkowitz.** *How to Be Your Own Best Friend.* New York, Ballantine Books, 1971. *How to Be Awake and Alive.* New York: Random House, 1975.
A husband-and-wife team of psychologists provide, in these two small books, affirmative advice to the person who is not living up to the best of his or her potential. The first book is really about enhancing one's self-esteem; the second delves into childhood sources of adult unhappiness.

Rogers, C., and **B. Stevens.** *Person to Person: The Problem of Being Human.* Lafayette, Calif.: Real People Press, 1967.
A good analysis of the dynamics of Rogers's approach to client-centered therapy.

Sheehy, G. *Passages.* New York: Bantam Books, 1976.
A fascinating presentation of the common and predictable crises in adult life. It encourages people to accept and make the most of changes in adulthood.

Szasz, T. S. *Ideology and Insanity.* Garden City, N.Y.: Doubleday, 1970.
A collection of essays by a controversial psychiatrist, this book presents a case for removing mental and emotional problems from the area of medicine and treating them instead as "problems in living." The essays cover a variety of related topics, from involuntary commitment to community psychiatry.

Zimbardo, P. G. *Shyness.* Reading, Mass.: Addison-Wesley, 1978.
An authoritative but down-to-earth attempt to understand and deal with the widespread problem of shyness.

Chapter 2
Stress and Health

Benson, H. *The Relaxation Response.* New York: Avon Books, 1975.
A discussion of those elements common to all leading relaxation methods. It also presents a simplified program for self-relaxation.

McQuade, W., and **A. Aikman.** *Stress.* New York: Dutton, 1974.
This popularly oriented book describes the effects of stress on human beings and provides means for dealing with stress.

Selye, H. *Stress Without Distress.* New York: Lippincott, 1974.
Dr. Selye applies his scientific discoveries and hypotheses on stress to daily living.

Chapter 3
Human Sexuality

Bem, S. "Androgyny vs. the Tight Little Lives of Fluffy Women and Chesty Men." *Psychology Today* 9 (September 1975), 58.
A brief treatise on the importance of escaping from the confines of rigid sex-role stereotypes.

Calderone, M. S. *Questions and Answers About Love and Sex.* New York: St. Martin's Press, 1979.
A book about human sexuality within ongoing relationships, written in a frank question-and-answer style.

Comfort, A. *The Joy of Sex.* New York: Simon & Schuster, 1972.
An explicit, honest, warm presentation of love-making techniques, illustrated with numerous line drawings.

Fisher, P. *The Gay Mystique.* Briarcliff Manor, N.Y.: Stein and Day, 1972.
The author describes the world of the male homosexual and in the process explodes many myths about the gay world.

Forisha, B. *Sex Roles and Personal Awareness.* Morristown, N.J.: General Learning Press, 1978.
An optimistic view of changing sex roles in modern American culture.

Hite, S. *The Hite Report.* New York: Dell, 1976.
This nationwide survey of female sexuality was based on questionnaire responses from 3,000 women. The many direct quotes from respondents reinforce the conclusions of this controversial report. The book is very informative and reassuring.

Hoffman, M. *The Gay World.* New York: Basic Books, 1968.
Hoffman combines the insights of psychiatry and the social sciences in his thoughtful and intelligent probing of the social and individual roots of homosexuality.

Hyde, J. T. *Understanding Human Sexuality.* New York: McGraw-Hill, 1979.
This comprehensive text on sexuality deals with a wide range of issues —from gender-role development to basic erotic processes.

McCary, J. L. *Human Sexuality.* 2nd ed. New York: Van Nostrand, 1973.
The author explores the psychological and sociological factors of human sexuality as well as the physiological.

Masters, W. H., and **V. E. Johnson.** *The Pleasure Bond.* Boston: Little, Brown, 1975.
The noted sex researchers bring their technological knowledge to bear on the problems of long-term sexual relationships and on the role of sex in marriage.

West, D. J. *Homosexuality.* Chicago: Aldine, 1968.
West utilizes the results of physiological and psychological research in his examination of the causes, social significance, and treatment of homosexuality.

Chapter 4
Reproduction and Health

Apgar, V., and **J. Beck.** *Is My Baby All Right?* New York: Trident Press, 1972.
A highly informative guide to birth defects: what causes them, the major defects, how they can be treated or prevented.

Berrill, L. J. *The Person in the Womb.* New York: Dodd, Mead, 1968.

In this beautifully written book, Berrill describes what takes place in the womb as a new individual develops. Aspects of human development from ovulation and genetic complications to the significance of prenatal individuality are discussed from both the scientific and humanistic perspectives.

Bing, E. *Moving Through Pregnancy.* New York: Bobbs-Merrill, 1975.
Bing, the woman who introduced the Lamaze method of natural childbirth to this country, emphasizes keeping an active life style while pregnant.

Consumer's Union. "Cutting the Risks of Childbirth After 35." *Consumer Reports* (May 1979), 302–306.
A dramatic account of the increasing risks of pregnancy and child rearing after the age of thirty-five. Includes suggestions for minimizing some of these risks.

Consumer's Union. "Test Yourself for Pregnancy." *Consumer Reports* (November 1978), 644–645.
A discussion of the self-testing kits for pregnancy and their drawbacks in terms both of expense and accuracy.

Greenblatt, A. *Heredity and You: How You Can Protect Your Family's Future.* New York: Coward, McCann & Geoghegan, 1974.
A useful guide to the causes, symptoms, diagnosis, and treatment of genetic disorders.

Lamaze, F. *Painless Childbirth.* Chicago: Contemporary Books, 1956.
The classical explanation of and guidelines for natural childbirth from the originator of the Lamaze technique.

Rugh, R., and **L. Shettles.** *From Conception to Birth: The Drama of Life's Beginnings.* New York: Harper & Row, 1971.
This book is a detailed account of embryonic and fetal development, including more than a dozen remarkable color photographs of the developing human fetus.

The Womanly Art of Breastfeeding. Franklin Park, Ill.: La Leche League International, 1963.
The La Leche League has prepared a comprehensive guide to the procedures involved in breastfeeding. The book also covers the rationale for breastfeeding and answers women's questions about the effects of breastfeeding on the mother's body.

Chapter 5
Birth Control

Arnstein, H. S. *What Every Woman Needs To Know About Abortion.* New York: Scribner's, 1973.
This comprehensive guide for the woman considering abortion covers the alternatives involved, medical care, legal aspects, emotional factors, and aftercare. It includes a list of helpful agencies.

Greenfield, M. *The Complete Reference Book on Vasectomy.* New York: Avon Books, 1973.
The author discusses the pros and cons of male sterilization, the procedures involved, and the availability of surgery. A list of clinics and hospitals providing vasectomies is included.

Guttmacher, A. F. *Birth Control and Love.* New York: Macmillan, 1969.
Unwanted pregnancy can bring disharmony to an already crowded family or disaster to a woman who will seek an illegal abortion. The author believes that pregnancy should result from decision rather than be a risk of sexual expression. This readable book details methods of contraception, discusses abortion, and covers the problem of infertility.

Chapter 6
Marriage and Parenthood

Beck, J. *How To Raise a Brighter Child.* New York: Simon & Schuster, 1967.
Beck presents the case for early cognitive stimulation of children and provides guidelines for rearing mentally well-functioning children.

Bernard, J. *The Future of Marriage.* New York: World, 1972.
In this classic work, Jesse Bernard distinguishes "his" marriage from "her" marriage and shows that, statistically, men have benefited from marriage whereas women may actually have been harmed by this institution.

Bird, C. *The Two-Paycheck Marriage.* New York: Rawson Wade, 1979.
A definitive report on the social revolution resulting from the increasing number of women entering the work place, and the consequences for marriage, child rearing, and the self-image of women.

Cable, M. *The Little Darlings: A History of Child-Rearing in America.* New York: Scribner's 1975.
Cable has produced a fascinating study of attitudes toward children over the years, starting with colonial times. She emphasizes the need for a recognition of the rights of children.

Dodson, F. *How To Parent.* Los Angeles: Nash, 1970.
This book is a complete guide to the emotional and intellectual development of children to six years of age. Avoiding generalities, the author offers specific advice for handling all phases of the development of the preschool child.

Edwards, M., and **E. Hoover.** *The Challenge of Being Single.* Los Angeles: Tarcher, 1974.
The authors demonstrate that there is nothing abnormal about choosing the single life; they probe the psychological factors involved in being single.

Epstein, J. *Divorced in America.* Baltimore, Md.: Penguin, 1974.
The author explores the sexual, legal, psychological, and economic aspects of divorce.

Erikson, E. *Identity, Youth and Crisis.* New York: W. W. Norton, 1968.
This book is heavy reading but of value for those interested in Erikson's idea that the adolescent identity crisis is the crucial influencing force on adult development.

Ginott, H. *Between Parent and Child.* New York: Macmillan, 1965.

This excellent book emphasizes the importance of regarding a child's behavior as a special way of communicating ideas the child may not be able to verbalize. The author provides practical advice on how parents and children can understand and get along with one another.

Gordon, T. *P.E.T.: Parent Effectiveness Training.* New York: New American Library, 1975.
The author proposes in this book a "no-lose" method of solving conflicts. Both parents and child take part in the decision-making process so that neither "wins" nor "loses."

Holt, J. *How Children Fail.* New York: Pitman, 1964.
This book is an important critique of American education. Holt is an advocate of the open-classroom situation.

Holt, J. *How Children Learn.* New York: Pitman, 1967.
In this sequel to *How Children Fail,* Holt shows how some children are able to learn on their own, experimentally or as a game.

Hunt, M. M. *The World of the Formerly Married.* New York: McGraw-Hill, 1966.
One out of every three contemporary marriages will end in divorce. The author surveyed the middle-class divorced population, and his account of their lives is interesting and informative.

James, M. *Marriage Is for Loving.* Reading, Mass.: Addison-Wesley, 1979.
A comprehensive guide to the art and science of marriage, this book includes a variety of learning exercises geared to facilitate understanding and success in marriage.

Krantzler, M. *Creative Divorce.* New York: Signet, 1974.
The thesis of this interesting book is that divorce can provide an opportunity for personal growth.

Laing, R. D. *The Politics of Experience.* New York: Ballantine Books, 1967.
Laing offers a probing exposé of the individual and the family—the methods that family members use to manipulate and exploit one another in the name of socialization and protection.

McCary, J. L. *Freedom and Growth in Marriage.* New York: Hamilton, 1975.
The author presents marriage as a relationship in which each member must work to develop his or her human potential.

O'Neill, N., and G. O'Neill. *Open Marriage.* New York: Evans, 1972.
In this controversial work the authors contend that current attitudes toward marriage do not meet individual needs and that couples need to reexamine their relationship and restructure it so that each partner's needs can be met.

Rogers, C. *Becoming Partners: Marriage and Its Alternatives.* New York: Dell, 1972.
Carl Rogers interviewed people involved in a number of different relationships—communes, triads, mixed marriages, and so on—and has included the case studies of many of these marriages in this book, complete with his own commentaries. Rogers draws on his long experience as a therapist and on his own fifty-year marriage to produce an insightful and involving probe of human interaction at its most intimate level.

Westermarck, E. *A Short History of Marriage.* New York: Humanities Press, 1968.
More than a simple history of marriage, this book explores the variety of marriage contracts and rituals across time and cultures.

Chapter 7
Aging and Facing Death

Ariès, P. *Western Attitudes Toward Death.* Baltimore, Md.: Johns Hopkins, 1974.
A noted sociologist describes the rituals and attitudes surrounding death in Western culture from the thirteenth century on.

deBeauvoir, S. *The Coming of Age.* New York: Warren Books, 1970.
A comprehensive and masterful work on human aging—past, present, and future.

Heifetz, M. D., with C. Mangel. *The Right to Die.* New York: Putnam, 1975.
Writing sensitively about all aspects of euthanasia, a physician examines the social and ethical issues involved and advocates allowing people to die in whatever manner they choose.

Kart, C. S. et al. *Aging and Health—Biological and Social Perspectives.* Reading, Mass.: Addison-Wesley, 1978.
A general text on the health problems specific to aging.

Kübler-Ross, E. *Death: The Final Stage of Growth.* New York: Spectrum, 1975.
This noted thanatologist describes death as an important psychological stage and as a potential source of emotional growth for the families and friends of the terminal patient. She also comes to grips with the institutionalized setting for death and the need for medical personnel to be trained to deal with death.

Kübler-Ross, E. *On Death and Dying.* New York: Macmillan, 1969. *Questions and Answers on Death and Dying.* New York: Macmillan, 1974.
In this classic work and its follow-up volume, Kübler-Ross probes the important needs of the dying person.

Langone, J. *Vital Signs: The Way We Die in America.* Boston: Little, Brown, 1974.
A journalist presents a shocking picture of what happens around deathbeds—the callousness of medical personnel, the blindness of friends and relatives, the fear and turmoil of the terminal patient.

Lifton, R. J., and E. Olson. *Living and Dying.* New York: Praeger, 1974.
The authors have written a long essay on the denial of death in American society and how it is manifested in our culture.

Mitford, J. *The American Way of Death.* New York: Fawcett, 1969.

Mitford's book is a classic exposé of the funeral industry.

Parkes, C. M. *Bereavement: Studies of Grief in Adult Life.* New York: International Universities Press, 1972.
This book is a presentation of Parkes's twelve years of research on the way people react to death.

Phipps, J. *Death's Single Privacy: Grieving and Personal Growth.* New York: Seabury Press, 1974.
Phipps tells her personal story of dealing with her husband's death, telling her children their father is gone, handling difficult financial problems, and coming out of the experience with a different sense of self and a different viewpoint on life.

Schneidman, E. W. "You and Death," *Psychology Today* 4 (August 1970), 67–72; and 5 (June 1971), 43–45, 73–80.
Schneidman developed a death questionnaire that was published in August 1970; the results were published in June 1971. Taking the questionnaire is a valuable experience; reading people's responses is almost as enlightening.

Weisman, A. D. *The Realization of Death.* New York: Aronson, 1974.
A noted thanatologist describes his pioneering methods for dealing with cancer patients and potential suicides.

Chapter 8
Nutrition

Bailey, H. *The Vitamin Pioneers.* New York: Pyramid, 1970.
This fascinating book records the discovery of various vitamins and describes their function in maintaining health.

Deutsch, R. M. *The New Nuts Among the Berries.* Palo Alto, Calif.: Bull Publishing, 1977.
An eye-opening exposé of the modern forms of nutritional quackery, firmly based on the principles of nutritional science.

Kirschmann, J. D. *The Nutrition Almanac.* New York: McGraw-Hill, 1975.
This comprehensive volume contains tables of food composition, discussion of the physiology of digestion and the role of nutrients, and description of the consequences of nutritional deficiency. The book is very readable.

Lappe, F. M. *Diet for a Small Planet.* New York: Ballantine Books, 1975.
A delightful, though scientific, exploration of foods and nutrition from an ecological perspective. Destined to become a classic in the field.

Mayer, J. *A Diet for Living.* New York: Pocket Books, 1976.
The nation's leading authority on nutrition presents a light-hearted approach to making eating one of life's pleasures and the key to good health.

Smith, N. J. *Food for Sport.* Palo Alto, Calif.: Bull Publishing, 1976.
A discussion of the nutritional aspects of physical performance and sport. Debunks some of the popular fallacies on the subject.

Stare, F. J., and **M. McWilliams.** *Living Nutrition.* New York: Wiley, 1975.
In addition to basic information about nutrition, the authors cover the role of technology in food production, global food problems, social and economic factors in food selection, and nutritional disorders.

Stare, F. J., and **E. Whelan.** *Eat OK Feel OK! Food Facts and Your Health.* North Quincy, Mass.: Christopher Publishing, 1978.
A presentation of the facts of nutrition by the former Chairperson of the Department of Nutrition at Harvard University.

Trager, J. *The Food Book.* New York: Avon, 1970.
Trager has put together a fascinating history of food—how various items came to be eaten by humans, the myths surrounding various foods, the role of food in medicine, food frauds and fads, and the "invention" of new foods in recent times.

Whelan, E., and **F. J. Stare.** *Panic in the Pantry.* New York: Atheneum, 1975.
The authors put food fads into perspective, debunk many food myths (including the myth of "organic foods"), and justify the use of food additives.

Chapter 9
Weight Management

Berland, T. *Rating the Diets.* Skokie, Ill.: Consumer Guide, 1975.
Actually an issue of *Consumer Guide* magazine, this handy paperback is an invaluable introduction to the various weight reduction plans, from Stillman to grapefruit to macrobiotic diets. The diets are evaluated for health considerations as well as for effectiveness.

Ferguson, J. M. *Habits, Not Diets: The Real Way to Weight Control.* Palo Alto, Calif.: Bull Publishing, 1976.
An application of behavior-modification techniques to weight management. The book includes day-by-day steps toward a change in one's eating habits.

Mayer, J. *Overweight: Causes, Cost, and Control.* Englewood Cliffs, N.J.: Prentice-Hall, 1968.
Mayer attempts to dispel misconceptions about obesity and presents physiological causes and effects of this condition. He takes a nutritional approach to weight control and provides information on the variety of medicinal treatments in current use.

Sharkey, B. J. *Physiological Fitness and Weight Control.* Missoula, Mont.: Mountain Press, 1974.
A competent presentation of how to achieve physiological fitness and successfully manage weight control.

Chapter 10
Physical Fitness

Astrand, P-O. *Health and Fitness.* Woodbury, N.Y.: Barron's, 1977.
A simplified explanation, by Europe's foremost fitness expert, of the scientific principles of exercise; includes guidelines for tailor-

ing a fitness program to individual needs.

Cooper, K. *The Aerobics Way.* New York: Bantam Books, 1977.
An updated and expanded treatment of cardiovascular and respiratory fitness training by the developer of the original aerobics training system.

Fixx, J. F. *The Complete Book of Running.* New York: Random House, 1977.
An encyclopedic reference on running for competition, fun, and fitness. The book draws richly from the most authoritative sources on running and the physiology of exercise.

Shepherd, R. J. (ed.). *Frontiers of Fitness.* Springfield, Ill.: Charles C Thomas, 1971.
Shepherd has collected the results of recent research in the physiology of exercise.

Chapter 11
Drug and Drug Use

Benowicz, R. J. *Non-Prescription Drugs and Their Side Effects.* New York: Grosset & Dunlap, 1977.
Guidelines for the appropriate and safe use of the various nonprescription drugs.

Blum, R. H., et al. *Society and Drugs.* San Francisco: Jossey-Bass, 1969.
The history and sociology of drugs are explored in this extremely well-documented and carefully researched work.

Brecher, E. M. *Licit and Illicit Drugs.* Boston: Little, Brown, 1972.
Brecher and the editors of *Consumer Reports* have put together a comprehensive guide to psychoactive drugs.

Cohen, S. *The Drug Dilemma.* New York: McGraw-Hill, 1969.
Drug taking is presented as a recurrent historical phenomenon precipitated by social and psychological problems. The author outlines the dangers of drug taking and describes the role of parents and teachers in providing youth with a clearer sense of the meaning of life.

Kaplan, J. *Marijuana—The New Prohibition.* New York: World, 1970.
Kaplan believes that the destructiveness of antimarijuana laws far outweighs their benefits to society and advocates radical changes in the structure of present drug laws.

Pawlak, V. *Conscientious Guide to Drug Abuse.* Hollywood: Do It Now Foundation (P.O. Box 3573), 1970.
This drug guide is particularly useful in providing information on helping people who are on bad trips, have overdosed on speed, or have otherwise suffered unpleasant effects from taking drugs.

Szasz, T. *Ceremonial Chemistry: The Ritual Persecution of Drugs, Addicts and Pushers.* Garden City, N.Y.: Doubleday, 1974.
A noted psychiatrist criticizes American attitudes toward drug use and abuse and makes a strong case for decriminalization of drugs.

Task Force on Women. *A Woman's Choice: Deciding About Drugs.* DHEW Publication, Number 4DM 79-820.
A guide to the intelligent use of drugs, this publication deals especially with those drugs most often used by women.

Chapter 12
Alcohol

Cahalan, D. *Problem Drinkers.* San Francisco: Jossey-Bass, 1970.
This book is the result of a national survey involving 1,359 respondents. The social and personality characteristics that distinguish problem drinkers from alcoholics and the means to predict problem drinking are among topics discussed in this well-documented book.

Department of Health, Education and Welfare. *Alcohol and Health.* New York: Scribner's, 1972.
Originally prepared as a report to Congress, this volume provides a wealth of material on the effects of alcohol consumption on health.

Fort, J. *Alcohol: Our Biggest Drug Problem.* New York: McGraw-Hill, 1973.
Fort demonstrates that alcohol abuse must be considered a major drug problem in the United States and that social sanctions play a major role in perpetuating abuse of this drug.

Only, M. *High: A Farewell to the Pain of Alcoholism.* Englewood Cliffs, N.J.: Prentice-Hall, 1974.
A candid and involving account of one man's twenty-five-year dependence on alcohol and his final successful struggle to free himself from the drug.

Plant, T. F. (ed.). *Alcohol Problems: A Report to the Nation.* New York: Oxford University Press, 1967.
This readable book, written by a commission of experts on alcoholism and noted scholars in relevant disciplines, surveys contemporary alcohol use and abuse and offers specific suggestions for future treatment and study.

Roueché, B. *The Neutral Spirit.* Boston: Little, Brown, 1960.
Roueché provides an interesting non-technical discussion of the most widely used intoxicant known to humans. He discusses the history of the development of alcoholic beverages, as well as the physical and emotional effects of moderate and excessive drinking.

Chapter 13
Smoking

Hunt, W. A. (ed.). *Learning Mechanisms in Smoking.* Chicago: Aldine, 1970.
This book is the edited proceedings of a conference sponsored by the American Cancer Society. Several aspects of habituation, tolerance, and the roles of psychological, social, and pharmacological factors in cigarette smoking are discussed.

Lichtenstein, E. "How to Quit Smoking," *Psychology Today* 4 (January 1971), 42, 44–45.
Lichtenstein examines the effectiveness of aversive conditioning, group therapy, emotional role playing, and "cold turkey" as approaches to helping people quit smoking.

Magnuson, W. G., and **J. Carper.** "Toward a Safer Cigarette," in W. G. Magnuson and J. Carper, *The Dark Side of the Market Place.* Englewood Cliffs, N.J.: Prentice-Hall, 1968, pp. 185–207.
This article deals with cigarette advertising and the reluctance of cigarette manufacturers to produce a safer product.

U.S. Department of Health, Education, and Welfare. *Smoking and Health: A Report of the Surgeon General.* Washington, D.C.: U.S. Government Printing Office, 1979.
This report contains a wealth of information on the relationship between smoking and health. It also deals with the behavioral, social, and economic components of cigarette smoking.

Zalman, A., et al. *Stop Smoking for Good: A Proven Seven-Week Program.* New York: Walker, 1976.
A presentation of an effective method and program to stop smoking.

Chapter 14
Communicable Diseases

Camp, J. *Magic, Myth and Medicine.* New York: Taplinger, 1974.
The author traces magical cures and folk medicines that have been used against illness from ancient times to the present. His approach makes one realize that many current practices, now seen as scientific, may in time be considered "folk medicine."

Cockburn, A. *The Evolution and Eradication of Infectious Diseases.* Baltimore, Md.: Johns Hopkins, 1963.
This book provides valuable background material for the study of epidemiology. It covers such aspects as the role of speculation in research, the evolution of infectious diseases, and the basic principles of disease eradication. Several diseases are discussed as examples of the principles presented in the first half of the book.

Dale, P. M. *Medical Biographies: The Ailments of Thirty-three Famous Persons.* Norman, Okla.: University of Oklahoma Press, 1952.
This is a collection of nontechnical medical biographies of selected famous persons from Buddha to Grover Cleveland. Although possibly inaccurate, these interesting vignettes illustrate the importance of health and medicine throughout history.

Dubos, R., and **J. Dubos.** *The White Plague: Tuberculosis, Man and Society.* Boston: Little, Brown, 1952.
The nature of tuberculosis and preventive and therapeutic procedures are discussed in this book. The authors conclude that human beings must incorporate what they know about biology into their social system and the workings of everyday life before we can seriously consider eradicating social diseases.

Fuller, J. G. *Fever! The Hunt for a New Killer Virus.* New York: Reader's Digest Press, 1974.
Fuller has written a true life mystery-suspense story about the outbreak of a mysterious killer disease in Africa and the attempts of scientists and public health officials to discover its nature and source.

Gallagher, R. *Diseases That Plague Modern Man.* Dobbs Ferry, N.Y.: Oceana, 1969.
This fascinating book contains brief histories of ten communicable diseases, along with profiles of the diseases and how they can be prevented. The international efforts that have been created to control cholera, influenza, leprosy, plague, syphilis, and tuberculosis are discussed.

Lasagna, L. *The VD Epidemic: How It Started, Where It's Going, and What To Do About It.* Philadelphia: Temple University Press, 1975.
A leading physician explains all aspects of the sexually transmitted diseases—their symptoms, diagnosis, and treatment.

Reid, R. *Microbes and Men.* New York: Dutton, 1975.
Reid delves into the lives of the great scientists who hunted microbes and made important medical breakthroughs in the last century.

Rosebury, T. *Life on Man.* New York: Viking, 1969.
This book is a fascinating account of humanity's aversion to "germs" and excrement and of their concomitant obsession with cleanliness. Rosebury, a bacteriologist, underscores the importance of the symbiotic relationship between humanity and their microbes by citing the hapless fate of laboratory animals kept in a germfree state. The presentation is witty and charming, yet scholarly.

Rosebury, T. *Microbes and Morals.* New York: Viking, 1971.
This book is an interesting discussion of the history of venereal disease. It also traces the development of societal attitudes toward the STDs and offers an explanation for the present epidemic proportions of the diseases.

Roueché, B. *Annals of Epidemiology.* Boston: Little, Brown, 1967.
The fascinating description of investigations into puzzling outbreaks of disease makes this book interesting.

Roueché, B. *The Incurable Wound.* New York: Berkley, 1958.
The author has made a career of writing narratives about great feats of medical detection; this volume contains six true stories of how public health officials become detectives to track down the sources of a disease and halt its spread.

Zinsser, H. *Rats, Lice, and History.* Boston: Little, Brown, 1935.
Supposedly concerned with the life history of typhus fever, this book becomes an interesting digression on the historical significance of disease and the impact of rats and lice on humanity.

Chapter 15
Cancer

Nobile, P. *King Cancer: The Good, the Bad, and the Cure of Cancer.* New York: Sheed & Ward, 1975.

An extremely well-written presentation of cancer case histories and current research into cancer and its cure.

Pilgrim, I. *The Topic of Cancer.* New York: Crowell, 1974.
The author covers not only the nature of cancer but the current federal "crash program" of cancer research and criticizes the government's approach to this vital area.

Shimkin, M. B. *Science and Cancer.* Rev. ed. Washington, D.C.: U.S. Government Printing Office, 1973.
This illustrated Public Health Service publication was written to inform the general public about the medical and biological aspects of cancer. It also discusses some recent research developments in the cause and treatment of cancer.

Strax, P. *Early Detection: Breast Cancer Is Curable.* New York: Harper & Row, 1974.
This short book covers everything a woman should know about breast cancer, with special emphasis on self-examination and early detection.

Chapter 16
Cardiovascular Disease

Amosoff, N. *The Open Heart.* G. St. George (tr.). New York: Simon & Schuster, 1966.
This book is a compassionate account of the emotional turmoil experienced by cardiovascular surgeons. The author explains in personal terms the processes involved in such operations as heart-valve transplants and other open-heart surgery.

Boyland, B. R. *The New Heart.* Philadelphia: Chilton, 1969.
This book presents the history of treatment of heart dysfunctions and carries the discussion to the present with a prognosis for the future. All of the surgical procedures are described in simple terms, making this book a good source for quick reference.

Carruthers, M. *The Western Way of Death: Stress, Tension and Heart Attacks.* New York: Pantheon, 1975.
In this concise book, an eminent heart expert zeros in on the stresses of modern life as major factors in coronary artery disease.

Friedman, M., and **R. H. Rosenman.** *Type A Behavior and Your Heart.* New York: Knopf, 1974.
Two doctors distinguish between major behavior patterns people can adopt and suggest that people who are "Type A" are more likely to suffer a heart attack.

Meyer, A. J., and **J. B. Henderson.** "Multiple Risk Factor Reduction in the Prevention of Cardiovascular Disease." *Preventive Medicine* 3 (1974), 225–236.
A discussion of the multiple risks implicated in cardiovascular disease and the ways in which to reduce them.

Chapter 17
Health in the Environment

Bernarde, M. A. *Our Precarious Habitat.* New York: W. W. Norton, 1970.
Bernarde discusses the various ways in which technological society affects the environment. He is also concerned with the political aspects of pollution.

Cailliet, G., P. Setzer, and **M. Love.** *Everyman's Guide to Ecological Living.* New York: Macmillan, 1971.
The authors provide advice and suggestions about activities that concerned people can undertake to relieve impending environmental crises.

Commoner, B. *The Closing Circle.* New York: Bantam Books, 1972.
The environmental crisis presented with a view toward positive solutions.

De Bell, G. (ed.). *Environmental Handbook.* New York: Ballantine, 1970.
This book contains articles on all aspects of pollution and the environment. Among the contributors are René Dubos, Paul Ehrlich, and Lewis Mumford. Also included is a section of suggestions for community action.

Dubos, R. *Man Adapting.* New Haven, Conn.: Yale University Press, 1965.
Dubos considers health and disease to be expressions of an organism's success or failure to adapt to a changing environment. Health thus means more than merely reacting through passive mechanisms to physiochemical conditions; rather, human health requires the ability of creatively responding to one's environment.

Dubos, R. *So Human an Animal.* New York: Scribner's, 1968.
This Pulitzer Prize-winning book explores the philosophical and moral issues involved in the interaction of humans with their environment.

Ehrlich, P., A. H. Ehrlich, and **J. P. Holdren.** *Human Ecology: Problems and Solutions.* San Francisco: W. H. Freeman, 1973.
The noted environmentalist and his associates have put together a comprehensive introduction to the biological and physical aspects of human ecology.

Fuller, R. B. *Utopia or Oblivion.* New York: Bantam Books, 1969.
This visionary book, written by the inventor of the geodesic dome, pleads for the use of science, technology, and creativity to produce utopian living environments. According to Fuller, such activity would help resolve many of our environmental and social problems.

Maddox, J. *The Doomsday Syndrome.* New York: McGraw-Hill, 1972.
Maddox takes certain environmentalists to task for using scare tactics and distorted information in their efforts to spur the government and individuals to action in environmental areas.

Shepard, P., and **D. McKinley** (eds.). *The Subversive Science.* Boston: Houghton Mifflin, 1969.
A collection of essays from a variety

of fields, this book surveys the perspectives of ecological investigations. The editors have included stimulating papers written by eminent authorities from the fields of biology, psychology, philosophy, anthropology, and history.

Smith, W. E., and A. M. Smith. *Minamata.* New York: Holt, Rinehart and Winston, 1975.
A famed photographer and his wife put together this volume-length photo essay on the aftermath of the tragic mercury poisonings of the early 1960s. The photos are haunting; the text is a compassionate study of Minamata villagers and their long struggle for retribution.

Taylor, R. *Noise.* Baltimore, Md.: Penguin, 1970.
Well-illustrated, this short paperback covers the process of hearing, the problem of noise, and possible solutions to noise pollution.

Wagner, R. H. *Environment and Man.* New York: W. W. Norton, 1971.
Wagner has put together a good, solid introduction to all aspects of the environment and people's interaction with it.

Chapter 18
Health Care and the Consumer

Aaron, J. E. *First Aid and Emergency Care.* 2nd ed. New York: Macmillan, 1979.
A useful personal and family guide to handling accidental injury and common illnesses.

Belsky, M.S. *How To Choose and Use Your Doctor: Beyond the Medical Mystique.* New York: Arbor House, 1975.
A noted physician contends that patients should not be afraid to ask their doctor numerous questions about their health and their treatment; he provides a list of questions to ask and also goes into the future of group practice.

Bennett, H. *Cold Comfort: Colds and Flu—Everybody's Guide to Self-Care.* New York: Potter, 1979.
This detailed guide to the self-care of common respiratory infections suggests when medical attention should be sought.

Colburn, H. N., and P. M. Baker. "Health Hazard Appraisal—A Possible Tool in Health Protection and Promotion." *Canadian Journal of Public Health* 64 (1973), 490–492.
This article presents a plan for determining the health risks of important behavioral, psychological, and environmental factors, and offers pertinent suggestions for intervention before pathology develops.

Consumer's Union. "Delusions of Vigor—Better Health by Mail." *Consumer Reports* 44 (January 1979), 50.
An exposé of mail-order advertising and the sale of health products that promise more than they can deliver.

Consumer's Union. *The Medicine Show.* New York: Pantheon, 1976.
A fascinating presentation of modern health quackery, plus guidelines for becoming an intelligent health consumer.

Crichton, M. *Five Patients: The Hospital Explained.* New York: Knopf, 1970.
Using the experiences of five patients at Massachusetts General Hospital, the author explains the benefits and drawbacks of the large teaching hospital, which has become the focal point for innovation in medical care. He examines the development of modern diagnostic and surgical techniques, takes a critical look at current teaching methods and rising hospital costs, and looks hopefully at some of the ways in which hospital services are being extended and improved through the use of television and computers.

DeGroot, L. J. (ed.). *Medical Care.* Springfield, Ill.: Charles C Thomas, 1969.
This comprehensive anthology provides an excellent overview of American health care. All aspects of medical care from a physician's education to hospital services, public medical care, and insurance policies are discussed in detail. This book could be a valuable aid to the student seeking reference on almost any aspect of health-care delivery.

Galton, L. *The Complete Book of Symptoms and What They Can Mean.* New York: Simon & Schuster, 1978.
Symptoms of common illnesses, their causes, and the appropriate action to take.

Garfield, S. *Teeth, Teeth, Teeth.* New York: Simon & Schuster, 1969.
Subtitled "A Treatise on Teeth and Related Parts of Man, Land, & Water Animals from Earth's Beginning to the Future of Time," this fun book covers everything one could ever possibly want to know about teeth and their care.

Glazier, W. H. "The Task of Medicine," *Scientific American* 228 (April 1973), 13–17.
Glazier examines the current American medical system and finds that it must reorient itself to deal with chronic illness instead of the current acute illness orientation.

Grossmann, J. "Do-It-Yourself Doctoring?" *Family Health* 11 (February 1979), 20, 22–24.
A brief discussion of the advantages, pitfalls, and limitations of the medical self-care movement.

Henderson, J. *Emergency Medical Guide.* New York: McGraw-Hill, 1978.
A comprehensive guide to dealing with medical emergencies, written for the layperson.

Illich, I. *The Medical Nemesis—The Expropriation of Health.* London: Marion Boyars, 1975.
A brilliant indictment of the medical-care establishment for making unjustified promises to resolve health problems.

James, B. (ed.). *The Health of Americans.* Englewood Cliffs, N.J.: Prentice-Hall, 1970.
Suggestions for the improvement of health and health care in the United States are outlined in this book.

Kosa, J., A. Antonovsky, and **I. K. Zola** (eds.). *Poverty and Health.* Cambridge, Mass.: Harvard University Press, 1969.

The authors contend that present-day health care is a middle-class luxury, but poverty and medical discrimination can be eliminated with the advanced state of American technology.

Magnuson, W. L., and **J. Carper.** "The New Quackery," in W. L. Magnuson and J. Carper, *The Dark Side of the Market Place.* Englewood Cliffs, N.J.: Prentice-Hall, 1968, pp. 156–184.

The new quacks wear white medical gowns, surround themselves with diplomas and electronic machinery, and are taking in more money per year than is spent in research on all diseases. This article discusses exploitation by phony practitioners.

McTaggert, A. C. *The Health Care Dilemma.* 2nd ed. Boston: Holbrook Press, 1976.

A comprehensive treatment of the realities of health-care delivery in the United States, which presents the vast problems we face, delineates possible alternatives, and speculates about the future.

Mueller, C. B., and **M. Rudolph.** *Light and Vision.* New York: Time-Life Books, 1970.

This beautifully illustrated book is an excellent introduction to eye function as well as to the nature of light and the photographic process.

Nolen, W. A. *Healing: A Doctor in Search of a Miracle.* New York: Random House, 1975.

The author has looked into nontraditional approaches to healing—ranging from acupuncture to faith healing—and has exposed unscientific methods, false cures, and the failure of modern medicine to provide the kind of emotional "healing" that nontraditional methods produce.

O'Neill, J. J. *The Hard of Hearing.* Englewood Cliffs, N. J.: Prentice-Hall, 1964.

The physiology of the ear and the physics of sound are explained as background material for this study of the diagnosis and treatment of hearing disorders.

Pappworth, M. H. *Human Guinea Pigs.* Boston: Beacon Press, 1968.

In this revealing book, Pappworth discusses the increasing tendency among physicians to use their patients in experiments, with or without their consent. After citing examples, he suggests principles and legislative changes that should apply to such situations.

Revere, P. *Dentistry and Its Victims.* New York: St. Martin's Press, 1970.

The author goes beyond descriptions of the care and problems of teeth and discusses the patient-dentist relationship: how to tell a good dentist from a bad one, what to expect from a dentist, what is wrong with the current dental-care delivery system. In an entertaining manner this "anonymous" dentist makes one realize the importance of teeth and of good dental care.

Robbins, L., and **J. Hall.** *How to Practice Prospective Medicine.* Indianapolis, Ind.: Methodist Hospital of Indiana, 1970.

The pioneering work on detecting precursors of disease before frank pathology manifests itself. Although it is designed for health professionals, it may be understood by the layperson.

Scott, B. "When a Doctor Needs a Doctor," *Today's Health* 48 (May 1970), 54–55, 64.

Scott discusses the various ways in which the medical field regulates the quality of its practitioners.

Sehnert, K. W., with **H. Eisenberg.** *How to Be Your Own Doctor—Sometimes.* New York: Grosset & Dunlap, 1975.

A popular and reputable text on self-care.

Selzer, R. *Mortal Lessons—Notes on the Art of Surgery.* New York: Simon & Schuster, 1976.

A fascinating treatment of the philosophy and art of surgery, presented with vision, faith, and hope.

Stevens, S. S., and **F. Warshofsky.** *Sound and Hearing.* New York: Time-Life Books, 1970.

Typical of the Time-Life series, this is a highly readable and well-illustrated book. It explores the nature of sound and the physiology of hearing by using data from numerous disciplines.

Young, J. H. *The Medical Messiahs.* Princeton, N.J.: Princeton University Press, 1967.

This book is a thoroughly fascinating history of medical quackery in the United States during the past century.

Glossary

A

abortion The termination of a pregnancy before the fetus is capable of living outside the mother's body.

abscess A pus-filled cavity formed by the destruction of tissue from a severe infection.

active immunity The immunity acquired through the production of antibodies after contact with live pathogens or vaccines. See also *immunity; passive immunity.*

addiction See *physical dependence.*

adenocarcinoma A form of cancer that originates in the glands of the body.

aerobic exercise Any form of exercise in which the demands of the body for oxygen are met by a sufficient supply; usually an extended exercise that does not involve extreme physical exertion. See also *anaerobic exercise.*

affective disorder A disorder of mood or feeling.

affective psychoses A group of psychoses characterized by a disorder of mood. See also *manic-depressive psychosis.*

alcoholism The chronic use of alcohol to the extent that its use contributes to sickness, accidents, or dependence on the drug to avoid withdrawal symptoms.

alleles Pairs of genes on homologous chromosomes that affect the same traits. When two alleles are identical, a person is said to be *homozygous* for that trait; when the alleles carry differing instructions, the trait is said to be *heterozygous.*

amniocentesis The process by which cells are removed for examination from the amniotic fluid surrounding a fetus during pregnancy.

amniotic sac The fluid-filled sac that encloses the fetus during prenatal development.

amphetamines Stimulant drugs used to combat fatigue and reduce appetite; known to abusers as "uppers."

anaerobic exercise Any form of exercise in which the body develops an oxygen deficiency; usually an extreme exertion over a short time period. See also *aerobic exercise.*

anal stage In Freud's theory, the stage in a child's development during which bowel control is achieved and pleasure is focused on the functions of elimination.

anaplastic The term for a cancer in which the cellular structure is so altered that it no longer resembles the tissue from which it originated.

androgyny The quality of having both male and female characteristics.

aneurysm A blood-filled pocket that bulges out from a weak spot in an arterial wall. If it bursts it may cause a cerebral hemorrhage.

angina pectoris Chest pains resulting from an insufficient supply of blood to the heart muscle.

antianxiety drugs Minor tranquilizers. See *benzodiazepines.*

antibiotic drugs Substances produced by microorganisms that, in dilute solution, can kill or inhibit other microorganisms.

antibody A class of proteins manufactured by the body to specifically destroy an invading bacterium, virus, or other such agent. See also *antigen.*

antidepressants Mood-elevating drugs that increase activity and drive.

antigen Any agent that provokes the production of a specific antibody.

antipsychotic drugs Major tranquilizers used to treat serious psychiatric illnesses, particularly schizophrenia.

antisocial personality See *sociopathic personality.*

anxiety A feeling of uneasiness, fear, or distress that arises when a person is faced with possible or imagined danger or misfortune.

aphasia Difficulties in comprehension and the ability to speak; often follows a stroke.

atherosclerosis The deposit of fat on the inside of the arteries and the subsequent hardening of the inner linings.

atrophy Withering of tissue from disuse.

autonomic nervous system The subsystem of the motor branch of the nervous system that regulates the glands and the smooth and cardiac muscles.

B

bacteria Unicellular microorganisms; the main groups are bacilli, cocci, and spirilla.

barbiturates Sedative-hypnotic drugs that act as central-nervous-system depressants; known to abusers as "downers."

basal cells Cells that underlie the surface cells of a tissue.

behavior modification A method of achieving a goal—weight loss, for example, by discovering the cues that prompt one's present behavior (say overeating) and attempting to remove, avoid, or change them.

behavior therapy A type of therapy based on conditioning methods; its purpose is to eliminate maladaptive behavior and promote adaptive behavior.

benzodiazepines A group of minor tranquilizers including Valium and Librium.

benzopyrene A carcinogen found in cigarette smoke.

biodegradable Capable of being broken into smaller parts by the action of microorganisms.

biopsy The microscopic examination of surgically removed tissue to aid in diagnosis.
blood alcohol level The concentration of alcohol carried by the blood to the brain.

C

Caesarean operation (Caesarean section) Delivery of a baby through an incision in the abdomen when normal delivery is impossible or inadvisable.
caffeine A central-nervous-system stimulant; the main active ingredient in coffee, tea, and cola drinks.
calorie A measure of the energy produced by a given amount of food when it is eaten and burned in the body.
cancer A condition of abnormal cellular growth.
Cannabis sativa The Indian hemp plant from which hashish and marijuana are derived.
carbohydrates Chemicals produced by living organisms from carbon, oxygen, and hydrogen; used for the distribution of chemically stored energy among living organisms or within the body. Common carbohydrates include cellulose, starch, glycogen, and the simple sugars.
carcinogenic Cancer-inducing.
carcinomas Cancers that arise from epithelial cells such as those in skin, glands, and the membrane linings of organs.
cardiac Pertaining to the heart.
cardiac arrest Any complete stoppage of the heart.
cardiopulmonary resuscitation (CPR) Cardiac massage and resuscitation that includes ventilating the lungs; used in the absence of immediate medical attention.
carrier An individual who harbors and trasmits disease-causing organisms or genes without showing any symptoms.
cerebral embolism A type of stroke in which a mass of abnormal material is carried by the bloodstream until it clogs a blood vessel in the brain.
cerebral hemorrhage A type of stroke that occurs when a diseased blood vessel bursts in the brain, causing uncontrolled bleeding.
cerebral thrombosis A type of stroke caused by a clot that forms in and blocks a blood vessel in the brain.
cerebrovascular accident See *stroke.*
cervix The narrow, necklike end of the uterus opening into the vagina.
chancre A lesion or open sore that appears at the site of a syphilitic infection.
chemoprevention The study of new drugs that will stop or inhibit cancer growth.
chemotherapy The use of drugs in the selective inhibition of agents of disease.
cholesterol A chemical compound found in the fatty parts of animal tissue; it is thought to be involved in atherosclerosis.
chromosomes Chainlike assemblies of nucleic acids and proteins located in the cell nucleus; they contain the program for all the inheritable properties of a cell, and they enable the cell to reproduce itself.
cilia Minute, hairlike structures found in the bronchi and other passages of the body that serve to move fluids by wavelike oscillations.
climacteric See *menopause.*
clitoris The female structure corresponding to the male penis; it is the focal point of sexual response in the female.
cocaine A stimulant extracted from the leaves of the South American coca bush.
cognitive reappraisal A process used to alter one's perceptions of a situation so that it becomes less stressful.
collateral circulation Growth of additional coronary blood vessels resulting from strenuous exercise; diminishes the chance of heart attacks.
color blindness A sex-linked trait that is marked by the inability to perceive certain colors correctly.
columnar cells Cells in the respiratory passageway that have hairlike projections to keep harmful materials out of the lungs.
communicable Capable of being passed from one individual to another through direct contact or through intermediary agents such as insects or foul water.
companionate marriage A relationship based on friendship and shared activities.
condom A thin rubber covering for the penis used as a contraceptive device and a prophylactic against sexually transmitted diseases.
congenital Present at birth.
control groups Those groups in an experiment not exposed to the factor being studied.
coronary Referring to the heart vessels.
coronary thrombosis Formation of a blood-obstructing clot within a coronary artery, leading to a heart attack.
cor pulmonale A heart condition that is induced by the high capillary resistance of diseased lungs.
cunnilingus Oral stimulation of the vagina, vulva, clitoris, or anus. See also *fellatio.*
cyanosis The characteristic blue color of skin resulting from oxygen deprivation.

D

decibel A unit of measure used in assessing the loudness or intensity of sounds.
delusion A false belief; sometimes a symptom of paranoid schizophrenia.
depression A pattern of sadness, anxiety, fatigue, insomnia, underactivity, and reduced ability to function and work with others.
detumescence A loss of swelling.
diaphragm A contraceptive device composed of a circular metal spring covered with rubber; it is inserted into the vagina and covers the opening to the cervix.
diastolic pressure Pressure of the blood within the arteries when the heart is resting between contractions. See also *systolic pressure.*
disease Disability caused by the incorrect functioning of an organ, part, structure, or system of the body.
distress A negative reaction to a stressor.
dose-response effect The pattern of identifiable effects that occur with increasing exposure to a drug, a chemical, or radiation.
Down's syndrome A genetic disease caused by the presence of an extra chromosome and characterized by mental retardation and several physical defects; also known as mongolism.
drug Any biologically active substance that is foreign to the body and is deliberately introduced to affect its functioning.
drug abuse The use of a drug to an extent that produces definite impairment of social, psychological, or physiological functioning.
dual-career marriage A marriage in which both husband and wife pursue careers seriously.

E

egalitarian marriage A relationship in which both spouses share household tasks and decision making.
embryo A developing human organism during the first three months of pregnancy. See also *fetus.*
emotion The physiological and psychological form in which one

experiences one's estimates of the harmful and helpful effects of stimuli.

emotional lability Sudden and extreme mood fluctuations or inappropriate emotional reactions; often follows a stroke.

endemic Of normal occurrence in a specific population.

endogenous Developing or growing from within. See also *exogenous.*

epidemic Referring to a disease that affects a larger number of people than it normally would in a given area. See also *pandemic.*

epidemiology The study of the frequency, distribution, causes, and control of diseases within a population.

episiotomy Surgical incision in the vagina during childbirth to prevent tearing in the vaginal walls.

Epstein-Barr virus The organism that causes the most common form of infectious mononucleosis.

essential fat Fat tissue that is necessary to normal physiological functioning.

essential hypertension Persistent high blood pressure of unknown cause.

estrogen A hormone produced by the ovaries that is responsible for the development of secondary female characteristics. See also *progesterone.*

euthanasia Painlessly putting someone to death who is suffering from an incurable disease.

eutrophication The profusion, death, and decay of plant life in a body of water. Especially applicable to proliferation of algae under high pollution, eventually resulting in oxygen depletion of the water.

exogenous Produced from without. See also *endogenous.*

F

Fallopian tubes The two ducts that transport ova from the ovaries into the uterus; also called oviducts.

family planning The voluntary determination by a couple of the number and spacing of their children.

fellatio Oral stimulation of the penis. See also *cunnilingus.*

fertilization The process that unites the sperm and the ovum.

fetal alcohol syndrome A pattern of birth defects resulting from a mother's heavy drinking during pregnancy.

fetus The developing human organism during the last six months of pregnancy. See also *embryo.*

fiber In the diet, foodstuffs of plant origin (such as cellulose) that are indigestible but that provide "roughage" to aid in digestion.

fibrillation Rapid, ineffective, nonrhythmic contractions of the heart.

fixation In Freudian theory, arrested development such that in later life the individual remains attached to persons, objects, events, feelings, or attitudes experienced in infancy or early childhood.

fluorocarbons Chemical compounds that were used in aerosol spray cans until growing evidence showed that they destroy the ozone layer surrounding the planet.

fortification The addition of one or more nutrients not originally present in a particular food.

fungi Parasitic plants that lack chlorophyll.

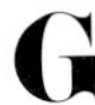

gamete A sex cell; an egg (ovum) or a sperm.

gamma globulins The class of blood proteins to which antibodies belong.

gender Biological sex, male or female.

gender identity The sense of oneself as masculine or feminine, resulting from psychosocial conditioning beginning at birth.

gender liberation The attempt to free both sexes from narrow and confining sex-role expectations.

gender role The behavior society considers appropriate for each sex.

genes The chromosomal units involved in the inheritance of a given trait.

genetic counseling Advice to prospective parents based on identifying the various possibilities of their conceiving a genetically abnormal child.

gerontology The study of aging and the aged.

glucose The simple sugar used by the body; other sugars are usually converted into glucose by enzymes in the body before they can be used as energy sources.

glycogen The form in which carbohydrates are stored in the liver.

Graafian follicles Small sacs inside the ovaries in which ova mature.

H

habituation The process of becoming accustomed to a particular set of circumstances or stimuli. In drug terminology, the state of psychological dependence on a drug. See also *physical dependence; tolerance.*

half-life The length of time required for half of any amount of a substance to decay and turn into another substance.

hallucination Sensory perception or experience for which there is no external stimulus.

hashish A drug consisting of a concentrated resin made from the leaves of the hemp plant.

hemophilia A genetic disease characterized by excessive bleeding due to the deficiency of certain blood components necessary for rapid blood clotting.

heroin An opiate derived from morphine.

high-density lipoprotein (HDL) The heaviest of the lipoproteins; it seems to be able to carry cholesterol to the liver and protect against heart disease and atherosclerosis.

holistic medicine Simultaneous attention to the many factors in a person's life contributory to disease or health.

homozygous See *alleles.*

host The recipient of foreign materials, such as infectious agents or tissue transplants.

human potential movement The theories, techniques, and programs that are aimed at improving one's health, happiness, and effectiveness.

hydrocarbons Pollutants that result from incomplete burning of fuel and are produced primarily by automobile emissions.

hymen Circular fold of tissue usually present at the entrance of the vagina in virginal females.

hyperplasia An abnormal increase in the number of cells in a given tissue; often associated with malignant tumors.

hypertension Persistent high blood pressure.

hypnotic Any drug that promotes sleep.

hypochondriasis Preoccupation with the body and with fear of diseases.

hysterical personality A personality trait characterized by the attempt to control relations with others by simulation of sickness.

hysterotomy A miniature Caesarean operation to abort a fetus after the twelfth week of pregnancy.

I

immune mechanism The manufacture of antibodies in response to a foreign substance or antigen, such as a disease-causing organism.

immunity The ability to resist infection or the development of a disease. See also *active immunity; passive immunity.*

immunoassay A pregnancy test involving the detection of HCG in a urine sample.

immunotherapy The use of the body's disease-fighting system against cancer or other diseases.
implantation The process by which the zygote burrows into the endometrium (lining of the uterine wall).
impotence The inability of a male to have or maintain an erection during intercourse.
incubation period The first phase of an infectious disease, in which the invading organisms multiply within the host.
infant mortality rate The number of infant deaths occurring before the age of one year per a given population.
infarct An area of tissue that has died because it has been denied its blood supply, often as a result of a blood clot.
infection The presence of pathogenic organisms in the body.
infectious disease A disease that is caused by an agent capable of reproducing within the host.
inflammation Redness, local warmth, swelling, and pain in body tissues resulting from intrusion of foreign matter.
interferon A protein produced by the body that inhibits the growth of viruses.
intrauterine device (IUD) A plastic or stainless-steel contraceptive device that is inserted into the uterus.
iron An important nutrient essential for hemoglobin production in the red blood cells.
isometric exercises Exercises that produce static muscular contractions that result from pushing or pulling against a stationary object.
isotonic exercises Exercises, such as calisthenics and weight training, that develop strength through repeated rhythmic movements.
IUD See *intrauterine device.*

L

labia majora The outer folds of skin on either side of the vagina.
labia minora The inner flaps of soft skin on either side of the vagina.
laetrile One of the best known quack cancer treatments. Also known as "vitamin B_{17}" or "aprikern."
Lamaze method Natural childbirth using special methods of breathing and relaxation.
laparoscopy Sterilization achieved by electrically severing the Fallopian tubes through a small abdominal incision.
latency stage According to Freud, the period of childhood corresponding to the grade-school years, in which sexual feelings become dormant.
leukemia Cancer of the white blood cells (leukocytes).
leukorrhea A vaginal discharge that is often a warning signal of genital infection.
life expectancy The average number of years a person may expect to live.
lipids Organic chemicals made up of carbon, oxygen, and hydrogen; unlike carbohydrates, they are poorly soluble in water; also used for energy storage and fuel. Commonly referred to as fats.
lipoproteins Substances containing both fat and protein that transport fat molecules; believed to be related to heart disease.
lithium An element that is used in drug form to treat persons diagnosed as manic or manic-depressive.
lymphocyte A type of white blood cell produced from lymphoid tissue.
lymphoma A cancerous tumor derived from lymphoid tissue and localized in the lymph nodes.
lymphosarcoma A cancer affecting both lymphoid and connective tissues.

M

macrophages Large phagocytes usually found in the tissues rather than in the bloodstream.
major tranquilizers Drugs used to treat psychosis; they alter the activity of certain neurotransmitters in the brain.
malignant Dangerous to health or life; cancerous.
malnutrition The lack or insufficiency of certain dietary ingredients.
manic-depressive psychosis A psychotic reaction characterized by extreme variations in mood, ranging from extreme elation to profound depression and back.
masturbation Sexual self-stimulation.
maternal mortality rate The number of pregnancy-related deaths occurring before, during, or after childbirth per a given population.
melanoma Cancer of the pigment-carrying cells of the skin.
menarche The onset of menstruation.
menopause The cessation of the menstrual cycle; also known as the climacteric.
menstruation A bloody discharge from the uterus at regular monthly intervals.
mescaline A hallucinogenic drug made from peyote, a type of cactus plant.
metapathologies Abraham Maslow's term for feelings such as alienation, anguish, apathy, and cynicism that result if metaneeds are not met. See also *metaneeds.*
metastases Sites of metastatic growth.
metastatic growth The spread of cancer from the original site to other parts of the body through the lymphatic or circulatory system, producing secondary growths.
methadone A synthetic opiate with no euphoric effect that is used to treat heroin abuse.
midwife A woman who assists a childbirth in the absence of a medical practitioner.
minerals Inorganic elements needed daily to help form tissues and various chemical substances in the body, to assist in nerve transmission and muscle contraction, and to help regulate fluid levels and the acid/base balance of the body.
Minimata disease Methyl mercury poisoning.
minor tranquilizer A drug, such as Valium or Librium, which calms or relaxes a person.
miscarriage Spontaneous abortion of an embryo or fetus.
mitosis A process of cell division involving the duplication of chromosomes and the production of two daughter cells identical to the original.
mongolism See *Down's syndrome.*
morphine The active ingredient in opium.
mortality Death; number of persons dying in a population, usually expressed as a ratio of the number of deaths per 100,000 persons. See also *morbidity.*
multifactors Two or more factors acting together to produce a particular disease condition, although neither will do so by itself.
multiphasic screening A type of health testing that combines a detailed computerized medical history and a series of diagnostic tests administered by paramedical personnel.
mutation The alternation of some portion of the DNA within the genes that leads to a change in genetic make-up.
myocardial infarction (heart attack) The damaging or death of a portion of the heart muscle as a result of reduction of the blood supply to that area.
myotonia Muscular tightness.

N

narcotic See *opiate.*
neoplasm A tumor or new growth of tissue.
neurosis A mental disorder that

prevents the victim from dealing effectively with reality; it is characterized by anxiety and partial impairment of functioning, although the neurotic individual can still carry on in most areas of his or her life. See also *psychosis.*

neurotransmitters Chemical substances that transmit nerve impulses within the brain.

nicotine The most prevalent drug in tobacco; it affects the nervous system and produces both habituation and tolerance.

nutrients The energy-yielding substances and building materials obtained from foods.

nutrition The science that relates the health and well-being of an organism to the food it consumes.

O

obesity A higher than average proportion of fat tissue in the body.

obsessive-compulsive behavior Behavior characterized by the persistent repetition of some thought or act.

occlusion A blood-vessel obstruction in the brain that can lead to a stroke.

Oedipal conflict According to Freud, a small boy's desire to possess his mother, coupled with hostility toward his father.

oopharectomy The removal of both ovaries.

open marriage A marriage that is based on flexibility and change to allow both partners to grow in ways that they need and want.

opiate Any drug of the opium family; also known as opiate alkaloids.

opium An opiate derived from the opium poppy whose active ingredient is morphine.

oral contraceptives Drugs taken orally to prevent conception.

oral stage According to Freud, the first stage of psychosexual development; during this early period, pleasure is focused in the mouth and in oral activities.

overexertion Exercising to the point of deep, lingering fatigue or injury to bones, joints, or muscles.

overweight Weight in excess of the average.

oviduct See *Fallopian tubes.*

P

pacemaker An area of specialized heart tissue that rhythmically triggers contraction of the heart muscle even in the absence of autonomic neural signals.

Papanicolaou test A diagnostic test to determine the presence of cancer of the cervix.

Pap smear See *Papanicolaou test.*

passive immunity An immunity acquired through means other than the production of antibodies, usually through transfer of antibodies from an actively immune person. See also *active immunity; immunity.*

pathogen A disease-producing organism.

peers Members of a given social category, such as a specific age group or social class.

personality disorder Any deeply ingrained maladaptive pattern of behavior. See also *hysterical personality; sociopathic personality.*

phagocytes A group of white blood cells that engulfs and digests bacteria and foreign particles.

phallic stage According to Freud, the stage in a young child's development during which pleasure is focused on the genitals; the Oedipal conflict arises during this stage.

pharmacology The study of the effects and mechanisms of action of drugs on living systems.

Phencyclidine A drug also known as PCP, Sernyl, or angel dust; it is unpredictable and can cause dangerous side effects and possibly death.

phenylketonuria (PKU) A genetic disease caused by the absence of the enzyme phenylalanine hydrozylase and characterized by progressive mental retardation.

phobia An irrational, strong fear.

phocomelia A condition characterized by congenitally stunted arms and legs.

photochemical smog A type of smog resulting from the interaction of exhaust, emissions from automobiles, and temperature inversion. Also called Los Angeles-type smog.

physical dependence A drug-induced condition in which a person requires frequent administration of the drug in order to avoid withdrawal. See also *habituation; tolerance.*

pion beam therapy A radiation device for detecting tumors while causing little or no damage to other organs.

placenta The organ that absorbs nutrients from the mother and distributes them to the developing child.

plaque The lipid deposits on an artery wall characteristic of atherosclerosis; also, a hardened composite of debris on the surface of a tooth, thought to play a role in tooth decay.

plasma The fluid portion of the blood.

pollution The release of biological, physical, and chemical wastes into the environment.

positive health The highest level of health possible within the limits set by heredity and environment. Also called optimal health.

premature ejaculation The tendency of some men to ejaculate before they or their partners would like.

prenatal care The medical supervision of pregnancy.

prepuce A flap of skin hooding the clitoris and penis.

primary impotence The lifelong inability of a man to achieve or maintain an erection.

primary orgasmic dysfunction A problem among women who have never experienced an orgasm through any means.

primary prevention Measures to reduce the incidence of mental disorders by preventing their development.

proctoscopy A procedure for conducting a rectal examination.

prodrome period The second phase of an infectious disease; it is a short interval characterized by headache, fever, nasal discharge, and other common symptoms, making diagnosis difficult.

progesterone A hormone secreted by the ovaries that plays an important role in embryonic development. See also *estrogen.*

progressive relaxation A technique for alleviating muscle tension.

prophylaxis Treatment for the prevention of a disease (adj. *prophylactic*).

proteins A category of vital organic chemicals that includes enzymes, hormones, and antibodies and constitutes one of the critical food substances.

psilocybin A psychedelic drug that comes from the Mexican mushroom, psilocybe; it is the safest of the hallucinogens.

psychedelic-hallucinogens Complex drugs that can produce excitement, agitation, hallucinations, depression, or other psychosis-like changes in mood, thinking, and behavior. Also called psychotogenics and psychotomimetics.

psychiatrist A medical doctor specializing in the study and treatment of mental and emotional disorders.

psychoactive Referring to any drug that produces a temporary change in a person's neurophysiological functions, affecting mood, thoughts, feelings, or behavior; also called psychotropic.

psychological dependence See *habituation.*

psychologist A specialist in the field of psychology, usually holding a master's degree or Ph.D. in psychology.
psychophysiological disorders The development of physical symptoms as a result of emotional imbalance; also known as psychosomatic disorders.
psychosis A severe mental disorder that prevents the individual from functioning in everyday life. See also *neurosis.*
psychosocial crisis Erik Erikson's term for a developmental struggle arising from a conflict between physiological, social, and psychological needs.
psychosomatic See *psychophysiological disorders.*
psychotomimetics See *psychedelic-hallucinogens.*
pubococcygeous muscles The muscles that surround the outer portion of the vagina.
pulmonary stenosis A congenital heart defect characterized by obstruction or narrowing of the valve between the right ventricle and the pulmonary artery.

quarantine The restriction on leaving or entering an area if an infectious disease has been diagnosed.

R

radiation sickness A serious illness caused by prolonged exposure to high levels of radiation; in its later stages it leads to hair loss, hemorrhaging, ulcers, and cataracts.
radioreceptor assay A pregnancy test involving the detection of HCG in a blood test.
retinoids Synthetic vitamins that have successfully reversed the cancer process in animals and are now being attempted in human therapy.
rhythm method A method of birth control based on determination of the time of ovulation and abstinence from coitus during the fertile period.
rickettsiae Bacteria-like organisms responsible for typhus fever and other diseases.
role confusion A conflict over one's sex role, occupational goals, or sense of identity.

S

safety Cognizance of the possibility of accidents and action to reduce their probability and to minimize their consequences.
saline abortion A method of abortion used after the twelfth week of pregnancy in which a salt solution is introduced into the uterus.
salpingitis Inflammation of the Fallopian tubes.
sarcoma Cancer arising in supportive tissue such as bones, cartilage, fat, or muscle.
saturated fats Fats that contain a maximum of hydrogen atoms in their chemical structure; they are usually animal fats. See also *unsaturated fats.*
schizophrenia A form of psychosis in which the patient suffers from disturbed thinking, moods, and behavior; hallucinations and delusions are common.
secondary impotence The inability of a man to achieve or maintain an erection in some or all sexual situations.
secondary orgasmic dysfunction A problem among women who experience orgasms sometimes but not whenever they would like.
secondary prevention The early detection and treatment of problems to prevent the worsening of mental disorders.
sedative Any drug that produces relaxation.
sedative-hypnotics Drugs that promote relaxation in small doses and sleep in large doses by depressing the activity of the central nervous system. See also *barbiturates; depressants.*
self-actualization The process of developing one's own true nature and fulfilling one's potentialities.
self-esteem The amount and quality of the regard people have toward themselves.
septum The muscular wall that separates the two halves of the heart. Septa are also present in the brain, nose, and elsewhere.
sex chromosomes The chromosomes that determine the sex of an organism. See also *autosome.*
sex-flush A redness spreading from the chest over the lower abdomen and shoulders that occurs during sexual excitement.
sexual dysfunction Any problem that prevents a person from engaging in sexual relations or from reaching orgasm during sex.
socialization The process of learning and conforming to the rules of one's culture.
social worker A counselor who holds a master's degree in social work.
sociopathic personality A personality trait characterized by repeated conflict with society; in the extreme form, the desire for self-gratification takes preference over all other values.
specificity The property of an antibody that enables it to recognize and combat only one type of foreign substance or organism.
sperm The male reproductive cells (gametes).
spermatogenesis The process of sperm formation.
spermatogonia Cells that will develop into sperm.
spermatozoa See *sperm.*
sphingolipidoses Genetic diseases characterized by the accumulation of sphingolipids (fatty substances) in various parts of the body, including the brain.
stamina The ability to mobilize energy to maintain movement over an extended period of time.
starch A chainlike assembly of many carbohydrate molecules.
strength The basic muscular force required for movement.
stress A strain or tension that disturbs a person's normal physical, mental, or emotional equilibrium.
stress mechanism The physiological adjustments the body makes in response to stressors. See also *stressor.*
stressor External stimuli such as loss of a job, an exam, or the death of a loved one that produce stress. See also *stress.*
stroke A sudden brain injury usually caused by an embolus or rupture of a blood vessel.
sucrose The form of sugar that occurs in sugar cane and sugar beets and is commonly known as table sugar.
sugar In the class of carbohydrates, straight chains of carbon rings.
suppleness The quality of muscles and joints that permits a full range of movement.
sympathetic system A branch of the autonomic nervous system that carries signals to activate such internal organs as the heart, liver, smooth muscles, and lungs.
synergism The joint action of a number of factors that greatly increase the effects of each.
systolic pressure The maximum pressure of the blood under the force of the contracting heart. See also *diastolic pressure.*

T

Tay-Sachs disease A genetically caused inability to metabolize certain fats; characterized by mental degradation, blindness, and death before the age of seven years.
temperature inversion A weather condition characterized by a layer of

cold air sandwiched between the surface air and a top layer of warm air, which tends to trap pollutants.

tertiary prevention Treatment and rehabilitation to prevent the severe effects of major mental disorders on the victim and on society.

tetralogy of Fallot A congenital heart defect involving the pulmonary artery, the aorta, the septum, and the right ventricle.

thanatology The study of death and dying.

thermography A diagnostic technique for breast cancer that uses no radiation.

thrombus A blood clot that forms inside the heart or blood vessels.

tolerance The bodily adaptation to a particular drug that necessitates an increased dosage of that drug in order to produce the same effect. See also *habituation; physical dependence.*

toxicity Potential for being poisonous.

toxin A poison produced by pathogenic bacteria.

toxoid A modified toxin used as a vaccine to induce antibody production.

tranquilizer A drug used to reduce anxiety and to induce relaxation.

transcatheter closure A surgical technique used to correct congenital heart defects.

transient ischemic attack A temporary attack with symptoms similar to a stroke; often precedes a stroke.

triglycerides Fatty acids in the body resulting from excess glucose that is neither burned as energy nor stored as glycogen.

trisomy A genetic abnormality in which three homologous chromosomes exist instead of the usual pair.

tubal ligation Sterilization achieved by surgically tying the Fallopian tubes.

tumor An abnormal mass of new tissue growing independent of its surrounding tissue structures.

U

ultrasound techniques Methods of locating tumors deep in the body without exposing normal tissue to radiation.

undernutrition Insufficient amounts of food.

unsaturated fats Fats that contain double-bonded carbon atoms and less than a full complement of hydrogen atoms in their chemical structure; they are usually vegetable fats rather than animal fats. See also *saturated fats.*

uterus (womb) A hollow muscular organ whose function is to hold and nourish the fetus.

V

vagina The canal leading from the vulva to the cervix.

vas deferens The duct leading from the epididymis to the urethra that carries sperm during ejaculation.

vasectomy A method of birth control for males in which the vas deferens is tied and severed, preventing sperm from leaving the testes.

vasocongestion The accumulation of blood in certain blood vessels.

virus A small disease agent or parasitic particle that is composed of a DNA core with a protein covering.

vitamins A group of organic chemicals essential in small amounts for normal metabolism.

W

withdrawal Psychologically, a form of defense mechanism in which a person retreats from reality in a stressful situation. In drug terminology, a temporary illness precipitated by the lack of a drug in the body of a physically dependent person.

Z

zygote The fertilized egg cell.

Index

A

Abdominal circumference test for overweight, 181
Abortion: as birth control, 107–109; spontaneous, 82
Abscess, 281
Absorption, alcohol, 243–246
Acceptance, and coping with death, 151
Accident prevention, 367–369
Acetaminophen, 235–236
Acid indigestion, 82
Acidulants, 172
Acrylonitrile, 340
Action, and emotion, 13
Active immunity, 282
Activity Level Guide, 185-186
Additives, food, 172–173
Adenocarcinomas, 302
Adjustment approach to mental disorders, 27
Adolescence, and parents, 129–130
Adoption, 132
Adrenal glands, 46
Adrenocorticotrophic hormone, 46–47
Aerobic exercise, 202–203
Aerosol spray cans, 341
Affective disorders, 29
Affective psychoses, 32–33
AFL-CIO, 340
Age: and attitudes toward death, 147–148; and heart disease, 317; and hypertension, 323; and rheumatic fever, 321; and sexual activity, 60; and smoking, 263, 264–265
Ageism, 146
Aging, 135–136; dealing with, 139–141; and exercise, 207–208; and nutrition, 175; process, 136–139; and sexuality, 62, 142–143; and social life, 144–146; *see also* Death
Air pollution, 341–342
Al-Anon, 255
Alateen, 255
Alarm stage, stress, 47
Alcohol, 7, 224-225, 241; and alcoholism, 251–255; in American society, 248–251; and cancer, 306; and congenital defects, 91; and multisubstance abuse, 219; physiological effects, 242–246; psychological effects, 246–248
Alcoholics, 251
Alcoholics Anonymous (AA), 255
Alcoholism, 251–255
Aldrin, 339–340
Algal blooms, 343
Ambulatory dying, 149–150
American Cancer Society, 267, 308, 372
American College of Surgeons, 310
American Hospital Association, 377
American Medical Association, 373–374, 376
American Petroleum Institute, 340
American Psychiatric Association, 63
The American Way of Death (Mitford), 155
Amniocentesis, 95, 96
Amnion, 79
Amphetamines, 229–230
Amytal, 225
Anaerobic exercise, 202–203
Anal stage of development, 18
Anaplastic cancer, 302
Anesthesia, and childbirth, 86
Aneurysm, 323
Anger, and coping with death, 151
Angina pectoris, 317–318
Annas, George J., 377
Antabuse, 255
Antacids, 236
Anthropometric measurements, 181
Antianxiety drugs, 228
Antibiotic drugs, 295
Antibodies, 281
Anticipatory grief, 153
Antidepressant drugs, 228–229
Antidiarrhea preparations, 237
Antigens, 281
Antihistamines, 236
Antioxidants, food, 172
Antipsychotic drugs, 228
Antisocial personalities, 33
Anxiety, 30–32
Aphasia, and stroke, 324
Appraisal, and emotion, 12
Approach-approach situation, 20
Approach-avoidance situation, 21
Arnold, Magda, 12–13
Arthritis, and quacks, 379
Arthur, Ransom J., 50
Asbestos, 305, 336–337, 340
Aspirin, 235–236, 284; and strokes, 325
Atherosclerosis, 317; and strokes, 323
Atria, heart, 319
Atrophy, 200
Automobiles: accidents, 367–368; and air pollution, 341, 342
Autonomic nervous system, 13–14, 46–47
Autonomy, 20
Avoidance-avoidance situation, 21

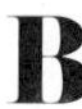

Baby: blue, 321; test tube, 90
Bacteria, 278
Barbiturates, 225–226, 246
Bargaining, and coping with death, 151
Basal cells, and smoking, 260
Bass technique, oral hygiene, 374
BCG, 311
Beach, Frank, 61
Behavior modification, and weight control, 187–188
Bell, Alan, 62–63
Bellock, Nedra B., 7
Benign tumor, 300

Benzedrine, 229
Benzodiazepines, 225–226
Benzopyrene, and cigarette smoke, 259
Bereaved, needs of, 153–154
Bernard, Jessie, 115, 116
Biodegradable substances, 341
Biopsy, 308
Birth. *See* Childbirth
Birth control, 99; abortion, 107–109; contraception, 100–101; family planning, 100; of future, 106–107; pills, 175; requiring no medical care, 101–104; requiring nonsurgical medical care, 104–106; requiring surgery, 106
Birth rate, 125–126, 347
Bisexuality, 63
Black Death, 273–274
Blacks, and sickle cell anemia, 92
Bleaches, food, 172
Block, heart, 319
Blood alcohol level, 243–246
Blood clot: and heart attack, 317; and stroke, 317
Blood examinations, during pregnancy, 82
Blood pressure, 375; high, 322–323
Blue baby, 321
Blue Cross/Blue Shield, 361
Body: composition, 180–181; defenses against communicable diseases, 279–281; and emotions, 13–14; weight, and alcohol, 245
Bowlby, John, 15
Brain, blood clot, and stroke, 317
Branden, Nathaniel, 16
Breads, 170–172
Breast feeding, 88–89
Breasts, 371
Breslow, Lester, 7
The Broken Heart: The Medical Consequences of Loneliness in America (Lynch), 16
Bronchitis, and smoking, 262
Brown, Louise, 90
Buddy system, in kicking the smoking habit, 266
Burns, 368
Butyrophenones, 228

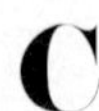

Caesarean operation, 86
Caffeine, 229
Calisthenics, 196, 201, 202
Calorie(s), 169, 185–188
Calorie Calculator and Activity Level Guide, 185–186
Cancer, 299–300; and quackery, 311, 379; causes, 302–304; and chemicals, 305, 336–340; detection and diagnosis, 307–308; and diet, 304; distribution 302; and drugs, 305; and heredity, 304; and immune mechanisms, 306; and nutrition, 176; and overweight, 184; and pollution, 305; prevention, 306–307; and radiation, 305; research, 311–312; and smoking, 260–261, 302, 304, 306; treatment, 308–311; types, 302; as uncontrolled growth, 300–302; and viruses, 305–306
Candidiasis, 290
Cannabis, 232–234, 249–250
Capillarization, 201
Carbohydrates and nutrition, 163–166
Carbon monoxide, 341
Carcinomas, 260, 302
Cardiac arrest, 319–320
Cardiopulmonary resuscitation (CPR), 320
Cardiovascular diseases, 315–317; atherosclerosis, 317; congenital heart disease, 321; heart attacks, 317–320; heart failure, 320–321; high blood pressure, 322–323; prevention, 330; rheumatic heart disease, 321–322; risk factors, 323–328; strokes, 323–325; surgery for, 328–330; *see also* Disease
Cardiovascular exercise, precautions, 204
Casals, Pablo, 139
Cereals, 170–172
Cerebral embolism, 323, 324
Cerebral hemorrhage, 323, 324
Cerebral palsy, 91
Cerebral thrombosis, 323, 324
Cell poisons, for cancer therapy, 310
Center for Disease Control, 191, 286
Cerebrovascular accidents, 323
Cervix, 63
Chafetz, Morris, 252
Chancre, 288
Chancroid, 291
Chemicals: and cancer, 305; environmental hazards, 336–340
Chemoprevention, 311
Chemotherapy, 295, 310
Child(ren): adoption, 132; and discipline, 127–129; and divorce, 123, 131; and elderly, 144; and exercise, 200; and marriage, 121; molestation, 143; nutritional needs, 173; relationship with parents, 126–129; spacing, 100; *see also* Childbirth; Parenthood
Child abuse, 130–131
Childbirth: and breast feeding, 88–89; and labor, 85–88; midwifery, 87–88; prepared, 83–85; stages, 86; test tube babies, 90; *see also* Child(ren); Parenthood
Chlordane, 340
Chlorine levels, water, 343
Cholesterol, 166–176
Chromates, 305
Chromosomes, 93; and gender, 58–59
Chronic diseases, 275–276
Cigarette smoking. *See* Smoking
Cilia, 280
Circulation, collateral, 326
Circumcision, 70
Climacteria, 78–79
Clinic, community, 355–356
Clinical disease stage, infection, 279
Clitoris, 64
Cocaine, 230–231
Coffee, 229
Cognitive reappraisal, 51
Cohabitation, 117–118
Coitus interruptus, 101
Cold, common, 283–284
Cold-packing, 329
Color-blindness, 94
Coloring agents, food, 173
Columnar cells, and smoking, 260
Communicable diseases, 273–274; analysis of, 274–275; body defenses against, 279–281; causes, 275–276; common, 282–286; control and prevention, 295–296; course of infection, 279; immunity, 281–282; infection agents, 276–278; patterns, 292–295; sexually transmitted, 286–292; spread of infection, 278–279; status of, 296–297; *see also* Disease
Community health care role, 355 356
Compensation, 21
Competence, 20
Conception, and prenatal development, 79–80
Condoms, 101, 103, 291
Conflicting emotions, 20–21
Congenital defects, 89–92
Congestive heart failure, 320–321
Consumers, and health care decisions, 377–378
Contraception. *See* Birth control
Contraceptives, oral, 104–105
Contracts, marriage, 117
Control: of communicable disease, 295–296; emotional, 21–23; of sexually transmitted diseases, 291–292; of stress responses, 50–52
Control groups, 275
Convalescence stage, infection, 279
Cooper, Kenneth H., 202–203
Coping with death, 151–153
Copper bracelet, and arthritis, 379
Coronary atherosclerosis, 317

Coronary thrombosis. *See* Heart attack
Cor pulmonale, 330
Corpus luteum, 78
Costs: of drugs, 215–217; of dying, 155; of health care, 357–360; of mental illness, 27–28; of surgery, 359
Cough drops, 284
Counseling: genetic, 85–96; marriage, 123
Creams, and birth control, 103–104
Creativity, and aging, 139
Crisis intervention, 37
Crisis medicine, 365
Crowding, and stress, 45
Crowding and Behavior (Freedman), 45
Cunnilingus, 61–62
Curing agents, food, 172–173
Cyanosis, and congenital heart disease, 321

D

D and C, 109
DDT, 339–340, 343
Deafness 90; and noise, 344–345
Death, 135–136; attitudes toward, 147–148; and bereaved, 153–154; coping with, 151–153; defined, 140–147; euthanasia, 150–151; and experience of dying, 148–149; and funeral rites, 154–156; and grief, 153; and needs of dying person, 149–150; *see also* Aging
Decibels, 344
Decline stage, infection, 279
Decongestants, 284
Defense mechanisms, 21
Deficiencies, diet, 177
Delaney Clause, 173
Delusions, 32
Delirium tremens (DTs), 219, 245
Demerol, 86
Dempsey, David, 154
Denial, 21; and coping with death, 151;
Dennis, Wayne, 139
Densimetric test, for overweight, 181
Deoxyribonucleic acid, 162
Dependence, on drugs, 218–219
Depressants, 224–228
Depression, 29–30, 37; and aging, 139; and coping with death, 151
DES, 91
Despair, 20; and aging, 141
DET, 232
Detection of cancer, 307–308
Detumscence, 67
Deviance approach to mental disorders, 26
Devices, fitness, 206
Dexedrine, 229
Diabetes, 163, 176; and cardiovascular disease, 326; and overweight, 184
Diagnosis of cancer, 307–308
Diaphragms, 105
Diastolic pressure, 322
Dicks, Henry, 123
Diet, balanced, 169–173; and cancer, 304, 306; as cardiovascular risk factor, 325–326; deficiencies, 177; fad, 190–192; and food fads, 164–165; low protein, 162–163
Diethylstilbestrol (DES), 91
Dieting. *See* Weight control
Dieldrin, 339–340
Dilation and curettage (D and C), 109
Directory of Medical Specialists, 373–374
Discipline, and parent-child relationship, 127–129
Disease: and aging, 138; building resistance to, 292; chronic, 275–276; and nutrition, 175–177; and smoking, 260–263; and stress, 47–49; *see also* Cardiovascular disease; Communicable disease
Displacement, 21
Distress, 42
Distribution: of cancer, 302; of health care, 360; of physicians, 356–357, 360
Divorce: and children, 123, 131; and marriage, 121–123
DMT, 231, 232
DNA, 162
Doctors. *See* Physicians
Dodson, Fitzhugh, 128–129
Dole, Vincent, 227, 228
Doriden, 225
Dosage, drug, 216
Dose-response effect, drug, 336
Doubt, 20
Douching, 78, 104
Down's syndrome, 94–95
Drinking. *See* Alcohol
Drownings, 369
Drug(s), 213–214; and alcohol, 246; antidepressants and Librium, 228–229; and cancer, 305; and congenital defects, 91; defined, 214; dependence, 218–219; depressants, 224–228; hazards and costs, 215–217; multisubstance abuse, 219; over-the-counter, 214, 234–237; physiological variables, 215–217; prescription, 237–238; psychedelic hallucinogens, 231–234; psychoactive, 224–234; stimulants, 229–231; for stress, 51; toxicity and interactions, 217; tranquilizers, 228; use behavior, 220–221; use causes, 221–224
Drug abuse, 214–215; causes, 221–224; multisubstance, 219
Drunkenness, 250–251
Dual career marriage, 116
Dumps, 343–344
Dying: ambulatory, 149–150; cost, 155; experience of, 148–149; at home, 150; needs of person, 149–150
Dysfunction, sexual, 68–70

E

Ectopic pregnancy, 77
EDITH (Exit Drills in the Home), 368
Education, and attitudes toward death, 148
Edwards, Robert, 90
Ejaculation, 69; premature, 70
Electrocardiogram, 319
Ellis, Albert, 119
Embolism, cerebral, 323, 324
Embolus, 323
Embryo, 79
Emetics, 237
Emergency treatment, for cardiac arrest, 319–320
Emotion(s), 11–12; and body, 13–14; control of, 21–23; dealing with, 20–23; defined, 11–13; development of, 18–20; Erikson's development theories, 18–20; Freud's development theories, 18; maturity, and mental health, 23–24; nature of, 12–13; and need for love, 14–16; and need for self-esteem, 16; and needs hierarchy, 16, 18
Emotional liability, 324
Emphysema, and smoking, 262
Emulsifiers, food, 172
Endemic disease, 275
Endocarditis, 227
Endocrine system, 46–47
Endogenous microbes, 276
Energy: nuclear, 345–347; solar, 348
Enrichment, food, 172
Environment: chemical hazards to, 336–340; pollution, 341–345; and population, 347–350; and radiation, 345–347; solving problems of, 350–351; and stress, 44
Environmental Protection Agency, 339–340
Epidemic, 274
Epidemiology, 274
Episiotomy, 85
Epstein-Barr virus, 286
Erikson, Erik, 112, 141, 146; emotional development stages, 18–20
Escape, 21
Escherichia coli, 278

Essential fat, 181–182
Essential hypertension, 323
Estrogen, 78, 79, 91, 104–105, 305
Eustress, 42
Euthanasia, 150–15
Eutrophication, 343
Excess fat, 182
Excitement phase: female sexual response, 64; male sexual response, 66
Exercise, 7; and aging, 207–208; as cardiovascular risk factor, 326; and health, 198–200; and overweight, 183; and stress, 51; and weight control, 187–188; *see also* Fitness
Exhaustion stage, stress, 47
Exhibitionism, 143
Exogenous organisms, 276–277
Experience, and alcohol use, 247–248
Extramarital intercourse, 61
Eyes, 370–371

F

Fabry's disease, 93
Fad: diet, 190–192; fitness, 206
Faddists, food, 164–165
Failure, 20
Fallopian tube, 76–77
Family: and aging, 142–144; and alcohol, 248; single parent, 131; *see also* Parenthood
Family planning. *See* Birth control
Fat, 166–167, 176
Fat clinics, 192
Fat tissue, 180–181, 182
Fear, 31
Fellatio, 60
Females, *See* Women
Feminine hygiene, 78
Fertilization, 76
Fertilizers, 349
Fetal alcohol syndrome, 91, 246
Fetus, 79
Fever, 281
Fiber, and nutrition, 168–169
Fibrillation, 319
Fires, in homes, 368–369
Firming agents, food, 172
Fitness: elements of, 196–198; and exercise, 198–203; extent of, 200–202; planning for, 203–208; role of, 195–196; *see also* Exercise
Fixations, 18
Flashbacks, 232
Flavoring agents, food, 173
Fluorocarbons, 341–342
Foams, and birth control, 103–104
Food: additives, 172–173; components, 162–166; energy equivalents and weight control, 188; fads, 164–165; groups, 169–172; labeling, 172; and population, 348–350; *see also* Nutrition
Food and Drug Administration, 79, 91, 104, 164, 236, 237; and diets, 191, 192; and food additives, 173
Food stamps, 175
Ford, Betty, 218
Ford, Clellan, 61
Fort, Joel, 221
Fortification, food, 172
Freedman, Jonathan, 22, 45
Freud, Sigmund, 21, 230; emotional development stages, 18
Friendship, and aging, 145–146
Fries, James F., 370, 375, 379
Frigidity, 68
Fromm, Erich, 69
Fructose, 163
Fruits, 170
Funeral rites, 154–156
Fungi, 278
The Future of Marriage (Bernard), 115

G

Gadgets, fitness, 206
Gametes, 75
Gamma globulin, 282
Garbage, 343–344
Gauchev's disease, 93
Gender identity, 55–57; and emotions, 21–23
Gender liberation, 57
Gender roles, 57
Generativity, 20
Genetic counseling, 95–96
Genetic disease, 92, 95
Genetic factors, in gender identity, 56
Genital herpes, 290
Genital stage of development, 18
Genital warts, 291
German measles, 91–92
Gerontology, 136
Glans penis, 67
Glasser, William, 200
Glaucoma test, 375
Glenn, John, 368
Glucose, 163
Glycogen, 163
Gonococci, 289
Gonorrhea, 92, 286–287, 289–290
Goodyear Co., 340
Gordon, Thomas, 130
Gould, Robert E., 63, 125
Graafian follicle, 77
Grant, Cary, 339
Green revolution, 349–350
Grief, and death, 153–154
Grief therapy, 154
Group Health Cooperative of Puget Sound, 361
Group marriage, 119
Group practice, 360–361
Growth needs, 16
Guilt, 20

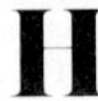

Habituation, drug, 218
Haldol, 228
Hallucinations, 32
Hallucinogens, 231–232
Hangover, 245–246
Happiness, 22
Harlow, Harry, 14–15
Hashish, 232
HCG, 192
Health: and aging, 138; defined, 4–5; determinants of, 5–6; and exercise, 198–200; hazards to, 7; holistic, 4–5; literature, 369–370; parenting for, 132; and population, 347–350; and radiation, 345–347; testing, 362; *see also* Fitness; Health Care; Nutrition
Health and Nutrition Examination, 180
Health care, 353; accident prevention, 367–373; community role in, 355–356; consumer decisions on, 377, 378; delivery of, 356–360; and doctor, 373–377; in future, 364; improving, 360–365; national health insurance and national health service, 363–365; and quackery, 311, 378–379; quality of, 360; right to, 354–355; scope of self-care, 364, 373; self-care movement, 365–367; vs. sickness care, 361–362; *see also* Fitness; Health; Nutrition
The Health Consequences of Smoking, 257
Health Insurance, 357, 363–365
Health Insurance Plan of Greater New York, 361
Health maintenance organization, 360, 361
Health spas, 192
The Healthy State (Sidel), 364–365
Hearing, and noise, 344–345
Heart, and exercise, 201–202, 206
Heart attacks: angina pectoris, 317–318; and blood clot in atherosclerotic coronary artery, 317; cardiac arrest and emergency treatment, 319–320; faltering heartbeat, 319; and fitness, 201–202; heart block, 319; myocardial infarction, 318–319; postcardiac rehabilitation, 320; warming signs, 318
Heartbeat, faltering, 319
Heart block, 319
Heartburn, 82

Heart disease, 176; congenital, 321; and overweight, 184; rheumatic, 321–322; and smoking, 261–262
Heart failure, 320–321
Heart-lung machine, 321
Heimlich technique, 372
Helping others, 26
Hemorrhage, cerebral, 323, 324
Hemorrhoids, 82
Hemoglobin, 92, 201
Hemophilia, 93–94
Hepatitis, 227, 285
Hepburn, Katharine, 119
Heptachlor, 340
Herbicides, 339–340, 349
Heredity: and cancer, 304; and overweight, 181
Heroin, 226, 228
Herpes simplex Type 2, 92, 286, 290, 306
Hex A, 93
High-density lipoprotein (HDL), 325
Hodgkins disease, 302
Holmes, Thomas H., 43, 45, 47–48
Home: accidents in, 368, 369; delivery of baby in, 87–88; dying at, 150
Homosexualities (Bell and Weinberg), 64–65
Homosexuality, 63–65
Hormonal factors, and gender identity, 56–57
Hormones: and cancer therapy, 310; and gender, 56–59; ovarian, 78; and stress, 46–47;
Horn, Daniel, 266
Hospice, 150
Hospitalization, costs, 357–358
Hot flashes, 79
Hot lines, crisis, 37
How to Be Your Own Doctor—Sometimes (Sehnert), 365
Human chorionic gonadotropin (HCG), 80–81
Human potential movement, 26
Humectants, food, 172
Hydrocarbons, 341
Hydrogenated fats, 166
Hygeine: and cancer prevention, 306–307; feminine, 78
Hymen, 63–64
Hyperplasia, and smoking, 260
Hypertension, 168, 322–323; and overweight, 184
Hypnosis, 52
Hypochondria, 32
Hypothalamus, 46
Hypnotic drugs, 225–226
Hypoglycemia, 163
Hypokinetic Disease (Raab and Kraus), 198
Hysterical personalities, 33
Hysterotomy, 109

I

Identification, 21
Identity, 20; gender, 57–59; and youth, 121–114
Identity, Youth, and Crisis (Erikson), 112
Immune mechanisms, 281; and cancer, 306
Immunity from disease, 281–282
Immunoassay, 80–81
Immunotherapy, 311
Implantation, 79
Impotence, 68
Incineration, 343
Incubation period, infection, 279
Indigestion, acid, 82
Infant mortality, 274
Infarct, 319
Infection, 277; agents of, 276–278; course of, 279; spread of, 278–279
Inferiority, 20
Infertility, 89
Inflammation, 280–281
Influenza, 284–285
Initiative, 20
Insanity, 27
Integrity, 20; and aging, 141
Intellectual skills, and aging, 138–139
Interaction, drug, 217, 219, 246
Intercourse, 60–61
Interferon, 281, 296, 311, 312
Intimacy, 20, 24; and marriage, 125
Intoxication, 250–251
Intrauterine devices, 105
Ionizing radiation, 305
Iron, 167
Ischemic attacks, transient, 324
Isolation, 20; and coping with death, 151
Isometric exercise, 196
Isotonic exercise, 196
IUDs, 105

J

Jackson, Don, 30
Jackson, Reggie, 119
Jacobson, Edmond, 51
Janis, Irving L., 49
Jellies, and birth control, 103–104
Jews, and Tay-Sachs disease, 93
Joan of Arc, 26
Jogging, 199–200
Johnson, Virginia, 58, 63–68, 69, 70, 142, 143
Judo, 52
Junk food, and overweight, 184

K

Kaiser Foundation, Medical Care Program, 361
Kane, Robert, 364
Kaplan, Helen Singer, 69, 70
Karate, 52
Kelly, Joan, 131
Kilocalories, 169
Kinsey, Alfred, 58, 61
Kissing, 59
Kissing disease, 285–286
Kostrubala, Thaddeus, 199–200
Kraus, Hans, 198
Kübler-Ross, Elizabeth, 149, 151–153
Kuhn, Maggie, 146
Kung fu, 52
Kwashiorkor, 162

L

Labeling: of food 172; and mental health, 27
Labia majora, 64
Labia minora, 64
Lability, emotional, 324
Labor, and birth, 85–86
Labor pains, 85
Lactose, 163
Laetrile, 311
Lamaze method, 85
Laparoscopy, 106
Last Chance Diet, 191
Latency stage of development, 18
Law, and mental disorders, 27
Laxatives, 236–237
Lead poisoning, 338–339, 355
Learning, 20
Leeuwenhoek, Anton van, 274
Leukemia, 302
Leukoplakia, and smoking, 260
Leukorrhea, 78
Levin, Lowell, 372
Levinson, Daniel, 125
Lewin, Kurt, 20–21
Librium, 225, 226
Life, everyday problems, 34–35
Life changes and stress, 43–44
Life expectancy, 3, 140, 274
Life style; and health, 7–8; and stress 52
Liking and Loving (Rubin), 114
Lipids, 166–167; storage diseases, 93
Lipoproteins, 325
Lithium, 228–229
Litter, 343
Loneliness, 16
Los Angeles Suicide Prevention Center, 37

Love: and marriage, 114; need for, 14–16; and sex, 69
Low-density lipoprotein (LDL), 325
LSD, 215, 216–217, 231–232, 243
Lung cancer, and smoking, 260
Lungs: and exercise, 206; ventilating in CPR, 320
Lymphocyte, 281
Lymphoma, 302
Lymphosarcoma, 302
Lynch, James J., 16

M

Macrophages, 280
Malaria, 92
Males. *See* Men
Malignant tumors, 300
Malpighi, Marcello, 274
Manic-depressive psychosis, 32–33, 229
MAO inhibitors, 228
Margin of safety for chemicals, 336
Marijuana, 232–234, 249–250
Marital Tensions (Dicks), 123
Marriage, 111–112; and aging, 142; alternatives to, 117–120; expectations, 115–117; and love, 114; making it work, 120, 123; myths about, 123–125; reasons for 112; and remarriage, 144; selecting partner 112–115; *see also* Parenthood
Marriage counseling, 123
Martial arts, 52
Maslow, Abraham, 16–18, 23–24
Massage, cardiac, 320
Masters, William, 58, 63, 65–68, 69, 70, 142, 143
Masturbation, 59
Matek, Stanley, 364
Maternal mortality, 274
Maturity,: and aging, 141; emotional, 23–24
Mayer, Jean, 181, 185, 216
Mead, Margaret, 112
Meat: in diet, 169–170; substitutes for, 162
Medicaid, 359, 363; and abortion, 108–109
Medicare, 359–363
Meditation, 51–52
Melanoma, 302
Mellaril, 228
Men: cancer in, 302; gender identity in, 55–57; gonorrhea in, 289; infertility in, 89; marriage expectations, 115; reproductive system, 75–76; sexual problems, 68–71; sexual response, 66–68
Menarche, 76
Menopause, 78–79
Menstruation, 76
Mental disorders: classification, 28–34; defined, 26–27; getting help for, 34–38; magnitude and cost, 27–28; signs of, 35–37
Mental health: criteria for, 5, 6; and emotional maturity, 23–24; facilitating 24–26
Mental retardation, and Down's syndrome, 95
Mercury pollution, 337–338
Merigan, Thomas C., 312
Mescaline, 231, 232
Mesothelioma, 305
Metabolic agents, for cancer therapy, 310
Metaneeds, 16–18
Metapathologies, 18
Metastases, 300
Methadone, 227, 228
Methedrine, 229
Microcephaly, 90, 91
Microvascular bypass surgery, 328
Midwifery, and childbirth at home, 87–88
Milk: breast feeding, 88–89; and diet, 170
Milk of magnesia, 236–237
Miller, Warren, 101
Miltown, 225
Minamata disease, 337–338
Minerals, 167
Mirror test, for overweight, 181
Miscarriage, 82
Mistrust versus trust, 20
Mitford, Jessica, 155
Mitosis, 306
Money, and marriage, 120–121
Mongolism, 94–95
Moniliasis, 290
Monoamine oxidase inhibitors, 228
Mononucleosis, 285–286
Monounsaturated fats, 166
Mood elevators, 228–229
Moody, Raymond, 149
Morning sickness, 82
Morphine, 226–228
Mortality, 3, 274, 347; and heart disease, 317; and smoking, 258, 259; *see also* Death
Moses, Grandma, 139
Motivation: for alcohol use, 247; for drug use, 221–222
Mouth-to-mouth resuscitation, 320, 366
Multiphasic screening, 362
Mutation, 92
Myocardial infarction, 318–319
Myotonia, 64

N

Nader, Ralph, 356, 365
National Academy of Sciences, 166, 174
National Academy of Sciences/ National Research Council, 169
National Center for Health Statistics, 179
National Center on Child Abuse and Neglect, 130
National Commission on Marijuana and Drug Use, 220
National health service, 363–365
National Health Survey, 372
National Highway Safety Traffic Administration, 250
National Institute of Mental Health, 29
National Institute on Alcohol Abuse and Alcoholism 250
National Institute on Drug Abuse, 219, 227, 228
National Institutes of Health (NIH), 139
National Safety Council, 367
National Survey on Drug Abuse, 231, 232, 233, 249
Native American Church, 232
Natural Childbirth, 83–85
Needs hierarchy, 16, 18
Nembutal, 225, 225
Neoplasm, 300
Neuroses, 30–32
Neurotransmitters, 29, 229
Nicotine, 259
Niemann Pick disease, 93
Nitrates, 343
Nitrites, 172–173
Nitrogen oxides, 341
No-Doz, 229
Noise pollution, 344–345
Non-biodegradable chemicals, 341
Nonemissive erection, 68
Nonsmokers, rights of, 267–268
Nonwhites, hypertension in, 323
North by Northwest, 339
Nuclear power, 345–347
Nurturance need, and marriage, 125
Nutrients, food, 172
Nutrition, 7, 161, 162; and carbohydrates, 163; and disease, 175–177; and food components, 162–169; special needs, 173–175; *see also* Diet; Fitness; Weight control
Nyswander, Marie, 227–228

Obesity: and cardiovascular diseases,

325, 326; and overweight, 180–181; *see also* Weight control
Obsessive-compulsive behaviors, 32
Occlusion, blood vessel, and stroke, 323
Occupational Safety and Health Administration (OSHA), 44, 340
Oedipal complex, 18
Oncogenes, 306
O'Neill, Nena and George, 116
Oopherectomy, 78
Open-heart surgery, 321
Open marriage, 116
Opiates, 226–228
Optimal health, 4
Oral contraceptives, 104, 105
Oral hygiene, 374
Oral stage of development, 18
Oral stimulation, 59–60
Orgasmic phase: female sexual response, 65; male sexual response, 67
Orgasmic platform, 65
Orthopedic integrity, and exercise, 201
Osteoarthritis, 208
Ovaries, 77–78
Overexertion, 204
Overnutrition, 175–177
Overpackaging, 351
Over-the-counter drugs, 214, 234–237
Overweight: causes, 181–184; and obesity, 180–181; *see also* Weight control
Oviducts, 76–77
Ovulation, 77
Oxygen, and exercise, 202–203
Ozone layer, 341–342

P

PABA, 307
Pacemaker, 319, 328
PAH, 305
Pandemic disease, 275
Pap smear, 308, 375
Paralysis, and stroke, 323
Parasites, 278
Parasympathetic nervous system, 13–14
Parent Effectiveness Training, 129–130
Parenthood, 111–112, 125–126; and adoption, 132; children and divorce 131; and health, 132; and parent-child relationship, 126–131; and single-parent families, 131
Parents Anonymous, 131
Parkes, Collin Murray, 153
Particulate matter, 341
Passive immunization, 282
Pathogens, 276
Patients and doctors, 373–377
Patient's Bill of Rights, 377
PCB, 341, 343
PCP, 231, 232
Pediculosis pubis, 291
Peer group pressures, and drug use, 223–224
Penicillin, 295
Penis, 66–68
Perception, and emotion, 12
Personality: and marriage, 120; disorders, 33
Pesticides, 339–340, 349
Pets, and needs of bereaved, 154
Petting, 59–60
Peyote, 231, 232
Phagocytes, 280
Phallic stage of development, 18
Pharmacological factors in smoking, 265
Pharmacology, 215–216, 366
Phenylalanine-hydroxylase, 93
Phenylketonuria (PKU), 93
Phencyclidine, 231, 232
Phenothiazines, 228
Phobias, 32
Phocomelia, 91
Phosphates, 343
Photochemical smog, 341, 342
Physical dependence, on drugs, 219
Physical examinations, 374–375; during pregnancy, 81–82
Physical fitness. *See* Fitness
Physical well-being, 5, 6
Physicians: distribution of, 356–357, 360; group practice, 360–361; and patient, 373–377
Physiology: and alcohol, 242–246; and drugs, 215–216; of sexuality, 63–68; of stress, 45–47
Pill: as cardiovascular risk factor, 326–327; and nutrition, 175; as oral contraceptive, 104–105; and smoking, 262
Pinch test for overweight, 181
Pion beam therapy, 310
Pituitary gland, 46–47
Pius XII, Pope, 151
Placebo effect, 378
Placenta, 79
Planned Parenthood Federation, 81
Planning: family, 100; for fitness, 203–208
Plaque, 166
Plasma cells, 281
Plateau phase: female sexual response, 64–65; male sexual response, 67
The Pleasure Bond (Masters and Johnson), 69
Plutonium, 345
Poisonings, 369
Pollution, 341–345; and cancer, 305
Polyunsaturated fats, 166
Population, 347–350
Positive health, 4
Postcardiac rehabilitation, 320
Potency, drug, 216–217
Pregnancy: and alcohol, 246; and blood examinations, 82; discomfort, 82; labor and birth, 85–86; nutritional needs during, 174–175; prepared childbirth, 83–85; and smoking, 262; and spontaneous abortion, 82; testing, 80–81
Preludin, 229
Premarital intercourse, 60
Premature ejaculation, 68
Prenatal care, 80
Prenatal development, 79–80
Prenatal diagnosis, 95
Prepared childbirth, 83–85
Prepuce, 64
Preservatives, in food, 172–173
President's Council on Fitness, 199
Pressure, handling, 50
Prevention: of cancer, 306–307; of cardiovascular diseases, 330; of communicable diseases, 295–296; of mental disorders, 37–38; of sexually transmitted diseases, 291–292
Primary impotence, 70
Primary orgasmic dysfunction, 70
Proctoscopy, 308
Prodrome stage of infection, 279
Productivity, and aging, 139
Progesterone, 78, 91, 106
Progestin, 104–105
Progressive relaxation, 51
Projection, 21
Prophylactic surgery, 307
Prospective medicine, 365
Protein, 162–163
Protozoa, 278
Psilocybin, 231, 232
Psychedelic drugs, 231–232
Psychoactive drugs, 214–234
Psychological effects, of alcohol, 246–248
Psychological factors: in drug use, 221–222; in smoking, 264–265
The Psychology of Self-Esteem (Branden), 16
Psychopaths, 33
Psychophysiological reactions, 33–34
Psychoses, 32–33
Psychosocial crisis, 18
Psychosomatic disease, 49
Psychosomatic reactions, 33–34
Psychotogenics, 231–232
Psychotomimetics, 231–232
Public Health Service, 91, 109, 223, 226, 246

Public Interest Research Group, 356
Pubococcygeous muscles, 63
Pulmonary stenosis, 321
Pulse, 371
Pus, 281

Quaalude, 225
Quackery, 311, 378–379
Quarantining, 273

R

Raab, Wilhelm, 198
Radiation, and cancer, 305, 307, 309–310
Radiation sickness, 346–347
Radioreceptor assay, 81
Rahe, Richard, 43, 45, 47–48, 50
Rationalization, 21
Reaction formation, 21
Reassurance of worth, and marriage, 125
Recommended Daily Allowance, 162, 169, 172
Recreational sports, 205, 206
Red Dye II, 173
Regression, 21
Rehabilitation: of alcoholic, 254; postcardiac, 320
Relaxation, and stress 51–52
Remarriage, 144
Report on Smoking and Health, 257
Repression, 21
Reproduction: and breast feeding, 88–89; conception and prenatal development, 79–80; congenital defects, 89–92; female system, 76–79; and genetic counseling, 95–96; and genetic disease, 92–95; and infertility, 89; labor and birth, 85–88; male contribution, 75–76; *see also* Pregnancy
Resistance stage, stress, 47
Resolution phase: female sexual response, 66; male sexual response, 67
Respiratory Distress Syndrome (RDS) 174
Resuscitation, cardiopulmonary, 320
Retinoids, 311
Rheumatic fever, 321–322
Rh test, 82
Rhythm method, birth control, 105–106
Ribonucleic acid, 162
Rickettsiae, 278
The Rights of Hospital Patients (Annas), 377
Risk factor, cardiovascular, 325–328
RNA, 162
Role, gender, 57
Role confusion, 20
Roosevelt, Eleanor, 139
Rougement, Denis de, 114
Rubella, and congenital defects, 91–92
Rubin, Zick, 114
Running, 199–200

St. Christopher's hospice, 150
Saline abortion, 109
Salpingitis, 77
Salt, and nutrition, 167–168
Sanity, 27
Sarcomas, 302
Saturated fat, 166, 176
Saunders, Cicely, 150
Scabies, 291
Schizophrenia, 32
Seconal, 225, 226
Secondary impotence, 68
Secondary orgasmic dysfunction, 68
Security need, and marriage, 125
Sedative, 51
Sedative-hypnotics, 225–226
Sehnert, Keith, 365, 370, 375
Self, sense of, 24
Self-actualization, 23–24
Self care: movement, 365–367; scope, 370–372
Self Care (Levin), 372
Self-esteem need, 16
Selye, Hans, 42, 47, 52
Seminal fluid, 76
Senility, 139
Serial monogamy, 123
Sernyl, 231, 232
Sequestrants, 172
Sex flush, 64, 67
Sex-linked genetic diseases, 93–94
Sex therapy, 70
Sexual dysfunction, 68–70
Sexuality: and aging, 142–143; bisexuality, 63; evolution of, 71; and gender identity, 55–57; homosexuality, 61–63; and marriage, 121; options, 61–63; physiology of, 63–68; revolution in, 57; and love, 69; problems, 68–71; study of, 58
Sexually transmitted diseases, 286–292
Sewage, 342–343
Shame, 20
Sharing need, and marriage, 125
Shyness, overcoming, 17
Shyness (Zimbardo), 17
Sickle-cell anemia, 92
Sickness care, vs. health care, 361–362
Sidel, Victor and Ruth, 364–365
Silent heart attack, 317
Single life, 119–120
Single-parent family, 131
Sleeping, 7
Smog, 341–342
Smoke, cigarette: components of, 259; as disease agent, 260–263
Smoker, profile, 263–264
Smoking, 7, 257–158; and cancer, 260–261, 302, 304, 306; as cardiovascular risk factor, 325; and congenital defects, 91; and heart attacks, 326–327, 328, 330; kicking the habit, 263, 266–267; as manufactured epidemic, 258–259; and Pill, 326–327; reasons for, 264–265; and rights of nonsmokers, 267–268
Sociability, 24
Social factors: in gender identity, 57; in smoking, 264–265
social life, and aging, 144–146
Social Readjustment Rating Scale, 43–45, 47–48
Social well-being, 5–6
Sociological factors, in drug use, 222–223
Sociopathic personalities, 33
Solar energy, 348
Solid wastes 343, 344
Solubility, drug, 217
Sopor, 225
Spastic cerebral palsy, 91
Spermatogenesis, 75–76
Spermatogonia, 75
Spermatozoa, 75–76
Spermicides, 103–104
Sphingolipids, 93
Spitz, Rene, 15
Spontaneous abortion, 82
Sports, recreational, 205–206
Spot reducing, 206
Sputum cytology, 308
Stabilizers, food, 172
Stagnation, 20
Stamina, and fitness, 196–197, 201–202
Starches, 163–166
Stenosis, pulmonary, 321
Steptol, Patrick, 90
Sterilization, 106
Stimulants, drug, 229–230
Stimulus, and stress, 42
STP, 232
Strength, 206; and fitness, 196–198, 200
Stress: as cardiovascular risk factor, 326; controlling responses to, 50–52; defined, 41–42; and disease, 47–49; and exercise, 199–200; and life changes, 43–44; and life style, 52; mechanism, 46–47; physiology,

45; positive effects, 42; and relaxation techniques, 51–52; response to, 45; signs of, 45–46; and stressors, 42–45
Stressors: crowding, 45; environmental, 44; response to, 45; variety of, 42–43
Strokes, 323–324; and blood clot on brain, 317; transient ischemic attacks, 324; treatment, 324–325; warning signs, 318
Sublimation, 21
Sucrose, 163
Suction curettage, 109
Suffocation, 369
Sugars, 163–166
Suicide, 29–30, 37
Sulfur oxides, 341, 342
Sunlight, and cancer, 301–302, 305, 307
Sunscreens, 305, 307
Suppleness, and fitness, 196–198, 201
Surgery: and birth control, 106; cardiovascular, 328–330; and congenital heart disease, 321; costs, 359
Suppleness, and exercise, 206
Supreme Court, and abortion, 107
Sweating, 192
Sympathetic nervous system, 13–14
Synergism, drug, 217
Synthesia, 231
Syphilis, 286, 287–289; and congenital defects, 92, 288
Systolic pressure, 322
Szasz, Thomas, 27

T

Tai chi, 52
Taking Care of Yourself (Fries and Vickery), 370
Tay-Sachs disease, 93
TB test, 375
Teen-agers: and drinking, 250; nutritional needs, 174
Teeth, 373–374; decay, 166
Temperature, 370
Temperature inversion, 342
Tension, and exercise, 199–200
Tests for fatness, 181
Test for pregnancy, 80–81
Test-tube babies, 90
Tetralogy of Fallot, 321
Thalidomide, 91
Thanatology, 135–136
THC, 232, 234
Thermal pollution, 343
Thickners, food, 172
Thinking, and emotions, 13
Thioxanthenes, 228
Thorazine, 228
Three Mile Island, 345–346
Throat, 370
Thrombosis, cerebral, 323, 324
Thrombus, 318
Thrush, 290
Timing, and congenital defects, 91
Tizard, Barbara, 132
Tobacco. *See* Smoking
Tolerance: for alcohol, 248; for drugs 218
Toxicity, drug, 216, 217
Toxins, 277
Toxoids, 282
Traffic accidents, and drunkenness, 251
Tranquilizers, 51, 219, 228–231
Transcatheter closure, 329
Transcendental Meditation (TM), 52
Transplant: artery, 328; heart, 329
Treatment: of alcoholism, 255; of cancer, 308–311; of cardiac arrest, 319–230; of strokes, 324–325; of syphilis, 288–289
Treponema pallidum, 287
Triage, 361–362
Trichomoniasis, 290
Triglycerides, 163
Trust versus mistrust, 20
Tubal ligation, 106
Tumor, 300
Twins, overweight studies on, 181

U

Ultrasound, 310
Undernutruition, 175
United Nations: campaign against pests, 340; ILO survey of marriage, 116
Unmedicated childbirth, 83–85
Uranium, 345–346
Urethra, 64
Uterus, 76

V

Vacuum aspiration, 109
Vagina, 63–64
Vaginal spermicides, 103–104
Vaginismus, 68
Valium, 225, 226
Values, and emotions, 13
Van Itallie, Theodore, 183
Vaporizer, 284
Varicose veins, 82
Vas deferens, 76
Vasectomy, 106
Vasocongestion, 64
Vegetables in diet, 170
Venereal disease, 286–287
Ventilation, lungs in CPR, 320
Ventricles, heart, 319
Vibrators, 379
Vickery, Donald M., 370, 375, 379
Vinyl chloride, 305, 340
Viruses, 278; and cancer, 305–306
Vitamins, 164–167; and colds, 284; deficiencies, 177 and food groups, 169–172; and Pill, 175

W

Wallerstein, Judith, 13
Warning signs, of heart attack and stroke, 318
Water: as food component, 168; pollution, 342–343; and weight control, 188, 192
Weight control, 7, 179, 185–187; and fad diets, 190–192; at fat clinics, 192; and exercise, 206; reasons for, 184–185; successful, 185–189; and sweating, 192; *see also* Diet; Fitness; Nutrition
Weight training, 196
Weil, Andrew T., 234
Weinberg, Martin, 62–63
Weiss, Robert S., 125
Widowhood, 143–144
Withdrawal, and birth control, 101
Withdrawal, drug, 227
Withdrawal syndrome, drug, 219
Womb, 76
Women: and cancer, 302; and cardiovascular disease, 315–316; and drug abuse, 219; gender identity, 57–59; gonorrhea in, 289; hypertension in, 323; infertility, 89; marriage expectations, 116; reproductive system, 76–79; sexual problems, 68–71; sexual response in, 65–68; and smoking, 262–263
Woodruff Diana S., 140
Work, productive, 24
World Health Organization (WHO), 88, 296; definition of health, 4
Worms (parasites), 278

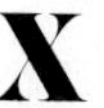

X-rays, 305, 307

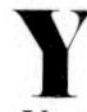

Yoga, 52
Youth: drinking among, 248–250; and identity, 112–114

Z

Zen Macrobiotic Diet, 192
Zimbardo, Philip, 17
Zinberg, Norman E., 234
Zygote, 79

Credits and Acknowledgments

Chapter 1 Mental Health
17—Adapted from *Shyness: What it is, What to do about it* by Philip Zimbardo, copyright © 1977, by permission of Addison-Wesley Publishing Co., Reading, Mass.

Chapter 3 Human Sexuality
64—Doug Armstrong, after Masters and Johnson, *Human Sexual Response,* Little, Brown and Company, 1966.

Chapter 4 Reproduction and Health
77—Edward Allgor; 83—John Dawson, after "Care During Pregnancy," *Story of Life,* 16, pp.434–435; 86—John Dawson; 95—John Dawson.

Chapter 5 Birth Control
108—Adapted from *Birth Control Handbook,* 7th ed., 1971.

Chapter 6 Marriage and Parenthood
127, 129—Howard Saunders.

Chapter 7 Aging and Facing Death
140—Reprinted with permission, Family Health Magazine, January 1975 © All rights reserved.

Chapter 8 Nutrition
164—Reprinted with permission, Family Health Magazine, June 1974 © All rights reserved.

Chapter 9 Weight Management
187—Taken from *Reduce and Be Happy* by Donald Hewitt, M.D., Pacific Press Publishing Assoc., 1955; 188—Copyright ©, The American Dietetic Association. Reprinted with permission.

Chapter 10 Physical Fitness
198—Table reprinted by permission of Heldref Publications, Washington, DC 20016; 205—From "Beyond Diet . . . Exercise Your Way to Fitness and Heart Health," by Lenore R. Zohman, M.D., CPC International, Inc., Englewood Cliffs, N.J. 1974.

Chapter 11 Drugs and Drug Use
216—Patty Peck; 235—Reprinted from *Take Care of Yourself: A Consumer's Guide to Medical Care* by Donald Vickery, M.D., and James Fries, M.D., copyright © 1976, by permission of Addison-Wesley Publishing Company, Reading Mass.

Chapter 12 Alcohol
253—Adapted from M.M. Glatt, "Group Therapy in Alcoholism," *The British Journal of Addiction,* Vol. 54, no. 2, January 1958.

Chapter 13 Smoking
259—Adapted by permission from *The New England Journal of Medicine,* Vol. 300, pp. 213–217, 1979; 261—Tom Lewis.

Chapter 14 Communicable Diseases
282—Tom Lewis; 287—Doug Armstrong; 293—*Demographic Yearbook,* 1976 (life expectancies—Population Reference Bureau, October 1978); 294—National Center for Health Statistics, *Vital Statistics Report,* March 1978; 295—Population Reference Bureau, *World Population Data Sheet.*

Chapter 15 Cancer
301—Tom Lewis; 303—American Cancer Society, *Cancer Facts and Figures—*1978; 307—Selection reprinted from *Preventing Cancer* by Dr. Elizabeth Whelan, with permission of W.W. Norton & Company, Inc. Copyright © 1978 by Elizabeth Whelan; 309—Tom Lewis.

Chapter 16 Cardiovascular Diseases
316—Edward Allgor; 318—Reprinted with permission of Macmillan Publishing

Co., Inc., from *Introduction to Public Health,* 7th Edition, by Daniel M. Wilner, Rosabelle Price Walkley, and Edward J. O'Neill. Copyright © by Macmillan Publishing Co., Inc. Adapted from American Heart Association, *Heart Facts,* 1975, p. 20; 324—Tom Lewis; 327—Copyright © 1978, *Medical Self-Care Magazine* (P.O. Box 717, Inverness, California 94937). Reprinted by permission.

Chapter 17 Health in the Environment

334–335—David Attie; 337—Fred Haynes; 344—Shirley Dethloff, after Bernards, *Our Precarious Habits,* Norton, 1970.

Chapter 18 Health Care and the Consumer

364—From *Urban Health,* Atlanta Georgia, October 1978. By permission; 366—From *You and Your Health* by William Fassbender. Copyright © 1977, John Wiley & Sons, Inc. Reprinted by permission of John Wiley & Sons, Inc.; 368—From The National Fire Protection Assoc., Boston, Mass., 02210. 369—From *Family Safety,* a National Safety Council Publication; 373—Tom Lewis; 376—Adapted from *How to be your own Doctor—Sometimes* by Keith W. Sehert with Howard Eisenberg. Copyright © 1975 by Keith W. Sehert, M.D. and Howard Eisenberg. All Rights reserved. Used by permission of Grosset & Dunlap, Inc.; 377—© 1975 by The American Hospital Assoc., 840 North Lake Shore Drive, Chicago, Illinois 60611.

Photo Credits

6—Jay Maisel/The Image Bank; 8—Clyde H. Smith/Peter Arnold, Inc..

10–11—Nicholas Foster/The Image Bank; 12—Mark A. Mittelman/Taurus Photos; 15—(left & right) Harry F. Harlow, University of Wisconsin Primate Laboratory; 16—Joel Gordon; 23—Martin Rogers/Woodfin Camp & Assoc..

28—(top left) Courtesy, Warner Brothers; (bottom and top right) Museum of Modern Art/Film Stills Archive; 43—(top) Sherry Suris; (center) Jim Anderson/Woodfin Camp & Assoc.; (bottom) Charles Harbutt/Magnum.

58—(top) Joseph Schuyler/Stock, Boston; (bottom) Marilyn Sanders/Peter Arnold, Inc.; 59—Timothy Eagan/Woodfin Camp & Assoc.; 60—Joel Gordon; 62 (left) Jack and Betty Cheetham/Magnum; (right) Sherry Suris; 71—Jeffrey Jay Foxx/Woodfin Camp & Assoc.

74–75—Elizabeth Wilcox; 81—Courtesy of the Carnegie Institution of Washington, Department of Embryology; 84—(top) Erika Stone/Photo Researchers, Inc.; (center) Mimi Forsyth/Monkmeyer Press Photo; (bottom) Ed Lettau/Photo Researchers, Inc.; 87—Elizabeth Wilcox; 88—Ken Heyman; 92—Gabriele Wunderlich; 94—Sybil Shelton/Monkmeyer Press Photo; 95—(center) Department of Neurosciences, University of California, San Diego.

98–99—Culver Pictures; 100—Mimi Forsyth/Monkmeyer Press Photo;

117—(left) American Standard/New York Public Library; (right) Michal Heron; 118—Rick Smolan; 119—(left) Museum of Modern Art/Film Stills Archive; (right) Peter Vandermark/Stock, Boston; 124—Christa Armstrong/Photo Researchers, Inc.; 126—David Austen/Woodfin Camp & Assoc.

134–135—C. Vergara/Photo Researchers, Inc.; 137—Bruce Davidson/Magnum; 139—Henle/Monkmeyer Press Photo; 141—(bottom left) E. F. Bernstein/Peter Arnold, Inc.; (top left) Joel Gordon; (top right) Ed Lettau/Photo Researchers, Inc.; 143—Joe Molnar; 147—Ginger Chih/Peter Arnold, Inc.; 150—Photo by Mark Jury; 154—Erika Stone/Peter Arnold, Inc.; 155—(left) Tony Ray Jones/Magnum; (right) M. Folco/Black Star; 156—Cornell Capa/Magnum.

160—Sol P. Steinberg Collection, New York; Courtesy, Harry N. Abrams; 174—Mimi Forsyth/Monkmeyer Press Photo; 176—Jeffery Foxx/Woodfin Camp & Assoc..

181—J. Schweiker/Photo Researchers, Inc.;

194–195—Jules Zalon/The Image Bank; 197—(top left) Michal Heron; (bottom left) Sylvia Johnson/Woodfin Camp & Assoc.; (right) Leif Skoogfors/Woodfin Camp & Assoc.;

197—(top left) Michal Heron; (bottom left) Sylvia Johnson/Woodfin Camp & Assoc,; (right) Leif Skoogfors/Woodfin Camp & Assoc.; 200—Guy Gilette/Photo Researchers, Inc.; 203—Rick Smolan; 207—Barbara Pfeffer/Peter Arnold, Inc.;

215—Tim Eagan/Woodfin Camp & Assoc.; 223—Ray Ellis/Rapho/Photo Researchers, Inc.; 226—National Audiovisual Center; 228—Cliff Feulner; 229—Courtesy, General Foods Corporation 231—Amy Meadow; 233—Sheri Suris; 244—Dr. Max E. Elliot/Univesity of California, San Diego; 247—Courtesy, Anheuser-Bush, Inc., St. Louis 249—Larry Mulvehill/Photo Researchers, Inc.; 250—Paul S. Conklin/Monkmeyer Press Photo; 254—Courtesy, Los Angeles Health Department, Alcoholism Rehabilitation Center.

256–257—Gerry Efinger; 260—Dr. Max E. Elliot/Univesity of California, San Diego; 262—American Cancer Society;

264—Courtesy of American Tobacco Company; 266—Bruce Roberts/Photo Researchers, Inc.; 268—Mimi Forsyth/Monkmeyer Press Photo.

272–273—Amy Meadow/Susan Schor; 276—Thomas Nebbia/DPI; 285—Lester V. Bergman & Assoc..

298–299—Courtesy, The American Cancer Society, N. Y.; 301—(top left) Dr. Max E. Elliot/U.S.C.D.; (top right) Patric Thurston/Transworld Feature Syndicate, Inc.; 310—The American Cancer Society.

314–315—V-Dia/Scala Fine Arts Publishers; 319—Scripps Memorial Hospital 320—Dan Budnik/Woodfin Camp & Assoc.; 328—Renald von Muchow; 329—Carl Roadman/Photo Researchers, Inc.

338—W. Eugene Smith/Magnum; 339—Museum of Modern Art/Film Stills Archive 342—Chuck O'Rear/Woodfin Camp & Assoc.; 346—Bill Pierce/Woodfin Camp & Assoc.; 350—Thomas Hopker/Woodfin Camp & Assoc.,

356—Bruce Roberts/Rapho/Photo Researchers, Inc.; 359—*(left)* Joel Gordon; *(right)* Woodfin Camp & Assoc; 363—Jon Brenneis Photographs; 370—Timothy Eagm/Woodfin Camp & Assoc.; 374—Gerry Efinger;